# Management Principles

## for Health Professionals

### EIGHTH EDITION

**Joan Gratto Liebler, MA, MPA**

Professor Emerita
Health Information Management
Temple University
Philadelphia, Pennsylvania

**Charles R. McConnell, MBA, CM**

Consultant
Human Resources and Health Care Management
Ontario, New York

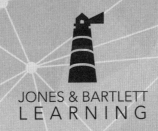

JONES & BARTLETT
L E A R N I N G

*World Headquarters*
Jones & Bartlett Learning
5 Wall Street
Burlington, MA 01803
978-443-5000
info@jblearning.com
www.jblearning.com

Jones & Bartlett Learning books and products are available through most bookstores and online booksellers. To contact Jones & Bartlett Learning directly, call 800-832-0034, fax 978-443-8000, or visit our website, www.jblearning.com.

19778-5

**Production Credits**
VP, Product Management: Amanda Martin
Director of Product Management: Laura Pagluica
Product Manager: Sophie Fleck Teague
Product Assistant: Tess Sackmann
Project Specialist: David Wile
Digital Project Specialist: Rachel DiMaggio
Senior Marketing Manager: Susanne Walker
Manufacturing and Inventory Control Supervisor:
    Therese Connell
Composition: codeMantra U.S. LLC
Project Management: codeMantra U.S. LLC
Cover Design: Theresa Manley
Text Design: Kristin E. Parker
Senior Media Development Editor: Troy Liston
Rights Specialist: Maria Leon Maimone
Cover Image (Title Page, Part Opener, Chapter Opener):
    © The Hornbills Studio/Shutterstock
Printing and Binding: McNaughton & Gunn

**Library of Congress Cataloging-in-Publication Data not available at time of printing**
Library of Congress Control Number: 2020930433

6048

Printed in the United States of America
24 23 22 21 20   10 9 8 7 6 5 4 3 2 1

*This Eighth Edition is dedicated to the memory of Charles R. (Chuck) McConnell.*

# Brief Contents

Preface                                        xvi

About the Authors                              xvii

What's New in the *Eighth Edition*             xviii

CHAPTER 1   The Dynamic Environment of Health Care .........1

CHAPTER 2   The Challenge of Change............................ 19

CHAPTER 3   Organizational Adaptation and Survival.......... 35

CHAPTER 4   Leadership and the Manager........................ 69

CHAPTER 5   Planning and Decision Making..................... 89

CHAPTER 6   Organizing and Staffing............................117

CHAPTER 7   Committees and Teams............................. 147

CHAPTER 8   Budget Planning and Implementation .......... 169

CHAPTER 9   Training and Development: The Backbone
            of Motivation and Retention ..................... 193

CHAPTER 10  Adaptation, Motivation, and Conflict
            Management .................................... 217

CHAPTER 11  Communication: The Glue That
            Binds Us Together .............................249

CHAPTER 12  Comprehensive Planning and
            Accountability Documentation ................267

CHAPTER 13  Quality Improvement and
            Control Processes..............................287

CHAPTER 14    **Human Resources Management:
A Line Manager's Perspective**......................303

CHAPTER 15    **Day-to-Day Management for the Health
Professional-as-Manager**.........................321

**Index**                                    **343**

# Contents

Preface . . . . . . . . . . . . . . . . . . . . . . . . . . . . xvi
About the Authors . . . . . . . . . . . . . . . . . . . .xvii
What's New in the *Eighth Edition* . . . . . . xviii

## CHAPTER 1 The Dynamic Environment of Health Care . . . . . . . 1

The Dynamic Environment of Health Care . . . . . 1
Client/Patient Characteristics. . . . . . . . . . . . . . 2
Trends Relating to Practitioners and
  Caregivers . . . . . . . . . . . . . . . . . . . . . . . . . . . . 3
  The Family as Caregiver . . . . . . . . . . . . . . . . . . . . 3
  Changes in Management Support Services. . . . . . . 3
  Patterns of Care . . . . . . . . . . . . . . . . . . . . . . . . . . . 4
The Healthcare Setting: Formal
  Organizational Patterns and Levels of Care . . . 4
  Provider Growth: Mergers, Joint Ventures,
    and Collaborative Partnerships. . . . . . . . . . . . . 4
  Clarification of Terms . . . . . . . . . . . . . . . . . . . . . . 4
  Range of Service and Levels of Care . . . . . . . . . . . 5
Laws, Regulations, and Accrediting
  Standards . . . . . . . . . . . . . . . . . . . . . . . . . . . . 6
  Regulations Stemming from Laws . . . . . . . . . . . . . 7
  Accrediting Standards . . . . . . . . . . . . . . . . . . . . . . 7
  Professional Association Standards
    and Guidelines. . . . . . . . . . . . . . . . . . . . . . . . . 7
  Sources of Information About Requirements . . . . . 7
The Impact of Technology . . . . . . . . . . . . . . . . . 8
  eHealth and Virtual Health . . . . . . . . . . . . . . . . . . 8
  Here Come the Robots. . . . . . . . . . . . . . . . . . . . . . 8
  The Personal Health Record. . . . . . . . . . . . . . . . . . 8
  Data Warehousing and Data Mining . . . . . . . . . . . 9
  Translational Medicine. . . . . . . . . . . . . . . . . . . . . . 9
  The Health Information Exchange . . . . . . . . . . . . . 9
  Privacy and Security Issues . . . . . . . . . . . . . . . . . . 9
  Informatics Standards and Common Language . . . . 9
  The Virtual Enterprise . . . . . . . . . . . . . . . . . . . . . 10
  Reimbursement and Patterns of Payment. . . . . . . 10
The Managed Care Era . . . . . . . . . . . . . . . . . . 11
  The Managed Care "Solution" and the
    Beginning of Restricted Access . . . . . . . . . . . . 11

The Annual Congressional Budget
  Allocations. . . . . . . . . . . . . . . . . . . . . . . . . . . 12
  Related Considerations . . . . . . . . . . . . . . . . . . . . 13
Reimbursement System Weaknesses . . . . . . . 14
Social and Ethical Factors. . . . . . . . . . . . . . . . . 14
The Role Set of the Healthcare
  Practitioner as Manager . . . . . . . . . . . . . . . . 15
  Classic Management Functions
    and Essential Competencies . . . . . . . . . . . . . . 15
Management as an Art and a Science . . . . . . . 16
  Characteristics of an Effective Manager . . . . . . . . 16
The Manager's Wheel Book . . . . . . . . . . . . . . . 17
  An Excerpt for a Manager's Wheel Book . . . . . . . . 17
  Format of Wheel Book . . . . . . . . . . . . . . . . . . . . . 18

## CHAPTER 2 The Challenge of Change . . . . . . . . . . . . . . . . . . . . . . 19

The Impact of Change . . . . . . . . . . . . . . . . . . . 19
The Manager as Change Agent. . . . . . . . . . . . . 19
Review of Successful Change . . . . . . . . . . . . . . 19
  Change as Opportunity: Y2K. . . . . . . . . . . . . . . . 20
  The Routinization of Change:
    The Patient Self-Determination
    Act of 1990 . . . . . . . . . . . . . . . . . . . . . . . . . . 20
  Extensive Change via Legislation:
    Health Insurance Portability and
    Accountability Act of 1996. . . . . . . . . . . . . . . . 21
  *Title II in the Spotlight.* . . . . . . . . . . . . . . . . . . . . 21
  *The Continuing Privacy Controversy.* . . . . . . . . . . . 22
  *Effects on an Organization.* . . . . . . . . . . . . . . . . . . 22
  *Physical Layout Considerations* . . . . . . . . . . . . . . . 23
  *The Privacy Official* . . . . . . . . . . . . . . . . . . . . . . . 23
  *The Department Manager and HIPAA* . . . . . . . . . . 23
  A Study in Proactive Change: Electronic
    Health Records. . . . . . . . . . . . . . . . . . . . . . . . 24
  *Individual Initiative.* . . . . . . . . . . . . . . . . . . . . . . . 24
  *Advocacy in the Public Arena.* . . . . . . . . . . . . . . . . 24
  *Partnerships with Key Stakeholders* . . . . . . . . . . . . 24
  *Outreach to Clients and Patients* . . . . . . . . . . . . . . 25
  *Continual Adjustments to Information Systems* . . . . . 25
  *Reassessing Health Information Management
    Job Roles and Credentialing* . . . . . . . . . . . . . . . 26

Economic and Market Forces:
  Anticipatory Readiness Through
  Organizational Restructuring . . . . . . . . . . . . . 26
Disruption in Personal Circumstances:
  Revitalization Through Career Development . . . 26
Change and Resistance to Change . . . . . . . . . 27
  The Collision of Constancy and Change . . . . . . . 27
  The Roots of Resistance . . . . . . . . . . . . . . . . . . . 27
  Primary Causes of Resistance . . . . . . . . . . . . . . . 28
    Organizational Changes . . . . . . . . . . . . . . . . . . . . . 28
    Management Changes . . . . . . . . . . . . . . . . . . . . . . 28
    Policy Changes . . . . . . . . . . . . . . . . . . . . . . . . . . 29
  Many Causes . . . . . . . . . . . . . . . . . . . . . . . . . . . . 29
  Meeting Change Head-On . . . . . . . . . . . . . . . . . . 29
  Flexibility and Adaptability . . . . . . . . . . . . . . . . . 29
  A Matter of Control . . . . . . . . . . . . . . . . . . . . . . . 29
  Addressing Resistance with Employees . . . . . . . . 30
    Tell Them . . . . . . . . . . . . . . . . . . . . . . . . . . . . . . . 30
    Convince Them . . . . . . . . . . . . . . . . . . . . . . . . . . . 30
    Involve Them . . . . . . . . . . . . . . . . . . . . . . . . . . . . 30
  Guidelines for Effective Management
    of Change . . . . . . . . . . . . . . . . . . . . . . . . . . . . . 31
  True Resistance . . . . . . . . . . . . . . . . . . . . . . . . . . 31
One More Challenge: The Patient Protection
  and Affordable Care Act of 2010 . . . . . . . . . 31
  A Template for Assessing Health
    Insurance Proposals . . . . . . . . . . . . . . . . . . . . . 33

**CHAPTER 3 Organizational
Adaptation and Survival . . . . . . . . 35**

The Organization as a Total System . . . . . . . . 35
The History of Management . . . . . . . . . . . . . . 36
  Scientific Management . . . . . . . . . . . . . . . . . . . . 36
  The Behavioralists and the Human Relations
    Approach . . . . . . . . . . . . . . . . . . . . . . . . . . . . . 36
  Structuralism . . . . . . . . . . . . . . . . . . . . . . . . . . . 37
  The Management Process School . . . . . . . . . . . . 37
  The Quantitative or Operations
    Research Approach . . . . . . . . . . . . . . . . . . . . . . 37
The Systems Approach . . . . . . . . . . . . . . . . . . 37
  Basic Systems Concepts and Definitions . . . . . . . 37
  The Nature of Inputs . . . . . . . . . . . . . . . . . . . . . . 38
  The Nature of Outputs . . . . . . . . . . . . . . . . . . . . 38
  Throughputs . . . . . . . . . . . . . . . . . . . . . . . . . . . . 39
  Feedback . . . . . . . . . . . . . . . . . . . . . . . . . . . . . . 39
Formal Versus Informal Organizations . . . . . . 40
Classification of Organizations . . . . . . . . . . . 41
  Prime Beneficiary . . . . . . . . . . . . . . . . . . . . . . . . 41
  Authority Structure . . . . . . . . . . . . . . . . . . . . . . 41
  Genotypic Characteristics . . . . . . . . . . . . . . . . . 41

Classification of Healthcare Organizations . . . 42
Classic Bureaucracy . . . . . . . . . . . . . . . . . . . . 43
Consequences of Organizational Form . . . . . . 44
The Clientele Network . . . . . . . . . . . . . . . . . . . 44
Clients . . . . . . . . . . . . . . . . . . . . . . . . . . . . . . . 45
Suppliers . . . . . . . . . . . . . . . . . . . . . . . . . . . . . 46
  Resource Suppliers . . . . . . . . . . . . . . . . . . . . . . 46
  Associates . . . . . . . . . . . . . . . . . . . . . . . . . . . . . 47
  Supporters . . . . . . . . . . . . . . . . . . . . . . . . . . . . . 48
Advisers . . . . . . . . . . . . . . . . . . . . . . . . . . . . . . 48
Controllers . . . . . . . . . . . . . . . . . . . . . . . . . . . . 49
Adversaries . . . . . . . . . . . . . . . . . . . . . . . . . . . . 49
Coalitions for Building Community
  and Client Involvement . . . . . . . . . . . . . . . . . 50
Example of Clientele Network for a
  Physical Therapy Unit . . . . . . . . . . . . . . . . . . 51
Introducing Organizational Survival
  Strategies . . . . . . . . . . . . . . . . . . . . . . . . . . . 52
Bureaucratic Imperialism . . . . . . . . . . . . . . . . 52
Co-Optation . . . . . . . . . . . . . . . . . . . . . . . . . . 54
  Formal Versus Informal Co-Optation . . . . . . . . . . 54
  Control of Co-Opted Groups . . . . . . . . . . . . . . . . 54
Hibernation and Adaptation . . . . . . . . . . . . . . 55
Goal Succession, Multiplication,
  and Expansion . . . . . . . . . . . . . . . . . . . . . . . . 56
The Corporate Culture . . . . . . . . . . . . . . . . . . 57
Organizational Life Cycle . . . . . . . . . . . . . . . . 58
  Gestation . . . . . . . . . . . . . . . . . . . . . . . . . . . . . . 58
  Youth . . . . . . . . . . . . . . . . . . . . . . . . . . . . . . . . . 58
  Middle Age . . . . . . . . . . . . . . . . . . . . . . . . . . . . 60
  Old Age . . . . . . . . . . . . . . . . . . . . . . . . . . . . . . . 61
Linking Theory and Practice:
  An Application of Organizational
  Analysis Using the Life Cycle Model . . . . . . . 63
The Management Reference Portfolio . . . . . . . 65
Appendix 3–A: Wheel Book Entries—Know
  Your Organization . . . . . . . . . . . . . . . . . . . . . 67
Notes . . . . . . . . . . . . . . . . . . . . . . . . . . . . . . . . 68

**CHAPTER 4 Leadership and
the Manager . . . . . . . . . . . . . . . . . . . 69**

Change and the Manager . . . . . . . . . . . . . . . . 69
Why Follow the Manager? . . . . . . . . . . . . . . . . 70
The Concept of Power . . . . . . . . . . . . . . . . . . . 70
The Concept of Influence . . . . . . . . . . . . . . . . 71

The Concept of Formal Authority . . . . . . . . . . 71

The Importance of Authority . . . . . . . . . . . . . 71

Sources of Power, Influence,
and Authority . . . . . . . . . . . . . . . . . . . . . . . 72

The Consent Theory of Authority . . . . . . . . . . . 72

The Theory of Formal Organizational
Authority . . . . . . . . . . . . . . . . . . . . . . . . . . . 73

Cultural Expectations . . . . . . . . . . . . . . . . . . . 74

Technical Competence and Expertise . . . . . . . . . 74

Characteristics of Authority Holders . . . . . . . . . 75

Authority by Default . . . . . . . . . . . . . . . . . . . . 75

The Manager's Use of Sources of Authority . . . . . 75

Restrictions on the Use of Authority . . . . . . . . 75

Importance of Delegation . . . . . . . . . . . . . . . 76

"Dos" and "Don'ts" of Delegation . . . . . . . . . . . 76

Effects of Good Delegation . . . . . . . . . . . . . . . 77

Leadership . . . . . . . . . . . . . . . . . . . . . . . . . . 78

Definition of Leadership . . . . . . . . . . . . . . . . . 78

Where Do "Leaders" Come From? . . . . . . . . . . . 78

What Drives People to Become Leaders? . . . . . . 79

Leadership Qualities . . . . . . . . . . . . . . . . . . . . 79

Leadership Functions . . . . . . . . . . . . . . . . . . . 80

From Theory to Practice: A Leader's
Plan of Action . . . . . . . . . . . . . . . . . . . . . . . 80

Styles of Leadership . . . . . . . . . . . . . . . . . . . . 81

*Autocratic Leadership* . . . . . . . . . . . . . . . . . . . 81

*Bureaucratic Leadership* . . . . . . . . . . . . . . . . . 81

*Participative Leadership* . . . . . . . . . . . . . . . . . 81

*Consultative Leadership* . . . . . . . . . . . . . . . . . 82

*Laissez-Faire Leadership* . . . . . . . . . . . . . . . . . 82

*Paternalistic Leadership* . . . . . . . . . . . . . . . . . 82

Continuum of Leadership Styles . . . . . . . . . . . . 82

Factors That Influence Leadership Style . . . . . . . 83

Communicating Your Own Managerial Style . . . . . 83

Situational Leadership and Adjustment . . . . . . . . 84

Some Final Thoughts About Authentic
Personal Leadership . . . . . . . . . . . . . . . . . . . 85

Value-Added Characteristics . . . . . . . . . . . . . . . 85

*Engaged, Conscious Living* . . . . . . . . . . . . . . . . 85

*Gracious Interpersonal Relationships* . . . . . . . . . 85

*Calm, Orderly Work Habits* . . . . . . . . . . . . . . . 85

*Embodiment of Values* . . . . . . . . . . . . . . . . . . 86

Growing in the Leadership Role;
Enhancing One's Career Path . . . . . . . . . . . 86

A Data-Driven Review . . . . . . . . . . . . . . . . . . . 86

Using the Manager's Wheel Book . . . . . . . . . . 87

Appendix 4–A: Wheel Book—Examples
Relating to Leadership Role . . . . . . . . . . . . 88

Notes . . . . . . . . . . . . . . . . . . . . . . . . . . . . . 88

**CHAPTER 5 Planning and
Decision Making . . . . . . . . . . . . . . . . 89**

Characteristics of Planning . . . . . . . . . . . . . . 89

Participants in Planning . . . . . . . . . . . . . . . . 90

The Planning Process . . . . . . . . . . . . . . . . . . 90

Planning Constraints or Boundaries . . . . . . . . 91

Strategic or Limiting Factors as Constraints . . . . . 92

Characteristics of Effective Plans . . . . . . . . . . 92

Anticipating Changes and Updates
in Existing Plans . . . . . . . . . . . . . . . . . . . . . 93

Planning for the Unknown . . . . . . . . . . . . . . . 94

Types of Plans . . . . . . . . . . . . . . . . . . . . . . . 94

Core Values, Philosophy, Heritage
Statement, and Mission . . . . . . . . . . . . . . . 94

Overall Goals . . . . . . . . . . . . . . . . . . . . . . . . 97

Objectives . . . . . . . . . . . . . . . . . . . . . . . . . . 97

Functional Objectives . . . . . . . . . . . . . . . . . . 98

Policies . . . . . . . . . . . . . . . . . . . . . . . . . . . . 99

Sources of Policy . . . . . . . . . . . . . . . . . . . . . 99

Wording of Policies . . . . . . . . . . . . . . . . . . . 100

Procedures . . . . . . . . . . . . . . . . . . . . . . . . 101

Procedure Manual Format . . . . . . . . . . . . . . 101

Development of the Procedure Manual . . . . . . 103

Methods . . . . . . . . . . . . . . . . . . . . . . . . . . 103

Rules . . . . . . . . . . . . . . . . . . . . . . . . . . . . . 103

Project Planning . . . . . . . . . . . . . . . . . . . . . 104

The Project Manager . . . . . . . . . . . . . . . . . . 104

Elements and Examples of
Major Projects . . . . . . . . . . . . . . . . . . . . . 104

Name of Project . . . . . . . . . . . . . . . . . . . . . 104

Focus and Scope of the Project . . . . . . . . . . . 104

Scope of Service . . . . . . . . . . . . . . . . . . . . . 105

Project Manager and
Project Team . . . . . . . . . . . . . . . . . . . . . . 105

Time Frame and Milestone Events . . . . . . . . . 105

Cost Factors . . . . . . . . . . . . . . . . . . . . . . . . 105

The Evaluation Process . . . . . . . . . . . . . . . . 105

The Plan and the Process . . . . . . . . . . . . . . 110

Decision Making . . . . . . . . . . . . . . . . . . . . 111

Evaluating a Decision's Importance . . . . . . . . 111

Evaluation of Alternatives . . . . . . . . . . . . . . 112

Root and Branch Decision Making . . . . . . . . . 112

Satisficing and Maximizing . . . . . . . . . . . . . 112

The Pareto Principle (Paretian Optimality) . . . . 113

Continuing Assessment of Decisions . . . . . . . 113

Analysis of Unanticipated
Consequences . . . . . . . . . . . . . . . . . . . . . 114

x **Contents**

Decision-Making Tools and Techniques..... 114
    Considered Opinion and Devil's Advocate...... 114
    The Factor Analysis Matrix ................ 114
    The Decision Tree ........................ 115
Notes.................................. 116

**CHAPTER 6 Organizing and Staffing ................... 117**

The Process of Organizing................ 117
Fundamental Concepts and Principles ..... 118
The Span of Management ................ 120
Line and Staff Relationships.............. 121
    The Relationship of Line and Staff Authority ..................... 122
    Line and Staff Interaction................. 122
    The Contractual Management Team.......... 122
The Dual Pyramid Form of Organization in Health Care............ 123
Basic Departmentation ................. 123
    Orphan Activities ..................... 124
    Deadly Parallel Arrangements ........... 125
Specific Scheduling ..................... 125
Flexibility in Organizational Structure ...... 126
    Matrix Organization .................. 126
    Temporary Departmentation ............ 126
    Temporary Agency Services.............. 127
    Outsourcing ......................... 127
    Contracted Services.................... 128
    Flexible Options for Worker Scheduling ....... 129
    Flextime ............................ 129
    Telecommuting ....................... 129
The Organizational Chart ............... 130
    Types of Charts ....................... 131
    General Arrangements and Conventions ....... 131
    Preparing the Organizational Chart .......... 132
The Job Description..................... 133
    Job Analysis.......................... 133
    Job Description Content and Format.......... 134
    Job Rating and Classification .............. 136
    Recruitment.......................... 137
    The Final Selection Process ............... 137
    Employee Development and Retention ........ 138
    Summary of Uses of the Job Description ....... 138
The Management Inventory............... 138
The Credentialed Practitioner as Consultant ...................... 139
The Independent Contractor.............. 139

Guidelines for Contracts and Reports ...... 139
    The Contract.......................... 139
    The Written Report ..................... 140
Sample Contract for a Health Information Consultant ................ 140
Consultant Agreement for Health Information Services ................. 140
Key Activities of Health Information Consultant (Addendum to February 1, 20N1, Contract)................. 141
Sample Cover Letter and Report .......... 142
Cover Letter ........................... 142
Quarterly Report: Health Information Services................ 143
    Dates of Site Visits and Primary Activities ...... 143
    Persons Interviewed During Site Visits......... 143
    Key Activities......................... 143

**CHAPTER 7 Committees and Teams...................... 147**

The Nature of Committees ............... 149
    The Plural Executive ................... 149
    The Task Force ....................... 150
The Purposes and Uses of Committees..... 150
    To Gain the Advantage of Group Deliberation...................... 150
    To Offset Decentralization and Consolidate Authority................. 151
    To Counterbalance Authority.............. 151
    To Provide Representation of Interest Groups....................... 151
    To Protect Due Process ................. 151
    To Promote Coordination and Cooperation ..... 152
    To Avoid Action....................... 152
    To Train Members ..................... 152
Limitations and Disadvantages of Committees......................... 152
Enhancement of Committee Effectiveness ...153
    Legitimization of Committee Activity.......... 153
    Logistical Support ..................... 153
    Scope, Function, and Authority............. 154
    Committee Size and Composition ........... 154
    Periodic Review of Committee Purpose and Function ...................... 155
The Committee Chairperson............. 156
    Selection and Duties ................... 156
    Chairing the Meeting................... 156
    Follow-Up Activity ..................... 157

Committee Member Orientation. . . . . . . . . . 158
Minutes and Proceedings . . . . . . . . . . . . . 158
    Preparation of Minutes . . . . . . . . . . . . . . . . . . . . 159
    Content of Minutes . . . . . . . . . . . . . . . . . . . . . . 159
Where Do Teams Fit In? . . . . . . . . . . . . . . 161
As Employee Involvement Increases . . . . . . . 162
Employee Teams and
    Their Future . . . . . . . . . . . . . . . . . . . . 163
    Avoiding "Committee Paralysis". . . . . . . . . . . . . 163
    Occasional Shortcomings of Teams . . . . . . . . . . 163
    What to Avoid in Using Employee Teams . . . . . . 164
    Proper Focus of Effective Employee Teams . . . . . 164
Guidelines for Group Deliberations . . . . . . . 165
    The Manager's Wheel Book Reflecting
        Committee and Team Activity . . . . . . . . . . . . 166
Appendix 7–A: Wheel Book Excerpts
    Reflecting Committee and
    Team Activity. . . . . . . . . . . . . . . . . . . . 167

**CHAPTER 8 Budget Planning
and Implementation . . . . . . . . . . 169**

The Revenue Cycle. . . . . . . . . . . . . . . . . . 170
    Revenue Sources . . . . . . . . . . . . . . . . . . . . . . 171
    Cash and the Revenue Cycle . . . . . . . . . . . . . . 171
The Budget. . . . . . . . . . . . . . . . . . . . . . 171
Uses of the Budget . . . . . . . . . . . . . . . . . 172
Budget Periods . . . . . . . . . . . . . . . . . . . 172
    Periodic Moving Budget . . . . . . . . . . . . . . . . . 173
    Milestone Budgeting . . . . . . . . . . . . . . . . . . . 173
Types of Budgets . . . . . . . . . . . . . . . . . . 173
    The Uniform System or Code of Accounts. . . . . . 174
    Cost Centers . . . . . . . . . . . . . . . . . . . . . . . . 174
    Responsibility Center. . . . . . . . . . . . . . . . . . . 175
Approaches to Budgeting . . . . . . . . . . . . . 175
The Budgetary Process. . . . . . . . . . . . . . . 176
    Initial Preparation . . . . . . . . . . . . . . . . . . . . 176
    The Budget Reference Portfolio . . . . . . . . . . . . 176
    The Review and Approval Process . . . . . . . . . . 177
    Implementation Phase. . . . . . . . . . . . . . . . . . 178
Capital Expenses . . . . . . . . . . . . . . . . . . 178
Supplies and Other Expenses. . . . . . . . . . . 180
    Maintenance and Repair . . . . . . . . . . . . . . . . 181
    Specialty References and Licensure Software . . . . 182
    Staff Development. . . . . . . . . . . . . . . . . . . . . 182
The Personnel Budget. . . . . . . . . . . . . . . 183
Direct and Indirect Expenses . . . . . . . . . . . 185

Budget Justification. . . . . . . . . . . . . . . . . 185
    The Budget Cut . . . . . . . . . . . . . . . . . . . . . . 186
    Cost Comparison. . . . . . . . . . . . . . . . . . . . . . 186
Budget Variances. . . . . . . . . . . . . . . . . . 186
    Example of Variance Analysis . . . . . . . . . . . . . 187
The General Audit . . . . . . . . . . . . . . . . . 188
    The Audit Committee . . . . . . . . . . . . . . . . . . 188
Sample Budget: Health Information
    Service. . . . . . . . . . . . . . . . . . . . . . . 188
Appendix 8–A: Sample Annual
    Budget—Health Information Service. . . . . . 189
    Health Information Department Budget. . . . . . . 190
      *Personnel Costs* . . . . . . . . . . . . . . . . . . . . 190
      *Equipment* . . . . . . . . . . . . . . . . . . . . . . . 190
      *Supplies*. . . . . . . . . . . . . . . . . . . . . . . . . 191
      *Services* . . . . . . . . . . . . . . . . . . . . . . . . 191
      *Cost Transfers*. . . . . . . . . . . . . . . . . . . . . 191
      *Summary*. . . . . . . . . . . . . . . . . . . . . . . . 191
Appendix 8–B: Wheel Book Excerpts—
    Budget Issues . . . . . . . . . . . . . . . . . . . 192

**CHAPTER 9 Training and
Development: The Backbone
of Motivation and Retention . . . . 193**

Employee Development. . . . . . . . . . . . . . . 193
    Relationship of Training and Development
      to the Basic Management Functions. . . . . . . . 194
Orientation . . . . . . . . . . . . . . . . . . . . . 194
    General Orientation. . . . . . . . . . . . . . . . . . . . 194
    Departmental Orientation . . . . . . . . . . . . . . . 195
    Of Special Concern: Standards
      of Conduct and Behavior . . . . . . . . . . . . . . 196
      *Conflict of Interest*. . . . . . . . . . . . . . . . . . . 196
      *Use of Organizational Assets and Information* . . . 197
      *Referral Practices* . . . . . . . . . . . . . . . . . . . 197
      *Political Activity* . . . . . . . . . . . . . . . . . . . . 198
      *Employee Privacy*. . . . . . . . . . . . . . . . . . . 198
      *Patient Confidentiality* . . . . . . . . . . . . . . . . 198
      *Employee Relationships*. . . . . . . . . . . . . . . . 198
    Contemporary Concerns: E-mail,
      the Internet, and Social Media . . . . . . . . . . . 198
      *Policy* . . . . . . . . . . . . . . . . . . . . . . . . . 199
Training. . . . . . . . . . . . . . . . . . . . . . . 200
    Identification of Training Needs. . . . . . . . . . . . 200
    Training Module Content. . . . . . . . . . . . . . . . 203
    Training Methods and Techniques . . . . . . . . . . 204
      *Job Rotation* . . . . . . . . . . . . . . . . . . . . . . 204
      *Formal Lecture Presentations*. . . . . . . . . . . . . 204
      *Seminars and Conferences*. . . . . . . . . . . . . . . 204

*Role Playing* .................................... 204
*Committee Assignments* ..................... 204
*Case Studies* .................................... 204
Program Implementation .................... 205
Evaluation of Outcomes ..................... 205
Resources for Training ........................ 205
Addressing Diversity .......................... 206
*Recognizing Differences* ..................... 206
*In the Manager–Employee Relationship* ........... 207
*What About Diversity Training?* ............. 207
Mentoring .......................................... 207
Network ............................................ 208
Peer Pals .......................................... 208
Clinical Affiliation/Clinical Practice
Program and Contract ...................... 208
Organizational Responsibility
and Coordination ......................... 208
Elements of the Clinical Affiliation Agreement ... 208
Appendix 9–A: Frequently Asked
Questions About Sexual Harassment ..... 210
Appendix 9–B: Training Design:
Release of Information ................... 213
Background Information and Needs
Assessment ................................. 213
The Redesign of the Training Program ..... 213
Phase One: Valuing Our Mission—Valuing
Your Role ................................... 214
Communication in Stressful Situations ..... 214
Phase Two—Release of Information Functions. . . 214
*Purpose* .......................................... 214
*Overall Training Objective* ................... 214
*Assumptions* .................................... 214
*Resources* ....................................... 214
*Training Sequence and Performance Level* ........ 215
*Methods* .......................................... 215

## CHAPTER 10 Adaptation, Motivation, and Conflict Management ........... 217

Adaptation and Motivation .................... 217
Adaptation to Organizational Life .......... 217
Techniques for Fostering Integration ........ 218
*Work Rules* ...................................... 218
*Incentives and Sanctions* ..................... 218
*Selection* ........................................ 218
*Training* .......................................... 218
*Identification with the Organization* ......... 219
*The Work Group* ................................ 219
Theories of Motivation ....................... 219
Bases of Motivation .......................... 219

Observation of Existing Work Situations ....... 219
Cultural Expectations about Work .......... 220
Motivational Theories ........................ 220
Practical Strategies for Employee
Motivation ................................... 220
Motivators ....................................... 220
Dissatisfiers ..................................... 221
Motivational Strategies ....................... 221
Motivation in Critical Incidents .......... 221
Appreciative Inquiry .......................... 222
The Appreciative Inquiry Process .......... 222
Motivational Aspects of
Appreciative Inquiry .................... 222
Motivation and Downsizing ................... 223
What Follows Downsizing? .................. 223
The Necessity of Reducing the Workforce ...... 224
The Employees Who Remain ............... 225
Immediate and Natural Reactions
to Downsizing ............................ 225
Employee Motivation Following Downsizing .... 225
Changes in Managers' Roles ................. 226
Conflict ............................................ 226
The Study of Conflict ........................ 227
Organizational Conflict ....................... 227
The Basic Conflict ........................... 227
*Overt Level* ..................................... 227
*The Hidden Agenda* .......................... 228
The Sources of Conflict ..................... 228
*The Nature of the Organization* ............. 228
*The Organizational Climate* .................. 228
*The Organizational Structure* ................ 229
*Individual Versus Organizational Needs* ......... 229
*Solutions to Previous Conflicts* .............. 229
The Participants ............................... 230
The Provision of an Arena ................... 231
The Development of Rules .................. 231
Strategies for Dealing with
Organizational Conflict ................. 231
Conflict Model Applied to Whistleblower
Action ....................................... 232
Discipline ......................................... 232
Progressive Disciplinary Action ............ 233
*Counseling* ..................................... 233
*Oral Warning* ................................... 233
*Written Warning* ............................... 234
*Before Suspension* ............................ 234
*Suspension and Discharge* ................... 234
Heading Off Infractions Before They Occur ..... 237
Appeal Procedure ............................ 237
Grievance Procedure ........................ 237

The Labor Union and the Collective
Bargaining Agreement . . . . . . . . . . . . . . . . . 238
Labor Unions in Health Care: Trends
and Indicators . . . . . . . . . . . . . . . . . . . . . . . 238
Appendix 10–A: Sample Collective
Bargaining Agreement . . . . . . . . . . . . . . . . . 240

# CHAPTER 11 Communication: The Glue That Binds Us Together . . . . . . . . . . . . . . . . . . . **249**

A Complex Process . . . . . . . . . . . . . . . . . . . . . . 249
Communication and the
Individual Manager . . . . . . . . . . . . . . . . . . . . 250
Face-to-Face . . . . . . . . . . . . . . . . . . . . . . . . . . . 250
The Telephone . . . . . . . . . . . . . . . . . . . . . . . . . 251
Voice Mail . . . . . . . . . . . . . . . . . . . . . . . . . . . . 251
Letters and Memos . . . . . . . . . . . . . . . . . . . . 251
E-mail and Instant Messaging . . . . . . . . . . . . 251
Verbal (Oral) Communication . . . . . . . . . . . . . 252
Nonverbal Communication . . . . . . . . . . . . . . 252
Components of Communication . . . . . . . . . . . 252
Methods of Improving Communication . . . . . . 252
Communication Barriers . . . . . . . . . . . . . . . . 253
Speaking to Groups . . . . . . . . . . . . . . . . . . . . 253
The Meeting . . . . . . . . . . . . . . . . . . . . . . . . . . 254
*The Staff Meeting* . . . . . . . . . . . . . . . . . . . . . . 254
*The General Meeting* . . . . . . . . . . . . . . . . . . . 254
Written Communication . . . . . . . . . . . . . . . . . . 255
The Importance of Written
Communication . . . . . . . . . . . . . . . . . . . . . . 255
E-mail: Helpful, but the Source of Many
Problems . . . . . . . . . . . . . . . . . . . . . . . . . . . . 255
Some Guidelines About Social Media
Policies and Practices . . . . . . . . . . . . . . . . . 256
Some Additional Considerations . . . . . . . . . . 257
Memos and Letters . . . . . . . . . . . . . . . . . . . . 258
*Write for a Specific Audience* . . . . . . . . . . . . . 258
*Avoid Unneeded Words* . . . . . . . . . . . . . . . . . 259
*Use Simple Words* . . . . . . . . . . . . . . . . . . . . . 259
*Edit and Rewrite* . . . . . . . . . . . . . . . . . . . . . . 260
*Change Old Habits* . . . . . . . . . . . . . . . . . . . . 260
*Sample Letter: Wrong and Right* . . . . . . . . . . 261
Formal Writing and Reporting . . . . . . . . . . . . 262
Communication in Organizations . . . . . . . . . . 262
Formal Communication . . . . . . . . . . . . . . . . . 262
*Verbal* . . . . . . . . . . . . . . . . . . . . . . . . . . . . . . 262
*Nonverbal* . . . . . . . . . . . . . . . . . . . . . . . . . . . 263
Informal Communication . . . . . . . . . . . . . . . . 263
Tools for Improving Communication . . . . . . . . 263
Barriers to Communication in Organizations . . . . 264
*Special Consideration: Directional Flow Barriers* . . . . . . 265
Orders and Directives . . . . . . . . . . . . . . . . . . . 266
Verbal Orders Versus Written Orders . . . . . . . . . 266
Making Orders Acceptable and Effective . . . . . . . 266

# CHAPTER 12 Comprehensive Planning and Accountability Documentation . . . . . . . . . . . . . . . . **267**

The Strategic Plan . . . . . . . . . . . . . . . . . . . . . . 268
Content of Strategic/Master Plans . . . . . . . . . . 268
*Vision and Mission Statement and Core Values* . . . . . . 268
*Strategic Overview of Current Status* . . . . . . . . . . . 268
*Major Strategic Goals and Action Plan or
Detailed Objectives* . . . . . . . . . . . . . . . . . . . . . 268
*Resources Needed and Their Probable Source* . . . . . . 268
*Evaluation Process* . . . . . . . . . . . . . . . . . . . . . . 269
The Strategic Planning Process . . . . . . . . . . . . 269
The Annual Report . . . . . . . . . . . . . . . . . . . . . . 270
The Executive Summary . . . . . . . . . . . . . . . . . 270
Major Project Proposal . . . . . . . . . . . . . . . . . . 271
The Development Officer . . . . . . . . . . . . . . . . . 271
Background Preparation . . . . . . . . . . . . . . . . . 271
Content of Project Proposals . . . . . . . . . . . . . . 271
Business Planning for Independent
Practice . . . . . . . . . . . . . . . . . . . . . . . . . . . . . 272
The Need for a Business Plan . . . . . . . . . . . . . 272
Three Reminders . . . . . . . . . . . . . . . . . . . . . . 273
Self-Employment Considerations: Income
and Taxes and Other Issues . . . . . . . . . . . . . 273
Articles of Incorporation and Bylaws . . . . . . . . 273
*Name of Organization* . . . . . . . . . . . . . . . . . . . 273
*Legal Status or Configuration* . . . . . . . . . . . . . . 273
*Service or Product* . . . . . . . . . . . . . . . . . . . . . . 274
*Board of Directors and Officers* . . . . . . . . . . . . . 274
*Executive Officer* . . . . . . . . . . . . . . . . . . . . . . 274
*Meetings* . . . . . . . . . . . . . . . . . . . . . . . . . . . . 274
*Finances* . . . . . . . . . . . . . . . . . . . . . . . . . . . . 274
*Formal Bylaws* . . . . . . . . . . . . . . . . . . . . . . . . 274
*Dissolution of the Business* . . . . . . . . . . . . . . . . 274
Content of the Business Plan . . . . . . . . . . . . . 274
The Due Diligence Review . . . . . . . . . . . . . . . . 274
Focus and Content of the Due Diligence
Review . . . . . . . . . . . . . . . . . . . . . . . . . . . . . 275
The Plan of Correction . . . . . . . . . . . . . . . . . . 275
Appendix 12–A: Newman Eldercare
Services, Inc.: Strategic Plan . . . . . . . . . . . 278
Mission . . . . . . . . . . . . . . . . . . . . . . . . . . . . . . 278
Core Values . . . . . . . . . . . . . . . . . . . . . . . . . . . 278

Strategic Overview........................ 278
SWOT Analysis .......................... 279
Goals and Objectives ..................... 279
Resources Needed and
  Their Provision ....................... 279
Action Plan............................. 280
Evaluation.............................. 280
Appendix 12–B: Annual Report
  of the Health Information Services ....... 281
Licensure and Accreditation ............... 281
Health Information Systems Review ....... 281
Client/Patient Outreach................... 281
Budget and Resource Allocation .......... 282
Staff Development and Training .......... 282
Professional Leadership ................. 282
Appendix 12–C: Executive Summary:
  Annual Report of the Health
  Information Services ................. 283
Appendix 12–D: Sample Project
  Proposal for Funding ................. 284
Need for Program Expansion ............. 284
Meeting the Need........................ 284
Timeline ............................... 285
    January 20n1........................ 285
    February 20n1....................... 285
Budget Considerations ................. 285
Plan to Become Self-Sustaining.......... 285
Program Evaluation..................... 286

## CHAPTER 13 Quality Improvement and Control Processes .....................287

Quality, Excellence, and Continuous
  Performance Improvement ............. 287
The Characteristics of a Thriving
  Organization ......................... 287
The Search for Excellence: A Long
  and Varied History.................... 288
    Quality Control, Quality Assurance,
      and Quality Management.............. 289
    The Common Driving Force ............. 289
    Performance Improvement Focus ........ 290
The Management Function of Controlling ... 292
    When Improvements Fail .............. 293
    Participants in the Planning—Controlling
      Process. .......................... 294

The Basic Control Process ............... 294
Characteristics of Adequate Controls ......... 294
Types of Standards....................... 295
The Intangible Nature of Service ........... 295
Selected Strategies ..................... 295
Benchmarking and Best Practices......... 296
    Sources of Benchmarking Measures .......... 297
    Sample Benchmarking Studies:
      Health Information Management .......... 297
Tools of Control ....................... 297
    Gantt Chart......................... 298
      Basic Components of Gantt Charts .......... 298
      Standard Symbols...................... 298
    The Flowchart....................... 299
      Uses of the Flowchart ................. 300
      Flowchart Symbols ................... 300
      Support Documentation.................. 300
    Total Quality Management Display Charts...... 301
      Run Chart ........................ 301
      Histogram ........................ 301
      Scattergram ...................... 301
      Cause–Effect Chart ("Fishbone Diagram"
        or Ishikawa Diagram).............. 301
      Pareto Chart ..................... 301
The Critical Cycle........................ 301

## CHAPTER 14 Human Resources Management: A Line Manager's Perspective ...303

"Personnel" Equals People............... 303
A Vital Staff Function ................... 304
A Service of Increasing Value ............. 304
Increase in Employee-Related Tasks....... 304
    Proliferation of Laws Related to Employment ... 305
    The Effects of Flattening ............... 305
    Some Directions in Human Resources ........ 305
Learning About Your Human Resources
  Department........................... 306
    The Nature of the Function: Staff
      Versus Line ....................... 306
    The Human Resources Reporting
      Relationship....................... 306
    The Human Resources Functions ........... 307
    Rounding Out Your Knowledge............. 308
Putting the Human Resources
  Department to Work................... 308
    A Universal Approach ................. 308
    Taking the Initiative.................. 309
Some Specific Action Steps.............. 309
    Finding New Employees ............... 309

Bringing Job Descriptions Up-to-Date . . . . . . . . 309
Evaluating Employees . . . . . . . . . . . . . . . . . . . . . 310
Disciplining Employees . . . . . . . . . . . . . . . . . . . . 310
Dealing with Training Needs . . . . . . . . . . . . . . . . 311
Further Use of Human Resources . . . . . . . . 311
Wanted: Well-Considered Input . . . . . . . . . . 311
Understanding Why As Well As What . . . . . . 311
Legal Guides for Managerial Behavior . . . . . . 312
Labor Relations . . . . . . . . . . . . . . . . . . . . . . . . . 313
Wages and Hours . . . . . . . . . . . . . . . . . . . . . . . 313
Equal Pay . . . . . . . . . . . . . . . . . . . . . . . . . . . . . 313
Civil Rights . . . . . . . . . . . . . . . . . . . . . . . . . . . . 314
Americans with Disabilities Act . . . . . . . . . . . . 314
Family and Medical Leave Act . . . . . . . . . . . . . 314
Sexual Harassment . . . . . . . . . . . . . . . . . . . . . . 314
Violence in the Workplace . . . . . . . . . . . . . . . . 315
An Increasingly Legalistic Environment . . . . . 316
The Work Environment: Hostile
or Supportive? . . . . . . . . . . . . . . . . . . . . . . . 316
The Supportive Work Environment . . . . . . . . . 317
Emphasis on Service . . . . . . . . . . . . . . . . . . . . 318
The Manager's Wheel Book and
The Management Reference Portfolio . . . . . . . 318
Appendix 14–A: The Manager's
Wheel Book . . . . . . . . . . . . . . . . . . . . . . . . 319
Appendix 14–B: The Management
Reference Portfolio . . . . . . . . . . . . . . . . . . . 320

**CHAPTER 15 Day-to-Day
Management for the Health
Professional-as-Manager . . . . . . . 321**

A Second and Parallel Career . . . . . . . . . . . . . 321
Two Hats: Specialist and Manager . . . . . . . . 321
A Constant Balancing Act . . . . . . . . . . . . . . . 324
The Ego Barrier . . . . . . . . . . . . . . . . . . . . . . . . 324

The Professional Managing the
Professional . . . . . . . . . . . . . . . . . . . . . . . . . 325
The Professional as a Scarce Resource . . . . . . . . 325
The High-Skill Professional: Some Special
Management Problems . . . . . . . . . . . . . . . . . . 326
Credibility of the Professional's Superior . . . . . . . 327
Leadership and the Professional . . . . . . . . . . 328
The Professional and Change . . . . . . . . . . . . . 329
The Basis for Resistance . . . . . . . . . . . . . . . . . . 330
The Manager's Approach . . . . . . . . . . . . . . . . . . 330
Organizational Change, the Manager,
and the Professional . . . . . . . . . . . . . . . . . . . 330
Methods Improvement . . . . . . . . . . . . . . . . . . 331
Employee Problems . . . . . . . . . . . . . . . . . . . . . 331
Communication and the Language
of the Professional . . . . . . . . . . . . . . . . . . . . 331
An Open-Ended Task . . . . . . . . . . . . . . . . . . . . 333
The Next Step? . . . . . . . . . . . . . . . . . . . . . . . . . 333
A Private and Personal Assessment . . . . . . . . . . 333
Careers: Ladders and Tracks . . . . . . . . . . . . . . . 334
*Upward Versus Downward* . . . . . . . . . . . . . . . . . 334
*Which Way?* . . . . . . . . . . . . . . . . . . . . . . . . . . . . 335
A Matter of Human Motivation . . . . . . . . . . . . . 335
Consolidate Before the Next Reach . . . . . . . . . . 335
Dedication—and the Balancing Act . . . . . . . . . . 335
Goal Alignment . . . . . . . . . . . . . . . . . . . . . . . . . 336
Some Unchanging Fundamentals . . . . . . . . . . . . 336
*Remember the Supporting Skills* . . . . . . . . . . . . . . 336
Become Valuable . . . . . . . . . . . . . . . . . . . . . . . . 337
Appendix 15–A: Comprehensive
Wheel Book . . . . . . . . . . . . . . . . . . . . . . . . . 338
Appendix 15–B: Calendar for Wheel Book
and Case Problems . . . . . . . . . . . . . . . . . . . 340

**Index . . . . . . . . . . . . . . . . . . . . . . . . . . . 343**

# Preface

This book is intended for healthcare professionals who regularly perform the classic functions of a manager as part of their job duties—planning, organizing, decision making, staffing, leading or directing, communicating, and motivating—yet have not had extensive management training. Healthcare practitioners may exercise these functions on a continuing basis in their roles as department directors or unit supervisors, or they may participate in only a few of these traditional functions, such as training and development of unit staff. In any case, knowledge of management theory is an essential element in professional training, because no single function is ever addressed independently of all others. Individuals who are trained in management theory but do not have healthcare experience will find an abundance of examples linking theory to the healthcare environment. A wide variety of settings are reflected in the many examples provided.

In this book, emphasis is placed on definitions of terms, clarification of concepts, and, in some cases, highly detailed explanations of processes and concepts. The examples reflect typical practices in the healthcare setting. However, all examples are fictitious and none are intended as legal, financial, or accreditation advice.

Every author must decide what material to include and what level of detail to provide. We have been guided by experience gained in the classroom, as well as in many training and development workshops for healthcare practitioners. Three basic objectives determined the final selection and development of material:

1. *Acquaint the healthcare practitioner with management concepts essential to the understanding of the organizational environment within which the functions of the manager are performed.* Some material challenges assumptions about such concepts as power, authority, influence, and leadership. Some of the discussions focus on relatively new concepts such as social media use, cultural proficiency and diversity training, changes in credentialing, and job duties of both professional and technical support personnel. Practitioners must keep abreast of developing trends in management, guarding against being "the last to know."

2. *Provide a base for further study of management concepts.* Therefore, the classic literature in the field is cited, major theorists are noted, and terms are defined, especially where there is a divergence of opinion in management literature. We all stand on the shoulders of the management "giants" who paved the way in the field; a return to original sources is encouraged.

3. *Provide sufficient detail in selected areas to enable the practitioner to apply the concepts in day-to-day situations.* Several tools of planning and control, such as budget preparation and justification, training design, project management, special reports (e.g., the annual report, a strategic plan, a due diligence assessment, a consultant's report), and labor union contracts, are explained in detail.

We have attempted to provide enough information to make it possible for the reader to use these tools with ease at their basic level. It is the authors' hope that the readers will contribute to the literature and practice of healthcare management as they grow in their professional practice and management roles. We are grateful to our many colleagues who have journeyed with us over the years and shared their ideas with us.

*Joan Gratto Liebler*
*Charles R. McConnell*

*It is with regret that Joan Gratto Liebler and Jones & Bartlett Learning note the passing of Charles R. McConnell in late 2019.*

# About the Authors

**Joan Gratto Liebler**, MA, MPA, is Professor Emerita, Health Information Management, Temple University, Philadelphia, Pennsylvania. She has more than 40 years of professional experience in teaching and research in healthcare settings. In addition to teaching, her work and consulting experience include engagement with community health centers; behavioral health settings, schools, industrial clinics, prisons; and long-term care, acute care, and hospice facilities. She has also been an active participant in area-wide healthcare planning, end-of-life care coalitions, and area-wide emergency and disaster planning.

Ms. Liebler is also the author of *Medical Records: Policies and Guidelines* and has authored numerous journal articles and contributed chapters relating to health information management.

Ms. Liebler holds the degrees of Master of Public Administration, Temple University, Philadelphia, PA, and Master of Arts (concentration in Medical Ethics), St. Charles Borromeo Seminary, Philadelphia, Pennsylvania.

**Charles R. McConnell**, MBA, CM, led a successful career as an independent healthcare management and human resources consultant and freelance writer specializing in business, management, and human resources topics. For 11 years he was active as a management engineering consultant with the Management and Planning Services (MAPS) division of the Hospital Association of New York State (HANYS), and he later spent 18 years as a hospital human resources manager. As author, coauthor, and anthology editor, he published more than 30 books and contributed several hundred articles to various publications. For 40 years, he was editor of the quarterly professional journal *The Health Care Manager*.

Mr. McConnell received a Master of Business Administration and a Bachelor of Science degree in Engineering from the State University of New York at Buffalo.

# What's New in the *Eighth Edition*

*Management Principles for Health Professionals, Eighth Edition*, continues to present foundational principles of management in the context of contemporary healthcare. The *Eighth Edition* reflects current issues and trends, linking them to basic principles. The corporate culture as an over-arching ethos is identified and then applied to various management functions; new and continuing legislative and accrediting mandates are included. Throughout the chapters, telemedicine and eHealth, the impact of technology, social media issues, and changes relating to reimbursement are noted as pervasive themes. A variety of formats are used to present material; these formats include the content of a topic, and provide examples of methods of presentation for use in training and workshops. Two major reference tools are presented and developed throughout the text: The Manager's Wheel Book and The Management Reference Portfolio.

Examples and exhibits have been updated to reflect a wide variety of settings and clients. Settings include the traditional inpatient hospital and related specialty clinics; expanded use of ER and observation units/clinical decision units; rehabilitation services, both inpatient and outpatient; expanded use of adult day care centers for respite/vacation care; expanded use of homecare, supported by telemedicine. Some other examples include such varied settings as truck stop dispensaries, industrial health correction care, and programs for the homeless population.

Changing aspects of job content are noted, including the development of the nurse navigator role; "always on" and required or expected availability; technological skills requirements,

## Specific Chapter Updates

Chapter 1, "The Dynamic Environment of Health Care," presents a template for analyzing megatrends in health care including telemedicine and eHealth, increasing use of technology, "Here Come the Robots,"

retainer-fee and concierge care, respite and vacation care of elderly, ER care by appointment, medical cost sharing, Accountable Care Organizations, in-network care. A major new feature is the Manager's Wheel Book, its content and uses.

Chapter 2, "The Challenge of Change," includes six examples of major change, followed by an analysis of the incremental changes associated with each. Suggested quality assurance analysis relating to HIPAA compliance and advance directive practices are provided. Interoperability features of EHR and data degrading issues are noted. ACA is updated. A template for analyzing health insurance proposals is included.

Chapter 3, "Organizational Adaptation and Survival," includes expanded discussion of issues such as: when clients become adversaries, how to reach remote clients and expand client base, changes in practitioners' roles, with emphasis on the nurse navigator as a counter-balance to bureaucratic features of large organizations. The corporate culture as an over-arching ethos is discussed in detail. To link theory and practice, a detailed analysis of life cycle concepts with the related survival strategies is presented. The concept of the Management Reference Portfolio is introduced. "Know Your Organization" is presented, using the manager's wheel book as an analytical tool.

Chapter 4, "Leadership and the Manager," features sections on "Growing in the Leadership Role" and "Enhancing One's Career Path." These include a data-driven review process for a manager's self-evaluation and for aligning one's career path with the goals of the organization. Excerpts from the manager's wheel book are included to reflect leadership and career development activities.

Chapter 5, "Planning and Decision Making," adds material reflecting the corporate culture as a primary factor in these processes. Examples for assessing planning constraints and factors include settings and client characteristics in traditional settings as well as adult day care/respite care centers, correction care, truck stop dispensaries, and healthcare outreach programs for the homeless population. Additional examples of mission and core values are included. Policy excerpts include Institutional Review Board consent practices. Decision-making discussion includes assessment of degree of impact and probability. Detailed use of the after-action-review and the analysis of unanticipated outcomes are described as means for evaluating decisions.

Chapter 6, "Organizing and Staffing," includes analysis of organizational structure as centralized vs. decentralized, "tall," or "flat" models. Succession plans are described; clarification of employee status relating to contractual and temporary workers is given; classifications as essential and non-essential, "always on" availability requirements, and flextime options are described. Additional elements and wording of job descriptions are given. The consultant report reflects several current issues in long-term care: increased use of respite/vacation care; bullying and the incident report requirements; pain management and opioid use; pros and cons of documenting a spiritual history; indicators of social isolation; changing patterns of length of stay. The use of telehealth/eHealth and the personal health record are also included.

Chapter 7, "Committees and Teams," includes an exposition of the over-all context for committee and team development. The corporate culture is given particular attention regarding committees and teams and the values of cooperation, transparency, corporate compliance, safety and security, and outreach initiatives. Guidelines for group deliberation are given, and then illustrated in the after-action review of a major disaster. The manager's wheel book entries relating to committee and team activity are reviewed.

Chapter 8, "Budget Planning and Implementation" are presented within the context of the corporate culture, plus laws, regulations and standards for fiscal planning. An in-depth discussion of shared responsibilities is given, with emphasis on board of trustee's root decisions. These include balancing "safety net" commitment, cost-shifting impact, and debt limits. Identification of new elements in billing is noted (e.g., charges associated with eVisits and other telemedicine interactions). A budget reference portfolio and additional budget justification statements are included. Examples of budget auditing findings are noted.

Chapter 9, "Training and Development: The Backbone of Motivation and Retention," reflects the corporate culture values of success and excellence. Orientation topics include clarification about employees being "always on" and modified operations schedules requirements and expectations. Orientation also includes expanded discussion of social media and internet use. The topic of sexual harassment is presented in a Frequently Asked Questions format, thus giving both the content of this topic and an example of a training method.

Chapter 10, "Adaptation, Motivation, and Conflict Management," includes additional examples of the sources of conflict; the conflict model is applied in detail to Whistleblower activity. Union trends and issues are noted, including concerns about the increased use of robots in replacing workers; the effects of the Supreme Court JANUS decision are described.

Chapter 11, "Communication: The Glue that Binds Us Together," provides information about social media and e-mail, texting, and instant messaging through an analysis of policy and practices, with particular emphasis on limits on management's prerogatives. Methods for enhancing communication effectiveness are noted, including the SBAR format.

Chapter 12, "Comprehensive Planning and Accountability Documentation," relates planning and review documents to the corporate culture and values of accountability, transparency, and shared responsibility. The standard reports have updated entries reflecting "By the Numbers" reporting; telemedicine and eHealth; the personal health record; closure of a facility details. A Plan of Correction as a mandated response to licensure or accreditation reviews is included. Excerpts from the manager's wheel book are given to illustrate the usefulness of these factual support materials for writing accurate reports.

Chapter 13, "Quality Improvement and Control Processes," has new material about the characteristics of a thriving organization. A variety of quality improvement topics are suggested, including readmission within 30 days, focused review of over/underuse of services, patterns of use regarding inpatient admissions from ER and Observation Unit, pain management, and opioid use.

Chapter 14, "Human Resources Management: A Line Manager's Perspective," includes aspects of online and social media recruiting; using the manager's wheel book to identify significant activity to include in employee evaluation; processes associated with both voluntary and involuntary separation from the organization. Particular emphasis is given to the work environment: hostile or supportive and practices that foster one or the other environment.

Chapter 15, "Day-to-Day Management for the Health Professional-as-Manager," provides additional material for self-assessment, career development and the review of personal and professional goals, and the necessity for aligning these with the organization's goals. The final appendix includes a complete wheel book for comprehensive analysis of the role and functions of the middle manager.

## CHAPTER 1

# The Dynamic Environment of Health Care

## CHAPTER OBJECTIVES

- Describe the healthcare environment as it has evolved since the middle to late 1960s, with attention to the dynamic interplay of key factors.
- Examine megatrends in the healthcare environment with attention to:
  - Client characteristics
  - Professional practitioners and caregivers
  - Healthcare marketplace and settings
  - Applicable laws, regulations, and standards
  - Impact of technology
  - Privacy and security considerations
  - Financing of health care
  - Social and cultural factors
- Identify the role set of the healthcare practitioner as manager.
- Review the classic functions of the manager and the related competencies.
- Introduce the concept of The Manager's Wheel Book, its content, and uses.
- Define and differentiate between management as an art and a science.
- Conceptualize the characteristics of an effective manager.

## ▶ The Dynamic Environment of Health Care

The contemporary healthcare environment is a dynamic one, combining enduring patterns of practice with evolving ones to meet the challenges and opportunities of changing times. The healthcare organization is a highly visible one in most communities. It is a fixture with deep roots in the social, religious, fraternal, and civic fabric of the society. It is a major economic force, accounting for approximately one-sixth of the national economy. In some local settings, the healthcare organization is one of the major employers, with the local economy tied to this sector. The image of the hospital is anchored in personal lives: it is the place of major life events, including birth and death, and episodes of care throughout one's life. Families recount the stories of "remember the time when we all rushed to the hospital …" and similar recollections. The hospital is anchored in the popular culture as a common frame of reference. People express, in ordinary terms, their stereotypic reference to the healthcare setting: "He works up at the hospital," "Oh yes, we made another trip to the emergency room," or "I have a doctor's appointment." Popular media also uses similar references; television shows regularly feature dramatic scenes in the acute care hospital, with the physician as an almost universally visible presence. Care is often depicted as happening in the emergency department.

On closer examination, one recognizes that, in fact, many changes have occurred in the healthcare environment. The traditional hospital remains an important hub of care but with many levels of care and physical locations. The physician continues to hold a major place on the healthcare team, but there has been a steady increase in the development and use of other practitioners (e.g., nurse midwife, physical therapist as independent agent, physician assistant) to complement and augment the physician's role. A casual conversation reflects such change; a person is just as likely to go to the mall to get a brief physical examination at a walk-in, franchised clinic as he or she would be to go to the traditional physician's office. One might get an annual "flu" shot at the grocery store or smoking cessation counseling from the pharmacist at a commercial drug store. One might have an appointment for care with a nurse practitioner instead of a physician. Instead of using an emergency service at a hospital, one might receive health care at a freestanding clinic or an urgent care service at a shopping mall. Within the emergency service setting there are changes: emergency service care by appointment. In this instance, the patient (or caregiver) arranges an arrival time and waits at home until the designated time. The purposes of this reservation process are reducing wait time in the emergency room (ER) and enhancing the general comfort of the patient in their home setting. Careful assessment is needed when using this approach; a patient might delay seeking care because they do not realize the seriousness of their condition. Another innovation in health care is that of boutique care, also called retainer-fee care or concierge care. The patient and primary care physician enter into a retainer arrangement, with the patient paying an annual fee for overall care; the physician agrees to limit the number of patients to increase a more personalized approach, decrease waiting times, and increase availability. Some practices charge additional fees for certain tests and services.

Although the setting and practitioners have developed and changed, the underlying theme remains: how to provide health care that is the best, most effective, accessible, and affordable, in a stable yet flexible delivery system? This is the enduring goal.

Those who manage healthcare organizations monitor trends and issues associated with the healthcare delivery system in order to reach this goal. Thus, a manager seeks to have thorough awareness and knowledge of the interplay of the dynamic forces. It is useful, therefore, to follow a systematic approach to identify, monitor, and respond to changes in the healthcare environment. The following template provides such a systematic approach. The starting point is the client/patient/recipient of care. This is followed in turn by considerations of the professional practitioners and caregivers; healthcare market place and settings; applicable laws, regulations, and standards; impact of technology; privacy and security considerations; financing; and social–cultural factors. These topics and trends are discussed more fully in the subsequent chapters.

# ▶ Client/Patient Characteristics

The demographic patterns of the overall population have a direct impact on the healthcare organization. For example, the increase in the number of older people requires more facilities and personnel specializing in care of this group, such as continuing care, skilled nursing care, and home care. Clinical conditions associated with aging also lead to the development of specialty programs, such as Alzheimer's disease and memory care, cardiac and stroke rehabilitation, and wellness programs to promote healthy aging. At the other end of the age spectrum, attention to neonatal care, healthy growth and development, and preventive care are points of focus. Particular attention is given to adolescents and young adults who engage in contact sports, where concussion, permanent brain injury, fractures, and sprains are common. In all age groups, there is a rising rate of obesity, type 2 diabetes, and addictions to substances, such as heroin, opioids, methadone, and assorted "street drugs." Medical marijuana use has become an acceptable element in pain management care, although there continues to be questions about conflict of federal versus state law about the legalization of this substance.

Diseases and illnesses are, of course, an ever-present consideration. Some diseases seem to have been conquered and eliminated through timely intervention. Some recur after long periods of absence. Tuberculosis, measles, mumps, polio, smallpox, and pertussis are examples of successes in disease management and prevention. Sometimes, however, new strains may develop or compliance with immunization mandates may decrease so that these types of communicable diseases reappear.

Decades of use of antibacterial medicines has given rise to superbugs, resistant to the usual treatment. Another element of concern is the appearance of an almost unknown disease entity (e.g., Ebola or a pandemic agent). New clinical conditions may also arise within certain age groups, necessitating fresh approaches to their care. By way of example, consider the rise in autism or childhood obesity.

Other characteristics of the client/patient population reflect patterns of usage and the associated costs of care. The identification of superusers—patients who have high readmission rates and/or longer than average lengths of stay or more complications—gives providers an insight into practices needing improvement (e.g., better discharge planning or increased patient education). The geographic region that constitutes the general catchment area of the facility should be analyzed to identify health conditions common to the area. Examples include rural farm regions, with associated injuries and illnesses; heavy industry, with work-related injuries; and winter resort areas, with injuries resulting from strenuous outdoor activity (e.g., fractures from skiing injuries).

## ▶ Trends Relating to Practitioners and Caregivers

The trends and issues relating to practitioners and caregivers cluster around the continuing expansion of scope of practice, with the related increase in education and credentialing. The traditional attending physician role has given way to the inpatient physician, the hospitalist. The one-to-one physician–patient role set continues to shift from solo practice to group practice and team coverage. Licensed, credentialed nonphysician practitioners continue to augment the care provided by the physician. These physician-extenders often specialize—for example, the physical therapist in sports-related care, the occupational therapist in autism programs, the nurse practitioner in wellness care for the frail elderly, the nurse midwife in high risk pregnancy care, the nurse case manager in transition care, the nurse navigator in coordinating discharge plans and after-care training, and the physician assistant in emergency care.

Educational requirements include advanced degrees in the designated field.

There is a related shift in the practice settings for these various practitioners. The move away from inpatient-based care leads to an increase in independent practice. Sometimes the franchise model is favored over self-employment. Regional and national franchises provide a turnkey practice environment with the additional benefits of a management support division.

## The Family as Caregiver

Although the provision of care by family members is a practice that long predates formal healthcare models, these caregivers are the focus of renewed attention. As shorter stays for inpatient care, or subacute care to reduce inpatient care, become the norm, the role of the family caretaker intensifies. The patient care plan, with emphasis on the discharge plan, necessarily includes instruction to family members about such elements as medication regimen, wound care, infection prevention, and injection processes. Long-term care facilities and adult day care centers have adopted programs for respite care to provide relief for family caregivers as well as to give frail elderly a variety of care.

If a patient does not have a family member who is able to assist in these ways, or if the patient (often a frail, elderly person) lives alone, coordination of services with a community agency or commercial company is needed. This gives rise to related issues. Can family members be reimbursed by insurance providers? If so, what is needed by way of documentation and billing? And there is yet another related issue: how can employers assist workers to meet the demands of work as well as help the family member? Practices such as flexible work hours and unpaid leave become both desirable and necessary elements.

## Changes in Management Support Services

Behind the scenes, there is the wide network of management support services within the healthcare organization. The trend toward specialization increases within these ranks, with new job categories being developed in response to related trends. With regard to finances and reimbursement, chief financial officers (or similar administrators) augment their teams with clinical reimbursement auditors, coding and billing compliance officers, physician coder-educators, and certified medical coders. The regulatory standards manager specializes in coordinating the many compliance factors flowing from laws, regulations, and standards. The chief information officer augments that role with specialized teams, including nurse informaticians, clinical information specialists, and information technology experts.

## Patterns of Care

Improvements in patient care services, the utilization of advanced technologies such as telemedicine, and the financial pressures to reduce the length of stay for inpatient care have resulted in shorter stays, more transitional care, and (possibly) a higher readmission rate. To offset a high readmission rate, additional attention is given to the discharge plan, including home care and telemedicine services. The increased use of the observation unit in the emergency department also helps reduce admission and readmission rate. These issues and trends lead to a discussion of the healthcare setting.

# ▶ The Healthcare Setting: Formal Organizational Patterns and Levels of Care

Each healthcare setting has a distinct pattern of organization and offers specific levels of care. Characteristics include ownership and sponsorship, nonprofit or for-profit corporate status, and distinct levels of care. These elements are specified in the license to operate as well as in the corporate charter. Ownership and sponsorship often reflect deep ties to the immediate community. A sector of the community, such as a fraternal organization, a religious association, or an academic institution, developed and funded the original hospital or clinic, almost always as nonprofit because of their own nonprofit status. These organizations purchased the land, had the buildings erected and equipped, and provided continued supplemental funding for the enterprise. Federal, state, city, and county units of government also own and sponsor certain facilities (e.g., facilities for veterans, state behavioral care facilities, county residential programs for the intellectually challenged). For-profit ownership and sponsorship include owner–investor hospital and clinic chains, long-term care facilities, and franchise operations for specialty care (e.g., eye care, rehabilitation centers, retail clinics in drugstores and big-box retailer stores). Over the past several decades, sponsorship by religious or fraternal organizations has diminished, with the resulting sale of these healthcare facilities to other entities. The original name is often retained because it is a familiar and respected designation in the community.

## Provider Growth: Mergers, Joint Ventures, and Collaborative Partnerships

Healthcare organizations periodically change or augment their service offerings, with a resulting change in corporate structure. This restructuring may take the form of a merger, a joint venture, or a collaborative partnership. Why do healthcare organizations seek restructuring? There are several reasons:

- The desire to express an overall value of promoting comprehensive, readily accessible care by shoring up smaller community-based facilities, keeping them from closure
- The need for improved efficiencies resulting from centralized administrative practices such as financial and health information resource streamlining or public relations and marketing intensification
- The desire and/or need to penetrate new markets to attract additional clients
- The desire and/or need to increase size so as to have greater clout in negotiations with managed care providers who tend to bypass smaller entities

As cost-containment pressure began to grow, providers—primarily hospitals—initially moved into mergers, mostly to secure economies of scale and other operating efficiencies and sometimes for reasons as basic as survival. The growth and expansion of managed care plans provided further incentive to merge among hospitals, which seems to have inspired health plan mergers in return. Each time a significant merger occurs, one side gains more leverage in negotiating contracts. The larger the managed care plan, the greater the clout in negotiating with hospitals and physicians and vice versa.

## Clarification of Terms

The term merger is used to describe the blending of two or more corporate entities to create one new organization with one licensure and one provider number for reimbursement purposes. One central board of trustees or directors is created, usually with representation from each of the merged facilities. Debts and assets are combined. For example, suppose a university medical center buys a smaller community-based hospital. Ownership and control is now shifted to the new organization. Sometimes the names of the original facilities are retained as part of public relations and marketing, as when a community group or religious-affiliated group has great loyalty and ties to the organization. Alternatively, a combined name is used, such as Mayfair Hospital of the University Medical System.

The joint venture differs from a merger in that each organization retains its own standing as a specific legal/corporate entity. A joint venture or affiliation is a formal agreement between or among member facilities to officially coordinate and share one or more activities. Ownership and control of each party remains distinct, but binding agreements, beneficial to all parties, are developed. Shared activities typically include managed care negotiations, group purchasing discounts, staff development and education offerings, and shared management services. Each organization keeps its own name with the addition of some reference to its affiliated status, as in the title: Port Martin Hospital, an affiliate of Vincent Medical Center.

A collaborative partnership is another interorganizational arrangement. As with the joint venture, each organization retains its own standing as a specific legal–corporate entity. The purpose of the collaborative partnership is to draw on the mutually beneficial resources of each party for a specific time period associated with the completion of agreed-on projects. An example from research illustrates this point: a university's neuroscience and psychology departments and a hospital pediatric service combine research efforts in the area of autism. A formal letter of agreement or mutual understanding is exchanged, outlining the essential aspects of the cooperative arrangement.

Such restructuring efforts, especially the formal merger, are preceded by mutual due diligence reviews in which operational, financial, and legal issues are assessed. Federal regulations and state licensing requirements must be followed. Details of the impact of the restructuring on operational levels are considered, with each manager providing reports, statistics, contractual information, leases (as of equipment), and staffing arrangements, including independent contractors and outsourced work.

In the instance of a full merger, practical considerations constitute major points of focus. Examples include redesigning forms, merging the master patient index and record system into one new system, merging finance and billing processes, and officially discharging and readmitting patients when the legally binding merger has taken place.

Present-day mergers and joint ventures can have a pronounced effect on the health professional entering a management position. Consider the example of a laboratory manager who must now oversee a geographically divided service because a two-hospital merger results in this person being responsible for two sites that are miles apart. There is far more to consider in managing a split department than in managing a single-site operation. The manager's job is made all the more difficult. Overall, however, mergers, joint ventures, and collaborative partnerships are an opportunity for the professional-as-manager, with greatly increased responsibility and accountability and a role of increasing complexity.

## Range of Service and Levels of Care

One of the most distinguishing features of a specific healthcare organization is the range of service, along with levels of care. This feature identifies the organization as a particular kind of organization, explicitly defined in its license to operate (e.g., an acute care hospital, an adult day care center, a hospice). An organization may offer many different services, both inpatient and outpatient. The range of service and levels of care are part of the overall definition of the organization; the specific types of care are delineated. Groups such as the American Hospital Association (AHA), The Joint Commission (TJC) and similar associations, and various designated federal and/or state agencies define types and levels of care. Thus, a hospital might develop its range of services at an advanced level, with a variety of specialty services, to meet the definition of tertiary care. A small, rural hospital might seek to meet the basic standards for a critical access facility (a Centers for Medicare and Medicaid Services designation), capitalizing on the flexibility such designation requires.

Clinics vary in their range of service from the relatively small, walk-in clinic to more complex services, such as an urgent care clinic or specialty clinic associated with a hospital. In this latter arrangement, the inpatient service coordinates care with its companion outpatient clinic. Examples include surgery, cardiac care, and prenatal and postnatal care.

Another way of noting the variety of care services is to group organizations by client characteristics and treatment needs: geriatric behavioral care, rapid treatment for drug-dependent clients, women's health, comprehensive cancer care, sports medicine, hospice care, and intensive day treatment for at-risk youth. Care of frail, elderly people has been and is a growth industry because of the simple fact of demographics—the increasing numbers of older individuals. The variety of levels of care includes independent living units; personal care assistance, including secured units for dementia care; skilled nursing care; and comprehensive continuing care facilities. Adult day care programs augment residential care.

Further details about the range of care can be found by identifying the organization's place in the overall continuum of care. For the purposes of this discussion, the acute care, inpatient facility will be placed at the center, with the continuum of care segmented as subacute and post-acute, although it should be noted that not all care involves inpatient admission. Thus, an organization might tailor its services to support transitional care, either temporary or permanent care, with a post-acute rehabilitation center, a long-term nursing care center, and assisted living and secured personal care for frail, elderly people. The continuing emphasis on reducing readmission rates for inpatient care gives new impetus to the development and/or expansion of these types of services. A traditional nursing home, specializing in "balance of life" care of frail, elderly people, might restructure its programs to add posthospitalization care, with the expectation that the length of stay will be weeks or (a few) months—not indeterminate and permanent. Home care programs have increased in prominence because of their place in the sequence of care. Shortened inpatient stays, outpatient same-day surgery, and transitional care from hospital to nursing home to the patient's personal residence intensify the need for home care by nurses, along with a variety of other caregivers (e.g., health aides, homemaker aides).

Hospice care represents a model of service that utilizes several levels of care. Care of the terminally ill (regardless of age) is rendered in the home, in the hospital when needed, and in a nursing care facility. A hospice might be owned and sponsored by an inpatient facility or operate as a stand-alone organization. One way to describe hospice care is this: the hospice program follows the patient and family as they move through the various changes in location.

In the continuing search for the best care, with flexibility and affordability, there has been renewed interest in domiciliary care for the elderly or developmentally disabled. The underlying idea is a return to home-like, individual care provided by paid caregivers, often in a patient's own homes. Some states have active programs to increase the number and quality of such arrangements, along with active plans to decrease the number of nursing home beds.

The group home for adolescents or developmentally challenged persons continues to be an area of change. The movement is away from large, institutional-based care to very small units (e.g., four to six clients in a family-like group home).

## ▶ Laws, Regulations, and Accrediting Standards

Laws, regulations, and accrediting standards are a major consideration in the delivery of health care. They affect every aspect of the healthcare system. The sheer volume of such requirements, some of which are in contradiction to others, has increased to the point that most organizations have a formally designated compliance officer. This high-level manager, assigned to the chief executive division, has the responsibility of assessing compliance with current requirements, monitoring proposed changes, and helping departments and services prepare for upcoming changes. Other responsibilities of this officer include the preparation of required reports and studies, the coordination of site visits, and the preparation of any follow-up action or plan of correction. In addition, this officer provides liaison with the Board of Trustee's corporate compliance committee. Managers at the operational level work closely with this office in order to comply—indeed excel—at meeting all requirements.

The operational level managers, while assisted by the compliance office, must take the initiative on their own to ensure that day-to-day practices and systems are in order. A systematic review of laws, regulations, and standards facilitates this practice. A manager can sort through the thicket of requirements by analyzing them in terms of several features:

- Setting. Licensure laws at the state level authorize the owner/sponsors to offer specific types of care (e.g., acute care hospital, behavioral care facility, rehabilitation center). The definitions and requirements in this fundamental law are the starting point; without meeting this set of binding elements, the organization would not be permitted to function. Changes in program offerings, including expansion, termination, or sale, trigger an update in licensure status.
- Patient/client group. Certain issues concerning definition of the patient/client must be

considered: when does the relationship begin; who is eligible for certain programs of care; what aspects of reimbursement for care apply; who may consent for care; and what, if any, special provisions attach to certain patient groups (e.g., any patients needing protective care).

- Professional practitioners and the support staff. Professional practitioners are required to have a license to practice. Both the individual and the organization's officials must be mindful of the necessity of meeting this set of rules. In addition to this requirement, there are many laws and regulations governing working conditions, hours and rates of pay, and nondiscrimination.
- Systems requirements. Specific aspects of the administrative and support systems are often laid out in detail, including time frames; requirements for record development and retention; and review processes relating to patient care, safety, and privacy. Required documentation of care is delineated in terms of content and time (e.g., development of plan of care, discharge plan, medication profile, restraint usage).

The sources of law are both state and federal governments. In addition to these, local units of government, such as counties and cities, have laws that apply to most or all formal organizations in their geographic jurisdiction. The usual ones are fire and safety codes, zoning regulations, environmental requirements, and traffic controls.

## Regulations Stemming from Laws

The usual practice in lawmaking is this: the basic law is developed and passed, with the lawmakers recognizing that further details will be needed. The specific law usually indicates which government department or agency is invested with this rule-making power. Healthcare providers are most familiar with the Department of Health and Human Services (DHHS) and its Centers for Medicare and Medicaid Services (CMS—formerly the Health Care Financing Administration) division that has the authority to develop Medicare rules and regulations. Other current "headliner" laws and companion regulations include the Health Information Technology for Economic and Clinical Health Act (HITECH), the Health Insurance Portability and Accountability Act (HIPAA) of 1996, and the Patient Protection and Affordable Care Act (PPACA) of 2010, now commonly referred to as the Affordable Care Act (ACA).

## Accrediting Standards

Although these standards or elements of performance are not required as such, most healthcare facilities seek to meet them and have official recognition by an appropriate accrediting agency. Some of the usual nationwide accrediting bodies are TJC, the Commission on Accreditation of Rehabilitation Facilities (CARF), and the Accrediting Commission for Health Care.

Within the accrediting process for the overall facility, there are additional criteria for certain programs, with the resulting assurance of quality care. By way of example, TJC has an additional approval rating for rehabilitation services. It also has disease-specific care certification.

## Professional Association Standards and Guidelines

Professional associations develop standards of practice and related guidelines in their area of expertise. These guidelines reflect best practices and provide practical methods of developing and implementing operational level systems. In addition to the practical aspect of meeting such optional standards, there is prestige value associated with gaining recognition by outside groups. Receiving magnet designation from the American Nurses' Credentialing Center illustrates this dual benefit.

## Sources of Information About Requirements

Managers face a challenge in trying to keep up to date regarding the many requirements. They must take a proactive stand, especially for those aspects relating to their department or service.

One's professional association is a reliable source of timely and thorough information. The umbrella organizations such as the AHA monitor current and prospective issues and make the information readily available. A useful practice for managers to adopt is the regular monitoring of the Federal Register for federal regulations, and the companion publication at the state level. These agencies publish agenda listings on a periodic basis (e.g., annually, semiannually) to alert the public about probable new regulations. This is augmented by an official Notice of Proposed Rulemaking about a specific topic.

Government agencies, public and private "think tanks," and other associations prepare position papers; national, state, or regional health initiatives proposals; and similar plans. The DHHS's national health goals or a state governor's long-range plans are examples of readily available documents to alert managers of trends and issues.

# ▶ The Impact of Technology

A survey of any health discipline would readily provide examples of the impact of technology. New treatment modalities emerge. For example, specialty care is taken to the patient (e.g., bedside anesthesia, mobile vans with chemotherapy, portable diagnostic equipment). There is rapid and constant adoption of computerized devices. Several areas of interest are highlighted here to illustrate the trends and issues of a high-tech world and its implications for healthcare delivery.

## eHealth and Virtual Health

This segment of health care has several names: eHealth, Virtual Health, and Digital Connectivity. The eVisit, wherein patient and provider communicate by means of technological interaction instead of face-to-face, in an office, has become commonplace. Telemedicine or telehealth is a broader and slightly older term, reflecting the same kind of interaction. Both methods utilize video conferencing, telephone systems, and computers. The eVisit by the patient with the clinician is a particularly good method for patients who are in rural areas without easy access to their primary care provider; it is useful in the same way for the homebound patient without transportation or whose chronic illness is exacerbated by going outside the home. Virtual counseling is another example of this kind of care; the sufferer of posttraumatic stress disorder or depression might find easier access to interventions and care because it is readily available through technology. Also, the eVisit is a useful alternative when inclement weather makes travel to on-site care unwise or impossible. In addition, remote monitoring provides real-time feedback to providers and patients, allowing them to make more timely interventions when indicated. Common applications include monitoring heart-related conditions, diabetes, and pulmonary hypertension.

Teleconferencing provides clinicians with ready access to specialists in another setting, thus providing the patient and care team with expert advice and avoiding the transfer of the patient. The telestroke program exemplifies this type of interaction where time is of the essence. The popular use of apps for self-monitoring, both for a clinical condition and wellness, provides clients and caregivers with some baseline information about a client's ongoing condition. The user can set up reminders about medication use, blood sugar levels, or blood pressure monitoring. Diet and exercise information can be tracked. Coupled with popular web searches for health information (e.g., getting a "second opinion" from a website), the consumer of health care generates his or her own personal health record (PHR).

## Here Come the Robots

Robotic technology is a growing one in most sectors, including health care; these technologies have had gradual implementation and have become a fixture, with greater use anticipated. Examples include transport and delivery of supplies; mixing and dispensing medications; surgical applications, especially in highly delicate care, such as eye surgery. Devices such as a robotic arm enhance care in rehabilitation units. For some aspects of robot utilization (e.g., transport and delivery), a cost savings tends to result, thus offsetting the cost of robot with reduced costs relating to personnel. There is, of course, some loss of personalization and this is a drawback; a caregiver picks up on both subtle and overt changes in a patient during routine care and in the conversational exchange; a patient often expresses important information such as an increase in discomfort or pain that would not be conveyed in the robotic intervention. This observational opportunity is lost in the high tech approach.

## The Personal Health Record

The PHR is not a new concept. Conscientious individuals routinely keep important health documents, including immunization records, summaries of episodes of care, and their own tracking notes about a chronic condition. Fitness application data and various self-testing (such as do-it-yourself EKG monitoring) have become common. What is new is the increased computerization of such notes. With the emphasis on developing and maintaining an electronic health record system, healthcare organizations encourage the incorporation of client-generated portfolios and the official documentation from healthcare providers into a comprehensive document. Patients' rights to access and receive a copy of their health records has been well established and is encouraged. This is a gradual change from the days when there was limited or no routine access. The PHR does not replace the legal record of the healthcare provider—the PHR is developed and maintained by the patient/client and the official record by the provider. There is a related trend: having the patient access the ongoing, official record through electronic systems. Providers make this possible through the development of secure portal access to the information and encourage its use through patient education about the process. Information includes access to test results, discharge instructions, procedure information, and similar data. The goal is to increase patients' involvement in their own care. The electronic health record is more fully discussed in the chapter on the challenges of change in the healthcare system.

## Data Warehousing and Data Mining

As the electronic data capture and retention and manipulation increase, so does the sheer volume of data. These electronic measures incorporate and enhance the more historical methods of the hard copy record, decentralized indexes and registries, and special studies. Data warehousing refers to the centralized depository of data collected from most or all aspects of the organization (e.g., patient demographics, financial/billing transactions, clinical decision making) gathered into one consistent computerized format. Easy connectivity to national and international data bases (e.g., National Library of Medicine, Medicare Providers Analysis and Review) is yet another feature of this process. Data mining is the analysis and extraction of data to find meaningful facts and trends for real-time interventions in clinical decision-making support, studies and oversight review of administrative and clinical practice by designated review groups, budget support, and related data usage. Trend analysis and predictive indicators (e.g., injury prediction outcomes in pediatric emergencies or predictions of impending arrhythmia and sudden death, mortality predictions) are readily available to clinicians. Data mining is also a business; a medical center, with its fast compilation of core data and specialty data elements, may sell nonidentifiable patient data to pharmaceutical, medical device, and biotech industries.

## Translational Medicine

With the ready availability of support data, clinicians seek to more effectively and rapidly complete the cycle of bench to bedside to bench. Translational medicine emerges as an area of intensified interest, with hospitals coordinating these efforts through a clinical innovation office headed by a physician with an appropriate support staff. This strengthens both research capabilities and clinical practice.

## The Health Information Exchange

The electronic health record enhances patient care within the organization because of its real-time, comprehensive features. But what of the situations in which care is given in more than one setting? The release of information process, using traditional hard copy or even electronic transmission, usually starts after the patient is admitted. Why not develop systems of interchange of information, regardless of the point of care? Such a system would facilitate communication among providers, reduce the number of unneeded tests, and provide a more comprehensive review of patients' past and ongoing care. Technology supports this concept; the electronic movement of health-related information is available. The coordinated efforts to make this a reality have led to the development of regional health information exchange of patient-consented information.

## Privacy and Security Issues

The positive aspects of technology as applied to health care are clear. But along with these positive benefits, there arise new concerns for privacy and security issues. Hackers can access and even destroy computerized data bases. Identifying theft, including medical identity, is an increasing problem for individuals and organizations. Consequently, safeguards are increased to secure the data, yet keep it easily accessible by legitimate users. There is a growing body of laws and regulations relating to these issues, foremost of which is HIPAA, mandating a variety of controls and practices to ensure patient privacy is protected. A more detailed discussion of this law and its requirements is in the chapter on the challenge of change.

## Informatics Standards and Common Language

The goals of data sharing in support of patient care are generally well accepted, with active implementation of systems. To make this effective, there is the continuing need for interoperability of systems along with informatics standards and common language. These efforts include the development of standard vocabulary and classification systems, such as the National Library of Medicine's Unified Medical Language System as well as the standards developed by the Institute of Electrical and Electronic Engineers and the Health Level-7 standards. HIPAA regulations require uniform protocols for electronic transactions for both format and content of data capture and transmission. The development of a national healthcare information infrastructure has the support of key advocates who support the development and implementation of national standards.

## The Virtual Enterprise

The concept of the virtual enterprise has emerged as a result of available technology in both the for-profit and nonprofit sectors. Organizations develop contractual partnerships with independent companies and individuals who provide goods and services. Instead of on-site departments, services, units, or direct employer–employee relationships, organizations outsource many functions. By way of example, consider the contemporary health information department that has outsourced several functions: transcription, billing and coding support, release of information, and document storage and retrieval. Another example, drawn from a direct patient care program, is reflected in a chronic disease management service within a home health agency. The home health agency coordinates services from other health providers who remain independent agents. This trend is so common that, in job descriptions and want ads, the job location is noted whether the setting is on-site or virtual.

## Reimbursement and Patterns of Payment

Patterns of payment for health care have changed in response to social, political, and economic pressures. Hospitals and clinics have deep historical roots in charitable, not-for-profit models; along with this early approach to care, there was also the fee-for-service approach as patients made payments directly to practitioners.

Health insurance programs, both nonprofit such as Blue Cross and Blue Shield and commercial insurance plans, emerged in the 1930s as partners in the payment for healthcare services. The form of insurance that many of these early plans offered was frequently referred to as "hospitalization" insurance; it covered costs when one was hospitalized, but the majority of early plans did not cover common ancillary services, such as visits to physicians.

The 1960s saw the introduction of federally funded care with the creation of Medicare coverage for the elderly and Medicaid, essentially a welfare program, to provide coverage for low-income persons and the indigent. Medicare and Medicaid were established by the same federal legislation, but they differ as sources of payment. Medicare reimbursement is fully federal, but Medicaid reimbursement is shared, with 50% coming from the federal government and the remaining 50% split between state and county. In some instances, the second 50% is split evenly between state and county; in others, the split is unequal (e.g., 34% state and 16% county).

Concern for healthcare costs has gathered momentum since the 1960s, as have efforts to control or reduce these costs. Costs clearly took a leap upward immediately following the introduction of Medicare and Medicaid; however, Medicare and Medicaid are not the sole cause of the cost escalation. Rather, costs have been driven up by a complex combination of forces that include the aforementioned programs and other government undertakings, private not-for-profit and commercial insurers, changes in medical practice and advancements in technology, proliferation of medical specialties, increases in physician fees, advances in pharmaceuticals, overexpansion of the country's hospital system, economic improvements in the lot of healthcare workers, and the desires and demands of the public. These and other forces have kept healthcare costs rising at a rate that has outpaced overall inflation two- or threefold in some years.

As concern for healthcare costs has spread, so have attempts to control costs without adversely affecting quality or hindering access. The final two decades of the 20th century and the beginning of this century have seen some significant dollar-driven phenomena that are dramatically changing the face of healthcare delivery. Specifically, these include the following:

- The rise of competition among providers in an industry that was long considered essentially devoid of competition
- Changes in the structure of care delivery, such as system shrinkage, as hospitals decertify beds; an increase in hospital closures, mergers, and other affiliations that catalyzed the growth of healthcare systems; and the proliferation of independent specialty practices
- The advent and growth and expansion of managed care

In one way or another, most modern societal concerns for health care relate directly to cost or, in some instances, to issues of access to health care, which in turn translate directly into concern for cost. Massive change in health care has become a way of life, and dollars are one of the principal drivers of this change.

# ▶ The Managed Care Era

## The Managed Care "Solution" and the Beginning of Restricted Access

Aside from technological advances, much of what has occurred in recent years in the organization of healthcare delivery and payment has been driven by concern for costs. Changes have been driven by the desire to stem alarming cost increases and, in some instances, to reduce costs overall. These efforts have been variously focused. Government and insurers have acted on the healthcare money supply, essentially forcing providers to find ways of operating on less money than they think they require. Provider organizations have taken steps to adjust expenditures to fall within the financial limitations they face. These steps have included closures, downsizing, formation of systems to take advantage of economies of scale, and otherwise seeking ways of delivering care more economically and efficiently. In this cost-conscious environment, managed care has evolved.

Managed care, consisting of a number of practices intended to reduce costs and improve quality, seemed, at least in concept, to offer workable solutions to the problem of providing reasonable access to quality care at an affordable cost. Managed care included economic incentives for physicians and patients, programs for reviewing the medical necessity of specific services, increased beneficiary cost-sharing, controls on hospital inpatient admissions and lengths of stay, cost-sharing incentives for outpatient surgery, selective contracting with providers, and management of high-cost cases.

The most commonly encountered form of managed care is the health maintenance organization (HMO). The HMO concept was initially proposed in the 1960s when healthcare costs began to increase all out of proportion to other costs and so-called "normal" inflation following the introduction of Medicare and Medicaid. The HMO was formally promoted as a remedy for rising healthcare costs by the Health Maintenance Organization Act of 1973. The full title of this legislation is "An Act to amend the Public Health Service Act to provide assistance and encouragement for the establishment and expansion of health maintenance organizations, and for other purposes." From today's perspective, it is interesting to note that in implementing the HMO Act, it was necessary to override laws in place in a number of states that actually forbade the establishment of such entities.

The HMO Act provided for grants and loans to be used for starting or expanding HMOs. Preempting state restrictions on the establishment and operation of federally qualified HMOs, it required employers with 25 or more employees to offer federally certified HMO options if they already offered traditional health insurance to employees. (It did not require employers to offer health insurance if they did not already do so.) To become federally certified, an HMO had to offer a comprehensive package of specific benefits, be available to a broadly representative population on an equitable basis, be available at the same or lower cost than traditional insurance coverage, and provide for increased participation by consumers. Portions of the HMO Act have been amended several times since its initial passage, most notably by HIPAA.

Specifically, an HMO is a managed care plan that incorporates financing and delivery of a defined set of healthcare services to persons who are enrolled in a service network.

For the first time in the history of American health care, the introduction of managed care placed significant restrictions on the use of services. The public was introduced to the concept of the primary care physician as the "gatekeeper" to control access to specialists and various other services. Formerly, an insured individual could go to a specialist at will, and insurance would usually pay for the service. But with the gatekeeper in place, a subscriber's visits to a specialist were covered only if the patient was properly referred by the primary care physician. Subscribers who went to specialists without referral suddenly found themselves billed for the entire cost of the specialists.

By placing restrictions on the services that would be paid for and under what circumstances they could be accessed, managed care plans exerted control over some health insurance premium costs for employers and subscribers. In return for controlled costs, users had to accept limitations on their choice of physicians, having to choose from among those who agreed to participate in a given plan and accept that plan's payments, accept limitations on what services would be available to them, and, in most instances, agree to pay specified deductibles and copayments.

Managed care organizations and governmental payers brought pressure to bear on hospitals as well. Hospitals and physicians were encouraged to reduce the length of hospital stays, reduce the use of most ancillary services, and meet more medical needs on an outpatient basis. Review processes were established, and hospitals were penalized financially if their costs were determined to be "too high" or their inpatient stays "too long." Eventually, payment became linked to a standard or target length of stay so that a given diagnosis was compensated at a predetermined amount regardless of how long the patient was hospitalized.

As managed care organizations grew larger and stronger, they began to negotiate with hospitals concerning the use of their services. Various plans negotiated contracts with hospitals that would provide the best price breaks for the plan's patients, and price competition between and among providers became a reality.

By the end of the 20th century, approximately 160 million Americans were enrolled in managed care plans, encompassing what many thought to be the majority of people who were suitable for managed care. In-and-out participation of some groups, such as the younger aging (people in their 60s or so) and Medicaid patients, was anticipated. However, the bulk of people on whom managed care plans could best make their money were supposedly already enrolled. But managed care continued to grow in a manner essentially consistent with the growth of the population overall.

Much of the movement into managed care was driven by corporate employers attempting to contain healthcare benefit costs. However, during this same period of growing managed care enrollment, the number of managed care plans experiencing financial problems also increased steadily.

Managed care was able to slow the rate of health insurance premium increases throughout most of the 1990s. However, early in the first decade of the 2000s, the cost of insurance coverage again began climbing at an alarming rate. The gradual unfolding of the ACA, with its increased premiums, added to this trend. The average middle-class subscribers and the public in general had reached a negative consensus about managed care. This caused some damage to the political viability of for-profit managed care, and it hurt managed care overall. Indeed, it seemed increasingly likely that managed care might not be financially affordable in the long run.

As they grew larger, managed care organizations began to deal directly with hospitals, negotiating the use of their services. As various plans contracted with hospitals that would give the best price breaks for the plan's patients, price competition between and among providers became a factor to be considered.

Although managed care provided cost-saving benefits at least for a time, it is evident that managed care plans have not been able to sustain their promises of delivering efficient and cost-effective care. An aging population, newer and more expensive technologies, newer and higher priced prescription drugs, new federal and state mandates, and pressure from healthcare providers for higher fees have essentially wiped out the savings from managed care for employers and subscribers alike. It is likely, however, that without managed care, costs and cost increases would be even more pronounced than at present. Essentially the managed care model became a permanent and common feature in the coordination of and payment for care.

Managed care groups as well as voluntary groups sometimes work together to achieve cost savings and improve coordination of care under such programs as CMS's accountable care organizations (ACO's). By working together within a designation region, these groups reduce cost by sharing information that, in turn, reduces duplicate testing, increases wellness care, and prevents medical errors. If cost savings are realized, Medicare returns a portion of the savings to the ACO's providers.

There have been on-going initiatives to develop programs to coordinate care and share the costs. In addition to those already discussed, there is an alternative to managed care, namely, the medical cost-sharing model. These organizations are somewhat like insurers, but are not, generally, regulated as such. They are usually sponsored by some non-profit group as a service to their members. The members who join the medical cost-sharing program agree to pay a specified amount into a general pool of money to pay the medical bills of members. When a member incurs medical costs (of a specified category), he or she submits the bill to his or her cost-sharing group, which then pays the bill. In order to keep costs down, the cost-sharing group has eligibility requirements. These include members' agreement to avoid high-risk behaviors (e.g., no smoking). Failure to comply with these requirements would result in non-payment by the cost-sharing organization.

## ▶ **The Annual Congressional Budget Allocations**

During the formulations and passage of the annual federal budget, additional requirements affecting managed care, Medicare and Medicaid, and other reimbursement program are developed. Some requirements are reduced or eliminated. The process is both a political one and a practical one: the allocation of funds must be incorporated into an overall budget, with mandatory federal debt limits. The political overlay reflects a variety of attempts to respond to constituency concerns. Thus, it is an annual process requiring careful attention by the healthcare reimbursement community. State-level budget processes require similar monitoring and input.

Payment for health care flows from a number of sources, some major and well known and some less recognizable and relatively specialized. A number of these sources can be grouped together under the heading of "government," the largest being, of course, Medicare and Medicaid. Yet in addition to Medicare and Medicaid, there are other government programs that reimburse for health care at both state and federal levels. There are, for example, specific programs for providing health services to the dependents and survivors of military personnel, and there is the health care for former military personnel provided by the hospital system of the Veterans Administration. Also, under "government" are a number of state programs, including Workers' Compensation, which pays for health care for sick or injured workers whose condition results from job-related conditions. The programs includes compensation for lost income. Many of the states also have unique programs designed to serve certain specific population segments. In addition to government programs, various programs can be gathered under the heading of private insurance. This collection of payers includes not-for-profit entities such as Blue Cross–Blue Shield, commercial (for-profit) insurance companies, and the many HMOs that comprise a large proportion of payers. These entities just named interlock to a considerable extent; for example, many managed care programs are operated by not-for-profits such as Blue Cross and Blue Shield, which also administer insurance programs designed to supplement Medicare benefits.

Much health care delivered by the HMOs and other insurers subjects users to deductibles and copays, making patients and families payers to a considerable extent. (A "deductible" is a designated amount a patient must pay before certain coverage kicks in, and a "copay"—common to essentially all programs to some extent—is a designated portion of the cost of a specific service that must be borne by the patient.)

Some larger organizations have essentially entered into the health insurance business by self-insuring for their employees. Practical (and permissible) for only sizable organizations with sufficient financial capability, these self-insurers pay their employees' claims directly using, in most instances, an administrative claim service to handle the transactions. However, most self-insurers also carry additional coverage against the possibility of catastrophic claims.

However, getting down to absolute basics, it is the population at large that pays for health care through taxes, through insurance premiums, and out of their own pockets.

## Related Considerations

A number of additional programs or practices in place or under active consideration affect payment for health care. To enumerate just a few:

- Network designation is the concept under which a patient's plan pays up to 100% of costs within one's network and the patient pays 100% of costs incurred outside of the network. Usually insurers and employers place a dollar limit on what the plan pays for expensive procedures, potentially resulting in some large medical bills for patients. Certain problems arise with out-of-network care; a patient does not always know that the provider or facility is not part of the network. For instance, in an emergency or accident, the patient is taken to the nearest facility which may not be in the network. The patient often is unable to participate in the decision due to their condition, or the patient's condition requires immediate care, regardless of network considerations.

- Regional pricing is another concept that has come under consideration in some quarters. In its simplest form, this is pricing that has its basis in the economy of a specified geographic area, suggesting that the same service may cost more in a "wealthier" region than in a "poorer" area.

- Although still evolving, the concept of the medical home offers financial incentives for providers to focus on the quality of patient outcomes rather than on the volume of services provided. The medical home can be a physical or virtual network of providers; the keys to its success are related to information technology and payment reform. The medical home is designed around patient needs and aims to improve access to care and improve communication in what is promoted as an innovative approach to delivering comprehensive patient-centered preventive and primary care. The ACA contains provisions that support use of the medical home model, including new payment policies.

- Built into the formal reimbursement methods of the principal programs and organizations that pay for healthcare services are numerous requirements and conditions; the purpose of which is cost containment. For example, there is the routine review for preventable readmission within 30 days under which some amount of reimbursement may be denied if a particular readmission within that time frame is considered not medically necessary. There is also the increased use of temporary admission to an observation unit rather than to a formal inpatient unit, reacting to the knowledge that the former, often associated with the emergency department, is less costly than a regular hospital admission and does not unnecessarily tie up a bed in an acute care unit.

- Another practice that serves both coordination of patient care and cost containment is the concept of bundling for continuum of care. This involves discharge planning and coordination of posthospital care and recognizes that acute hospital care is but one step in addressing a patient's needs. The continuum of care model recognizes that complete recovery requires organized posthospital follow-up to ensure return to health and to minimize the chances of readmission.
- A fairly long-standing practice relating to both quality of care and cost containment is utilization review. Hospital discharges are examined in detail to identify unnecessary treatments, excessive lengths of stay, and quality issues, with the intent of potentially improving quality of care while containing costs.

In general, virtually all of the reimbursement practices of the payers for health care have built-in rules, regulations, and requirements that place limits on certain practices (e.g., limiting length of hospital stays for specific diagnoses) and attendant penalties in the form of reduced or denied reimbursement.

# ▶ Reimbursement System Weaknesses

It generally holds true that the larger and more complex a system or program, the greater the chances of error and the more opportunity there is for misuse or mistreatment of the process itself. The overall healthcare reimbursement structure is both large and complex. There are many chances for the occurrence of honest errors, and there are many opportunities for deliberate fraud and abuse. Here are a few examples:

- Double billing or false billing by providers, perhaps billing twice for certain procedures,

or—rather common among fraud cases—billing for services never rendered
- Billing for more service than was rendered, as in billing for more treatment than was actually provided and billing payers for appointments that patients had actually canceled (consider the case of the provider who actually billed as much as 33 hours in a single day)
- Billing for services that are actually not covered under the prevailing reimbursement mechanism
- "Double dipping" in Medicaid programs by individuals using addresses in two states and collecting benefits from both for the same care
- Stringent efforts to combat fraud and abuse include both internal and external audits of reimbursement and the documentation to support claims.

# ▶ Social and Ethical Factors

The use of technology, privacy concerns, and continuing issues related to healthcare availability and financing give rise to new debates about social and ethical factors. These norms have always been a part of the healthcare ethos, but from time to time, more urgent considerations are required. As noted previously, a technological breakthrough occasions such renewed interest. At another time, a new legislative mandate, such as the Patient Self-Determination Act, brings about fresh consideration of enduring concerns. Increased sensitivity to patient or consumer wishes is yet another source of attentiveness to social and ethical issues. For example, the increased use by patients of alternative therapies and interventions has reopened the question about proper integration of nontraditional care with the more standardized modes. The debate reaches into the questions of reimbursement as well; healthcare plans are increasingly approving some alternative or complementary intervention as reimbursable costs. Another ethical issue in healthcare financing stems from a new practice: the embedded nurse, one who is an employee of the insurance company but assigned to the direct care team within a healthcare facility. Whose agent is this employee? What ethical dilemmas does this worker face? Do patients know that their care is being rendered by one whose assignment includes cost-effectiveness as a direct part of his or her work? Rationing of health care is yet another area of continuing discussion, including "quality-adjusted remaining years" indicators and "complete lives" measures. Finally, the use of marijuana for medical purposes showcases another example of societal norms shifting to greater acceptance of such substances.

Ethical considerations such as these result in the increased use of the ethics review committee, the institutional review board, and similar clinical and administrative review groups.

## ▶ The Role Set of the Healthcare Practitioner as Manager

The dynamic setting of healthcare organizations constitutes the environment of the manager, specifically the healthcare practitioner as manager. Often unseen by the patient or the public, the managers of departments and services work behind the scenes to support direct patient care interactions. In this specialized environment of a healthcare organization, qualified professional practitioners may assume the role of unit supervisors, project managers, or department heads. The role may emerge gradually as the numbers of patients increase, as the number and type of services expand, and as specialization occurs within a profession. The role of manager begins to emerge as budget preparations need to be made, job descriptions need to be updated and refined, and staffing patterns need to be reassessed and expanded.

For example, a physical therapy staff specialist may develop a successful program for patients with spinal cord injuries. As the practitioner most directly involved in the work, this individual may be given full administrative responsibility for that program.

Alternatively, an occupational therapist may find that a small program in home care flourishes and is subsequently made into a specialized division. Again, this credentialed practitioner in a healthcare profession may be given a managerial role. Practitioners who develop their own independent practices assume the role of manager for their business enterprises. The role of the practitioner as manager is reinforced further by various legal, regulatory, and accrediting agencies, which often require chiefs of service or department heads to be qualified practitioners in their distinct disciplines.

### Classic Management Functions and Essential Competencies

The healthcare practitioner–manager engages in traditional management activities—the circle of actions in which each component (e.g., planning, decision making) leads to the next. These activities are a mix of routine, repeated activities of an ongoing nature, along with periodic major activities such as preparation for and participating in accreditation processes, or major projects such as a complete systems overhaul. **Figure 1–1** illustrates the interrelationships of management functions. **Table 1–1** provides examples of daily activities of the professional practitioner as manager.

Management functions typically include the following:

- Planning: the selection of objectives, the establishment of goals, and the factual determination of the existing situation and the desired future state.

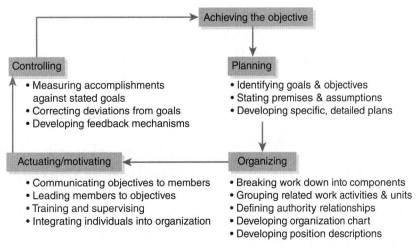

**Figure 1–1** Interrelationship of Management Functions.

**Table 1-1** The Chief of Service as Manager: Example of Daily Activities

| Activity | Management Function Reflected |
|---|---|
| Readjust staffing pattern for the day because of employee absenteeism | Staffing |
| Review cases with staff, encouraging staff members to assume greater responsibility | Controlling<br>Planning<br>Leading/motivating/actuating |
| Counsel employee with habitual lateness problem | Controlling<br>Leading/motivating/actuating |
| Present departmental quality assurance plan for approval of risk management/quality assurance committee | Planning<br>Leadership |
| Conduct research to improve treatment techniques | Planning<br>Leadership |
| Dialogue with third-party reimbursement manager about coverage for innovative services | Planning<br>Leadership |

- Decision making: part of the planning process in that a commitment to one of the several alternatives (decisions) must be made. Others may assist in planning, but decision making is the privilege and burden of managers. Decision making includes the development of alternatives, conscious choice, and commitment.
- Organizing: the design of a pattern of roles and relationships that contribute to the goal. Roles are assigned, authority and responsibility are determined, and provision is made for coordination. Organization typically involves the development of the organization chart, job descriptions, and statements of work flow.
- Staffing: the determination of personnel needs and the selection, orientation, training, and continuing evaluation of the individuals who hold the required positions identified in the organizing process.
- Directing or actuating: the provision of guidance and leadership so that the work performed is goal oriented. It is the exercise of the manager's influence as well as the process of teaching, coaching, and motivating workers.
- Controlling: the determination of what is being accomplished, the assessment of performance as it relates to the accomplishment of the organizational goals, and the initiation of corrective actions. In contemporary management practice, the larger concepts of performance improvement and total quality management include controlling.

Essential competencies and characteristics of an effective manager are discussed in the next section.

## ▶ Management as an Art and a Science

Management has been defined as the process of getting things done through and with people. It is the planning and directing of effort and the organizing and employing of resources (both human and material) to accomplish some predetermined objective. Management is both an art and a science. Especially in its early years of development at the turn of the 20th century, management's scientific aspects were emphasized. This scientific approach included and continues to include research and studies about the most efficient methods, leadership styles, and patterns of organization. However, management science tends to lack the distinct characteristics of an exact discipline, such as chemistry or mathematics. A more intuitive and nuanced set of elements reflect management as an art as well as a science. One speaks of the art of leadership and motivation. One relies on intuition and experience in situation of conflict or crisis.

Managers seek to combine the best of both approaches, striving to become effective managers.

## Characteristics of an Effective Manager

The classic functions of a manager have been noted in the previous section. The highlighting of the characteristics of the effective manager augments this role set; they reflect the essential competencies of a manager. Five major characteristics of effective managers are:

1. They know the internal structure and characteristics of their organization:
   - Its overall mission
   - Its client characteristics and needs
   - Its specific products or services offered to meet these needs
   - Its specific setting or combination of settings and formal organizational category (e.g., acute care, freestanding clinic)
   - Its specific laws, regulations, and accrediting standards applicable to each type of health-care unit
2. They know the internal and external dynamics of their organization:
   - The organization's strengths
   - The challenges to its survival
   - The areas requiring adaptation and innovation
   - Its life cycle
   - Its network of internal and external relationships
   - Its survival strategies
3. They lead and motivate the workforce by doing the following:
   - Developing and maintaining a positive workplace environment
   - Reducing conflict
   - Increasing worker satisfaction through training and ongoing development and the provision of proper wages and benefits
   - Maintaining effective communication
4. They engage in the search for excellence through continuous quality improvement.
5. They remain aware of and respond to the following:
   - Trends (e.g., changes in technology, patterns of reimbursement, social issues)
   - The challenge of change and the necessity of being a change agent and a leader

The manger's responsibility to identify and respond to change is the focus of the following chapter.

## ▶ The Manager's Wheel Book

This concept is drawn from the maritime world. The captain of the ship holds the primary position of authority, plans the course, directs the crew, and makes necessary adjustments to the course. To accomplish these activities, a captain's log, the wheel book, is maintained. It contains factual information: distances travelled, weather conditions, supplies obtained, information about unplanned events. If someone had to take the captain's place in an emergency, the wheel book entries would provide immediate information for use by the person replacing the captain. As the responsibility holders for their departments, managers could use a similar concept, a manager's wheel book, showing simple, factual entries by date. Its uses are several:

1. As a quick reference to recall date and action, such as when renewal of vendor contract occurred
2. Planning: comparing a plan to actual performance (e.g., budget preparation, planning long range initiatives)
3. Identify orientation and training needs
4. Orienting a clinical affiliation student to the role of manager and aspects of the particular setting
5. Preparing major reports such as the annual report
6. Preparing employee evaluations by reviewing the past year's critical incidents
7. Preparing policy and procedure updates
8. Analysis of one's duties, activities, and preparing one's self-evaluation

The wheel book contents, reflecting one or several years, help managers identify trends and separate out the one or two situations from those that have moved beyond a popular trend into enduring elements. It also helps a manager in those challenging moments when one might be tempted to make an emotional response: "Why is this always happening in your unit?" "That vendor never delivers on time!" These might surface as quick responses to a pressing situation, but a quick check through the daily log does not support the momentary impression.

Of primary importance is its use to assist others who might need to take over, such as in an emergency and/or a manager's unavailability due to leave of absence, illness, vacation, or conference attendance.

## An Excerpt for a Manager's Wheel Book

The log is a simple one: date; activity; note column

Additional examples of entries are given throughout this text, illustrating its use and content.

| Date | Activity | Notes |
|---|---|---|
| April 17 | Reviewed vacation coverage plan for July–August | |
| | Monthly meeting with peer group; discussed ICD-11 status | |
| | Met with Supply Chain assistant director about reducing variety of brand-specific supplies | |

| Date | Activity | Notes |
|------|----------|-------|
|  | Employee (N)—end of probationary period; completed HR documents to move employee from probationary to full status |  |
|  | Annual evaluation reports—preliminary preparation; reviewed January–March weather-related closure; critical incident response; availability |  |
|  | Met with HR department re: current status of March 17 whistleblower report |  |
|  | Unplanned visit from colleagues from neighboring state |  |
|  | False alarm—fire alarm in remote storage area |  |
|  | Unexpected resignation notice from assistant director |  |

A comprehensive wheel book example is provided at the end of the final chapter.

A manager's day is often a mix of planned activity (e.g., a monthly meeting, completion of personnel forms) with the unplanned occurences (e.g., unplanned visit from colleagues, fire alarm). Notice that it is not a TO DO list; the log contains what did happen. It will be the basis of a TO DO list, but the emphasis is the capture of day-to-day activity. Many of the entries will be a repeat of early ones. In maritime language, "Continuing as Before" was a common phrase to indicate that no new events occurred and the ship was proceeding on course. In this adaptation of the wheel book, a manager would not take a short cut to entries lest this lead to a loss of background information. Seemingly repetitious entries (e.g., certain regular meetings, employee matters) are common; they reflect a stable, routine, well-ordered environment. The entries need not be long; brief notation is sufficient.

## Format of Wheel Book

One might want to choose to simply add this type of information to one's calendar. Meetings, for example, are already listed. A prompt column for TO DO is often included on business calendars. Personal information is often listed in one's calendar. Using the existing personal/business calendar might seem convenient, but there is a drawback to this method: when the manager leaves, or is temporarily unavailable, the information in personal/desk calendar goes with him or her. The wheel book and simple logging of date and activity of what actually happened are a straightforward alternative.

The log entries do not show details; the related documents serve that purpose (e.g., minutes of meeting, completed evaluation form, equipment inventory and specifications file).

Along with the Manager's Reference Portfolio (discussed in Chapter 3), the Manager's Wheel Book provides a useful source of information about planned, seasonal, and ordinary activity along with the unplanned events that make up a manager's work.

## CHAPTER 2

# The Challenge of Change

## CHAPTER OBJECTIVES

- Identify the impact of change on organizational life.
- Identify the manager's role as change agent.
- Review examples of successful change.
- Examine a major change having ongoing impact.
- Describe the organizational change process.
- Identify specific strategies for dealing with resistance to change.

## ▶ The Impact of Change

Change in the healthcare environment is continuous and challenging; the trends and issues in the healthcare setting reflect the reality in every stage of the life cycle of the organization, as well as in its attendant survival strategies. Trends and issues intensify, becoming mandates for change in patient care, setting, and administrative support. This affects workers at all levels. Such changes consume financial and administrative resources; they have the potential of draining emotional and physical energy away from primary goals. Thus, the managers accept the role of change agent, seeking to stabilize the organization in the face of change.

## ▶ The Manager as Change Agent

Managers, as the visible leaders of their units, assume the function of change agents. This change agent role involves moving the trend or issue from challenge to stable and routine. This is accomplished in several ways:

- Mediating imposed change through adjusting patterns of practice, staffing, and administrative routines
- Monitoring horizon events through active assessment of trends and issues
- Creating a change-ready environment
- Taking the lead in accepting change

## ▶ Review of Successful Change

Managers foster a change-ready environment by reminding the work group of successful changes. This raises the comfort level of the group and provides insight into strategies for achieving desired outcomes. Six examples are provided here to illustrate the process of successful change, along with ongoing responses. They reflect the move from major, rapid change to incremental, continuous adjustment.

- Year 2000 (Y2K): change as opportunity
- Patient Self-Determination Act (PSDA): routinization of change
- Health Insurance Portability and Accountability Act (HIPAA): extensive change via legislation

- Electronic health records: proactive change
- Economic and market forces: anticipatory readiness through organizational restructuring
- Disruption in personal circumstances: revitalization through career development

## Change as Opportunity: Y2K

Recall the transition to the new century: Y2K. The phrase alone reminds us of successful responses to an inevitable change. It also reminds us of the pre-Y2K concerns about technology-dependent systems: would they work? Faced with the possibility of massive systems failure, managers carefully defined the characteristics of this anticipated change:

1. A definitive event with an exact timetable
2. Well known ahead of time (3- or 4-year run-up)
3. Unknowns or uncertainty mixed with known technical aspects: which systems might fail, what would the resulting impact be (e.g., failure of power grids, communication disruption, financial infrastructure chaos)

During the run-up to Y2K, managers assessed the potential impact and planned accordingly. Furthermore, many managers seized the opportunity to make even bigger changes. When the cost of upgrading some existing systems was compared with adopting new systems, managers chose to spend the money and time on a comprehensive overhaul.

Funding such a major project became part of the challenge. Many chose a combination of borrowing, along with "bare bones" budgets, with deferred maintenance and elimination of discretionary projects (e.g., refurbishing) to meet this need. The end result in many organizations was the adoption of new, well-integrated computerized systems. This overall plan of upgrading was supplemented with contingency planning closer to the December 31, 1999, deadline. Managers took such practical steps as:

- Eliminating all backlogs (e.g., coding, billing, transcription)
- Preregistering selected patient groups (e.g., prenatal care patients)
- Obtaining and warehousing extra supplies
- Adjusting staffing patterns for the eve of Y2K and the days immediately following it, with workers available and trained to carry out manual backup for critical functions

Managers also took the opportunity to review and update the emergency preparedness and disaster plans for the healthcare organization. Again, the anticipated Y2K change was the catalytic agent for renewed efforts in these areas. Y2K came and ran its course; this major change was absorbed with relative ease because of careful planning. Two decades later, some of the issues remain because the nature of the basic concern remains. Is it time for a complete overhaul of the technology system? Is incremental change no longer effective? The threats to the system from electromagnetic pulse impact failure of the power grid, or disasters are ongoing concerns, requiring ongoing monitoring and incremental change.

## The Routinization of Change: The Patient Self-Determination Act of 1990

End-of-life care and related decisions have always been a part of the healthcare environment. However, technological change (e.g., advances in life support systems) along with definitive court cases (e.g., *Quinlan, Cruzan, Conroy*) led to a renewed interest in these issues. This interest, in turn, resulted in the passage of the PSDA, which had implications for patient care as well as the administrative support systems.

The response to this change was orderly and timely because the healthcare providers and the administrative teams assessed the change in a systematic manner. This strategy of absorbing change through rapid routinization into existing modes of practice included the following:

1. Outreach to clients or patients and their families, along with the public at large, to provide information and guidance about healthcare proxies, advance directives, and living wills. Information about support services such as social service, chaplaincy, and hospice care was included as part of the regular client/patient education programs.
2. Review and update of do not resuscitate (DNR) orders and related protocols for full or selected therapeutic efforts.
3. Review of plan of care protocols for "balance of life" admissions.
4. Increased emphasis on spiritual and psychological considerations of patients and families, with documentation through values history or similar assessments.
5. Renewed involvement of the ethics committee of the medical staff to provide the healthcare practitioner, patient, and family with guidance. The committee also adopted review protocols to assess patterns of compliance with advance directives and end-of-life care.
6. Documentation and related administrative processes augmented to reflect the details of this

sequence of care (e.g., documentation that an advance directive was made, movement of the document with the patient as he or she changed location, flagging the chart to indicate the presence of the directive). Existing policies and procedures were updated to reflect these additional practices.

The changes stemming from the PSDA were easily managed through systematic review and adjustment of existing, well-established routines. However, there is a potential downside to routinizing change: the changes might become so well accepted that they are more or less ignored. For example, the living will become just another piece of paper or data entry, checked off as being available but not truly part of the care plan. A thorough quality assurance or improvement review of actual practice relating to advance directives highlights the need for ongoing attention to this issue. As a practical matter, there remains a need to ensure the availability of the official advance directive. If a patient is receiving care from more than one healthcare professional, and/or hospital or clinic, the patient usually needs to give each provider an official copy, not a photocopy, or at least indicate that he or she has an official directive and where it is located. However, without the document per se, the provider can only proceed with generally accepted treatment protocols. In an emergency episode, and even in planned encounters, patients rarely carry an advance directive. In a similar situation, that of a patient traveling from their home state to another state (e.g., on business or personal matters), the advance directive may not apply. Even with interstate compact agreements, this issue is still not settled.

At a more basic level, a patient might ask for a sample form to fill in. Unless one is consulting a lawyer, one might accept the simplified check-list version, completing it as part of an intake process while sitting in a waiting area. There is the possibility of inadvertently checking the wrong box, not understanding the terminology, or simply leaving most options unchecked. Finally, there is the remote possibility of someone else later on altering the document by changing the checkmark—checkoff lists are easily altered. There is a need for continued education of the general public as well as patients about this important topic. The original impetus to adopt advance directives has lessened somewhat. The larger cultural and ethical aspects of life-and-death issues currently focus on assisted suicide.

Because response to legislated change is often required, it is useful to examine yet another such mandate. A consideration of HIPAA reflects a different dynamic in the organizational process of responding to new requirements.

## Extensive Change via Legislation: Health Insurance Portability and Accountability Act of 1996

This act, known commonly by the acronym HIPAA (Public Law Number 104 of the 191st Congress) (PL 104-191), was enacted in 1996. When it was a newly passed law, its most visible portion was broadly described by the name of the law, addressing primarily "portability" of employee health insurance.

The intent of HIPAA was to enable workers to change jobs without fear of losing healthcare coverage. It enabled workers to move from one employer's plan to another's without gaps in coverage and without encountering restrictions based on preexisting conditions. It specified that a worker could move from plan to plan without disruption of coverage.

At first, many healthcare managers were not concerned with HIPAA. Human resources managers became most aware of the new law because it concerned their benefits plans, but the burden of notification was borne mostly by the employers' health insurance carriers, so there was little to do other than answering employees' questions. For many managers, the employer had no concerns about HIPAA beyond ensuring health insurance portability. Additional clarifications and guidelines have been promulgated over the years, resulting in routine, incremental change. For example, employer-sponsored wellness programs have gained popularity; does HIPAA apply? Yes, if the program is part of the employer-sponsored group health plan. The employer may not access workers' information about participation in, or details of, wellness program results even though the employer pays for the program.

Managers continue to respond to the ongoing mandates of this law, consisting of five sections: titles I, II, III, IV, and V.

### *Title II in the Spotlight*

Titles I, III, IV, and V of HIPAA deal with employee health insurance, promoting medical savings accounts, and setting standards for covering long-term care. Title II is the section driving most HIPAA-related change. This section is called "Preventing Health Care Fraud and Abuse, Administrative Simplification, and Medical Liability Reform" under the standard regulatory term *Administrative Simplification*.

Administrative Simplification includes several requirements designated for implementation at differing times. Compliance with the Privacy Rule, the most contentious part of HIPAA, was required by April 14, 2003. Compliance with the Transactions and Code Sets (TCS) Rule was required by October 16, 2003, and the Security Rule was set for implementation in April 2005. The Centers for Medicare and Medicaid Services have issued, and continue to issue, a wide variety of rules and guidelines, with managers implementing these routinely. HIPAA has become a fixed feature in healthcare systems.

Controversy over the intent versus the reality of HIPAA involves the Privacy Rule. In trying to strike a balance between the accessibility of personal health information by those who truly need it and matters of patient privacy, portions of HIPAA have created considerable work and expense for healthcare providers and organizations that do business with them, not to mention creating inconvenience and frustration for patients and others.

### The Continuing Privacy Controversy

Reactions to the Privacy Rule have been numerous. Patients and their advocates claimed that these new requirements were forcing a choice between access to medical care and control of their personal medical information. Government, however, claimed that the rules would successfully balance patient privacy against the needs of the healthcare industry for information for research promoting public health objectives and improving the quality of care.

When HIPAA's privacy regulations first received widespread exposure, hospitals, insurers, health maintenance organizations, and others claimed that the Privacy Rule would impose costly new burdens on the industry. At the same time, Congress was claiming that HIPAA's protections were immensely popular with consumers. Consumer advocates hailed the Privacy Rule as a major step toward comprehensive standards for medical privacy while suggesting that it did not go far enough.

To comply with the Privacy Rule, affected organizations were required to

- Publish policies and procedures addressing the handling of patient medical information
- Train employees in the proper handling of protected health information
- Monitor compliance with all requirements for handling protected health information
- Maintain documented proof that all pertinent requirements for information handling requirements are fulfilled

The HIPAA privacy requirements has caused frustration for patients and others. For example, a spouse who has to help obtain a referral or follow up on a test result cannot do so without the signed authorization of the patient (unless the patient is a minor). Anyone other than a minor or a legally incapable or incapacitated individual must give written permission for anyone else to receive any of his or her personal medical information.

There are a number of instances in which personal medical information can be used without patient consent. These instances, along with all patients' rights concerning personal medical information, must be delineated in the Privacy Notice that every provider organization must provide to every patient.

### Effects on an Organization

All healthcare plans and providers must comply with HIPAA. Provider organizations include physicians' and dentists' offices; hospitals, nursing homes, and hospices; home health providers; clinical laboratories; imaging services; pharmacies, clinics, and freestanding surgical centers and urgent care centers. In addition, such organizations include any other entities that provide health-related services to individuals. Also required to comply are other organizations that serve the direct providers of health care (e.g., billing services and medical equipment dealers). All affected organizations must

- Protect patient information from unauthorized use or distribution and from malfeasance and misuse
- Implement specific data formats and code sets for consistency of information processing and preservation
- Set up audit mechanisms to safeguard against fraud and abuse

All subcontractors, suppliers, or others coming into contact with protected patient information are also required to comply with the HIPAA Privacy Rule. In addition, all arrangements with such entities must define the acceptable uses of patient information.

Depending on organization size and structure, compliance with the HIPAA Privacy Rule could involve several departments (as in a mid-size to large hospital), a few people (as in a small hospital or nursing home), or a single person (as in a small medical office). Overall, whether compliance is accomplished by separate departments or just a person or two, compliance can involve a number of activities, including information technology, health information management, social services, finance, administration, and ancillary or supporting services.

The necessary changes have been numerous and have added to the workload in every affected area.

Providers routinely obtain written consent from patients or their legal representatives for the use or disclosure of information in their medical records, as had been the standard practice. However, renewed attention has been focused on release of information practices. Also, providers are now legally required to disclose when patient information has been improperly accessed or disclosed.

The Privacy Rule created a widespread need for healthcare providers to revise their systems to protect patient information and combat misuse and abuse. Providers now must protect patient information in all forms, implement specific data formats and code sets, monitor compliance within their organizations, implement appropriate policies and procedures, provide training all in HIPAA's privacy requirements, and require the organization's outside business partners to return or destroy protected information once it is no longer needed. Also, it is not enough simply to do everything that is supposed to be done: there are also a number of documentation requirements as well. Even a provider organization's telecommuting or home-based program must be HIPAA compliant.

## *Physical Layout Considerations*

The HIPAA Privacy Rule has necessitated changes in physical arrangements to ensure that no one other than the patient and caregiver or other legitimately involved person knows the nature of the patient's problem—or even, for that matter, that the specific individual is a patient. Medical orders or information about an individual's condition must be conveyed with a guarantee of privacy. Numerous organizations had to move desks or workstations, erect privacy partitions, provide soundproofing, and make other alterations so that no one other than those who are legally entitled to hear may overhear what passes between patient or representative and a legitimately concerned party. As with the advance directive topic, a quality assurance/improvement study about this aspect of privacy might yield information about unintended breaches. Consider the common situation of check-in at the reception area of a physician's office or clinic. Or even a pharmacy. The receptionist asks for name, date of birth, and reason for visit/whom are you seeing, or what medication are you obtaining. This transaction often occurs within hearing distance of others in the waiting area or, in the case of a commercial pharmacy, at the cash register area. While further intake assessment is done in properly arranged locations, the check-in/check-out area might not meet privacy requirements.

## *The Privacy Official*

Every healthcare provider organization must have a person designated to oversee HIPAA compliance. In a large organization, this position could be filled by a full-time HIPAA coordinator. In a small organization, such as a medical office, the task might be an additional responsibility of the office manager. This person must monitor all aspects of compliance and ensure that appropriate policies and procedures are maintained and kept current. Professional associations, including the American Health Information Management Association (AHIMA), have developed detailed position descriptions and guidelines for privacy officers.

## *The Department Manager and HIPAA*

Depending on the nature of a department's activity, HIPAA's requirements could significantly affect the manager's role. For example, health information management must be concerned with the release of information. A manager within information technology or information systems will be significantly concerned with the Security Rule because of its relevance for information stored or transmitted electronically.

As with other laws affecting the workplace, there is much more to compliance with HIPAA than simply putting policies, procedures, and systems in place. Some HIPAA regulations are complex, and in the most heavily affected areas of an organization, considerable training can be required. Also, HIPAA necessitates some training for most staff regardless of department; any person who comes into contact with protected patient information must receive privacy training. As a consequence, most managers will be both trainees and trainers, learning HIPAA's privacy requirements, remaining up to date, and communicating them to employees.

Some HIPAA requirements continue to be amplified, and it is clear that the law's basic privacy requirements are here to stay in one form or another. Privacy rules will continue to affect every physician, patient, hospital, pharmacy, healthcare provider, and all other entities having contact with patient medical information in any form. The American Recovery and Reinvestment Act of 2009 and the related Health Information Technology for Economic and Clinical Health Act amplify privacy practices, with particular emphasis on breach notification. The breach notification provisions include detailed regulations touching on the following issues:

- Notification of individuals if there is significant risk of financial, reputational, or other harm

- Time frames and manner of notification
- Tracking and reporting
- Internal compliance monitoring systems

As an unexpected positive outcome of HIPAA-related actions, the health information management environment has been primed to undertake major efforts in expanding electronic health records.

# A Study in Proactive Change: Electronic Health Records

Implementation of electronic health records reflects a proactive approach to change. The application of technology to enhance the creation and use of health-care information has been a welcome advance. The migration from hard copy records and systems to automated ones represents change, both incremental and rapid. Data gathering and analysis via punched cards in the early 1960s was a precursor of advances to come. As the country became accustomed to electronic capture, exchange, and use of information as a result of the new technology (the credit card—easy to use, easy to carry), smart cards with embedded personal health information were a highlight in the early 1970s. Why not apply the same idea to one's personal information? Applications of smart cards in the late 1980s included patient's use of interactive behavioral healthcare protocols. Throughout this period, automated and outsourced administrative processes were adopted readily. The Y2K events occasioned a thorough review of systems. Advances in technology, plus related legislation in favor of electronic health records, have resulted in rapid change and a cascade of changes. Note, by way of example, the adoption of Health Level-7 standards, the creation of a national health information technology coordinator and the national health information technology plan, and such specific legislation as the Medical Modernization Act and its mandates concerning electronic prescription systems.

The electronic health record incentive program provided an additional catalyst for the adoption of this massive system change. Yes, the technology is continually evolving, but the underlying principle is enduring: quality health information for use in patient care, research, and administrative support. Legislative mandates requiring universal adoption of electronic health records further reinforce this ongoing professional mission.

Health information practitioners have taken leadership roles in their workplaces and through their national association, AHIMA, along with its state component organizations. A strategy for proactive engagement with these changes was developed and continues to be applied as the migration from hard copy to electronic information systems unfolds. The overall strategy has six features:

1. Individual initiative within the workplace
2. Advocacy in the public arena
3. Partnership with key stakeholders
4. Outreach to clients and patients
5. Continual adjustments to information systems
6. Reassessment of health information management job roles and credentialing

## Individual Initiative

Within the workplace, individual health information managers have steadily adopted computer technology to support basic operations. Workflow and processes have been gradually converted over time, including automated master patient indexes, coding and reimbursement processes, digital imaging, and speech recognition dictation. Internal administrative systems have served as building blocks for the expansion of computerized systems to include electronic health records. Although individual initiative continues to be an important facet of this transition, fostering change through advocacy has been primarily an organized group effort through the national association, AHIMA.

## Advocacy in the Public Arena

External forces, particularly law and regulation, are affecting the process of developing electronic health records. It is essential, then, that professional practitioners help shape the debate, contributing their knowledge and expertise through organized efforts. Regular interaction with lawmakers and regulatory agency officials has been central to this process. Participation in work groups, task forces, and special initiatives has been steady. Landmark events bear the imprint of such involvement, including the Centers for Disease Control and Prevention's Public Health Information Network to implement the Consolidated Health Informatics standards, the Public Health Data Standards Consortium, the Department of Health and Human Services (DHHS), the American Health Information Community and its initiatives toward creating a national health information network, and the Certification Commission for Healthcare Information Technology.

## Partnerships with Key Stakeholders

The health information profession has long been the authoritative source of practice standards. With the advent of electronic health records, many of the questions that have arisen are variations of issues with which health information management practitioners have successfully dealt. Those experiences have prepared these practitioners to offer guidance in such areas as documentation content and standardization, authentication of documentation, informed consent, accuracy of patient information, access and authorized use of data, and data security.

AHIMA has developed a series of position papers, statements of best practices, and guidelines for these and related topics. This organization has strengthened its efforts through partnership with key stakeholders, as the following examples demonstrate

- American Health Information Community (DHHS): standards for electronic health data
- American Medical Informatics Association: data standards
- Medical Group Management Association: performance improvements and need for consistent data standards
- National Library of Medicine: data mapping (e.g., Systematized Nomenclature of Medicine and International Classification of Disease interface)
- American Society for Testing and Materials and its committee on health informatics: core data elements and definitions
- Corporate partner industry briefings: cosponsored exchange sessions
- As major initiatives move forward with the implementation of the EHR, AHIMA has partnered with governmental and private groups to develop guidelines regarding the interoperability of systems. Issues relating to digital degrading over time (an unknown factor) also constitute areas of common interest. Some of the organizations are Work group for Electronic Data Exchange (WEDI), The Institute of Electrical and Electronic Engineers and their continuing project on Health Level–7 standards, The American Medical Informatics Association, and the CMS's guidelines on Promoting Interoperability Program. IT vendors associations also constitute active participants.
- Regional Health Information Exchanges (RHIE) provide coordination among healthcare providers (e.g., physicians, hospitals, nursing homes) who enter into an agreement to share electronic health records among the RHIE. Having obtained patient consent to share information in this manner helps to foster rapid access to their information, avoid duplication of testing, and

enhance coordination of care. AHIMA members participate in RHIE activities and help promulgate its benefits through patient education regarding consent for release of information.

Through these and similar outreach efforts, AHIMA makes available valuable guidance to those involved in adopting electronic health records.

Another major initiative by AHIMA has been the move toward open membership. In recognition of the important partnership with information technology specialists, clinicians, and others with a shared interest in health information, as well as to foster even greater teamwork, the AHIMA members voted to eliminate associate membership, moving this group into the active membership category. An open, inclusive membership provides additional strength to the association in its efforts to support the electronic health record initiative.

## Outreach to Clients and Patients

Consumers are an important partner in the effective use of electronic health records. AHIMA has developed an initiative to raise public awareness of these personal health records. As part of this initiative, individual health information practitioners, using AHIMA-created presentations, interact at local and regional levels with consumer groups such as local chambers of commerce, health fair coordinators, and specialty support groups (e.g., cancer support groups). Presentations and articles by health information management professionals concerning the health information exchange or "how to" explanations about accessing an electronic health record for one's personal use have fostered patient engagement in this unfolding endeavor.

An important adjunct to this outreach is advocacy. Clients and patients must continue to have trust in the process of revealing their personal information fully and truthfully during healthcare interactions. AHIMA continues to press for specific protective legislation with a nondiscrimination focus: protect the patient from any discriminatory action stemming from documented information about patient care encounters.

## Continual Adjustments to Information Systems

In summary, electronic health record initiatives reflect the best in proactive involvement by managers in facing major change. As the transition from paper to electronic records continues, AHIMA has provided position papers, best practices guidelines, and training materials including document imaging to link paper documents to electronic health records, along with retention guidelines for postscanning management of data; "copy and paste" guidelines; making corrections, amendments, and deletions to ensure record integrity; the definition of the legal record; and e-discovery rules under federal rules of civil procedures. The transition to fully electronic records has not been accomplished. The sheer cost of a complete changeover is a prohibitive factor; however, incremental change continues. Smaller organizations such as a physician's and dentist's office might choose to continue the hybrid system until there is a natural migration to the EHR as new patients enter the system. Inpatient facilities continue to use short-form summaries, such as a discharge binder or an expanded SBAR form to facilitate the exchange of information when a patient is moved to another unit or transferred to another facility.

## Reassessing Health Information Management Job Roles and Credentialing

The changing landscape of health information management job roles and functions has produced associations that periodically review this work. Such evaluation has become a more urgent priority as attention to the need to reassess both traditional jobs as well as emerging ones. Logical steps have included identifying the new configuration of jobs and role sets, identifying the associated knowledge and competencies, and developing and expanding the educational preparatory levels (associate, bachelor's, and master's degrees, as well as graduate certificate in healthcare informatics). The credentialing process has also been expanded to include new categories of specialization (e.g., Certified Documentation Improvement Practitioner, Certification in Healthcare Privacy and Security).

## Economic and Market Forces: Anticipatory Readiness Through Organizational Restructuring

Sometimes an organization as a whole faces severe circumstances caused by economic and market forces. Consider the situation of a facility offering two levels of care for frail, elderly people: personal care and assisted living. This facility opened 40 years ago and has been in the same physical building since then. It has had a history of modest but steady success. An analysis of the balance sheet reflected breakeven points for 11 of the 40 years and 14 years of modest profit.

Only the first few years showed yearly losses, primarily because of startup costs. Then, most recently, there was a 5-year run of steady loss and increased debt, due to increased competition in local market and to the need for expensive renovations to the 40-year old physical facility. Decreasing reimbursement rates from third-party payers added to this erosion of revenue.

To reverse this trend, the management team undertook the process of preparing the organization to survive and thrive in a new era. The team restructured the organization. It also anticipated probable changes in state law, including those leading to a decrease in skilled care beds through a buy-back provision. Decreased reimbursement for this level of care gave the organization an additional reason to convert some units to increase the size of its dementia care service. Assisted living care was discontinued. The assisted living building was converted to additional personal care and respite care, plus an adult day care center with respite care included. Telemedicine access was added to the day care component, thus providing clients easily accessible communication with physicians and other healthcare providers. Tele-appointments became an attractive feature of the center. Hours of care were expanded to cover 6:30 A.M. through 7:00 P.M., and weekend and holiday hours were offered. Comprehensive home care services, using a contractual provider, rounded out the reconfigured services. Through all of these efforts, the organization emerged from its threatened state and became a leading provider in its geographic region.

## Disruption in Personal Circumstances: Revitalization Through Career Development

The individual is certainly not immune to the pressure of change. Consider the situation of the health information professional whose family circumstances require increased income over the next several years. This credentialed practitioner had been working part-time as a coding specialist in a community hospital. There were no anticipated resignations in the department management team, and internal advancement was unlikely. Furthermore, this woman needed to remain in the region for family reasons. Recognizing the constraints in her situation, she made and implemented a plan for advancement. First, she utilized the AHIMA career development and self-assessment program to identify competencies needing upgrading. While continuing to work, she undertook master's degree studies in health informatics and participated in several projects. These projects included research in correctional facilities, juvenile detention centers, and protective service agencies. Through this health information professional's involvement in local civic activity, an opportunity developed for her to work in first local, and then regional, correctional facilities. She worked first as a part-time consultant and then as the full-time director of the health information department. Both her personal and professional goals were met.

Using the foregoing examples as background, let us now consider the theoretical aspects of organizational change.

## ▶ Change and Resistance to Change

Change is inevitable, but change can also be chaotic and painful. Alfred North Whitehead once said, "The art of progress is to preserve order amid change and to preserve change amid order." That statement captures the essence of change and its effects on all of life. Much change is beneficial, even necessary, but change is often upsetting and unsettling and thus must be controlled. For good or ill, change is inevitable. So, too, is resistance to change inevitable.

This section addresses the inevitability of change, including how, as individuals, we tend to deal with change and how, as managers, we can deal with employee resistance to change. In discussing this topic, it is necessary to look at individual attitudes toward change, those of both managers and employees alike, because resistance is a human reaction that can arise in anyone regardless of organizational position. In other words, the manager who is expected to be a change agent and supportive of inevitable change may initially experience feelings of resistance equivalent to those of the employee. It is also necessary to consider how to meet change when it occurs and how to make change work.

### The Collision of Constancy and Change

Up until a few decades ago, an individual could adopt a career and with few exceptions expect to remain in that career for a lifetime. The effects of the knowledge explosion and the Industrial Revolution that preceded it, however, included changes that rendered some occupations obsolete or changed them dramatically. Occupations that had existed for several generations all but vanished as machines took over work that had long been done by hand. Entire industries

disappeared. For example, whaling, once an economic mainstay of the northeastern United States, shriveled and died as petroleum products replaced whale oil. Many individuals have seen their jobs and careers disappear as a consequence of change that continues to accelerate to this day.

Those working in the delivery of health care have seen and are seeing new medical technologies arise to either replace or augment existing technologies, in some instances making it necessary for workers to learn new skills or seek new occupations. Some individuals still working in diagnostic imaging were first employed when imaging was entirely X-ray; they have seen the addition of the computerized axial tomography (CAT) scan, magnetic resonance imaging (MRI), positron emission tomography (PET) scan, and other technologies. One technologist who had been employed in a hospital laboratory for 30 years observed that more than 80% of the tests she performed on a routine basis did not exist when she first entered the field. People have been conditioned by centuries of change to desire constancy or near-constancy. That, plus a natural tendency to seek equilibrium with the surroundings, conditions many people to be automatic resisters of change. They are continually attempting to preserve equilibrium with the environment, and whenever it is disturbed, they tend to take steps to reestablish that equilibrium—to return to a "comfort zone." Certainly not all people behave in the same manner, but it is likely that most people seek equilibrium with their surroundings and tend to equate security with constancy. Indeed, security was once likely to be found in adopting an occupation and doing it well for life or in remaining a loyal employee of one organization for life. No longer, however, is there security in constancy; rather, today's security, to the extent that it may exist, lies in flexibility and adaptability.

### The Roots of Resistance

The principal cause of most resistance to change is the disturbance of the previously mentioned equilibrium. Resistance will, of course, be influenced considerably by one's knowledge of where a given change is coming from. It is unlikely that a person will resist a change with which he or she wholeheartedly agrees or one that is his or her own idea to begin with. The person does not resist such a change because it is welcome and, therefore, does not threaten one's equilibrium. Thus, it is not change itself that people resist but rather *being changed*—being made to change by forces or circumstances outside of themselves.

A secondary major cause of resistance lies in the inability of people to mentally conceive of certain possibilities or think beyond the boundaries of what they presently know or believe. The limitations imposed by what people know and what they believe can provide significant barriers to creativity and progress. Ideas that are today deemed revolutionary were not originally welcomed with open minds. Many people we have come to think of as innovators and visionaries were, in their day, regarded as dreamers, charlatans, or crackpots. Here are four examples.

1. Barely 2 months before the Wright brothers flew, a noted scientist publicly explained why a heavier-than-air flying machine could never work. However, the brothers went ahead and flew anyway; they had an advantage in not knowing "it couldn't be done."
2. A device called a "telephone" was branded a fraud, with an "expert" proclaiming that even if it were possible to transmit human voice over wires, the device would have no practical value.
3. When television was new, the head of a major Hollywood studio proclaimed that people would soon get tired of staring at a plywood box every night.
4. Even in the field of medicine, change has often been thought impossible: in 1837, leading British surgeon Sir John Erichson stated that the abdomen, the chest, and the brain would "forever be shut from the intrusion of the wise and humane surgeon." Note as well that many people alive today once thought that surgery on a living heart would never be possible.

To a considerable extent, then, the roots of resistance to change are within human beings themselves.

# Primary Causes of Resistance

Concerning change that occurs in the workplace, people tend to be thrown off balance by changes that are thrust on them and especially by the way in which many of these changes are introduced. Common sources of change in the work organization occur in many areas:

- Organizational structure, when departments are altered or interdepartmental relationships or management reporting relationships are changed, including the changes that result from merger, affiliation, or system formation
- Management, whether in a department, a division, or an entire organization
- Product or service lines, as services are added, dropped, or altered significantly

- Introduction of new technology, bringing with it new equipment that employees must learn to use
- Job restructuring, altering the duties of particular jobs, such as combining jobs that were formerly separate
- Methods and procedures, requiring workers to learn new ways of doing their jobs
- The organization's policies, especially personnel policies affecting terms and conditions of employment

Consider how much—or perhaps how little—control the average rank-and-file employee or the typical department manager can exert over the foregoing changes. In most instances, the individual is essentially powerless. Managers and some employees might perhaps have a voice in restructuring jobs and altering methods and procedures, and perhaps they might be involved in selecting or recommending new equipment, but chances are they have little or no voice in the decisions necessitating such changes. It is doubtful that many employees or managers below the level of executive management have any influence on changes in products or services. And concerning the remainder of the major sources of change described—significant sources of stress and resistance for managers and employees alike—rank-and-file employees and their department managers are powerless.

## *Organizational Changes*

Depending on the extent of reorganization, structural changes within a healthcare organization, such as combining departments or groups or realigning departments under different executives, can engender ill feelings and generate considerable resistance. Most department managers and their employees are well aware that reorganizing under any name—reengineering or downsizing—often means that some people will lose their jobs, so fear and insecurity and thus resistance increase while productivity inevitably decreases. Even more likely to upset employees are the changes accompanying merger or other form of affiliation, acquisition by a larger organization, or health system formation.

## *Management Changes*

Changes in management are among the most potentially upsetting changes employees can experience. The stress of a management change, and thus the resistance to it, is concentrated within the hierarchy beneath the management position that is turning over; therefore, a change in department manager will affect primarily that department, whereas a change in chief executive officer will affect the entire organization. A change in management almost always involves exchanging a known quantity for a complete or partial unknown, and it is fear and apprehension concerning the unknown that causes most initial resistance to management changes.

### Policy Changes

Major changes in the policies of the organization, especially personnel policies affecting terms and conditions of employment, are likely to spark a certain amount of employee resistance, especially if employees perceive they are losing something. In these years of fiscal belt-tightening, it is not uncommon to see, for example, employers in health care and elsewhere shifting an increasing portion of ever-growing health insurance costs to employees, or reducing the corporate contribution to defined-contribution retirement plans or other investment plans, or reducing the sick-time benefit and combining the remainder with vacation and personal time in "paid time off" plans. Such policy changes have inspired so much resistance for some employers that they have become major issues in union organizing campaigns and labor contract negotiations.

## Many Causes

Resistance can occur anywhere, resulting from almost any change within an organization, often arising in situations that no one had thought would prompt any objections. Times of relative turmoil in health care, with all of the fallout of "merger mania" and all of the cost-reducing and cost-saving pressures brought to bear on the healthcare delivery system, finds the healthcare worker—and the healthcare manager as well—working in an environment of intensifying change and an eroding sense of security.

## Meeting Change Head-On

The healthcare department manager is in a uniquely difficult position relative to change that has an impact on the healthcare organization. As an employee, the manager is just as affected by change as the rank-and-file employees and is just as likely to feel helpless, demoralized, and resistant. Yet it is up to the manager to try to minimize the negative reactions of the work group and attempt to raise employee morale and ensure continued productivity. If the manager openly projects doom, gloom, and resistance, the staff will be all the more likely to become more deeply mired in doom, gloom, and resistance themselves, ensuring

that morale and productivity both suffer. It can be a most difficult role for the manager to function as "cheerleader" when there seems to be nothing to cheer about. Yet the manager must make a conscious effort to rise above all the negative thinking. Succeeding at doing so is largely a matter of attitude, including the willingness to take a moderate amount of risk.

## Flexibility and Adaptability

As noted, people can no longer find security in constancy, maintaining loyalty to the same ideas, concepts, and institutions for life. Rather, security, to whatever extent it exists today, is more likely found in flexibility and adaptability. The manager who remains rooted in place, with a fixed set of ideas and an unchanging concept of the job, will not be particularly successful; however, the manager who can move about, who can flex and adapt as circumstances change, stands a much greater chance of success. Also, to enhance the department's chances of success in adjusting to changing circumstances, the manager must be a role model for flexibility and adaptability.

A department manager may be able to help some employees increase their flexibility by instituting cross-training wherever possible. For cross-training to be effective, it is necessary that there be a number of employees distributed across multiple jobs of approximately the same skill or grade level; thus, it is not possible in every department. When cross-training is possible, however, there are benefits for employee, department, and organization alike. With people trained in multiple activities, coverage for vacations and other absences is more readily accomplished, employees get the advantages of task variety, and employees may become more secure during times of readjustment by being capable of moving into certain other jobs, already trained and competent.

## A Matter of Control

The department manager who becomes caught up in a sea of change should immediately learn the difference between what can be controlled and what cannot be controlled. Much energy is wasted in trying to control that which is uncontrollable. For example, a manager may be greatly stressed about an impending merger and subsequent combination of departments, but there is nothing that the manager can do about it; it will happen whether he or she wishes it or not.

Stress as a response to change, both real and impending, is an emotional reaction. An important early step in gaining a measure of control over one's circumstances is learning to control one's emotions.

A person may have little or no control over the changes themselves; however, he or she has complete control over how one's *response* to the changes.

Fortunately, there are usually a few factors that the individual department manager can control to some extent. Reorganizing or reengineering frequently results in the need to combine positions and restructure a number of jobs—that is, change job descriptions, assignments, crew or team sizes, equipment, or later services. These actions usually entail changes in methods and procedures, changes that can be determined in detail within the department by the manager, often with the participation of the employees.

## Addressing Resistance with Employees

A manager responsible for implementing change has three available avenues along which to approach employees regarding a specific change. The manager can (1) simply tell them what to do, (2) convince them of the necessity for doing it, or (3) involve them in planning for the change.

### Tell Them

The use of specific orders or commands is one of the hallmarks of the autocratic or authoritarian leader. The boss is the boss, a giver of orders who either makes a decision and orders its implementation or relays without expansion or clarification the mandate from above.

The authoritarian approach is sometimes necessary; occasionally, it is the only option available under urgent or completely unanticipated circumstances. However, in most situations the "tell-them" approach is the approach most likely to generate resistance, so it should be used in only those rare instances when it is the only means available.

### Convince Them

In most instances, including those in which the change in question is an absolute mandate from top management, the individual manager has room for explanation and persuasion. At the very least, there is the opportunity to try making each employee aware of the reasons for the change and the necessity for its implementation. It may be necessary for the manager to champion the cause of something clearly distasteful to all concerned (except, most likely, to those mandating compliance) because it may be good for the institution overall or good for patients, or even perhaps because it is mandated by new government regulations. The employees may not like what they are called on to do, but they are more likely to respond as needed if they know and understand why the change must be implemented.

The employees deserve all the information available, and this information often serves the manager well because it can remove the shadow of the unknown from the employees and thus lessen their resistance. Few, if any, changes cannot be approached by this means. The authoritarian "tell-them" approach should be reserved as a last resort to be used on those occasions when employees clearly cannot be "sold" on the change.

### Involve Them

Whenever possible, and especially if it affects the way they do their assigned jobs, employees should become involved in shaping the details of any particular change. It has been repeatedly demonstrated that employees are far more likely to understand and comply when they have a voice in determining the form and substance of the change. For example, if new equipment is under consideration and there is sufficient lead time, it is helpful to obtain the input of the people who will have to work with the equipment once it is in place. This sort of involvement not only enhances employee cooperation but often leads to a better decision because of the perspective of the people doing the hands-on work. When expansion or remodeling will change the characteristics of the department, employee input in the planning stages will bring the workers' perspective into determining optimal layout and work flow. Through involvement, change can become a positive force. Employees will be more likely to comply because they own part of the change; in effect, a piece of it is their idea.

There is another potential benefit to involvement as well: employee knowledge of the details of the work in ways the manager may never have. The manager supervises a number of tasks, some of which he or she may have once done personally. However, the employees regularly perform in hands-on fashion the tasks the manager only oversees. Thus, the employees usually know the details of the work far better than the manager and are in a better position to provide the basis for positive change in task performance.

The numerous sources of management advice that promote the value of employee involvement are correct. The participative and consultative approaches to management are the best ways of getting things done through employees. The most effective ways of reducing or removing the fear of the unknown make full use of communication and involvement.

# Guidelines for Effective Management of Change

To secure employee cooperation and participation and successfully manage change in the workplace, it is necessary for the manager to take the following steps:

- *Plan thoroughly.* Fully evaluate the potential change and examine all implications of its potential impact on the department and the total organization.
- *Communicate fully.* Completely communicate the change, starting early, ensuring that the employees are not taken by surprise. This should ideally be two-way communication, preparing the way for employees' involvement by soliciting their comments or suggestions.
- *Convince employees.* As necessary, take steps to sell employees on the value and benefits of the proposed change. When possible, appeal to employees' self-interest, letting them know how they stand to benefit from the change and how it might make their work easier.
- *Involve employees when possible.* It is not possible to completely involve employees in all matters, but involvement is nevertheless possible on many occasions. Be especially aware of the value of employees as a source of job knowledge, and tap this source not only for the acceptance of change but also for the development of improvements.
- *Monitor implementation.* As with the implementation of any decision, monitor the implementation of any change until the new way is established as part of the accepted work pattern. A new work method, dependent for its success on willing adoption by individual employees, can be introduced in a burst of enthusiasm. Do not let it die of its own weight as the novelty wears off and old habits return. New habits are not easily formed, and the employees need all the help the manager can furnish through conscientious follow-up.

## True Resistance

Resistance to change will never be completely eliminated. People possess differing degrees of flexibility and exhibit varying degrees of acceptance of ideas that are not purely their own. However, involvement helps, and the manager will eventually discover, if not already having done so, that most employees are willing to cooperate and genuinely want to contribute.

Beyond involvement, however, continuing communication is the key. Full knowledge and understanding of what is happening and why it is happening are the strongest forces the manager can bring to bear on the problems of resistance to change. Ultimately, one will discover that it is not change that people resist so much as they resist *being changed.*

In addition to applying the foregoing strategies, managers facilitate their response to change by

1. Recommitting to the full spectrum of their role through a review of the enduring functions of the manager
2. Remaining attentive to
   - Developments in the history of management and the ways in which managers adjusted their focus from time to time
   - Shifts in organizational life from informal to formal, stable organizational patterns
   - Opportunities for building a strong network of internal and external relationships

# ▶ One More Challenge: The Patient Protection and Affordable Care Act of 2010

The major legislation known as the Patient Protection and Affordable Care Act of 2010 (PPAC), more commonly referred to as the Affordable Care Act (ACA), affects the healthcare system at all levels. Middle managers often need to use the strategies described in this chapter to deal with the massive changes associated with this legislation focusing on the provision of affordable care and healthcare reform. They need to take into account the political aspects of the legislation's passage, which has led to further amendments, deletions, and changes in its implementation time frame. The federal mandates, in turn, generated companion state-level legislation. More than 100 regulatory agencies, boards, and councils are empowered to issue guidelines and mandatory regulations. The designated time frame for the implementation of the federal law was from 2010 to 2018. Thus, there has been an almost decade-long period of sustained change, with continuing change being a regular feature going forward.

The manager who has a positive attitude will more easily respond to these challenges than one who is resistant. Flexibility, creativity, and attentiveness to the unfolding mandates—these traits will serve the manager well. A commitment to factual analysis will lead the manager to develop a system for monitoring the details of this law. For guidance, the manager should turn to trusted sources, such as professional associations—especially these organizations' legislative divisions, which monitor primary documents such as federal and state regulation publications. The manager might partner with several peers in the work setting to study the unfolding mandates and share insight about their impact.

Following is a suggested template for use in tracking these changes. A few examples are included under the headings as a starter.

- Impact on the organizational setting
  - Increase in community health centers
  - Development of independence-at-home programs
  - Creation of community-based transition programs for Medicare patients at high risk for readmission to acute care
  - Phasing out of physician-owned specialty hospitals
  - Increase in use of observation units as a bridge between emergency care and admission/readmission to inpatient care
- Patterns of care
  - Increase in use of outcome measurement for clinical effectiveness research
  - Implementation of wellness programs and preventive care (e.g., smoking cessation counseling)
  - Wellness care incentives
  - Increased emphasis on coordination of care for all stages of care, with particular attention to discharge planning and reduction of preventable readmission within 30 days
  - Creation of medical homes or health homes programs (i.e., a decentralized coordinator of care) for chronic illness care. (*Note*: The term *homes* is not used to denote a place to live; in this context, it means the primary caregiver who coordinates various aspects of care including referrals to specialists.) The expanded role of the nurse navigator as coordinator of posthospital care is associated with the medical home or medical hub concept.
- Practitioners
  - Increased funding for training
  - Increased utilization of physician assistants and nurse practitioners

- Increased roles for pharmacists in direct counseling of patients concerning medication management
- Clients
  - Increased numbers as individuals come under new health insurance coverage
  - Surge in demand for specific services as coverage for these services unfolds (e.g., free annual physical examination)
  - Increased need for client education about the details of coverage and the time frames associated with various benefits (e.g., preexisting conditions coverage and its limits)
  - Increased need to capture eligibility data (e.g., income levels, prescription medication expenses for the benefit period, Medicare or Medicaid coverage)
  - Increased sensitivity to patients' concerns about their coverage and their continued access to care. This involves the development of trusted adviser contacts who assist clients with their understanding of their eligibility for, and coverage options, with regard to healthcare insurance plans
- Employees
  - Need for timely information about changes in health insurance coverage, copayments, and deductibles
  - Need for annual information (on W-2 forms) about the dollar value of the health insurance fringe benefit
  - Concern for job security when the organizational setting changes
  - Questions about job rotation (e.g., if mergers occur or if community-based programs are developed, will the employee be obliged to rotate among various geographic locations?)
  - Need for more frequent continuing education (e.g., intake processing and health insurance questions)
- Specific systems impact
  - Budget adjustments to include resources for more frequent continuing education
  - Increase in fraud detection processes
  - Increase in patient-centered outcomes standards research and studies
  - Increase in monitoring of discharge planning, coordination of care, readmission rates, and supportive rationale

## A Template for Assessing Health Insurance Proposals

Health insurance proposals will be offered with predictable regularity such as during national election candidate selection. Associations involved in healthcare provision will continue their efforts at health insurance reform. In assessing proposals, and their potential impact on the managers' responsibilities and concerns, a useful template to follow is this.

1. *Extent of coverage*: inpatient care; outpatient care both hospital-sponsored and free-standing; telemedicine/e-health interactions; long-term care, rehabilitation, hospice, home care; comprehensive coverage from prenatal to end of life; catastrophic care only
2. *Method of financing*: general taxation; payroll tax, similar to Social Security; tax credits; surcharge on natural resources; luxury tax; copayments and deductibles
3. *Federal-state government relationship*: Worker Compensation model; Medicare-Medicaid model
4. *Relationship to existing programs*: all phased out completely and replaced with an entirely new system; building on/expanding and coordination with existing programs such as private insurance, managed care, medical sharing groups, and county and city hospitals and clinics; Medicare and Medicaid
5. *Methods of review and control*: utilization review; quality monitoring; financial audits; healthcare planning agencies, with approval/disapproval power; cost-containment requirements; uniform billing
6. *Organizational form to administer the over-all program*: existing framework (e.g., DHHS, or CMS); government-sponsored HMO; the public utility model with franchises and licensure and rate-control features; public corporation

The manager constantly attends to change, meets it through managing the organization through its life cycle, uses strategies for organizational adaptation and survival, and strengthens the organization's relationships with key constituents and stakeholders. These concepts are discussed in subsequent chapters.

## CHAPTER 3

# Organizational Adaptation and Survival

## CHAPTER OBJECTIVES

- Present the concept of the organization as a total system.
- Describe the evolution of the total system approach to management.
- Describe the development and characteristics of the formal organization.
- Identify the approaches to the classification of organizations and apply these to the healthcare organization.
- Introduce the concept of the clientele network and describe the application of these components to the healthcare organization.
- Identify the need for organizational survival as a fundamental goal of organizational effort.
- Describe selected management strategies used to enhance organizational survival.
- Analyze the phases of the organizational life cycle and relate these to the functions of the manager.
- Describe the development and characteristics of corporate culture and its relationship to organizational life cycles.
- Provide information for developing a management reference portfolio.

## ▶ The Organization as a Total System

The manager's environment is the formal organization, with its multiple aspects and ever-changing dynamics. The effective manager knows the internal and external dynamics of the organization: its strengths and vulnerabilities, challenges to its survival, areas requiring adaptation and innovation, its life cycle, its network of internal and external relationships, and its survival strategies.

There is a subtlety to the interaction of these dimensions of organizational life. Although much is written down in the organization's major documents (e.g., its formal history, mission statement, policies, procedures, organizational charts), there are other layers of interaction about which the manager has both an interest and a concern. There is a kind of "tribal knowledge" within an organization; there are early warning cues about conflict, change, and opportunity. A manager does not want to miss these important signals or be blind-sided. Thus, the astute manager drills down into the fabric of the organization, using the tools mentioned above. The manager observes both the broad characteristics of the organization along with noting the fine details. In addition, the manager views the organization as a total system: the work per se, the workers, the clients, the internal and external mandates and requirements, and the interaction of the public-at-large with the organization.

An organization does not exist in a static world; rather, it is in a continual state of transaction with its environment. As an open system, the organization receives inputs from its environment, acts on them and is acted on by them, and produces outputs such as goods and services (and even organizational survival, which can be considered an essential output.) Consequently, the organizational environment consists of both internal and external components. The specific functions of the manager are modified by the organizational environment (i.e., the specific attributes of the given work setting).

Classical organizational theory provides the manager with concepts to assess the organizational environment, including the following:

- Examination of its characteristics and components through a typology of organizations
- Analysis of its clientele network
- Review of its life cycle

Managers are enabled, through continual monitoring of the environment, to anticipate change and prepare for it rather than dealing with it through reactive responses. A short review of the history of management is a starting place for identifying past practice and current trends.

# ▶ The History of Management

Knowledge of the history of management provides a framework within which contemporary managerial challenges may be reviewed. Modern managers benefit from the experiences of their predecessors. They may assess current problems and plan solutions by using theories that have been developed and tested over time. Contemporary executives may take from past approaches the elements that have been proved successful and seek to integrate them into a unified system of modern management practice.[1]

In an examination of the phases in management history, it must be remembered that history is not completely linear. Any period in history involves the interplay of components that cannot be separated into distinct elements, and each period is part of a continuum of events. The specific features of management history phases given here are intended to exemplify the predominant emphasis within each period and are only highlights.

Another cautionary note is warranted in regard to assigning dates to various periods. The dates given here are intended as guides. There is no precise day and year when one school of thought or predominant approach began or ended. As in any study of history, the dates suggest approximate periods when particular practices were developed and applied with sufficient regularity as to constitute a school of management thought or a predominant approach. The classic

concepts presented here provide a base for ongoing research and study about formal organizations.

## Scientific Management

The work of Frederick Taylor (1865–1915) forms the commonly accepted basis of scientific management. Taylor started as a day laborer in a steel mill, advanced to foreman, and experienced the struggles of middle management as workers resisted top executives' efforts to achieve more productivity. He faced the basic question: what is a fair day's work? With Carl G. L. Barth (1860–1939) and Henry L. Gantt (1861–1919), Taylor made a scientific study of workers, machines, and the workplace. These pioneers originated modern industrial practices of standardization of parts, uniformity of work methods, and the assembly line. In addition, Frank Gilbreth (1868–1924) and Lillian Gilbreth (1878–1972) developed a classification system for fundamental motions to facilitate the study of work methods. Lillian Gilbreth may be of particular interest to occupational therapists because much of her later work concerned the efficiency of physically handicapped women in the management of their homes. The concept of scientific management continues to be the basis for continuous quality improvement, productivity studies, and cost containment.

## The Behavioralists and the Human Relations Approach

Although the major figures in the development of scientific management emphasized the work rather than the worker, concern for the latter was apparent. Lillian Gilbreth, a psychologist, tended to stress the needs of the employee. Frank Gilbreth developed a model promotion plan that emphasized regular meetings between employee and the individual responsible for evaluating the employee's work. The behavioralists increased the focus on the worker, applying the behavioral sciences to worker productivity and interaction. There remains to this day the shorthand reference to this era: the *Hawthorne effect,* in which positive change in productivity, reduction of conflict and the like are attributed to the increase in human interaction as much as they are to streamlining the work and introducing efficiency measure. The term stems from the work of Elton Mayo and F. J. Roethlisberger at Western Electric's Hawthorne works. Through these studies, the importance of the informal group and the social and motivational needs of workers were recognized. The behavioral science and human relations approaches may be linked because both emphasize the worker's social and psychological needs and stress group dynamics, psychology, and sociology. The emphasis on quality circles and total quality management, as well as the contemporary use of appreciative inquiry methods of assessing the strengths of an organization, are examples of this approach.

## Structuralism

Because work is done within specific organizational patterns and because the worker-superior roles imply authority relationships, the structure or framework within which these patterns occur has been studied. Structuralism is based on Max Weber's theory of bureaucracy or formal organization. Major theorists in the structuralist school of thought (e.g., Robert K. Merton, Philip Selznik, Peter Blau) have given particular attention to line and staff relationships, authority structure, the decision-making process, and the effect of organizational life on the individual worker. These issues continue to this day. Note, for example, the renewed discussions of best organizational pattern: specialized units or the "silo" pattern versus a "flatter" organizational pattern, with teams of workers and fewer authority layers.

## The Management Process School

This approach focuses on the managerial functions: the work of the chief executive and those in leadership–authority roles. Henri Fayol (1841–1925) is credited with having developed the concept of the functions of the manager. The basic processes and functions of management, including the universality of these elements, was the focus of study in the late 1930s and early 1940s. The manager as leader and leadership styles, and the role of middle managers, continue to be the focus of research.

## The Quantitative or Operations Research Approach

Problem solving and decision making with the aid of mathematical models and the use of probability and statistical inference characterize the quantitative or operations research approach to management. Also called the management science school, this approach includes various quantitative approaches to executive processes and is characterized by an interdisciplinary systems approach. The urgency of the problems in World War II and in the space program hastened the development of mathematical models and computer technology for problem solving. The current

adoption of the Six Sigma approach to continuous quality improvement relies on statistical analysis as one of its main elements of assessing organizational performance. The current emphasis on data-driven, evidenced-based patterns of patient care reflect the overall concept of quantitative analysis.

## ▶ The Systems Approach

Each school of management thought tends to emphasize one major feature of an organization:

1. Scientific management focuses on the work.
2. Human relations and behavioralism stress the worker and worker–manager relationship.
3. Structuralism emphasizes organizational design.
4. Management process theory focuses on the functions of the manager.
5. Management science theory adds computer technology to the scientific approach.

The search for a management method that takes into account each of these essential features led to the systems approach. This focuses on the organization as a whole, its internal and external components, the people in the organization, the work processes, and the organizational environment. The total environment of the organization, and the interrelationship of all of its parts, is seen as a continuous cycle of absorbing inputs from the organizational environment, processing these as throughputs, resulting in productive output. This cycle (input–throughput–output) may be applied to the organization as a whole or to any of its divisions. The changes in the organizational environment can be assessed continually in a structured manner to determine the impact of change and to make necessary adjustments.

Management theorists turned to biology and related sciences (e.g., L. von Bertalanffy, Kenneth E. Boulding) to develop this ecological approach to the study of organizations.[2] A change in any one aspect of the environment has an impact on other components. The specifics are analyzed—always in terms of the whole. The organization or formal institution is considered an entity that lives in a specific environment and has essential parts that are interdependent.

## Basic Systems Concepts and Definitions

A system may be defined as an assemblage or combination of things or parts forming a complex or unitary whole—a set of interaction units. The essential focus of the systems approach is the relationship and interdependence of the parts. The systems approach moves beyond structure or function (e.g., organization charts, departmentation) to emphasize the flow of information, the work, the inputs and the outputs. Systems add horizontal relationships to the vertical ones contained in traditional organizational theory. The systems model is made up of four basic components: inputs, throughputs or processes, outputs, and feedback. These components are considered within the overall environment.

## The Nature of Inputs

Inputs are the elements the system must accept because they are imposed by outside forces. The many constraints on organizational processes, such as government regulation and economic factors, are typical inputs imposed by outside groups. Certain inputs are needed to achieve organizational goals; for example, the inputs often are the raw materials that are processed to produce some object or service. The concepts of inputs may be expanded to include the demands made on the system, such as deadlines, priorities, or conflicting pressures. Goodwill toward the organization and general support (of the lack of these) also may be included as inputs.

A systematic review of inputs for a healthcare organization or one of its departments could include the following elements:

- Characteristics of the clients: average length of stay, diagnostic categories, payment status
- Legal and accrediting agency requirements: federal Medicare provisions, institutional licensure, certification of healthcare practitioners
- Federal and state laws concerning employment: collective bargaining legislation, the Occupational Safety and Health Act, workers' compensation legislation, Civil Rights Act
- Multiple goals: patient care, teaching, research

For more examples of inputs, recall the earlier discussion of the overall setting of healthcare organizations.

## The Nature of Outputs

Outputs are the goods and services that the organization (or subdivision or unit) must produce. These outputs may be routine, frequently predictable, and somewhat easy to identify. The stated purpose of the organization contains information on its basic, obvious outputs. For example, a fire department provides fire protection, a hospital offers patient care, a department store sells goods, a factory produces items, and an airline supplies transportation. Managers control routine outputs through the planning process.

Other necessary outputs are infrequent but predictable. By careful analysis of organizational data over a relatively long period, a manager can usually identify these infrequent outputs. For example, hospitals and programs are reaccredited periodically, and plans can be made for this predictable event. An organization that is tied directly to political sponsorship could take the cycle of presidential or congressional elections into account. Again, proper planning through identification and anticipation of such special periodic demands on the systems leads to greater control and, consequently, stability.

Most managers must deal with a third category of outputs: the nonpredictable ones for which they can and must plan. Certain demands on the system are made with sufficient regularity that although the exact numbers and times cannot be calculated, estimates can be made. This is an essential aspect of planning and controlling. In an outpatient clinic, for example, the number of walk-in and emergency patients is not completely predictable. To plan for these relatively random demands on the system, the manager can study patterns: times of arrival, purpose of the visit, or new or continuing client status. Some patient education would probably be done to help clients take advantage of orderly scheduling. Staffing patterns would be adjusted to meet the anticipated needs. The planning is designed to shift the nonpredictable to predictable. Other examples of nonpredictable outputs for which plans can be developed include employee turnover rates, seasonal demand for care (e.g., physical examinations for the upcoming school year). Even natural disasters associated with weather patterns (e.g., hurricane season, winter snowstorms) can be anticipated. Disaster planning, for example, is a required part of institutional planning. The renewed emphasis on disaster planning in light of bioterrorism, new strains of diseases (e.g., Ebola, flu strains), or periodic social–political disruption (riots) has added urgency to such planning.

Some outputs of a healthcare institution are as follows:

- Maintenance of licensure and accreditation status
- Compliance with special federal programs concerning quality assurance
- Provisions of acute care services for medical, surgical, obstetrics, and pediatric patients
- Provision of comprehensive wellness and preventive health services for clients in a specific geographic area

Outputs may be refined further by adding specific time or quality factors, or other statements of expected performance:

- One hundred percent follow-up on all patients who fail to keep appointments
- Processing of specified laboratory tests within (*n*) hours of receipt of specimen
- Retrieval of hard copy record from remote storage within (*n*) minutes of receipt of request

It may be useful to group outputs with related inputs by formulating an input–output analysis. It should be noted, however, that not every input generates a direct output; there is no one-to-one relationship in some instances. For example, the goal (output) of retrieving a hard copy record requires considerations (inputs) of accuracy of identification of the record, its location, and the delivery system procedures.

## Throughputs

Throughputs are the structures or processes by which inputs are converted to outputs. Physical plant, workflow, methods and procedures, and staffing patterns are throughputs. Inputs originate in the environment. Throughputs, as the term implies, are contained within the organization. Throughputs are analyzed by work sampling, simplification and methods improvement, lean management studies, reviews of staffing patterns, and physical layout.

Managers may be severely limited in their ability to control inputs, but the processes, structures, organizational patterns, and procedures that constitute throughputs are normally areas of management prerogative. In a specialized service, the control of throughputs is directly related to the manager's professional knowledge. For example, the procedures for processing patient flow within a clinic are developed by the head of the specific service because of that person's knowledge of patient care procedures, priorities, and the interrelationships among components of the treatment plan. The policies and procedures for the release of information from patients' health records are aspects of highly technical processes that are the domain of the professional health information specialist.

In some cases, elements that usually belong to the throughput category are considered inputs. These elements are imposed by the internal environment of the organization. Middle managers may not be able to exert direct control over some aspects of the work (e.g., physical space allocations, budget cuts, personnel vacancies). These elements are, essentially, inputs that must be accepted.

## Feedback

Changes in the input–output mix must be anticipated. To respond to these changes, managers need feedback on the acceptability and adequacy of the outputs. It is through the feedback process that inputs and throughputs are adjusted to produce better outputs. The communication network and control processes are the usual sources of organized feedback. Routine, orderly feedback is provided by such activities as market research and forecasting, client surveys, periodic accrediting agency reviews, and periodic employee evaluations in the work group.

The management by objectives process, short interval scheduling, program evaluation–review techniques, and various audits (e.g., safety, financial, infection control) constitute specific management tools of planning and controlling that include structured, factual feedback. If there is an absence of planned feedback, if the communication process is not sufficiently developed to permit safe and acceptable avenues for feedback, or if the feedback actually received is ignored, a certain amount of feedback will occur spontaneously. In this case, the feedback tends to take a negative form, such as a client outburst of anger; a precipitous lawsuit; a slew of anonymous, negative letters to local news media complaining about the organization; a wildcat strike; a consumer boycott; or an epidemic. Spontaneous feedback could take a positive form, of course, such as the acclamation of a hero or leader after a crisis, or an unsolicited letter of satisfaction from a client.

Some feedback is tacit, and the manager may assume that because there is no overt evidence to the contrary, all outputs are fine. The danger in such an assumption is that problems and difficulties may not come to light until a crisis occurs. The planning process is undermined because there are no reliable data that can be used to assess the impact of change and to implement the necessary adjustments. The overall system constantly seeks a balanced state. The management functions of decision making, leadership, and particularly correction of deviation from organizational goals are necessary for the detection, identification, and proper response to changes in the organizational environment. Through the systems approach, the manager focuses on the organization as a whole, attending to each particular unit in relation to the whole. Every organization can be studied through a review of its organizational environment, its degree of formal organizational and bureaucratic characteristics and its placement in traditional classification of organizations.

For more information about these concepts, see **Table 3–1**.

**Table 3–1** Relationship of Classic Management Functions and Systems Concepts

| Systems Concept | Predominant Management Function |
|---|---|
| Input analysis | |
|   Identification of constraints | |
|   Assessment of client characteristics | Planning |
|   Assessment of physical space | |
|   Budget allocation analysis | |
| Throughput determination | |
|   Development of policies, procedures, methods | Planning and controlling |
|   Development of detailed departmental layout | |
|   Specification of staffing pattern | Staffing |
|   Methods of worker productivity enhancement | Controlling, leadership, and motivation |
| Output analysis | |
|   Goal formulation | Planning |
|   Statement of objectives | |
|   Development of management by objectives plan | Planning and controlling |
| Feedback mechanisms | Controlling, communicating, and resolving conflict |
|   Development of feedback processes | Renewing planning cycle |
|   Adjustment of inputs and outputs in light of feedback | |
|   Adjustment of internal throughputs | |

# ▶ Formal Versus Informal Organizations

An organization is a basic social unit that has been established for the purpose of achieving a goal. A formal organization is characterized by several distinct features:

- A common goal; an accepted pattern of purpose
- A set of shared values or common beliefs that give individuals a sense of identification and belonging
- Continuity of goal-oriented interaction
- A division of labor deliberately planned to achieve the goal
- A system of authority or a chain of command to achieve conscious integration of the group and conscious coordination of efforts to reach the goal

An informal organization may be characterized by some of the features of formal organizations, but it necessarily lacks one or more of these features. Individuals who share a common value may meet regularly to foster some goal, and this group may become a recognizable

formal organization. Some informal groups never develop the consistent characteristics of a formal organization, however, and simply remain informal.

Formal organizations almost inevitably give rise to informal organizations. Such informal groups may be viewed as spontaneous organizations that emerge because individuals are brought together in a common workplace to pursue a common goal, which makes social interaction inescapable. Informal organizations arise as a means of easing the restrictions of formal structures, as in the cooperative communication and coordination that may occur outside of the officially mandated channels of authority. Through an informal organization's communication network, individuals may gain valuable information that supplements or clarifies formal communications. Also, informal groups help to integrate individuals into the organization and socialize them to accept their specific organizational roles. A manager must remain aware of the existence and composition of informal groups in the organization so that their functioning affects the formal structure in positive rather than negative ways.

# ▶ Classification of Organizations

When an organization's managers understand and accept its nature, organizational conflict can be reduced and organizational viability increased, because the managers function in a manner consistent with the type of organization shaping the interactions. Personal conflict can be reduced. Should an individual be unwilling or unable to accept certain aspects of a particular organizational type, that individual may decide to move to a different organizational climate. For example, if an individual practitioner prefers not to function in a highly structured, bureaucratic setting, it is better to recognize this before accepting employment in a government-sponsored healthcare institution. An individual who believes that health care should not be "for profit" would do well to seek employment in healthcare settings that are not predicated on the business model. An individual may gain an insight into the climate of a particular organization through the use of organizational classifications based on prime beneficiary, authority structure, and genotypic characteristics.

## Prime Beneficiary

Peter Blau and W. R. Scott presented a classification of organizations based on the prime beneficiary.[3] Their suggested model for the analysis of organizations focuses on the question: who benefits from the existence of the organization? Four types of organizations result from the application of this criterion:

1. Mutual benefit associations, where the members are the prime beneficiaries (e.g., professional association, credit union, collective bargaining unit)
2. Business concerns, where the owners are the prime beneficiaries
3. Service organizations, where the clients are the prime beneficiaries
4. Commonweal organizations, where the public at large is the prime beneficiary (e.g., police department, fire department)

Managers may formulate goals, establish priorities, and monitor activities to determine the effectiveness of the organization in meeting the needs of the prime beneficiary. Actions that do not foster such goals are eliminated, and proper priorities are formulated. Because the clients are the prime beneficiaries of a service organization, decisions about hours of service, the scope of services offered, and similar matters are made with the needs of clients in mind. In health care, the growing development of home care, flexible hours in outpatient clinics, and alternatives to full hospitalization are attempts at meeting the needs of the prime beneficiaries—the patients and their families. At the same time, healthcare worker units involved in collective bargaining can be considered mutual benefit associations. Managers in healthcare settings must balance the demands made by both types of organizational forms within one organization.

## Authority Structure

The organizational environment can also be classified according to the modes of authority that are operative in the institution. Managers must adopt leadership styles, develop procedures and methods for worker interaction, and determine client interactions in a manner that is consistent with the predominant authority structure. Healthcare organizations tend to embody more than one pattern of authority structure; for example, there are few limits on the activities of professional staff and more limits on the activities of semiskilled and unskilled workers. The work of Amatai Etzioni provides a typology of organizations based on the authority structure predominant in the institution.[4] The classification that results from this approach may be summarized as follows:

1. Predominantly coercive authority: prisons, concentration camps, custodial mental institutions, or coercive unions
2. Predominantly utilitarian, rational–legal authority: use of economic rewards; businesses, industry, unions, and the military in peacetime
3. Predominantly normative authority: use of membership, status, intrinsic values; religious organizations, universities, professional associations, mutual benefit associations, fraternal and philanthropic associations
4. Mixed structures: normative–coercive (e.g., combat units); utilitarian–normative (e.g., most labor unions); utilitarian–coercive (e.g., some early industries, some farms, company towns, ships)

## Genotypic Characteristics

Like the prime beneficiary concept, the classification of organizations by genotype is based on an analysis of their fundamental roots and purposes. Daniel Katz and Robert Kahn viewed organizations as subsystems of the larger society that carry out basic functions of that larger society. These basic functions are the focal point in this system of classification. The typology of organizations developed by Katz and Kahn is based on genotypes, or first-order characteristics. What is the most basic function that the organization carries out in terms of society?[5] The mission of the organization stems from this fundamental concept. These first-order, basic functions are as follows:

1. Productive or economic functions: the creation of wealth or goods as occurs in businesses
2. Maintenance of society: the socialization and general care of people as occurs in education, training, indoctrination, and health care
3. Adaptive functions: the creation of knowledge as occurs in universities and as a result of research and artistic endeavors
4. Managerial/political functions: the adjudication and coordination functions and control of resources and people as occur in court systems, police departments, political parties, interest groups, and government agencies

The charter, articles of incorporation, and statement of purpose are official documents of the organization that can be used to classify the organization according to this typology.

Goal statements are derived and priorities set in terms of primary function. Managers can monitor organizational change when the actual function performed differs from the stated function. When a social service agency spends a great deal of effort determining eligibility of patients for service under a variety of government programs, it is assuming some of the characteristics of a managerial/political organization. Sometimes this adjudication interferes with the delivery of the healthcare service; managers must make decisions in the light of this conflict. If priority is given to research and education over direct patient care, the healthcare practitioner must again come to terms with the true nature of the organization.

# ▶ Classification of Healthcare Organizations

When a healthcare organization is classified according to these typologies, the complexity of the setting becomes apparent. Classification by prime beneficiary offers several possibilities. In terms of direct patient care, for example, the healthcare organization can be classified as a typical service organization. Conversely, if it is a for-profit institution, classification as a business organization is more appropriate. If the healthcare organization has mixed goals, as does a teaching hospital associated with a medical school, it can be defined as a service organization with respect to its

clients—both the physicians to be educated and the patients to be treated. The potentially conflicting priorities of teaching and direct patient care underlie the selection of patients for treatment, however; preference may be given to those patients who are "interesting" cases for teaching purposes. Even when a healthcare institution is not directly associated with a medical school, a variety of clinical affiliation arrangements may be developed to meet the needs of such practitioners as occupational and physical therapists, medical technologists, social workers, health information administrators, dietitians, and other groups that require clinical practice as part of their educational sequence. In developing goal statements for a department, the chief of service must keep this secondary goal in mind.

A healthcare organization also is a commonweal organization insofar as it protects the public interest in matters of general community health, such as the benefits of the facility's research efforts for the public at large. In addition, healthcare institutions offer a variety of free health monitoring programs as a means of fostering health maintenance in the community.

Etzioni included the hospital as an example of a normative authority structure. This point could be argued, however, depending on the focus of organizational analysis. Professional staff members tend to function in the normative mode; their codes of ethics, their professional training, and the general level of behavior expected of them modify their individual participation in the organization as much as, if not more than, the formal bylaws and contractual arrangements. In this sense, the normative authority structure predominates. When the healthcare organization is viewed from another perspective, it seems to function more as a mixed normative–utilitarian structure. Given the business orientation and the increasing unionization of workers in the healthcare field, the utilitarian model seems to be a more appropriate category.

A coercive element is sometimes introduced into the healthcare setting, as when individuals are assigned to healthcare jobs in wartime as an alternative to military service or when hospital volunteer work is given as part of a court sentence. In such cases, a mix of normative–utilitarian–coercive authority is required, and the manager must adopt a variety of leadership and motivational styles in working with the different groups in the organization. Worker or member motivation and the source of the manager's authority differ for these different groups.

In the Katz and Kahn genotypic classification, the healthcare organization fits two categories, again indicating the mixed mandates of such entities. As an organization concerned with restoration, the health-care establishment functions to maintain society. It also performs adaptive functions when higher education and research are major goals.

# ▶ **Classic Bureaucracy**

Bureaucracy is such a common aspect of organizational life that it is often treated as synonymous with formal organization. The study of bureaucracy in its pure form was the work of the structuralists in management history: Max Weber, Peter Blau and W. Richard Scott, and Robert K. Merton. Weber's work is pivotal, as it presented the chief characteristics of bureaucracy in its pure form. Weber regarded the bureaucratic form as an ideal type and described the theoretically perfect organization.[6] In effect, he codified the major characteristics of formal organizations in which rational decision making and administrative efficiency are maximized. He did not include the dysfunctional aspects or the aberrations that occur when any characteristics are exaggerated, as in the popular equating of bureaucracy with "red tape." From the works of Weber and others, a composite set of characteristics or descriptive statements may be derived concerning the formal organization or bureaucracy.

1. Size
   a. Large scale of operations, large number of clients, high volume of work, and wide geographical dispersion
   b. Communication beyond face-to-face, personal interaction
2. Division of labor
   a. Systematic division of labor
   b. Clear limits and boundaries of work units
3. Specialization
   a. A result of division of labor
   b. Each unit's pursuit of its goal without conflict because of clear boundaries
   c. Areas of specialization and division of labor that correspond with official jurisdictional areas
   d. Specific sphere of competence for each incumbent
   e. Promotion of staff expertise
   f. Technical qualifications for officeholders
4. Official jurisdictional areas
   a. Fixed by rules, laws, or administrative regulation
   b. Specific official duties for each office

5. Rational–legal authority
   a. Formal authority attached to the official position or office
   b. Authority delegated in a stable way
   c. Clear rules delineating the use of authority
   d. Depersonalization of office: emphasis on the position, not the person
6. Principle of hierarchy
   a. Firmly ordered system of supervision and subordination
   b. Each lower office or position under the control and supervision of a higher one
   c. Systematic checking and reinforcing of compliance
7. Rules
   a. Providing continuity of operations
   b. Promoting stability, regardless of changing personnel
   c. Routinizing the work
   d. Generating "red tape" to foster conformity of behavior and orderliness of processes
8. Impersonality
   a. Impersonal orientation by officials
   b. Emphasis on the rules and regulations
   c. Disregard of personal considerations in clients and employees
   d. Rational judgments free of personal feeling
   e. Social distance among successive levels of the hierarchy
   f. Social distance from clients
9. The bureaucrat
   a. Career with system of promotion to reward loyalty and service
   b. Special training required because of specialization, division of labor, or technical rules
   c. Separation of manager from owner
   d. Compensation by salary, not direct payment by clients
10. The bureau (or office or administrative unit)
    a. Formulation and recording of all administrative acts, decisions, and rules
    b. Enhancement of systematic interpretation of norms and enforcement of rules
    c. Written documents, equipment, and support staff employed to maintain records
    d. Office management based on expert, specialized training
    e. Physical property, equipment, and supplies clearly separate from personal belongings and domicile of the officeholder

These characteristics are interwoven, each flowing from the others. For example, the growing size necessitates a division of labor, which in turn fosters specialization.

One of the dreams of many direct patient care practitioners is a healthcare delivery system that does not become bogged down in formalities. The private practice model seems to offer the solution. If the private practice or small group practice flourishes, however, the characteristics of formal organizations inevitably begin to emerge—for example, specialization and division of labor, procedures for uniformity, some form of authority structure, and a variety of rules. The wisest approach seems to involve taking the best features of formal bureaucracy and making particular efforts to avoid the negative elements, such as impersonality. Family-centered approaches to health care or the team approach are models that tend to offset the impersonalization associated with large healthcare organizations.

# ▶ Consequences of Organizational Form

Managers work in specific organizational environments, and their specific functions are shaped and modified by the organizational form, structure, and authority climate. Some specific consequences concern the following organizational characteristics:

- *Size.* The more layers in the hierarchy, the greater (potentially) the limits on managers' freedom in decision making. Their decisions may be subject to review at several levels, and more decisions may be imposed from these higher levels.
- *Organizational climate.* The degree to which clients, workers, and other managers participate in planning and decision-making processes is determined in part by the authority climate. Managers may have to modify their management or leadership style if it is inconsistent with the organization's authority structure. The basis of motivation may vary. In the highly normative setting, for example, members willingly participate; in the coercive organization, the basis of motivation tends to rest on the avoidance of punishment.
- *Degree of bureaucracy.* A highly bureaucratic organization may be associated with great predictability in routine practices but less innovation and more resistance to change. Efforts to offset distortion caused by layering in communication may constitute a large portion of the activities of a manager in a highly bureaucratic organization.

- *Phase in the life cycle.* The openness to innovation and the vigorous, aggressive undertakings through goal expansion and multiplication that characterize some stages of the life cycle may permit the manager to undertake a variety of activities that are precluded by concerns for organizational survival in other phases of the life cycle.

For these reasons, managers must assess the organizational setting and their own roles. Sometimes a new role-set for a practitioner develops, or a traditional one greatly expands, to offset increasing formalization and bureaucracy. The development of an ombudsman, either internal or external (as in a state's regulations for long-term care), is one example. A second example is that of a nurse navigator. This practitioner's duties include overall coordination of services for a patient (e.g., scheduling of tests, making appointments with specialists) and assisting family/caregivers with carrying out a care plan. They identify and help arrange contact with community support groups and resources. They explain options (e.g., respite care for hospice, vacation care in an older adult day care program). They identify barriers to care and provide information for dealing with these (e.g., need for transportation, questions about insurance coverage for a procedure). They provide educational materials.

The major concepts of the clientele network, organizational life cycle, and analysis of organizational goals are tools for such assessments. Their active use fosters in the manager an awareness of the overall organizational dynamics that shape managerial practice, worker interaction, and client services.

# ▶ The Clientele Network

Managers must devote constant attention to the web of relationships reflecting the needs and interests of individuals and groups both internal and external to the organization. Common terms used to describe these relationships include critical partners, stakeholders, champions, superusers, and communities of interest.

A major charge given implicitly to any manager is the building of internal and external relationships and developing a framework for partnership. This framework connects the people of the organization with one another and with the larger communities of interest. To do this, the manager must identify critical relationships, develop satisfactory working relationships with the several key individuals and groups involved, and, finally, work at maintaining these relationships. With the conservation of organizational resources, time, money, and personnel as a mandate, the manager seeks to capitalize on available external sources of power, influence, advice, and support as well as to identify those areas of potential difficulty, such as competition and rivalry, erosion of client goodwill, and shifting client demand and loyalty. In an era of increasing regulation of health care, the contemporary manager in the healthcare setting must identify and comply with multiple sets of changing regulations and guidelines issued by federal and state government agencies as well as by the various accrediting agencies.

Like a living organism, an organization exists in a dynamic environment to which it must continually adapt. The manager identifies these units and constructs a network of the pattern of interrelationships. Bertram Gross has developed the concept of the clientele network, noting that any organization is usually surrounded by a complex array of people, units, and other organizations that interrelate with it on the basis of various roles. He has provided a framework for analyzing these key relationships, using the categories of client, suppliers, advisers, controllers, and adversaries.[7] The following discussion applies Gross's concepts to the healthcare organization.

Wherever the concept of organization is used, a department manager could well substitute individual service or department. Although such a department or service is obviously a part of the organization, the development of the clientele network for a unit within the organization yields information about the critical relationships, clients, adversaries, and supporters of that department. Department-level managers must be aware of the unique environment of their departments or services as well as the overall environment of their organization. Note that a unit of an organization, or the organization as a whole, is sometimes categorized in more than one aspect of the clientele network. For example, a healthcare organization is a secondary client of the third-party payers; without the healthcare organization providing the necessary services, the insurers would not have a market for their insurance coverage offering. (The primary client group for the insurers are the patients per se.) At the same time, the third-party payers are also categorized as controllers in that they specify a variety of parameters that the care providers must meet (e.g., coverage of specific conditions, or time frames and formats for billing). Another example is that of a patient group, that is the primary client of a community-based healthcare center. This same group might become an opponent when they seek to limit the physical expansion of

the hospital (e.g., concerns over traffic congestion) or take action to prevent certain services from being offered (e.g., drug-addiction treatment) in the immediate geographic community. The supportive, caring clinic might be perceived by clients as an opponent when collection agency methods are used to obtain payment for services.

## ▶ Clients

The most obvious and immediate individuals and groups who make significant demands on the organization are the clients. Gross used the term clients in a broad sense—that is, to refer to those for whom goods and services are provided by the organization. Immediate, visible clients in health care, both for the organization and for any department directly involved in patient care services, are the patients.

The providers of direct healthcare services are immediate, visible clients for certain units within the organizations. The billing and accounts receivable office, the legal staff, and the health information service offer support services to assist physicians, nurses, and social workers in the provision of patient care. Given the traditional and historical development of the modern hospital, it could be said that the physicians are a special class of clients in that the organization of the hospital or clinic gives them the necessary support personnel and services for patient care. Physicians in different specialties are clients of each other, because they depend on each other for consultative services and referrals.

Certain services may be placed into the client category vis-à-vis each other. Some service units, such as physical therapy, are income producing; because the resources obtained are used on behalf of the whole organization, other units may be considered clients of the income-producing units. The billing and accounts receivable office relies on the health information service to supply certain documentation to satisfy financial claims, and the safety committee relies on the several patient care and administrative departments to supply the information necessary to perform its function.

The use of the broadest possible definition of "client" alerts the manager to the subtle facets of organizational relationships. The manager who recognizes the number of distinct client groups can more effectively monitor their several and sometimes conflicting demands for services.

Although one step removed from the immediate services or goods offered by the organization, less visible clients are nonetheless legitimate users of the services or goods. By identifying these secondary clients, the manager has a key to the primary and secondary goals of the organization or unit. In the many educational programs offered within healthcare organizations, for example, the sponsoring institutions (e.g., a college or university), the health professionals, and the technical students are secondary, less visible clients. Hospitals traditionally have direct patient care as a primary goal, with teaching and research as secondary goals. The ordering of priorities should stem from recognition of the multilevel client demands.

Family and caregivers are secondary clients; the postdischarge care plan, for example, includes clear identification of the designated caregivers, with their contact information recorded in the patient's official medical record. Appropriate training (e.g., medication administration, wound site care) for these individuals is usually a part of this plan. Formal caregiver programs have become a feature of contemporary health care.

The same physicians who are immediate clients in terms of their need for support services for their direct patient care activities are less visible clients in terms of their need for opportunities for education and research. The employees of the organizations are, in a sense, less visible clients, given that one of the organizational outputs is the provision of jobs. Occasionally, in health care the provision of jobs is an explicit goal. For example, the neighborhood health centers sponsored by the federal government were intended not only to provide healthcare services but also to afford job opportunities to area residents. Employees also depend on the employer for important resources (e.g., wellness programs, health insurance, retirement plans, continuing education) to advance in their careers. There is also the less tangible need: the need for recognition—being valued, celebrated, motivated.

Clients twice removed from the immediate goal of the organization may be termed *remote clients*. Many of these individuals and groups do not even know they are being served. In addition to patient care, teaching, and research, a third goal of healthcare organizations is generally given as the protection of the public at large—that is, remote clients. Remote clients of the healthcare organization benefit from the research done by the physicians and related research teams. For example, remote client benefits can be seen in immunization outreach programs. The maintenance of herd immunity is taken for granted by the public; healthcare providers are proactive in ensuring this protection through intensive efforts regarding immunization. Outreach efforts are carried out regarding many other topics (e.g., Lyme disease prevention, stroke, cancer, and wellness

initiatives). Public lectures, free screening, educational materials—all are common means of reaching remote clients. Focused outreach programs are developed to educate the public about an organization's programs. Typical outreach efforts to transfer remote clients into active, primary clients are an open house of veterans and their families, a social event with educational resources and speakers about a particular topic (e.g., women and stroke prevention), a heart-healthy supermarket shopping tour, or physicians and physical therapists assisting with high school sports teams as volunteers.

Managers, in assessing the stated and implied goals, may readily identify them by analyzing the needs of primary, visible clients as well as those of the less visible and remote clients. If the client demand is relatively stable, planning, organizing, and staffing needs may be assessed in a stable manner. The net effect is efficiency in the allocation of resources of money, space, and personnel.

There is within the client group a potential capacity to control the organization. On the one hand, when a business has only one major purchaser of its goods or an agency has only one group to serve, the clients could easily take charge of the organization, limiting its independence. On the other hand, the organization with multiple clients must set priorities, balance conflicting demands, and maneuver so as to satisfy several groups.

The manager maintains continuous awareness of potential new clients and their needs; for example, the ever-growing leisure culture and amateur sports creates an increased need for physical therapy services. The aging of the "baby boomer" population and increased longevity will lead to an increase in the need for such services as subacute care, caregiver support groups, and adult respite care. Managers reach out to such potential clients in a variety of ways such as participating in community-sponsored events (e.g., blood drives, weight loss seminars, preventive health initiatives). Managers also get involved with the many support groups (e.g., for kidney disease, breast cancer, arthritis, and autism), offering space for their meetings and presenting educational lectures.

# ▶ Suppliers

Three categories of suppliers are identified by Gross: resource suppliers, associates, and supporters.

## Resource Suppliers

Because no organization is totally self-sufficient, it must take in the necessary resources, raw material, money, and goodwill that it needs to survive and function. In this sense, the organization is the client of other organizations.

Within the given organization, one department or service is the supplier of another. In assessing workflow patterns, this concept is useful in identifying which aspects of the work are within the unit's immediate control and which originate in one or several other departments. For example, the health information service is the client of several other units in this sense. The proper gathering of patient identification information is the work of the several admissions and intake units; a health information department is dependent on these units for that part of the workflow. A centralized, computerized information technology system is dependent in the same way. The laboratory, medical imaging department, physical therapy department, and occupational therapy department all depend on the nursing service (or other unit that has the task of coordinating patient transportation in-house) to bring, send, or prepare patients so that the service/unit can proceed with its own work in a predictable manner. Essential information for the formulation of job descriptions concerning interdepartmental relationships or for the development of cross-training programs within the organization is obtained from an awareness of those organizational components that act as resource suppliers to each other.

In the same sense, the chief executive officer can be seen as a resource supplier, making the final adjudication in the allocation of space, money, and personnel to the units. The manager of the department or service should know the needs of other departments and should develop strategic alliances in the competition for scarce resources.

Resource suppliers are often external to the organization. Companies making specialty products or offering specialty services have a unique relationship to the healthcare organization. Such suppliers may be limited in number; in fact, there may be only one such supplier in a geographic area. The viability of such an organization is of interest and concern for the manager who relies on these products or services. Furthermore, with the implementation of such federal regulations as the Health Insurance Portability and Accountability Act and with issues relating to risk management, the healthcare organization that contracts with one or another such resource supplier needs to work with that resource supplier to ensure that it, too, follows the specific regulations. These considerations include policies, procedures, and safeguards relating to patient privacy and confidentiality. Chain-of-trust agreements are required for organizations dealing directly with

patient care information (such as an outsourced transcription service or a medical billing service). The healthcare manager will attend to the quality of products and services from external sources because these become part of the services offered by the healthcare organization.

In addition, there are points of vulnerability in the relationships between the organization and its resource suppliers. If a supplier goes out of business, with or without notice, the organization must find a new, reliable provider and look into reclamation of the organization's resources (e.g., documents stored or processed off-site). If there is a long-term, locked-in contract with a supplier, the organization may not be able to take advantage of another supplier who can provide needed goods on more favorable terms. If there is little or no competition among many suppliers, the few suppliers hold the power in negotiations. Finally, if a department manager finds that a supplier will not continue to provide the goods or services until a bill is paid, an awkward, indeed, difficult situation may develop; the payment process within an organization might be slow, or even fraught with problems, all of which are beyond the middle manager's ability to solve.

Managers take opportunities to partner with resource suppliers in special project development. For example, health information educators work with vendors to create virtual laboratory modules for use in educational institutions as well as for in-service training in healthcare settings. Another example is found in the partnerships of university-based departments of physical and rehabilitation medicine and a research and training program in life skills adjustment.

## Associates

Individuals or groups outside the organization who work cooperatively with the organization in a joint effort are associates of the organization. Associates have a common interest and common work that unites them with the organization. The manager who recognizes the efforts of associates will actively obtain their cooperation. Through informal sharing of ideas among themselves, the various healthcare practitioners frequently act as associates to one another. The health information practitioners from several area hospitals may collaborate informally on release of information concerns and work to publicize the regional health information exchange. The communities of practice and related sharing of best practices sponsored by the American Health Information Management Association (AHIMA) is yet another example of associate activity. A joint position statement on health information confidentiality, developed by health information organizations and agencies, is yet another example of associate interaction. The discussion about electronic health records in Chapter 2 contains a listing of groups who partner in this major joint effort.

Associate interaction is a useful as an ongoing activity, especially when a new demand on the system arises (e.g., the adoption of a new coding/classification system). When an organization is challenged by the requirements of meeting accrediting standards, the accrediting agency (usually categorized as a controller) provides associate-style interaction with the healthcare partner, providing a staff coach to the organization when it applies for accreditation. It coordinates peer review groups to give even further assistance.

## Supporters

Various politically, socially, and economically powerful individuals and groups in the society may be supporters of the organization. They mobilize "friendly power" for the organization, giving it encouragement and developing a climate of goodwill toward the organization. Such supporters can coordinate major activities, such as fund-raising, public relations, and intermediate services for the organization. This type of support helps the organization conserve its own resources for direct application to immediate goals, such as providing direct patient care. Individual organizations may quite simply lack the power to mobilize certain political or economic resources on their own behalf and may depend on a "friend in the castle" to help in these matters. The traditional pattern of appointing the political, social, and economic elite to the board of trustees in healthcare organizations is often an effort to mobilize such power on behalf of these organizations. Professional associations foster this relationship through regularly scheduled interaction with both state and federal lawmakers. For example, Capitol Hill Day, usually coordinated at the national level by the professional associations, is one such endeavor. Members of the association use this opportunity for face-to-face interaction with their elected officials, calling attention to issues of interest and concern. Testimony at hearings or availability for expert review on relevant topics are other examples of this type of interaction.

Occasionally, a nationally prominent figure demonstrates a particular interest in health care because of some personal experience with a particular health problem. In a sense, poliomyelitis, heart disease, and breast cancer received more attention because they affected a president or a member of his family. Leading political figures may work toward the passage of legislation on behalf of some specific healthcare need. A number of well-known entertainers and sports figures have supported fund-raising activities for certain healthcare issues. Such individuals command resources unavailable to a single institution.

The Lions Club programs to support eye care, the Easter Seals program in fund-raising and coordination of volunteers to work with developmentally challenged persons, and the Shriners' traditional support of health care for children with disabilities illustrate the typical activity of supporters. The traditional hospital auxiliary is yet another example of a support group. Its fund-raising activities may facilitate the development of special programs such as wound care surgery equipment, cataract surgery, or breast-health screening at no cost for those unable to pay, or the "No One Dies Alone" project. Supporters may help coordinate activities to the mutual benefit of all participants, offsetting the destructive aspect of competition and facilitating compliance with standards set by controllers by making resources available for use by the organization.

Although an organization may not actively declare itself a supporter, the net effect of its activities may provide support. Advocacy groups for privacy in general, for example, have helped raise the social consciousness of the public toward all issues concerning privacy, thus helping healthcare institutions to develop guidelines for the restrictive release of information. In such situations, collaboration in the development of and lobbying for pertinent state legislation becomes possible.

Sometimes a client group takes on the dual roles of both supporter and resource supplier, as in the case of hospice care. Some requirements for hospice programs include the mandate that a certain minimum amount of hospice care be given by volunteers. Clients become volunteers, thereby helping the organization meet this mandate.

## ▶ Advisers

Although they are like supporters in some ways, advisers have more specific activities that tend to set trends for the industry. They provide a particular form of resource or support through their advice. Gross stressed an important difference between supporters and advisers; the assistance and support of advisers help the organization use its resources and the support it receives from other sources. Advisers stand apart from the organization and often have a more impersonal relationship with the organization than do supporters.

The advice may be in the form of overall guidelines, position papers, data analysis, sample procedures and methods, best practices and benchmarking, or model legislation. The various professional organizations provide abundant resources for use. Sometimes an external organization has legal and accrediting authority over the organization; this is discussed in the next section on controllers. These same controllers occasionally take on the additional role of adviser because they want the licensed/accredited group to succeed. Thus, the controlling organization becomes an adviser through the provision of interpretive guidelines, sample policies and practices, educational material, and training sessions. If the accrediting process is too unwieldy, punitive, or costly, an organization may forgo it. Although it must meet licensure standards, accreditation is voluntary. The accrediting agencies stand to lose if they do not encourage and assist their constituency.

# ▶ Controllers

Those individuals or groups who have power over the organization are controllers. Healthcare organizations must comply with the regulations of several federal and state government agencies as well as with the mandates of the various accrediting agencies. A multispecialty healthcare organization is required to meet detailed regulations from different state agencies as a condition for licensure. For example, social service agencies must meet a variety of regulations from the following government agencies:

- Adoption and foster care: Office of Children, Youth, and Families
- Residential school and outpatient psychiatric clinic: Behavioral Care/Mental Health and Substance Abuse Services
- Personal care home: Office of Social Programs
- Skilled nursing facility: Department of Health

Several organizations and agencies have such control power. The level of detail varies greatly, ranging from the optimal standards stated by The Joint Commission to the highly detailed regulations (e.g., required room size) in a state law. Chapter 1 contains a discussion of settings, laws, regulations, and standards.

Certain controllers are internal to the organization and yet constitute a kind of separate organization. Workers as individuals are a part of the organization, but the unions that represent them stand outside the organization, exerting specific pressure on it through collective bargaining. The governing board is an integral part of the hierarchical structure, but in some ways the board of trustees is separate from the line managers, who are controlled by the decisions made by the top-level management group. The assessment of the net effect of such controllers' input gives the manager a sense of clear boundaries for planning and decision making. However innovative an idea might be, for example, the manager must still keep management practices in line with these constraints.

Controllers may also impose conflicting regulations on the institution, such as the mandate of the federal government to maintain almost absolute confidentiality of alcohol and drug abuse records and the mandate of third-party payers to provide satisfactory evidence of treatment for reimbursement. Managers may be forced to change their managerial style as a result of certain constraints imposed by a controller (e.g., the details of a union contract may limit severely the use of the laissez-faire style of management). By means of survey questionnaires and site visits, the manager may assess the net effect of these multiple regulations on workflow, services offered, staffing patterns mandated, and job descriptions restricted and refined.

# ▶ Adversaries

Health care traditionally carries overtones of great compassion and deep charitable roots. However, healthcare organizations, like many other organizations, have opponents and enemies as well as competitors and rivals. The rising cost of healthcare tends to be a source of conflict for healthcare professionals and the organizations in which they work.

Indeed, clients themselves at times take an adversarial stance because of small, cumulative changes in the organization. These are listed below:

- As the organization grows and assumes more and more impersonal characteristics, clients may become disaffected. Instead of speaking to a person, one may reach an answering machine, or instead of going to a familiar location, one must go to an off-site clinic or even to a newly acquired facility in another town.
- Patients may sense that they are second-class citizens because they do not participate in the health system's managed care insurance plan. Being reminded that a certain aspect of care would be paid for more readily if one has a "gold level" membership is disconcerting and erodes trust.
- The use of the electronic health system leads to inadvertent impersonalization. Here a clinician must look at the computer screen more than at the patient, or instead of a short but personable

set of interactions at registration, a patient checks-in using a personal computer.

- A patient may bring a full-scale, formal malpractice lawsuit.
- The healthcare organization's interaction with third-party payers may lead to an adversarial relationship. Denial of claims is the arena for this dynamic. The effect of denials spills over into the organization's relationship with its primary clients, the patients, with an attendant loss of goodwill. When final billing is received by the patient many months after the care event, or the billing is broken down into the care and the unreimbursed support services (facilities, supplies), patients become alienated.

Also, current and former employees sometimes take an adversarial role as whistle-blowers; this behavior may flow from good intentions or result from some negative experience. Employees who face reduction in staffing or many changes resulting from lean management initiatives may feel threatened by job loss or the disturbance of familiar relationships and routines.

All of this leads to shifting loyalty. Identifying and reducing, even eliminating, adversarial relationships remains an important managerial duty. Managers seek to offset disaffection by clients through processes such as risk management, customer/patient satisfaction surveys, development of ombudsman programs, and the use of expert advisers to assist with insurance claim issues.

Outright opponents or enemies are those individuals or groups who seek actively and aggressively to limit the organization in its activity. These opponents or enemies may have the power to bring an activity to a halt or to prohibit an activity from being started. For example, clients do not wish to have certain facilities, such as drug treatment centers or group homes for the developmentally challenged, too close to their homes. Furthermore, they may want ample parking and easy access to their hospital, but they do not want to disturb local housing units or business areas. Zoning codes may be enforced to prevent the development of alternative treatment facilities or the expansion of existing facilities. Clients may withdraw financial support as evidence of displeasure. In this high-tech age, organizations must deal with hackers, identity theft operatives, and systems hijackers. This threat to the organization requires diligent attention regarding detection and prevention, as well as processes to deal with the aftermath when a disruptive event occurs.

The concept of competition is well understood and accepted in the economic arena. Within reasonable boundaries, competition is favorable for clients because it forces providers to make products or services better or more accessible. The sharp edge of competition is also evident in healthcare delivery, possibly because certain factors in contemporary culture are producing shifts in client loyalty. These factors include erosion of strong ethnic and religious ties to one hospital or health center along with urban and suburban migration patterns.

Given a dropping inpatient census, a hospital may compete actively with a freestanding medical clinic by offering its own outpatient clinic services. To attract patients, one obstetrics unit may offer the latest in fetal monitoring, whereas another may stress family-centered childbirth. An urban medical school or medical center may offer the benefits of highly specialized techniques to offset a census drop because certain clients seek to avoid the city. A hospital seeking financial bond approval for an expanded facility or for some special activity may engage in active outreach to increase its patient population. To expand its customer base, a drug store might offer hearing aid services, basic eye care assessment, and blood pressure monitoring. A grocery store might offer flu shots; a school system might offer formal day-care programs for the summer recess. All these examples reflect competition between and among organizations.

Rivals, according to Gross, are those who produce different products but compete for resources, assistance, and support. In the healthcare setting, specialty hospitals could be considered the rivals of general hospitals (e.g., a children's hospital versus a pediatric unit in a general hospital, a birthing center versus an obstetrics unit). When the emphasis in definition is placed on competition for the same resources, there is evidence of rivalry among healthcare institutions for scarce personnel (e.g., registered nurses for the 3:00–11:00 P.M. shift, trained coding specialists, physicians for the emergency department).

Within an organization, one department may be cast as rival to another for needed space, additional personnel, and special funds. Managers may find that the same departments that are clients may also be supporters and rivals.

## ▶ Coalitions for Building Community and Client Involvement

The analysis of an organization through the application of the clientele network illustrates the intertwining of the organization with its local community. Healthcare organizations generally command respect; communities rely on them not only for health care but also for employment. The organization's management team is viewed as a major part of community leadership. In turn, the concerns of the community have an impact on the healthcare organization—job losses or gains, crime, and infrastructure development, to name a few salient issues.

Helping the community build alliances is an aspect of leadership. How is this best accomplished? There are some tried-and-true steps in community building. First, the management/leadership team clarifies, internally, the level of its involvement in community affairs. The prudent course in one situation might be simply starting the conversation—that is, helping raise the issue in a general way. In another situation, the organization might commit to a highly visible leadership role, or the provision of physical space for meetings and the loan of staff. Identification of the specific issue of focus (e.g., need for area-wide transportation, need for more elder care programs, economic development) is part of this process.

With this focus clarified, the team then starts its outreach efforts to the communities of interest and stakeholders. Team members devote efforts to developing and supporting community-based leadership, with the continuing offer of support. The leadership team, now expanded to include community members, sharpens its focus again, determining which specific problem to solve, which alternatives are available, how to select the best alternative, and how to develop a program of action. In many situations, the program of action involves local, state, or federal government entities. A healthcare organization, through its board of trustees, usually has one or more individuals who are power holders in their own right and whose influence can be used to advance the cause. Sometimes special funding is available through private or public grants; the healthcare organization, through its research and development division, might be the most effective agent to apply for and receive such funding.

As with any program, during its implementation and again at its conclusion, a variety of processes are used to provide feedback during this process. Community building and the development of ongoing alliances are mutually supportive endeavors. These skills are part of the manager's portfolio.

# ▶ Example of Clientele Network for a Physical Therapy Unit

A tabulation method can be used to analyze a departmental clientele network. The development of such a reference tool for the internal environment of the organization provides the manager with much information concerning relationships to be developed, aspects of the workflow to be considered, and regulations and guidelines that must be satisfied. The following is the clientele network of a spinal cord treatment service in a physical therapy department:

I. Clients
  A. Immediate clients
    1. Patients of the spinal cord injury service
    2. Hospital personnel assigned to the spinal cord injury service
  B. Secondary clients
    1. Family members
    2. Hospital medical staff for in-service education and clarification of policies and procedures
    3. Physical therapy students on clinical affiliation
    4. Local hospitals requesting information on special programs dealing with treatment of the spinal cord–injured patient
  C. Remote clients
    1. Local hospitals not yet a part of referral network
    2. Home health agencies
    3. School systems (sports injury care)
II. Suppliers
  A. Resources
    1. Physicians within the hospital who refer patients to the spinal cord injury unit
    2. Medical supply companies that supply equipment for both the patients and the department
    3. Bureau of Vocational Rehabilitation, which helps cover the cost of treatment and equipment
    4. Hospital transport system
  B. Associates
    1. National spinal cord treatment centers
    2. Other direct patient services (e.g., nursing, occupational therapy, speech, psychology, social services)
    3. Home health agencies
    4. Professional association educational materials
  C. Supporters
    1. Hospital physicians and residents
    2. Community service organizations
    3. Auxiliary organizations serving the spinal cord service
    4. Medical supply companies

5. County wheelchair sports association
6. Public relations department of the hospital

III. Advisers
   A. American Physical Therapy Association
   B. Hospital administrators
   C. Other direct patient care services within the hospital
   D. Insurance companies

IV. Controllers
   A. Accreditation agencies
      1. The Joint Commission
      2. Specialty accreditation agencies for rehabilitation facilities
   B. Federal government
      1. Medicare reimbursement regulations
      2. Equal employment opportunity
      3. Working conditions
   C. State government
      1. Licensing regulations for physical therapists
      2. Medicaid reimbursement regulations
   D. County hospital association
   E. Professional association codes of ethics
   F. Unions
   G. Hospital policies
   H. Third-party payers

V. Adversaries
   A. Opponents and enemies
      1. Neighborhood groups who oppose clinic expansion in a residential area
      2. Hospital personnel resistant to change
   B. Rivals and competitors
      1. Other local rehabilitation centers sharing the same clientele network
      2. Independent group practices specializing in rehabilitation

## ▶ Introducing Organizational Survival Strategies

Organizational survival and growth are implicit goals requiring the investment of energy and resources. Normally, only higher levels of management need give attention to organizational survival; it may be taken for granted by most employees or members, some of whom may even take actions that threaten the organization's survival (e.g., a prolonged strike). There may be an unwillingness to admit the legitimacy of survival as a goal because it seems self-serving. However,

managers disregard the concept of organizational survival—whether the whole corporation or just a department or unit—at their own peril.

So fundamental is the goal of organizational survival that it underpins all other goals. Fostering this goal contributes to the satisfaction of the more explicit goals of the group or organization. Survival is articulated as a goal in certain phases of organizational development—for example, when competition threatens. The clientele network includes competitors, rivals, enemies, and opponents that must be faced. Certain threats to organizational survival may be identified:

- Lack of strong, formal leadership after the early charismatic leadership of the founders
- Too-rapid change either within or outside the organization
- Shifting client demand, either with the loss of clients or with the increased exercise of control by clients
- Competition from stronger organizations
- High turnover rate in either the rank and file or the leadership
- Failure to recognize and accept organizational survival as a legitimate, although not the sole, organizational purpose

These factors drain from the organization the energy that should be goal-directed.

An organization ensures its survival through certain strategies and processes, such as bureaucratic imperialism, co-optation, patterns of adaptation, goal multiplication and expansion, use of organizational roles, conflict limitation, and integration of the individual into the organization. Astute managers recognize such patterns of organizational behavior and assess them realistically. A weak organization or unit cannot pull together the money, resources, and power to serve its clients effectively.

## ▶ Bureaucratic Imperialism

An organization develops to pursue a particular goal, serve a specific client group, or promote the good of a certain group. In effect, an organization stakes out its territory. Thus, a professional association seeks to represent the interests of members who have something in common, such as specific academic training and professional practice. A hospital or home health agency seeks to serve a particular area. A union focuses on the needs of one or several categories of workers.

A political party attempts to bring in members who hold a particular political philosophy. A government agency seeks to serve a specific constituency.

The classic definition of bureaucratic imperialism reflects the idea that a bureaucratic organization exerts a kind of pressure to develop a particular client group and then to expand it. It becomes imperialistic in the underlying power struggle and competition that ensues when any other group seeks to deal with the same clients, members, or area of jurisdiction. Matthew Holden, Jr., coined the term bureaucratic imperialism and defined it in the context of federal government agencies that must consider such factors as clients to be served, political aspects to be assessed, and benefits to be shared among administrative officials and key political clients. According to Holden's definition of the concept, bureaucratic imperialism is "a matter of interagency conflict in which two or more agencies try to assert permanent control over the same jurisdiction, or in which one agency actually seeks to take over another agency as well as the jurisdiction of that agency."[8] The idea of agency can be expanded to include any organization, the various components of the clientele network can be substituted for the constituency, and the role of manager can replace that of the administrative politician in those organizations that are not in the formal political setting.

Managers in many organizations can recognize the elements of this competitive mode of interaction among organizations. There may even be such competition among departments and units within an organization. In the healthcare field, competition may be seen in the areas of professional licensure and practice, accreditation processes for the organizations as a whole, the delineation of clients to be served, and similar areas.

Professional licensure has the effect of annexing specific "territory" as the proper domain of a given professional group, but other groups may seek to carry out the same, or at least similar, activities. For example, there is the question of the role of chiropractors in traditional healthcare settings. Is the use of medical imaging techniques the exclusive jurisdiction of physicians and trained medical imaging technicians or should the law be changed to permit chiropractors greater use of these techniques? Psychiatrists question the expanding role of others who have entered the field of behavioral health. As each healthcare profession develops, the question of jurisdiction emerges.

The accreditation process in health care reflects similar struggles for jurisdiction. Which shall be the definitive accreditation process for behavioral care facilities—that approved by the American Psychiatric Association or that approved by The Joint Commission? Should all of these processes be set aside, leaving only state governments to exercise such control through the licensure of institutions? Long-established professional associations (e.g., AHIMA) have developed sound examination and credentialing processes, only to see the rise of for-profit organizations that develop their own categories and provide certification.

Other examples may be drawn from the healthcare setting. There has been a jurisdictional dispute over blood banking between the American Red Cross and other blood bank procurement groups as well as competition among health maintenance organizations, or HMOs, with the more traditional Blue Cross–Blue Shield-type plans and commercial medical insurance companies.

Certain trends have occasioned the development of new organizational positions (e.g., chief privacy officer, chief compliance officer, chief information officer, health informatician). Are these new professions or do they fall under the education and credentialing of existing professional organizations? To state this question another way—whose organizational territory encompasses information technology? Within an organization, which department or service will be the designated leader for information technology application? No doubt the tasks will remain shared among several departments, with each continuing to exert its own prerogatives.

Another example may be drawn for the development and implementation of electronic health records—which agency or organization will be the final arbiter of core data elements, formats, standards, and technological aspects of the system? The Health Level-7 International has relatively universal acceptance. The Joint Commission has its elements of practice, AHIMA has its information governance principles, and ECRI (formerly the Emergency Care Research Institute) has clinical standards for core content as well as support technology as does the American Society for Testing and Measurement. The Institute of Medicine promulgates core functions for electronic health records. Managers must attend to these competing groups, which in turn must cooperate with one another.

Although the charitable nature of health care has been emphasized traditionally, the elements of competition and underlying conflict must be recognized. With shifts in patient populations and changes in each healthcare profession, healthcare managers must assess the effects of bureaucratic imperialism in a realistic manner. The competition engendered by bureaucratic imperialism and the resultant total or partial "colonization" of an organizational unit or client group may be functional. Holden noted that conflict not only forces organizational regrouping by clarifying client loyalty and wishes but also sharpens support for the agency or unit that "wins." Furthermore, it disrupts the bureaucratic form from time to time, causing a healthy review of client need, organizational purpose, and structural pattern.

# ▶ Co-Optation

Another method that organizations use to help ensure their survival is *co-optation*, an organizational strategy for adapting and responding to change. Philip Selznick described and labeled this strategy, which is viewed as both cooperative and adaptive. He defined co-optation as "an adaptive response on the part of the organization in response to the social forces in its environment; by this means, the organization averts threats to its stability by absorbing new elements into the leadership of the organization".[9] The organization, in effect, shares organizational power by absorbing these new elements. Selznick called it a realistic adjustment to the centers of institutional strength.

## Formal Versus Informal Co-Optation

Informal co-optation, the symbols of authority and administrative burdens are shared, but no substantial power is transferred. The organization does not permit the co-opted group to interfere with organizational unity of command. Normal bureaucratic processes tend to provide sufficient checks and balances on any co-opted group, just as they tend to restrict the actions of managers. Through formal co-optation, however, the organization seeks to demonstrate its accessibility to its various publics.

In health care, the co-optation process is suggested by the practice of appointing "ordinary" citizens to the board of trustees. Community behavioral care health centers and some neighborhood health centers tend to emphasize consumer or community representation. Health planning agencies include both providers and consumers in planning for health care on a regional or statewide basis. The formalization of nursing home ombudsmen or patient/resident councils is still another example of this process.

Professional associations in those disciplines that have technical-level practitioners have sought to open their governing processes in response to the growing strength of the technical-level group. Increases in numbers, greater degree of training, further specialization, and a general emphasis on the democratic process and provision of rights for all members have fostered changes in these associations. Open membership, such as that adopted by AHIMA, is an example of positive co-optation; the rapid developments in the wider field of information technology gave impetus to including the information technology specialists in the existing health information arena. Without cooperative adaptation to such internal changes, there is a risk that additional associations will be formed, possibly weakening the parent organization.

When an organization seeks to deal less overtly with shifting centers of power and to maintain the legitimacy of its own power, co-optation may be informal in nature. For example, managers may meet unofficially with informally delegated representatives of clients, employees, or outside groups. Organizational leaders may deal regularly with some groups, but there are no visible changes in the official leadership structures. No new positions are created; committee membership remains intact. Informal co-optation may be more important than formal co-optation because of its emphasis on true power, although each form serves its unique purpose. An organization can blend formal and informal co-optation processes, as they are not mutually exclusive.

## Control of Co-Opted Groups

Although the co-opted group could gain strength and attempt to consolidate power, this does not happen frequently for several reasons. First, the organization has the means of controlling participation. For example, only limited support may be given to the group; there may be no physical space, money, or staff available to give to the co-opted group, or management could simply withhold support. Another possible course is to assign so much activity to the co-opted group that it cannot succeed easily. With this approach, key leaders of the co-opted group generally retain their regular work assignments but now have additional projects and tasks relating to their special causes. Co-opted leaders also become the buffer individuals in the organization, because the group has placed its trust in them and looks for results faster than they can be produced. Such leaders may find their base of action eroded and their activity turning into a thankless task.

In a more Machiavellian approach, organizational authorities could schedule meetings at inconvenient hours or control their agendas in such a way that issues of significance to the co-opted group are too far down on the list of discussion items to be dealt with under the time constraints. Absolute insistence on parliamentary procedure may also be used as a weapon of control; a novice in the use of *Robert's Rules of Order* is at a distinct disadvantage when compared with a seasoned expert.

The subtle psychological process that occurs in the co-opted individual who is taken into the formal organization as a distinct outsider acts as another controlling measure. The person suddenly becomes, for this moment, one of the power holders and derives new status. Certain perquisites also are granted. A consumer representative, for example, may find his or her way paid, quite legitimately, for a special conference or fact-finding trip to study a problem. The individual, in becoming privy to more data and sometimes to confidential data, may start to "see things" from the organization's point of view. Also, certain subtle social barriers may make the co-opted individual uncomfortable, even though they may not be raised intentionally and may be part of the normal course of action for the group.

Individuals representing pressure groups find that their own time and energies are limited, even if they desire power. Other activities continue to demand their energies. In addition, certain issues lose popularity, and pressure groups may find their power base has eroded. Finally, the agenda items that were causes of conflict may become the recurring business of the organization. The conflict may become a routine, and the structure to deal with it may become a part of the formal organization. In the collective bargaining process, for example, the union is a part of the organization, and its leaders have built-in protection from factors that erode effective participation. Labor union officials commonly have certain reductions in workload so that they may attend to union business, space may be provided for their offices or meetings, and they may seek meetings with management as often as executives seek sessions with them. Co-optation has occurred in such a case, but without a loss of identity of the co-opted group. In healthcare organizations, consumer participation has become part of the organizations' continuing activity through the development of a more stable process for consumer input, such as the community governing board models.

## ▸ Hibernation and Adaptation

To maintain its equilibrium, an organization must adapt to changing inputs. This adjustment may take the passive form of *hibernation*, in which the institution enters a phase of retrenchment. Cutting losses may be the sensible option. If efforts to maintain an acceptable census in certain hospital units, such as obstetrics or pediatrics, are unsuccessful, there may be an administrative decision to close those units and concentrate on providing quality patient care in the remaining services. An organization may adjust or adapt to changing inputs more actively by anticipating them. Staff specialists may be brought in, equipment and physical facilities updated, and goals restated. Finally, the overall corporate form may be restructured as a permanent reorganization that formalizes the cumulative effects of changes. A hospital may move from private sponsorship to a state-related affiliated status, or a healthcare center may become the intake and referral service for behavioral care programs in the area. An assisted living facility may regroup as a personal care facility. Recall the example from an earlier discussion under adaptation to change.

The relationships among the concepts of hibernation, adaptation, and permanent change can be seen in the following case history of a state behavioral care hospital. After the state legislature cut the budget of all such state hospitals, the institution director began to set priorities for services so that the institution could survive. The least productive departments were asked to decrease their staff. The rehabilitation department lost two aide positions. The institution director had to force the organization into a state of hibernation to accomplish some essential conservation of resources. The director of rehabilitation services revised the department goals to improve the chances of departmental survival. After closing ancillary services, the director concentrated staff on visible areas of the hospital and asked them to make their work particularly praiseworthy. At the same time, the director emphasized the need to document services so that patients' progress in therapy programs could be demonstrated. The director adapted to the change in the organization.

The program changes proved successful. The director of the rehabilitation department consolidated the changes and modified the department's goals. Instead of offering periodic programs to adolescent, neurological, geriatric, and acute care patients, the staff would concentrate on acutely ill geriatric patients. The staff applied for funds that were available to treat this population. At the same time, the staff determined that the adolescent unit could benefit from their services. Although funds were shrinking, the staff serviced this unit because needs in that area were unmet. The director and the staff decided to apply for private funds to service neurological and acute care cases so that these programs could also continue. By adopting a combined strategy of hibernation and adaptation, with alternate plans for expansion, the department director was able to foster not only departmental survival but, ultimately, departmental growth.

Another example of hibernation as a survival strategy is illustrated by the response of a continuing care or retirement community to several challenges. Planning assumptions, budget projections, short- and long-term investments, and fee structures were based on expectations of a modest to robust profit. Unfortunately, a prolonged economic downturn reduced the rate of return on investments with no concomitant decrease in costs. Credit lines became more difficult to obtain and came with much higher interest rates. An increase in regulatory requirements for the assisted living component of the facility would have required major renovations that were cost prohibitive. As a response to these factors, the assisted living component was eliminated and other expansion plans were put on hold. Plans to seek additional, voluntary accreditation were also postponed until the organization had evidence that such accreditation would enhance its attractiveness as a care facility, with a resulting increase in admissions.

# ▶ Goal Succession, Multiplication, and Expansion

Because an organization that effectively serves multiple client groups can attract money, materials, and personnel more readily than an organization with a more limited constituency, leaders may actively seek to expand the original goals of the organization. In addition to the pressures in the organizational environment that may force the organization to modify its goals as an adaptive response, success in reaching organizational goals may enable managers to focus on expanded or even new goals. The terms *goal succession*, *goal expansion*, and *goal multiplication* are used to describe the process in which goals are modified, usually in a positive manner.

Amatai Etzioni described this tendency of organizations to find new goals when old ones have been realized or cannot be attained.[10] In goal succession, one goal is reached and is succeeded by a new one. One example is the March of Dimes, which began as a formal organization with the goal of eradicating polio; this objective was achieved. The organization had strong support and a well-developed formal structure. Rather than disband, the organization celebrated its achievement and undertook a new goal: the prevention of birth defects through a healthy babies initiative. Another example of this pattern involves the actions of a group of local merchants. They formed a cooperative group to coordinate clean-up efforts after catastrophic flooding—a goal that was met. However, a strong cooperative group had been formed and solid administrative structures had been developed; community and regional support was strong. Rather than disband after meeting its original goal, the group took on new goals of fostering economic development and promoting tourism. In addition, sometimes an organization takes on additional goals because the original goals are relatively unattainable. For example, a church may add a variety of social services to attract members when the worship services and doctrinal substance per se do not increase the church's membership. A missionary group may offer a variety of healthcare or educational services when its direct evangelical methods cannot be used. The original goal is not abandoned, but it is sought indirectly; more tangible goals of service and outreach succeed this primary goal.

Goal expansion is the process in which the original goal is retained and enlarged with variations. Many examples can be described:

- A college or university includes continuing education as well as traditional classes.
- An acute care facility may open a rehabilitation unit, including respite care, as an adjunct to its short-stay services.
- A medical center opens a specialty division just for the comprehensive care of senior citizens.
- A special day program for people with fetal alcohol spectrum disorder (FASD) adds an emergency overnight or short-stay unit. This same program partners with the National Association of Counsel for Children, which focuses on judicial proceedings affecting the client group (adolescents with FASD) common to both organizations.
- The Joint Commission continues to focus primarily on inpatient acute care hospital accreditation but has expanded its standards and accreditation process to include home care, outpatient, and emergency care units.
- A collective bargaining unit negotiates specific benefits for its workers and takes on the administrative processing of certain elements, such as the pension fund. The basic goal of improving the circumstances of the workers is retained and expanded beyond immediate economic benefits.
- A long-term care (skilled care) facility expands its goals to provide a new service: a memory care or Alzheimer's disease unit.

- The Easter Seals Association reflects a history of goal expansion, beginning with services for children with disabilities and currently offering additional services to families affected by autism. In response to the growing number of military service members who are returning from active duty with disabilities, the organization has broadened its client group to serve them.
- A community pharmacy implements comprehensive medication review for its customers.
- The Red Cross, which was originally organized to provide disaster relief in World War I, subsequently assists in coordinating relief from all disasters, regardless of cause. In recent years, this same agency has expanded its child care safety training to include grandparents who have become increasingly common caretakers of the young.
- Another example can be found in the personal care setting, where some of these facilities offer respite care in a secure unit for patients with dementia, thus providing family members the opportunity to take a break.

Note that in all of these examples, the basic goals are retained, and the new ones are derived from them. The new goals are closely related and are essentially extensions of the original goals.

Goal multiplication is also a process in which an original goal is retained and new ones added. In this case, however, the new goals reflect the organization's effort to diversify. Goal multiplication is often the natural outgrowth of success. A hospital may offer patient care as its traditional, primary goal. To this it may add the goal of education of physicians, nurses, and other healthcare professionals. Because excellence in education is frequently related to the adequacy of the institution's research programs, research may subsequently become a goal. The hospital may take on a goal of participating in social reform, seeking to undertake affirmative action hiring plans and to foster employment within its neighborhood. It may offer special training programs for those who are unemployed in its area or for those who are physically or developmentally impaired. It may coordinate extensive social services in an effort to assist patients and their families with both immediate healthcare problems and the larger social and economic problems they face. Large medical centers may take on activities such as real estate ventures, because (1) they need housing for visiting fellows, associates, and students in training, and (2) they view such pursuits as income-producing ventures. A nonprofit, community service organization provided general social service assistance in its designated geographic area. It added an additional goal, that of economic development initiatives to break the cycle of poverty.

Similar examples can be found in the business sector. A large hotel–motel corporation, with its resources for dealing with temporary living quarters, may go into the nursing home industry or the drug and alcohol treatment facility business by offering food, laundry, and housekeeping services; it may even operate a chain of convalescent or alcohol and drug rehabilitation centers. Several real estate firms might consolidate their efforts in direct sale of homes and then offer mortgage services as an additional program. Organizations may take on a variety of goals as a means of diversification; resources are directed toward satisfaction of all the goals. Such multiplication of goals is seen as a positive state of organizational growth.

## ▶ The Corporate Culture

As an organization moves through its life cycle, from inception to ending, there is an over-arching ethos, the corporate culture. At first, the elements of the organization's way of being are rather implicit. It will become increasingly explicit as the formal organization develops. These core values are reflected in the central activities as planning, decision making, organizational pattern, and development of support resources. Aspects of corporate culture include:

- *accountability*—financial audits, supply chain controls, review committees, annual reports;
- *transparency*—well-known plans, information about wages, salaries and benefits, long-range plans, and related evaluations of progress;
- *Innovation*—commitment to research, implementation of alternate care sites, extensive use of telemedicine, and other eHealth initiatives;
- *success and excellence*—seeking accreditation from independent, external bodies, achieving identifiable and publicized ratings from regulatory agencies, employee award system, pervasive quality assurance, and improvement processes;
- *compassionate and humane approaches to client and worker needs*—patient and family/caregiver support programs, navigator assistance, free screening for those unable to pay, agreeing to be a "safety net" hospital, flextime, remote work site options, day care on premises, "latch key" contact system for working parents;
- *Fairness*—balancing the compassion associated with free or subsidized care with avoidance of cost-shifting onto those who pay;

- *cooperation toward internal participants as well as external organizations*—internally through teams and group projects, participative leadership style, and externally through joint ventures, shared resources, affiliations;
- *community outreach*—civic organization membership, sponsorship of community events, making space and resources available for community meetings.

Managers are expected to know the corporate culture and reflect it in their activities.

# ▶ Organizational Life Cycle

Organizational change can be monitored through the analysis of an organization's *life cycle*. This concept is drawn from the pattern seen in living organisms. In management and administrative literature, the development of this model stems from the work of Marver Bernstein, who analyzed the stages of evolution and growth of independent federal regulatory commissions.[11] This model of the life cycle can be applied to advantage by any manager who wishes to analyze a particular management setting. The following material presents an application of this model to the healthcare setting.

The organization is assessed not in chronological years but in phases of growth and development. No absolute number of years can be assigned to each phase, and any attempt to do so to predict characteristics would force and possibly distort the model. The value of organizational analysis by means of the life cycle lies in its emphasis on characteristics of the stages rather than the years. For example, the neighborhood health centers established in the 1960s under Office of Economic Opportunity sponsorship had a relatively short life span in comparison with the life span of some large urban hospitals that are approaching a century or more of service. Both types of organizations have experienced the phases of the life cycle, with the former having completed the entire phase through decline and—in its original form—extinction.

The phases of the organizational life cycle usually meld into one another, just as they do in the biological model. Human beings do not suddenly become adolescents, adults, or senior citizens. So, too, organizations normally move from one phase to another at an imperceptible rate with some blurring of boundaries. Finally, not every organization reflects in detail every characteristic of each phase. The emphasis is on the cluster of characteristics that are predominant

at a specific time. By way of a detailed example, the AHIMA Life Cycle is an analysis of a professional organization and its development from gestation to its current stage (robust middle age); this example is provided in the concluding section of this chapter.

## Gestation

In this early formative stage, there is a gradual recognition and articulation of need or shared purpose. This stage often predates the formal organization; indeed, a major characteristic of this period is the movement from informal to formal organization. The impetus for organizing is strong, as it is necessary to bring together in an organized way the prime movers of the fledgling organization, its members (workers), and its clients.

Leadership tends to be strong and committed, and members are willing to work hard. Members' identification with organizational goals is strong because the members are in the unique situation of actualizing their internalized goals; in contrast, those who become part of the institution later must subsequently internalize the institution's objectives. Members of the management team find innovation the order of the day. Creative ideas meet with ready acceptance, because there is no precedent to act as a barrier to innovation. If there is a precedent in a parent organization, it may be cast off easily as part of the rejection of the old organization. A self-selection process also occurs, with individuals leaving if they do not agree with the form the organizational entity is taking. This is largely a flexible process, free of the formal resignation and separation procedures that come later.

## Youth

The early enthusiasm of the gestational phase carries over into the development of a formal organization. Idealism and high hopes continue to dominate the psychological atmosphere. The creativity of the gestational period is channeled toward developing an organization that will be free of the problems of similar institutions. There is a strong camaraderie among the original group of leaders and members. Organizational patterns exhibit a certain inevitability, however. If a creative new organization is successful, it is likely to experience an increase in clients that will force it to formalize policies and procedures rapidly so as to handle the greater demand for service.

Some crisis may occur that precipitates expansion earlier than planned. A health center may have a plan for gradual neighborhood outreach, for example, but a sudden epidemic of "flu" may bring an influx of clients before it is staffed adequately. Management must make rapid adjustments in clinic hours and staffing patterns to meet the demand for specific services and, at the same time, to continue its plan for comprehensive health screening. A center for the developmentally challenged may schedule one opening date, but a court order to vacate a large, decaying facility may require the new center to accept the immediate transfer of many patients. Routine, recurring situations are met by increasingly complex procedures and rules. Additional staff is needed, recruited, and brought into the organization, perhaps even in a crash program rather than through the gradual integration of new members.

At this point, a new generation of worker enters the organization. These workers are one phase removed from the era of idealism and deeply shared commitment to the organization's goals. The organizational structure (e.g., workflow, job descriptions, line and staff relationships, and roles and authority) is tested. For the newcomer brought in at the management level, formal position or hierarchical office is the primary base of authority. Other members of the management team, as the pioneers, know one another's strengths and weaknesses intimately, but these managers may need to test the newcomer's personal attributes and technical competence. Sometimes, because the new organization attempts to deal with some problem in an innovative manner, an individual healthcare practitioner is hired in a nontraditional role; not only the professional and technical competence, but also the managerial competence of that individual, are tested.

Communication networks are essential in any organization. During an organization's youth, it is necessary to rely on formal communication because the informal patterns are not yet well developed, except within the core group. This lack of an easy, anonymous, informal communication network forces individuals to communicate mainly along formal lines of authority. The core group may become more and more closed, more and more "in," relying on well-developed, secure relationships that stem from a shared history in the developing organization, while the newcomers form a distinct "out" group.

The jockeying for power and position may be intense. If managers hold an innovative office, those who oppose such creative organizational patterns may exert significant pressure to acquire jurisdiction or to force a return to traditional ways. Because there may have been much innovation in the overall organizational pattern during the gestation–youth transition stage, managers have little or no precedent against which they can measure their actions.

Certain problems center on the implementation of the original plans. The planners may start to experience frustration with managers who enter the organization during this period of formalization. Perhaps the original plans need modification; perhaps the innovative, ideal approach of the original group is not working, largely because of the change in the size of the organization. The line managers find themselves in the difficult situation of seeming to fail at the task on the one hand and being unable to make the original planners change their view on the other hand. The promise of innovation becomes empty, however, if the original planners guard innovation as their prerogative and refuse to accept other ideas.

In the youth phase of an organization, more time must be devoted to orientation and similar formal processes of integrating new individuals into the organization. Certain difficulties may be encountered in recruiting additional supervisors and professional practitioners. For example, there may be no secure retirement funds, only minimal group medical and life insurance, and a lack of benefits that are predicated on long-term investments and large membership. Salary ranges may be modest in comparison with those of more established organizations simply because insufficient time has passed for the development of adequate resources. The strong normative sense of idealism may have a negative effect on potential workers as well as a positive one; a certain dedication to the organization's cause may be expected, and it may also be assumed that personnel should be willing to work hard without being rewarded monetarily.

During these early years, a subtle cueing system emerges—what is valued, what is rewarded. There is a need to develop the customary external markers associated with motivation: awards and recognition events. Although it is important to develop these, managers must avoid trivializing this process by over-rewarding accomplishment (e.g., a 1-year pin). Managers should focus instead on markers such as safety records, number of client encounters (e.g., 1000), or certain goals the (e.g., training 100% of employees in a specific topic). These elements foster a sense of organizational stability and decrease worker concerns about job security.

The dynamics of bureaucratic imperialism are evident at this early stage. The youthful organization is exerting its claim in the marketplace of health care, trying to operate from a place of strength. Meanwhile, an existing organization may compete intensively for clients and resources. The new organization, with its limited resources, may become less innovative because it is not sure of its strength. It may choose to fight only those battles in which victory is certain. In a healthcare organization, the new unit may be treated as a stepchild of related healthcare institutions. A new community behavioral health center or a home care organization, for example, may have to choose between competing with older, traditional units within the parent organization and being completely independent, still competing for resources but with less legitimacy of claim. A struggle not unlike the classic parent–adolescent conflict may emerge. Thus, organizational energy may go into an internal struggle for survival rather than into serving clients and expanding goals.

If the client groups are well defined and no other group or institution is offering the same service, a youthful organization may flourish. A burn unit in a hospital may have an excellent chance of survival as an organization because of the specificity of its clients as compared, for example, with the chance of a general medical clinic's survival. A similar positive climate may foster the development of units for treatment of spinal cord injury or for rehabilitation of the hand as specialized services. In effect, a highly specialized client group may afford a unit or an organization a virtual monopoly, which will tend to place the unit or organization in a position of strength.

A particularly challenging aspect of the transition from gestation to youth is the necessary development of articles of incorporation and related bylaws. The closely knit group of founders must make plans to anticipate difficulties, conflicts, and the possibility of failure. Provision for removal of board members or officers, auditing of business records, succession plans to replace themselves, and the disposition of assets if the venture fails are concepts seemingly at odds with the idealism of this stage.

## Middle Age

The multiple constraints on the organization at middle age are compounded by several factors. In addition to the external influences that shape the work of the organization, internal factors must be dealt with, such as the organizational pattern, the growing bureaucratic form, the weight of decision by precedent, and an increasing number of traditions.

However, the organization also reaps many benefits from middle age. Many activities are routine and predictable; roles are clear; and communication, both formal and informal, is relatively reliable. These years are potentially stable and productive. There is a reasonable receptivity to new ideas, but middle age is not usually a time of constant massive or rapid change and disruption, even the positive disruption resulting from major innovation. The manager in an organization in its middle age performs the basic traditional management processes in a relatively predictable manner. Assessing change and adapting to it has become well established.

Periods of rejuvenation are precipitated by a variety of events. A new leader may act as a catalytic agent, bringing new vision to the organization; for example, the president of a corporation may push for goal expansion by introducing a new line of products, or an aggressive hospital administrator may push for the development of an alternative healthcare service model. Mergers and affiliations with new and developing types of healthcare institutions, such as community health centers and home care programs, may be the catalyst. Although primarily negative events, the fiscal chaos associated with bankruptcy or the loss of accreditation as a hospital may cause the organization to reassess its goals and restructure its form, thereby giving itself a new lease on life. Sheer competition, coupled with a strong belief in its mission of comprehensive care, might cause a community hospital to add services in specialties such as sports medicine and rehabilitation, cardiac treatment, behavioral health for older teenagers, and on-site comprehensive imaging and laboratory services.

Some external crisis or change of articulated values in the larger society may make the organization vital once again. The recent emergence of alternative modes of communal living reflects individuals' search for a mode of living that combats the alienation of urban society; organizations that provide alternative modes of living can be revitalized because of this new interest in shared living arrangements. The renewed interest in domiciliary care of the elderly reflects this trend. The effect of war on the vitality of the military is an obvious example of crisis as a catalytic agent that causes a spurt of new growth for an organization. The growth of consumer and environmental agencies is another organizational response to change or crisis in the larger society.

In health care, family practice has developed as a specialty in response to patients' wishes for a more comprehensive, more personal type of medical care. The hospice concept for the terminally ill became an alternative to the highly specialized setting of the acute care hospital.

An organization may experience a significant surge of vitality because of some internal activity, such as unionization of workers. During the covert as well as the overt stage of unionization, management may take steps to "get the house in order," including greater emphasis on worker–management cooperation in reaching the fundamental goals of the organization. Client groups may become more active, both to focus attention on the institution's primary purpose and to mobilize client goodwill in the face of the potential adversary (i.e., the union).

Yet another catalytic agent for revitalization of an organization is change in its sponsorship. Although such change (decreased presence of members of the sponsoring group, such as religious sisters) may alienate sectors of the original client group (those with strong ties to the founding sponsors), survival strategies already noted may be used to offset this potential loss of goodwill. Thus, celebration of the organization's milestones, its history, its long-term clients, along with formal and informal co-optation, helps restrengthen these ties. A strategy that can be used to advantage at such times of transition involves the temporary use of an outside management group. This management team, focusing on transition and/or turnaround efforts, has the advantage of objectivity. It can become also the target of the unhappiness of clients about changes, thus absorbing the negative energy of the passing phase. The middle managers are shielded from the negativity and thus they are able to focus on motivating and leading the workers and clients through the changing era.

In addition, legislation of massive scope, particularly at the federal level, may have a rejuvenating effect. The infusion of money into the healthcare system via Medicare and Medicaid is partly responsible for the growth of the long-term care industry, although population trends and sociological patterns for care of the aged outside of the family setting are contributing factors. The passage of government-sponsored healthcare planning and resource development initiatives rejuvenated some of the existing health planning agencies; their gradual phasing out of such initiatives, of course, has had the opposite effect in some instances by forcing a decline in certain planning groups. Changes in state professional licensure laws may bring certain professional groups into a season of new vigor because their scope of practice has been enlarged.

The bureaucratic hierarchy protects managers who derive authority from a position that traditionally is well defined by the organization's middle age. Planning and decision making are shared responsibilities, subject to several hierarchical levels of review. The same events that may spur rejuvenation also may hurl the organization into a state of decline, the major characteristic of the final stage: old age.

## Old Age

Staid routines, resistance to change, a long history of "how we do things," little or no innovation, and concern with survival are the obvious characteristics of an organization in decline. There may be feeble attempts to maintain the status quo or to serve clients in a minimal fashion, but the greater organizational energy is directed toward efforts to survive. If the end is inevitable, resources are guarded so that the institution can fulfill its obligations to its contractual suppliers and to its past and present employees (e.g., through vested pension funds, severance pay, related termination benefits). There may even be a well-organized, overt process of seeking job placement for employees. Time and resources may be made available to such individuals. This stage is a delicate one: members are competing for the same jobs in the same, or closely related, organizations and/or in the same geographic region. Employees become competitors with one another. Workers who keep applying for jobs, only to be rejected, become demoralized and anxious.

Because of an organization's dwindling resources, it may no longer serve clients well, and all but the most loyal clients will look to other organizations to meet their needs. The organization in decline cannot attract new clients; the cycle is broken. Without clients, the organization cannot mobilize financial and political resources to maintain its physical facilities, expand services, respond to technological change, or remain in compliance with new licensure or regulatory mandates. The end, which may come swiftly, may be brought about by a decision to close and a specific plan to do so in an orderly way. For example, a department store might announce a liquidation sale that ends with the closing date. Only the internal details of closing need attention; as far as clients are concerned, the organization has died.

A final closing date may be imposed on an organization. In a bankruptcy, for example, the date may be determined in the course of legal proceedings. Legislation that initially establishes certain programs may include a termination date, although the date is more commonly set when legislation to continue funding the program fails. The changes in medical care evaluation under professional standards review organizations, and the federally funded neighborhood health centers are examples in the healthcare field of programs that moved into a state of decline or closure when funding was no longer available through federal, state, or county legislation.

The closing decision may be a more passive one; there may be a gradual diminution of services and selective plant shutdowns and layoffs, as may occur in manufacturing corporations that rely primarily on military or space contracts. Bankruptcy is costly in economic and political terms in some cases, so the decision is implemented slowly. Indeed, it sometimes seems that no one actually makes a decision in some institutions that decline. Because of its unpopularity, the decision to close certain services, such as healthcare services, may be made in a somewhat passive way; however, the seemingly gradual slipping away of clients and the deterioration or outright closing of urban hospitals may be accompanied by the emergence of competitive forms of health care, such as home care units, neighborhood health centers, and mobile clinics.

Some organizations cease to exist entirely; others may change form or exist under new sponsorship. For example, some of the neighborhood health centers under specialty grant sponsorship have been absorbed into other federal government systems of health clinics. Some hospitals that had been owned and controlled by religious orders have become community-based, nonprofit institutions. Some organizations seem only to change title and official sponsorship. The various types of agencies for healthcare planning have included regional medical programs and regional comprehensive health planning programs. Other state agencies, such as departments of health, may find themselves in a caretaker role for the phased-out health planning agencies; the organizational structure, not the total mandate, of these planning agencies has changed or been eliminated.

Managers overseeing the closing stages of an organization face both challenges and opportunities. To end well becomes an unspoken goal and a goal that must be made explicit. Managers must come to terms with the realities associated with phasing out an organization. It will be a stressful time for all, and managers need to attend to personal well-being. Yes, there is a personal goal of being a "class act" right to the end. This starts with a decision—to stay to the end or to leave earlier. If a manager does not have a contractual obligation to stay, he or she might leave as soon as possible and plan accordingly. Ambivalence, lack of enthusiasm, and anxiety surface and contribute to poor leadership at this critical stage. Proceeding with forthrightness and directness is usually the best choice. But if a manager chooses to stay to the end, his or her attitude should flow from this unspoken mandate, that of ending well. There is much work to accomplish in the closure of an organization. Here are some of the main features of management concerns and activities; the values of transparency and accountability, as expressed in the corporate culture, are reflected in the following activities:

- Adopt and communicate a positive attitude about the unfolding events.
- Develop robust communication processes to offset rumors and uncertainties and to maintain the trust of workers and clients.

- Attend to the needs of the clients/patients by providing:
    a. Notice of closing and related information
    b. Continuity of care plans and referrals
    c. Detailed information about alternate points of care
    d. Detailed information about accessing/obtaining health records and information about final billing and claims
- Give timely notice to secondary clients (e.g., clinical affiliation agreements with colleges and university educational programs, on-the-job training programs with community-based groups).
- Attend to the needs of the workers:
    a. Give clear, timely information about the phases of the closure.
    b. State policy and procedures for using sick leave, vacation time, or compensation time, and any related options if available (e.g., additional pay instead of taking time off).
    c. State the policy and procedure for requesting time off for job interviews.
    d. Develop opportunities for lateral transfer to obtain additional job experience.
    e. Make sure awards and recognition deadlines are met.
    f. Work with human relations department to ensure workers understand their benefits and the associated requirements (e.g., health insurance coverage).
- Attend to the relationships with resource suppliers and supporter:
    a. Give timely notice and accurate information about the upcoming closure.
    b. Renegotiate contracts to phase out the arrangement, or, in some cases, to extend it (e.g., outsourced billing and coding, off-site storage, leased equipment).

Managers must develop plans to phase out essential activity and also prepare for the associated costs:

1. Payment of pensions, retirement funds, severance pay, escrow accounts (e.g., as in the case of continuing care facilities)
2. Continuance of health insurance, worker compensation, and unemployment insurance plans for the period mandated by law
3. Retention of, and access to, business and healthcare records
4. Renegotiation contracts for outsourced functions or leased equipment

5. Development a plan for maintaining essential functions (on site or outsourced) such as final billing and claims processing, storage of records
6. Arrangement of coverage by hiring temporary workers to offset the increased worker unavailability time due to increased use of vacation time, etc.
7. Participation in the final due diligence review, usually carried out by external consultants and auditors

One final activity flows from the need for psychological and symbolic closure. The many constituents of the organization, both internal and external, observe how well or how poorly this is accomplished. Thus, managers explicitly arrange for the retirement of organizational symbols such as logo, motto, and colors; items of historical meaning are honored and disposed of with care; and traditional fund-raising events are passed on to the new organization. The final closing event is more than a formality. It is public relations at its best. An old saying provides some guiding wisdom here: if it is done right, it is right forever.

Paradoxically, this may be a time of great opportunity for managers. Middle managers may have an opportunity to participate in activities outside their normal scope as the executive team grows thin. This may be the ideal time for middle managers to try their hand at related jobs, because failure may be ascribed to the situation rather than to inexperience or even incompetence. The same holds true for employees; managers can use this opportunity to motivate the remaining workers by giving them new opportunities to gain experience and to enhance their résumés. Valuable experience may be gained because this may also be a time of great creativity as the gestational phase begins for a new organization with its unique opportunities, challenges, and frustrations. Throughout the life cycle of the organization, strong leadership is needed. The next section contains a discussion of the manager as leader.

# ► Linking Theory and Practice: An Application of Organizational Analysis Using the Life Cycle Model

An analysis of a successful organization provides managers with insights into the coalescence of organizational survival strategies along with phases in the life cycle. AHIMA is an example of a strong, thriving, and vibrant organization, one reflecting the characteristics of stability and success associated with the middle-age phase in the life cycle. Organizational survival is not accidental; it takes purposeful action by leadership and a responsive membership or constituency to develop and thrive. Reviewing the history of an organization such as AHIMA links theoretical concepts to an identifiable, observable entity. When seeking to identify points of weakness in an organization, along with strategies used to enhance its success, a manager is well-served by such a detailed analysis, although it is a painstaking and time-consuming activity. A typical starting point is the gestational phase. For AHIMA, its gestational phase (early 20th century) developed from a specific need: readily available, well-documented medical records for use in direct patient care, research, and education. The catalytic agent for this interest was the ever-increasing specialty care by surgeons, especially in large, urban-based, inpatient hospitals. The collaboration of surgeons, medical records archivists (as many were called at that time), and major hospitals set the overall culture as one of cooperation and mutual assistance.

This characteristic remains constant throughout AHIMA's history. Because the need was a continuing and growing one, visionary leaders in medical information management realized the value of creating a formal association, the American Association of Medical Record Librarians. As is usual in a new organization, selecting a name is central to the identification and branding of the enterprise. Specific designation as medical record librarians reflected the practices of the time: just as books are acquired, retained for use, and accessed in a predictable manner in a library, so too are medical records—thus, the choice of well-understood designation, medical records librarians. Over the years, the name has changed, each time reflecting changes in health care: medical information expanded to health information to reflect both illness and wellness services; records (implying hard copy documents) give way to information, and currently, informatics, as the designation in order to reflect a broader concept, namely, that information is captured in both hard copy and digital forms. The current use of the term "clinical documentation" reflects the original and enduring focus of the profession's initiatives.

Along with the branding associated with selecting the name, the development of related materials and practices reinforce organizational identity: an official logo, motto, designated colors. The celebration of organizational founding, with attention to building identification with the organization by its members, also provides opportunity to reach the general public and thereby gain support. Thus, 10-year, 25-year, and so on milestone events are noted. The organization has survived the initial move from gestation to youth and then, as is the case with AHIMA, currently looks ahead to the 100th year event. These decisions are not superfluous or incidental; they are effective means of enhancing survival and growth.

Four processes are interrelated in the development of a stable organization: (1) identification of likely membership, (2) their credentialing, (3) their educational preparation, and (4) accreditation of educational programs. Successful organizations tend to focus on a specific potential membership; there is a natural cohesion among members with common needs, interests, and goals. The resources of the organization can be marshalled to support these. The young organization does not become over-stretched in its use of resources, making it vulnerable to failure. Initially, AHIMA membership was characterized as open, simply because the founding group was seeking members with a common interest. It would have been premature to close off membership in the gestational phase. The growth of the organization, its development into a formal one, and its increasing membership led to categorization of membership, tied to the credentialing process. The organization was for, and about, professionalization of the work. Structured membership (credentialed members as active members with voting privileges and office-holding eligibility) included additional categories for individuals and groups who wished to be formally included in the organization. Rather than shut the door on these interested parties and run the risk of losing their support and/or their developing their own (potentially rival) organization, the leaders with membership assent offered additional categories for associated members (e.g., vendors, representatives from various agencies, and students). These associate members did not have voting rights, nor were they eligible for holding office or committee positions. For many years, this was a settled question. Again, the resources of the organization could be focused on growth and expansion of its influence. Conflict over the issue did not drain the developing organization of energy as stability continued to be enhanced. One notable challenge to aspects of membership occurred well into the stable, middle-age phase: that of the concerns of the accredited technical practitioners and their eligibility for committee and office holding. As a highly normative organization, and one with a history of responsiveness to member concerns, adjustments were made to the internal structure to permit greater involvement by all credentialed members. Today's

environment—that of a high-tech world, informatics, information specialists—has led to a revisiting of membership categories, a shift back to open membership. This is another aspect of stable, flourishing organizations, such as AHIMA, namely the capacity to adjust to changing circumstances and interests while maintaining the central purpose of the organization.

One of the characteristics of a profession is the identification and development of a unique body of knowledge as this is reflective of the concept of bureaucratic imperialism: this is our "territory"; we are the definitive and authoritative body. Credentialing of individuals to certify that they meet standards of education and training in the specific field, and the accreditation of educational programs are interrelated. The credentialing process strengthened the early AHIMA by providing its members with a meaningful and identifiable role set. Uniformity of practice became routine and widespread. In its gestational and early-youth stage, AHIMA education initiatives developed through the use of the apprenticeship model. As the body of knowledge solidified, college-level programs, leading to official academic degrees, became common. For the technical level, correspondence courses were developed, which helped meet the needs of practitioners living and working in more rural areas. The advent of the community college system as well as an increase in the body of knowledge needed for effective practice led to the replacement of correspondence courses with associate degree preparation. Apprenticeships, well-regulated, are again offered as an adjunct to formal education.

A successful organization, over many years, will necessarily revisit root decisions, such as those associated with credentialing. The control over requirements, based on research and analysis of a profession's purview, is a continuing one. What are the outer limits of credentialing? Should every subset of the role have its own credential? Also, when practitioners have several such initials after their names, there is the possibility of loss of meaning.

With the increased content in the body of knowledge, the master's level degree in a broader category, namely, informatics, is becoming a growing feature of professional education. Continuing education requirements augment the basic entry-level certifications and foster respect for the credential as well as ensuring competency of practitioners.

The accrediting process for the profession reflects both the history of the organization (as noted, stemming from its close relationship with medical field) and the eventual move to greater independence from medical association approval. The physical therapy profession began this move toward greater independence, with other professions following this practice.

All of these indicators (well-established purpose, goals, membership, and credentials) reflect early- to middle-stage developments in formal organizations. AHIMA's growth tended to be steady, with no pronounced stage of hibernation. The World War II era necessarily caused some limits to activity, but AHIMA has not faced the necessity of falling back and waiting out challenges for its survival. It has continued to reflect the best characteristics of formal organizations, namely goal maintenance and then expansion. With an adaptive style of response through conscious goal expansion, AHIMA has developed educational materials, publications, specialty groups, and workshops for various nonacute care settings as they develop, including behavioral care, long-term care/nursing home, hospice, clinics, and so forth.

A quick review of adaptive responses to changing technology shows a pattern of effective response, and one that continues. When a new technology emerges that has an impact on health information content and systems, some of the same basic questions arise. AHIMA has a positive track record in this regard. Starting with one of the first technological inventions that had such an impact—the telephone—note the familiar themes. This example, from a 21st-century vantage point, might seem quaint, but notice the underlying legal and administrative questions. How to verify the identification and legitimacy of the sender of the communication; how to enter accurate and timely documentation; how to authenticate it; what elements constitute the official record? The early medical-record pioneers formulated and dealt with these considerations, taking the lead in developing the necessary standards and guidelines. As the technologies developed, including fax transmissions, electronic entries, and others, AHIMA developed appropriate guidance material to incorporate the changes.

Similar issues surface concerning record retention media—hard copy; microfilm, microfiche, digital methods; what is permitted by state or federal agencies; what is the legal ramification; what measures are needed to prevent data disintegration? These examples reflect the larger concept of AHIMA as the authoritative source regarding information documentation and processing. Knowing an organization's history helps us appreciate and learn from their experience.

Some features of its clientele network can be easily identified. It has built effective relationships with secondary clients—healthcare providers, health insurance companies; resource suppliers such as vendors, manufacturers, government, and private agencies;

supporters, including political and legislative groups, without itself becoming political; and controllers such as state and federal licensing and accrediting groups. Its rivals and opponents are generally brought into cooperative relationships, with conflict kept to a minimum. AHIMA has grown into a stable, vigorous, and enduring organization, with no signs of the characteristics of an organization in decline.

# ▶ The Management Reference Portfolio

In addition to using an analytical model, a manager has another useful tool for facilitating effective plans and decisions, the management reference portfolio. This notebook (hard copy or digital) contains a concise, easy-to-identify listing of materials that a manager needs to cite on day-to-day operations and more in-depth reports and projects. It is developed by the manager and reflects the specifics relating to the organization. One could characterize this reference portfolio as a kind of table of contents or index to existing laws and regulations, documents, and guidelines that are kept complete in specific files. Here are some examples of its use. A manager is working on a project proposal relating to the acute care organization's hospice program. Which laws, regulations, standards, and organizational policies apply? A quick review of the portfolio's listing under hospice shows the exact citations; these, in turn, are accessed. The reference listing itself does not contain the detailed content of, for example, the regulations, but the manager now has a roadmap for locating the necessary information. By way of an additional example, note how the manager would use such a reference. For example, a manager in day-to-day department administration is asked a quick question about holiday and over-time pay. Instead of half-guessing, giving a generalized answer, or postponing a response, the manager quickly checks his or her topical index and finds the applicable reference: Overtime Pay: see employee handbook, section 18; see also union contract—sections 11 and 20; see January 9, 20n2 HR memorandum. In another working situation, perhaps a manager with two assistant directors are working on policy updates and a question comes up concerning committee requirements. The team could (typically) have one member look it up later, add it to one's to-do list, and get back to the team at a subsequent meeting during which the policy is finalized. Or, more simply, the team could quickly check the reference portfolio, find the necessary item, access it, and finalize the discussion—no to-do list, no additional meeting, and no delay in finalizing the task. Reference portfolios are time-savers.

At a less obvious level, for example, a manager needs to maintain credibility after making a seemingly simple mistake (e.g., writing a report or making a presentation and not properly identifying the organization by its new title under reorganization or restructuring initiatives), which can erode his or her credibility as a factual error like this suggests that, perhaps this manager does not know other essential information.

Some of the major entries would include the entries listed below. Additional examples are included in the sections on planning, organizing, and budgeting, and the summary chapter on day-to-day management.

1. *A factual listing of essential information about the organization:* its current official title in full, its short title, its prior names. If mergers or restructuring has occurred the names and dates are listed.
2. *A current listing of governing board composition and names:* titles and names of top-level management; the organizational chart in detail.
3. *Employee matters:* employee handbook; union contract; HR memoranda;
4. *Systems and equipment:* equipment inventory; leases; supply-chain guidelines
5. *Laws, regulations, standards, listed by exact title:* dates of last site visit and upcoming reports and site visits. A cross-referenced listing of these requirements is developed by the manager showing, by topic, the various requirements (e.g., record retention standards of federal, state, accrediting agencies).
6. *Budget:* current and previous years; guidelines; working notes
7. *An analysis of the organization:* using the clientele network, life cycle, and adaptive strategies.

A manager's activities relating to understanding the dynamics of the healthcare environment, responding to change, and knowing one's organization are reflected in **Appendix 3–A**. This utilizes entries from the manager's wheel book and the reference portfolio.

# Appendix 3–A

# Wheel Book Entries—Know Your Organization

Background information: the setting for this fictitious example is a 100 year hospital, founded as an acute care, inpatient facility. Over the years, additional services were added, including outpatient clinics, observation units, and short stay transitional care. There were two mergers with other facilities, resulting in changes in ownership and sponsorship. Several members of the current management team expressed a need for a comprehensive reference manual reflecting past and current information. One department manager agreed to head up a working group to compile a "Know Your Organization" reference manual. Other department managers, along with representatives from public relations and human resources, volunteered to participate. They agreed to work on this project from November 1 through December 7.

Here are some typical wheel book entries reflecting the work group coordinator's activities.

| | |
|---|---|
| November 1 | Convened "Know Your Organization" working group; tasks, responsibilities and due dates agreed upon. References and resources provided. |
| Week of November 4 | Focused on life cycle of organization: original name, mission, sponsorship and ownership; subsequent changes in these items. |
| | Listing of current and past licensure and accrediting agencies. |
| | Listing of current and past federal and state agencies which regulated reimbursement and related quality improvement practices. |

| | |
|---|---|
| | Developed detailed, cross-reference matrix of laws, regulations, standards by topic (e.g., disaster plan; required reports). |
| Week of November 11 | Focused on clientele network: identification of original and current stakeholders within each category of the network (e.g., supporters, associates, competitors). |
| November 16 | Work group presentations of findings to date. |
| Week of November 18 | Focused on Organizational Survival: |
| | Goal succession and expansion, hibernation and adaptation, past and current competitors. |
| | Review of changes in client characteristics (e.g., demographics, mortality and morbidity, payment patterns). |
| Week of November 25 | Focused on compilation of all findings into "Know Your Organization" reference. |
| November 26 | Work group presentations re: organizational survival. |
| November 30 | All day wrap-up sessions; final presentations by each work group. |
| Week of December 1 | Compilations, editing, and distribution of draft of reference manual. |
| Week of December 7 | Final edit and distribution of "Know Your Organization" reference manual. |

## Notes

1. For additional reading about the early development of the history of management, see:
   a. Luther Gulick and Lyndall F. Urwick, eds., *Papers of the Science of Administration* (New York: Institute of Public Administration, 1929).
   b. Henri Fayol, *General and Industrial Administration* (Geneva, Switzerland: International Management Institute, 1929).
   c. Chester Bernard, *The Functions of the Executive* (Cambridge, MA: Harvard University Press, 1968).
   d. James Mooney and Alan C. Reiley, *The Principles of Organizations* (New York: Harper, 1939).
2. Ludwig von Bertalanffy, "General Systems Theory: A Critical Review," *General System* 7 (1962): 1–20; and Kenneth F. Boulding, "General Systems Theory: The Skeleton of Science," *Management Science* 2 (1956): 197–208.
3. Peter Blau and William Richard Scott, *Formal Organization* (San Francisco, CA: Chandler, 1962), 42.
4. Amatai Etzioni, *A Comparative Analysis of Complex Organizations* (Glencoe, IL: Free Press, 1961).
5. Daniel Katz and Robert L. Kahn, *The Social Psychology of Organizations* (New York: John Wiley & Sons, 1967), 11.
6. Max Weber, *The Theory of Social and Economic Organization*, trans. A. M. Henderson and Talcott Parsons; ed. Talcott Parsons (Glencoe, IL: Free Press, 1947), 324–386.
7. Bertram Gross, *Organizations and Their Managing* (New York: Free Press, 1968), 114–132 passim.
8. Matthew Holden, Jr., "Imperialism in Bureaucracy," *American Political Science Review* (December 1966): 943.
9. Philip Selznick, *TVA and the Grass Roots* (New York: Harper Torchbooks, 1966), *13*, 260–261.
10. Amatai Etzioni, *Modern Organizations* (Englewood Cliffs, NJ: Prentice-Hall, 1964), 13–14.
11. Marver Bernstein, *Regulating Business by Independent Commission* (Princeton, NJ: Princeton University Press, 1955).

## CHAPTER 4

# Leadership and the Manager

## CHAPTER OBJECTIVES

- Address the role of the manager as a principal agent of change.
- Differentiate among the terms *power, influence,* and *authority.*
- Recognize the importance of authority for organizational stability.
- Identify the sources of power, influence, and authority.
- Relate the sources of power, influence, and authority to the organizational position of the line manager.
- Recognize the limits placed on the use of power and authority in organizational settings.
- Recognize the importance of delegation of authority.
- Explore the nature of leadership and the reasons why individuals seek leadership positions.
- Identify the styles of leadership, their characteristics, and the circumstances under which they are applied.

## ▶ Change and the Manager

The healthcare setting of today is a highly dynamic environment in which the individual manager must embrace the reality of constant change and accept and fulfill the role of change agent within the organization. It is only through addressing essential change and truly leading employees in its acceptance and implementation that the manager can be successful in the long term. Denying or resisting change does not merely mean standing still but losing ground and actually going backward relative to technology and society as they race ahead.

The department manager must be able to deal with employee resistance to change, including the most frequently encountered causes of resistance and how best to approach resistance to change with employees. However, this implies that the manager is already completely on board with the necessity for a particular change. It is now appropriate to acknowledge that the manager may well be fully as susceptible to resistance as the employees. Who is the manger but simply another employee? He or she can be just as affected by misgivings and uncertainty about impending change as the rank-and-file staff.

Thus, the manager may have a difficult task up front in the implementation of change, especially change mandated "from on high" or forced by external circumstances, because the manager has nearly the same potential for resistance as the employees. Even the knowledge that a certain change is inevitable regardless of what it entails does not necessarily guarantee that the manager will be a willing advocate for the change.

Of course the manager, and just about everyone else for that matter, is likely to champion a change that was his or her own idea. But when ideas or directives or other requirements come from elsewhere, the manager, who may experience some feeling of resistance, must deliberately strive to overcome that feeling and become champion of the change. It is often extremely difficult for the manager who feels some personal misgivings to go forward as the driver of change.

We are told repeatedly that the manager can address change with the employees in three ways: tell them what to do, convince them of what must be done, or involve them in determining what must be done. This third approach, involving them, is all well and good—but often it cannot be used. The first approach, the tell-them-what-to-do route, is avoided if possible because it does little to temper resistance. This leaves the second approach, the need for the manager to convince the employees of what must be done. Clearly, many employees are more likely to get on board with a particular change if they know *why* it must be done. And an honest *why* is not simply telling the employees that it is "orders from administration" or blaming it on the ever-present yet never identifiable "they" as in "they are making me do it."

The central point of this brief discussion is that if the manager is to be a true agent of change and an honest and effective catalyst for change, the first person to be accepting and supportive of change is the manager. So if you, the manager, experience doubts or misgivings about some change that lies ahead, work these out within yourself and with your superiors as necessary. Your employees should be able to see you as a true agent of change who is there to support their efforts in implementing change and helping them through it such that everyone, yourself included, achieves a new comfort zone as essential change becomes part of the norm.

Additional discussion about implementing change is provided in Chapter 2, The Challenge of Change.

## ▶ Why Follow the Manager?

The manager issues an order or directive, and the result is compliance. But why do employees obey? Is it even appropriate to use the term *obey* to describe this compliance? Which bases of authority are operative in superior–subordinate transactions? What are the limits of a manager's authority? What if a particular supervisor is seen as a weak manager? Are there remedies available for addressing problems related to weak or ineffective management leadership? Of what value to the organization is the authority structure? What are the consequences for life within the organization if there is not general, unchallenged compliance most of the time? When actions of compliance are described, which term provides the proper point of reference—*power, authority,* or *influence*? Are these terms mutually exclusive or are they synonymous when used in the context of organizational relationships? These questions arise when discussion of authority in organizations is undertaken.

Organizational behavior is controlled behavior, behavior that is directed toward goal attainment. The authority structure is created to ensure adherence to organizational norms, to suppress spontaneous or random behavior, and to induce purposeful behavior consistent with the aims of the organization. No matter how the work within the organization is divided, no matter the extent to which specialization, departmentation, centralization, or decentralization is formalized, there must be some measure of legitimate authority if the organization is to be effective. The concept of formal authority is supported by the two related concepts of *power* and *influence.* These concepts may be separated for analytical purposes; in actual practice, however, the concepts of authority, power, and influence are intertwined.

## ▶ The Concept of Power

Power is the ability to obtain compliance by means of some form of coercion, whether blatant or subtle; one's own will prevail even in the face of resistance. Power is force or naked strength; it is a mental hold over another. Like authority and influence, power is aimed at encouraging compliance, but it does not seek consensus or agreement as a condition of that compliance.

Power is always relational. An individual who has power over another person can narrow that person's range of choices and obtain compliance. The power holder does not necessarily force compliance by physical acts but rather may operate in more subtle ways, such as an implied threat to apply sanctions. Latent power is frequently as effective as an overt show of power. Power attaches to people, not to official positions. The formal authority holder (i.e., the person who has the official title, organizational position, and grant of authority) may or may not have power in addition to this formal grant of authority.

An imbalance in superior–subordinate relationships can occur when a nonofficeholder has more power than the official officeholder. This can even be seen in family life. For example, when a 2-year-old boy shows signs of an incipient temper tantrum in the middle of the annual family gathering, the power balance clearly is in favor of the child if the tantrum pattern has developed. The child does not have to carry out the explosive behavior; the mere threat of the possibility brings about some desired behavior from the parent caught in the situation.

Workers often have some degree of power over line supervisors and managers. A worker with specific technical knowledge can withhold key information from a manager or can develop a relationship that is personally favorable. Information may not actually be withheld; the mere possibility that the manager cannot rely on an individual is enough to shift the balance, at least temporarily, in favor of the worker. Groups of workers can control a manager when it is known that the manager is responsible for meeting a deadline or filling a quota; the manager's ability to do so is dependent on the cooperation of the workers. Normal, steady output may be produced routinely, but the ability to make that extra push needed to surpass the quota or reach a special level of output rests more with the workers than with the manager. Strikes by workers are classic examples of mobilized power, but the power shifts back in favor of management if striking workers go without pay for a prolonged period or if they lose the goodwill and support of the community.

When an individual can supply something that a person values and cannot obtain elsewhere in an accepted manner, or when the individual can deprive one of something valued, then there is a power relationship. This implicit or explicit power relationship may or may not be perceived by one or both parties.

# ▶ The Concept of Influence

Like power, influence is the capacity to produce effects on others or obtain compliance from others, but it differs from power in the manner in which compliance is evoked. Power is coercive, but influence is accepted voluntarily. Influence is the capacity to obtain compliance without relying on formal actions, rules, or force. In relationships governed by influence, not only compliance but also consensus and agreement are sought; persuasion rather than latent or overt force is the major factor in influence. Influence supplements power, and it is sometimes difficult to distinguish latent power from influence in a given situation. Does the individual comply because of a relationship of influence or because of the latent power factor? Together, power and influence supplement formal authority.

# ▶ The Concept of Formal Authority

Authority may be described as legitimate power. It is the right to issue orders, to direct action, and to command or exact compliance. It is the right given to a manager to employ resources, make commitments, and exercise control. By a grant of formal authority, the manager is entitled, empowered, and authorized to act; thus, the manager incurs a *responsibility* to act. Authority may be expressed by direct command or instruction or, more commonly, by request or suggestion. Through the delegation of authority, coordination is established in the organization.

The authority mandate is delineated, communicated, and reinforced in several ways, including organizational charts, job descriptions, procedure manuals, and work rules. Although the exercise of authority in many situations tends to be similar to transactions of influence, authority differs from influence in that authority is clearly vested in the formal chain of command. Individuals are given specific grants of authority as a result of organizational position. Power and influence may be exercised by an individual authority holder, but they may also be exercised by individuals who do not have specific grants of authority.

Authority is both complemented and supplemented by power on the one hand and influence on the other hand. It is within the realm of formal authority to exact compliance by the threat of firing a person for failure to comply; however, this may be such a rare occurrence in an organization that such a threat is really an application of power more than an exercise of authority. However, formal aspects of authority may be so well developed that the major transactions remain at the level of influence, with the influence based largely on the holding of formal office. The infrequent use of formal authoritative directives to evoke compliance may indicate organizational health; that is, people know what to do and perform willingly.

# ▶ The Importance of Authority

When a subordinate refuses to accept the orders of a superior, the superior has several choices, each of which carries potentially negative consequences for the attainment of organizational goals. The superior can accept the insubordination, withdraw the order, and call on others to carry out the directive. This action would probably further weaken authority, however, because the superior would most likely be perceived as lacking the subtle blend of power and authority needed to exact compliance on a predictable basis. A chain reaction of insubordination could occur. If other workers are asked to carry out a directive that had been refused by one worker, resentment could build up and produce negative consequences. If the order is withdrawn completely, of course, the work will not be accomplished.

The manager who decides to enforce compliance may suspend or fire the insubordinate worker, but the superior still must find a worker to carry out the directive. If there is a chain reaction of insubordination, it may become impractical to suspend or fire the entire work force. In such circumstances, the situation moves from one of authority to one of power. Therefore, managers must identify and widen their bases of authority to help ensure a stable work climate.

# ▶ Sources of Power, Influence, and Authority

The manager's organizational relationships flow along the continuum of power, influence, and authority, varying in emphasis at different times and in different situations. To more fully understand the dynamics of the power–influence–authority triad, it is useful to examine the sources or bases of authority in formal organizations. The wider the base of authority, the stronger the manager's position; with a broad base of authority, the manager can work in the realm of influence and need not rely only on the formal grant of authority that attaches to organizational position.

The sources of formal authority have been studied by several theorists in the disciplines of social psychology, management, and political science. A review of the classic works from the Structuralist school of thought provides foundational concepts and terms relating to the sources or bases of authority: (1) acceptance or consent, (2) patterns of formal organization, (3) cultural expectations, (4) technical competence and expertise, and (5) characteristics of authority holders. The limits or weaknesses of each theory are offset by the approach taken in another.

## The Consent Theory of Authority

The belief that authority involves a subordinate's acceptance of a superior's decision is the basis for the acceptance or consent theory of formal authority.

A superior has authority only insofar as the subordinate accepts it. This theory implies that members of the organization have a choice concerning compliance, even when often they do not. It remains important to recognize the concepts of acceptance and consent to identify the centers of more subtle and diffuse resistance to authority, even when there is no overt and massive insubordination.

The zone of indifference and the zone of acceptance are two similar concepts in the acceptance or consent theory of authority. Chester Barnard used the term *zone of indifference* to describe that area in which an individual accepts an order without conscious questioning.[1] Barnard noted that the manager establishes an overall setting by means of preliminary education, prior persuasive efforts, and known inducements for compliance. The order then lies within the range that is more or less anticipated by the subordinate, who accepts it without conscious questioning or resistance because it is consistent with the overall organizational framework. Herbert Simon used the term *zone of acceptance* to reflect the same authority relationship. The zone of acceptance, according to Simon, is an area established by subordinates within which they are willing to accept the decisions made for them by their superior.[2] Simon noted that this zone is modified by positive and negative sanctions in the authority relationship, as well as by such factors as community of purpose, habit, and leadership.

Coupled with the foregoing factors is the concept of the rule of anticipated reactions, which Simon included in his discussion of the zone of acceptance.[3] According to this rule, subordinates seek to act in a manner that is acceptable to their superior, even when there has been no explicit command. The authority system, including anticipated review of actions, is so well developed that the superior needs only to review actions rather than issue commands. The past organizational history in which positive and negative sanctions were enforced is recalled; the expectation of the review of actions is fostered so that the subordinates' zone of acceptance is expanded.

Another approach to the concept of authority as a relationship between organizational leaders and their followers is described by Robert Presthus, who posited a transactional view of authority in which there is reciprocity among individuals at different levels in the hierarchy.[4] Compliance with authority is in some way rewarding to the individual, and the individual, therefore, plays an active role in defining and accepting authority. Everyone has formal authority, in that each person has a formal role in the organization. There is, Presthus stated, an implicit bargaining and exchange of authority, with each individual deferring to the other.

The notion of reciprocal expectations in authority relationships is further supported in Edgar Schein's discussion of the psychological contract.[5] As in Barnard's concept of the zone of indifference and in Simon's rule of anticipated reactions, the premise of member acceptance of organizational authority and its attendant control system is basic to the psychological contract. The workers' acceptance of authority constitutes a realm of upward influence; in turn, the workers expect the authority holders to honor the implicit restrictions on their grant of authority. The workers expect the authority holders to refrain from ordering actions that are inconsistent with the general climate of the given organization and from taking advantage of the workers' acceptance of authority. The workers also expect as part of this psychological contract the rewards of compliance (i.e., positive sanctions readily given and negative sanctions kept at a minimum).

## The Theory of Formal Organizational Authority

In his classic study of bureaucracies, Max Weber discussed three forms of authority: charismatic, traditional, and rational–legal. Charisma, as defined by Weber, is a "certain quality of an individual personality by virtue of which he is set apart from ordinary men and treated as endowed with supernatural, superhuman, or at least specifically exceptional qualities."[6] The social, religious, and political groups that form around charismatic leaders tend to lack formal role structure. The routines of bureaucratic structure are not developed and may even be disdained by the group. Charismatic authority figures function as revolutionary forces against established systems of leadership and authority. Such authority is not bound by explicit rules but rather remains invested in the key charismatic individual. Personal devotion to the leader or what might be termed an almost irrational faith in the leader bind the members of the group to one another and to the leader.

Because charismatic authority is linked to the individual leader, the organization's survival is similarly linked. If the organization is to endure, it must take on some of the characteristics of formal organizations, including a formalized authority pattern. In this area, two developments are possible. Charismatic leadership may evolve into a traditional system of authority, or it may develop into the rational–legal system of formal authority. In traditionalism, a pattern of succession is developed. A successor may be designated by the leader or hereditary/kinship succession may be established; then a system of transferring the leadership to the legitimately designated individual or heir must be developed. This, in turn, leads to a system of roles and formal authority. Weber uses the term *routinization of charisma* to describe this transformation of charismatic authority into, first, traditional authority, and then rational–legal authority.

Rational–legal authority is the authority predicated in formal organizations. It is generally assumed that formal organizations come into being and derive legitimacy from an overall social and legal system. Individuals accept authority within the formal organizational structure because the rights and duties of members of the organization are consistent with the more abstract rules that individuals in the larger society accept as legitimate and rational.

Within the formal organization, a system of roles and authority relationships is carefully constructed to enable the organization to survive and move toward its formal goal on a continuing, stable basis. Authority has its basis in the organizational position, not in any individual. Weber described in detail the major characteristics of bureaucratic structures; the following characteristics relate to the rational–legal authority structure[7]:

1. The principle of fixed and official jurisdictional areas means that areas are generally ordered by rules—that is, by laws or administrative regulations.
   a. The regular activities required for the purposes of the bureaucratically governed structure are distributed in a fixed way as official duties.
   b. The authority to give the commands required for the discharge of these duties is distributed in a stable way and is strictly delimited in a fixed way as official duties.
   c. Methodical provision is made for the regular and continuous fulfillment of these duties and for the execution of the corresponding rights; only persons who have generally regulated qualifications to serve are employed.
2. The principles of office hierarchy and of levels of graded authority mean that there is a firmly ordered system of superiority and subordination in which supervision of the lower offices is carried out by the higher ones.

The theory of formal organizational authority rests on this rational–legal system of formal office, impersonality of the officeholder, and a system of rules and regulations to constrain the grant of authority. Delegation of formal authority from top management to each successive level of management is the basis of formal organizational authority. Authority is derived from official position and is circumscribed by the limits imposed by the hierarchical order.

## Cultural Expectations

Both the consent theory of authority and the theory of formal organizational authority include an implicit assumption that individuals in a society are culturally induced to accept authority. Furthermore, the acceptable use of authority in organizations is defined in part by the larger societal mores as well as by union contract, corporate law, and state and federal law and regulation.

Acceptance of the status system in a society is learned as part of the general socialization process. General deference to authority is ingrained early in psychosocial development, and social roles with their sanctions are accepted and reinforced throughout life. The role of employee carries with it both formal and informal sanctions; insubordination is not generally condoned. Even as a group cheers the occasional rebel, there is attendant discomfort because something is out of order in the relationship. When the insubordination of an individual begins to threaten the economic security of the group, there is counterpressure on that individual to bring about reacceptance of authority. Fear of authority may bring about a similar response of renewed acceptance of authority and counterpressure on any dissidents.

The expected zone of acceptance or zone of indifference varies with different social roles. These variables are rarely spelled out in great detail; they are learned as much through the pervasive cultural formation process as through the formal orientation process in any one organization. There is a kind of "group mind" that includes the general realization that a particular behavior pattern is part of a given role, and the entire role set reinforces this general acceptance of authority.

## Technical Competence and Expertise

Three terms reflect the organizational authority that is derived from or based on the technical competence and expertise of the individual, regardless of which office or position the individual holds in the organization. These terms are *functional authority, law of the situation,* and *authority of facts.*

Functional authority is the limited right that line or staff members (or departments) may exercise over specified activities for which they are responsible.

Functional authority is given to the line or staff member as an exception to the principle of unity of command. For purposes of this discussion on the sources of authority, it is useful to emphasize the special character of functional authority, which is given to a line or staff member primarily because that individual has specialized knowledge and technical competence. For example, the human resources manager normally assists all other department heads in matters of employee relations, although this manager has no authority to intervene directly in manager–employee relations. The situation changes when there is a legally binding collective bargaining agreement: the human resources manager, with special training in labor relations, may be given functional authority over all matters stemming from the union contract because of specialized knowledge. Another example is that of information technology support staff who, because of technical competence, are given authority to make final decisions over certain aspects of data collection. The authority is granted because of the technical competence of the staff members.

Mary Parker Follett, a pioneer in management thought, introduced the terms *law of the situation* and *authority of facts.*[8] Follett described the ideal authority relationship as that stemming from the situation as a whole. Each participant in the organization who is assumed to have the necessary qualifications for the position held has authority associated with that position. Orders become depersonalized in that each participant in the process studies and accepts the factors in the situation as a whole. Follett stated that one person should not give orders to another person but rather both should agree to take their orders from the situation.[9] She developed this concept further: both the employer and the employee should study the situation and should apply their specialized knowledge and technical competence through the principles of scientific management. The emphasis shifts, in Follett's approach, from authority derived from one's official position or office to authority derived from the situation. The individual who has the most knowledge and competence to make the decision and issue the order in a particular situation has the authority to do so. The staff assistant or a key employee potentially has as much authority in a particular situation as does the holder of a hierarchical office. The incident command system used in hospital disaster management is an example of law of the situation, with command passing from unit manager, clinical specialist, or safety officer as the circumstance requires.

Closely tied to the concept of law of the situation is that of authority of facts. Follett stressed that, in modern organizations, individuals exercise authority and leadership because of their expert knowledge.[10] Again, leadership and authority shift from the hierarchical position to the situation. The person with the knowledge demanded by the situation tends to exercise effective authority.

Both of these concepts place emphasis on the depersonalization of orders. At the same time, the source of the authority is highly personal, in that knowledge and competence for the exercise of authority belong to an individual. Underlying the concepts of functional authority, law of the situation, and authority of facts is the theme that authority is derived from the technical competence and knowledge of individuals in the organization who do not necessarily hold formal office in the line hierarchy.

## Characteristics of Authority Holders

Authority rests in individuals. The talents and traits of the individual may become the source of authority, as in the case of the charismatic leader. A person holding power may use this as a base for gaining legitimate authority, or a group may invest the person of power with legitimate authority as a protective measure and seek to impose the limits and customs of authority. They may also accept the power holder as formal officeholder as a means of accepting the situation without further conflict. Technical competence and knowledge are also personal characteristics that become the basis of authority in certain situations.

## Authority by Default

A weak form of authority stems from situations in which the group members, either by conscious decision or by lack of attention to authority–leadership succession, do not develop strong, clear, authority patterns. A professional organization, for example, might decide to rotate authority–leadership roles through a nomination process that limits the choice of candidates from specific geographic regions. In another organization, the committee chair role might be simply rotated through all the members in turn, either because members do not wish to have any one department as dominant or simply because the task is seen as a chore. In another organization, provision for succession might be weakened because the same few members hold officer positions for years, so no new leadership is developed.

Of course, the time invariably comes when a long-term authority holder is no longer able to continue. A vacuum then arises, and a newer member is prevailed on to assume the office. When such occurs, authority by default is the rule. The officeholder must attend to building up the office or accept the realities of the situation, as he or she has only a limited authority mandate.

## The Manager's Use of Sources of Authority

In practice, managers should recognize all the potential sources of authority and weigh the contribution of each theory to obtain as complete a picture of the authority nexus as possible. They should assess their own grants of authority and try to determine which elements tend to strengthen their authority and which tend to erode it.

The base of authority shifts from time to time. As an example, suppose an individual is offered the position of department head of a health information service because of that individual's competence in the administration of health information systems; this specialized knowledge and technical competence is the first pillar of authority. When the individual accepts the position, the formal authority mandate of that official position is added. This authority, in turn, is shaped by the prevailing organizational climate, which includes either a wide or narrow zone of acceptance on the part of employees. The personal traits of the authority holder complete the authority base for that office.

The individual with a participative management style may emphasize those aspects of authority that widen the zone of acceptance. The setting itself may dictate the predominant authority base, as in the law of the situation; in a highly technical setting, those persons with the most technical knowledge use this knowledge as the base of authority. Although there is a tendency to downplay internal politics in organizations such as healthcare institutions, some individual managers may use power as a major source of authority. Astute managers regularly assess the several bases of authority available to them to enhance the authority relationships and thereby contribute more effectively to the achievement of organizational goals.

## ▶ Restrictions on the Use of Authority

Several factors restrict the use of authority. Some constraints stem from internal factors, such as the limits placed on authority at each organizational level; others stem from external factors, such as laws, regulations, and ethical considerations. The following is a systematic summary of these factors:

1. *Organizational position.* Each holder of authority receives a limited delegation of authority consistent with the position held in the organization. An individual has no legitimate formal authority beyond that accorded to the organizational position.
2. *Legal and contractual mandates.* Authority is limited by federal, state, and municipal laws and regulations relating to safety, work hours, licensure, and scope of practice; by internal corporate charter and bylaws; and by union contract.
3. *Social limitations.* The social codes, mores, and values of society at large include both implicit and explicit limits on the behavior of individuals. Authority holders are expected to act in a manner consistent with the predominant value system of the society. These social limitations are major factors in shaping the zone of acceptance and the general cultural deference of individuals who are members of organizations.
4. *Physical limits.* An authority holder can neither force a person to do something that is simply beyond that person's physical capabilities nor escape the natural limits of the physical environment, such as climate or physical laws.
5. *Technological constraints.* The advances and the limitations of the state of the art must be considered in the exercise of authority; no amount of power or authority can bring about a result that is beyond the technical ability of the individuals.
6. *Economic constraints.* The scarcity of needed resources limits the behavior of formal authority holders.
7. *Zone of acceptance of organization members.* Both authority and power have their limits in that the net cost of using either must be calculated. When a weak manager is faced with a strong employee group, perhaps as encountered in a strong union setting, the cost of using even legitimate authority may be too high; the authority grant is actually diminished.

Although many employees do not have complete freedom to choose what they will or will not do, they may resist authority in subtle ways, such as adherence to job duties exactly as stated in the job description, passive resistance, and failure to take initiative in any area not specifically designated by the supervisor. The manager must move into a distinct leadership position to develop a wide zone of acceptance with leadership becoming an essential adjunct to the exercise of authority.

## ▶ Importance of Delegation

Although the manager retains overall responsibility and authority for the work of the department or service, he or she must necessarily delegate authority to specific workers under his or her jurisdiction. Simply put, it is not possible for the manager to carry out every task. Therefore, each worker receives delegated authority from the manager to proceed on a day-to-day basis. Empowerment of the workers is essential.

Managers set up the parameters for action through several means: the development of policies and procedures, the promulgation of work rules and codes of behavior, the development of job descriptions with job duties and expectations well delineated, and the presentations of formal orientation and training programs associated with job duties. The manager consciously selects an appropriate style of leadership and communication to further enhance an atmosphere in which workers accept responsibility for their part in meeting the organizational goals.

A manager who is new to the role may experience some uneasiness with delegating. First, there is simply that natural tendency to think, "I can do this better or faster myself." Second, a manager may harbor some fears. For instance, if the worker fails at the task, the responsibility still rests with the manager; it is the manager who will take the heat, so to speak. There is also a certain loss of satisfaction and recognition; managers are often removed from day-to-day interaction with patients and their families and their own professional peers who remain in the arena of active, hands-on practice. Recognition of these inner barriers to delegation is the first step to overcoming resistance to this necessary aspect of authority.

## "Dos" and "Don'ts" of Delegation

*Know when to delegate.* In most day-to-day circumstances, delegation of authority is the norm. Routine tasks such as employee scheduling, for example, are easily accomplished by the supervisor closest to the unit. Certain highly specialized tasks such as revenue-cycle/compliance reviews are best delegated to a member of the department team who specializes in the area. Such a person would have the most up-to-date knowledge related to the topic. Workflow coordination and routine problem solving between or among working units are best accomplished by the immediate unit supervisors who are in continual interaction. Delegation is also a part of team development; the manager builds capability and confidence in the assistant managers, unit supervisors, and specialists. Delegation is part of the intentional training and mentoring goals of the manager.

*Know when not to delegate.* Certain activities remain the primary responsibility of the manager and normally are not delegated, such as hiring, disciplinary action, and termination. Generally, any task that falls under the heading of personnel management cannot be delegated; no nonmanagement employee must ever be empowered to make personnel decisions that affect other nonmanagement employees. Throughout each process, there will be input from unit managers and supervisors, but the final action is that of the manager. Complex or volatile employee or client situations sometimes arise; these, too, are the manager's responsibility. Overall systems and workflow, along with equipment and layout, are the manager's concerns, although there is input from unit managers and supervisors.

*Avoid common pitfalls associated with delegation.* Two common pitfalls can occur inadvertently; the prudent manager takes care to avoid these. First, a manager might undermine a unit supervisor by countermanding, even informally, a decision made by the first-line supervisor. For example, a unit supervisor might deny a request for a schedule change by an employee because of workflow or staffing considerations. The employee might informally ask the manager to approve the desired schedule change. Managers who allow themselves to override a subordinate manager's decisions undercut the authority and responsibility grant of this manager. (This is not the same thing as the normal grievance or appeal process during which an employee may meet with a higher-level manager at designated steps in the course of the seeking resolution.) Second, a manager, with the best of intentions, solicits information on a regular basis, perhaps daily, from unit managers. The casual but purposeful question, "How are things going in your unit today?" may lead to on-the-spot reports of one or another workflow or staffing problem. The concerned manager might readily respond, "I'll look into that and get back to you," instead of involving the subordinate supervisor in solving the problem.

*Interact with workers regularly.* It is necessary to set up a balanced system of availability and support. The manager remains available to unit supervisors through a mix of formal and informal interactions, such as the following:

- Formal, periodic meetings with individual supervisors for in-depth feedback about a specific

activity. These meetings focus on workflow and related problem solving.
- Formal development meetings with individual supervisors or the team of supervisors. The focus is development of supervisory skills, mentoring, and career path development.
- Informal day-to-day "prn" interaction.
- A combination of formal and informal daily briefing, sometimes referred to as "the huddle."

The huddle involves a brief daily meeting, about 15 minutes in length, held sometime between the early morning and midday. By this time, any immediate concerns will have surfaced, yet there is sufficient time remaining in the day to solve most problems that arise. The team usually remains standing while each supervisor summarizes the particular concerns in his or her functional unit, allowing each member of the team to become aware of workflow impact, employee issues, and "news of the day." Team members are able to make immediate plans to deal with intradepartmental concerns without the manager's having to mediate such coordination. An administrative assistant also attends, bringing materials for distribution on the spot, which eliminates the accumulation of materials in the inbox for each team member. The manager comments on such materials if follow-up is required. The assistant's presence also facilitates actions that keep things moving without further instruction—for example, he or she will follow up on a purchase order or check on a question relating to a payroll matter.

The manager typically rotates the location of the huddle among the different units of the department unless confidential information is involved. In the latter case, the unit supervisor of that department leads a roundtable briefing. This action provides visibility of the authority–responsibility mandate entrusted to that supervisor. The employees of the unit see their unit supervisor as a member of the team. Furthermore, this experience of leading a roundtable briefing provides additional training in leadership for each team member. The huddle takes place daily, even when the manager is unable to attend, thereby reinforcing the role set of the supervisors as designated agents of the manager. This practice empowers the unit supervisors by enabling them to take the lead.

## Effects of Good Delegation

Recognition of the benefits of proper delegation and, conversely, awareness of the consequences of poor delegation further enhance a manager's ability to delegate. Just as proper delegation increases the zone of acceptance on the part of employees, so failure to delegate demoralizes workers, thereby shrinking their field of cooperation. Morale suffers, turnover rates increase, and loss of productivity results. When workers in regular contact with clients cannot easily take immediate and effective action, client groups become alienated and unhappy and seek services elsewhere. The organization develops a reputation for being wrapped in bureaucratic red tape.

Finally, without proper delegation, a manager must remain constantly present to authorize action; this is time consuming and wasteful of managerial resources. It is also unrealistic because a manager's duties frequently require being out of the department or office and even away from the premises. With a manager's commitment to delegation in place, and with, the day-to-day activities flow toward accomplishing the overall mission of the organization.

# ▶ Leadership

Frequently, when professionals describe a leader as a powerful person who has made it to the top of his or her field, they use the expression "industry leader" or another similar label. The successful health professional does not seem to share familiar and common habits with the average practitioner. People imagine the person as a super-human figure when, in fact, leaders' day-to-day activities reflect a rather routine existence. Yet leadership is vital for the future growth and development of health professions. This section is designed to address the leadership qualities that everyone has buried within. Rather than define leadership as distant and unusual, this section describes it as a set of characteristics that emerge from individuals who are able to get things done within an organization.

"Natural leaders" do exist, but it is likely that they are few and far between. For the most part leaders are not born; they develop. In fact, leaders are not extraordinary in any way except that they can match organizational goals to the abilities and interests of their work groups. This talent is mercurial; some leaders are effective in one set of circumstances but not in others. Leadership is not based on impossible characteristics possessed by few; rather, it is a collection of abilities that successful managers have carefully cultivated.

## Definition of Leadership

A leader is a person who can organize tasks and make things happen through the efforts of a group of people. Using the unique interests and needs of every member of the work group, the effective leader inspires goal-directed behavior that is consistent and efficient. The leader cajoles, rewards, punishes, organizes, stimulates, strengthens, communicates, and motivates. There is no set standard for leadership behavior, as individuals must match their own characteristics to the needs of the organization.

The personal characteristics common to many leaders are a strong self-image, a vision of the future, a firm belief in the goals of the organization, the ability to influence the behavior of subordinates, and the ability to relate to and influence individuals in parallel or superior positions of authority.

Leadership exists both informally and formally. Informal leadership is exerted in many settings, including formal organizations. Within any formal organization, there are subunits and even para-organizations, such as collective bargaining units, that are led by individuals who do not hold formal hierarchical office. Leadership is implied, even explicitly included, in the role of the manager whose function is to achieve organizational objectives by coordinating, motivating, and directing the work group. For the remainder of this discussion on formal leadership, it is presumed that the manager is a leader in addition to being a holder of formal authority.

## Where Do "Leaders" Come From?

The word "leaders" in this subheading stands in quotes because not all persons in leadership positions are truly leaders.

In organizational life, leaders are "acquired" in two ways: they are promoted from the ranks of employees, and they are recruited from outside of the organization. Both means have their advantages and disadvantages. The leader promoted from within ordinarily knows the organization and its structure and workings, understands the policies and practices of the organization, knows about the processes he or she will oversee, and is familiar with the staff. But the leader promoted from within usually has drawbacks to overcome in the form of interpersonal relationships that can hamper the transition into a leadership role, especially, as frequently occurs, when one is promoted to managing a department in which he or she was one of the employees.

The leader recruited from outside usually comes in with no knowledge of the personalities already in place. Depending on conditions existing before the new leader's arrival, this person may be cautiously welcomed by the staff as one who can improve certain conditions or may be regarded with apprehension as a potential "new broom" who will make changes. So whether a new "leader"—whether first-line manager, middle manager, or whatever—rises from within or comes from outside, there are pluses and minuses associated with the appointment.

Anyone who has been part of a work organization for any length of time has learned that the best rank-and-file employees, those who are most knowledgeable and successful, do not necessarily make the best leaders. Yet there is a certain amount of logic in the promotion of the technically best employees into management. After all, promoting weak or even mediocre workers into management is surely not a consideration. But many leadership positions are filled by individuals who have had little or no education in the management of people. This is a large area of concern in many organizations, and it is often addressed through management development programs.

In addition to considering where leaders come from, it is important to probe a related question that says a great deal about many individuals who enter leadership. Why do many individuals seek leadership positions?

## What Drives People to Become Leaders?

There is an informal exercise that is worth conducting with a group of employees, especially with people in a supervisory development program who wish to become supervisors or have already been promoted to supervision. Lead them in a brainstorming exercise using this instruction; *list any or all reasons a given individual might have for seeking a leadership position.* Do not let the participants note just a few of the supposedly standard reasons, and do not be concerned with similarities and overlaps among reasons. Without too much prodding, a group of 10 or more people can come up with literally dozens of reasons why individuals seek leadership positions. Then have the group sort these reasons into two broad categories: (1) those addressing the true needs of leadership and (2) those addressing primarily an individual's needs or desires.

It does not take too long to discover that the reasons addressing an individual's needs or desires far outweigh the reasons that address the needs of the organization or entity that requires leadership. On the "up" side will be *to make a difference, to serve the customer, to implement my ideas, to improve the organization, to motivate and encourage employees, to solve some long-standing problems,* and a number of other similarly noble statements. On the "down" side, always the much longer list coming from this exercise, will be

*to make more money, to obtain better benefits, to acquire standing as a manager, to acquire power, to exert influence, to position myself to grow further,* and other essentially selfish reasons. If asked, of course, one who is seeking a leadership position will never articulate any of the selfish reasons but will surely state a couple of the organization-positive reasons.

Consider the public arena in which we obtain leaders by voting for them. Candidates will tell us what they stand for and what they propose to do if elected. A candidate for public office will always articulate some variation on *I only want to serve.* But consider this question: would this individual still "want to serve" if doing so did not entail acquiring money, benefits, position, power, prestige, influence, acclaim, and such?

Thus, people seek leadership positions for both positive and negative reasons, and many of these reasons are driven by selfishness. It is possible that many of the best potential leaders are buried in the general population; these are people who have or could develop the requisite skills but experience none of the selfish urges or who simply do not want the responsibility of what they may see as a thankless job. Once in a while, in the face of an emergent situation when others have failed or become incapacitated, one of these potential leaders will step into the breach and take charge, but this does not often happen. However, seldom do these best potential leaders step forward and seek leadership positions.

## Leadership Qualities

To influence and induce others to strive toward a goal, the leader must possess not only a strong vision of that goal but also the ability to render the goal meaningful to the group. The knowledge, insight, and skill of the leader are greater than those of other members of the group. At an obvious level, the leader leads but does not drag, coerce, or push the group. Group members are steadily induced to move toward the goal; they are influenced in a pervasive way so that the overall goal becomes their own goal. The leader does not achieve the work alone but instead successfully coordinates the work of the group. The leader inspires confidence through both emotional and knowledge ties with the followers. Indeed, a major factor that characterizes a truly successful leader is the willing acceptance of that leadership by the followers.

It is possible to generate a fairly lengthy list of qualities and characteristics that some would say "define" a leader. However, there are a couple of problems related to the creation of such a list. One difficulty, surely minor in the long run, is that no one person's list is ever complete in the eyes of another person, and it approaches the impossible to get even a few people to agree on which qualities and characteristics are more important than the others. But the greater difficulty with any list of "essential qualities and characteristics of a leader" is that no matter what quality or characteristic is cited as "essential," we can nevertheless point to some supposedly very successful "leaders" who are lacking in such. Many successful leaders are lacking, for example, in honesty, compassion, analytical ability, and numerous other qualities. So any attempt to define a leader by listing qualities and characteristics simply takes us back to the single characteristic that always holds true: the acceptance of the followers. One who is not accorded the acceptance of the followers does not truly lead but rather pushes.

## Leadership Functions

In formal organizations, the leader has certain functions that are tied to the organizational need for leadership. The leader is expected to influence, persuade, and in general control the group. As an individual with vision, the leader is expected to take calculated risks and to act as a catalyst in the change process.

The leader carries out important functions on behalf of group members through the role of representative. For example, employees look to their unit or department head to speak for them and to seek or to obtain advantages for them. The leader may be cast in several roles by followers, especially at the symbolic level, and may even be seen as the father or mother figure who shields the individual from difficulties. The leader may also be the scapegoat. As the management representative closest to the rank-and-file worker, the first-line leader–manager bears the brunt of anger when the organizational situation is less than optimal.

The leader is presumed to embody the values of the group. As such, the leader becomes the focal point in the motivational process. He or she fosters the development of the climate and conditions that favor individual involvement in group effort. Leadership is a process more than a structure; the leader fosters the climate for change so that the organization will possess the adaptability required for long-term survival.

## From Theory to Practice: A Leader's Plan of Action

The manager must make a conscious commitment to the exercise of leadership through specific actions. Leadership activity clusters in natural groupings and to a considerable extent are intertwined. Here are some examples of leadership action relating to health information management:

1. The leader starts and sustains the conversation. By being out in front of the trends, the leader studies the big challenges, "digests them," "talks them up," and translates them into action plans within the organization. Examples include encouraging employee development through the attainment of additional specialty credentials and promoting participation in regional health information projects and ongoing e-health initiatives.

2. The leader uses professional and technical competence to promote the health information professionals as the authoritative sources for clinical documentation systems and practices. Activities would typically include monitoring the federal initiatives concerning the electronic health record (EHR) initiative, the dissemination of information about the current changes in electronic discovery civil rule and the related topic of the definition of the electronic legal record, and serving as EHR project manager or team member.

3. The leader partners with key players in the organization. The leader identifies individuals whose support is critical to successful implementation of major systems—for example, the EHR, speech recognition technology, or computerized provider order entry. The leader takes the initiative in interdepartmental collaborative action such as:
   - Policy and procedure affecting joint action
   - Clinical pertinence review protocols
   - In-service training needs and partnering with external, affiliated, educational organizations needing clinical practice placements
   - Compliance reviews and billing audits
   - Risk management reviews
   - Interorganizational peer review

4. The leader is actively engaged in the life of the organization. The leader recognizes and accepts that necessary work extends beyond the routine 9–5 day and beyond the borders of the department. The leader's attitude is one of loyalty to and enthusiasm for the work of the organization. This visible support of the mission might take on a variety of forms:
   - Participation in organizational events to honor employees or volunteers—for example, employee recognition ceremonies and receptions
   - Participation in outreach activities such as career days, health fairs, and fund-raising events

- Attendance at events sponsored by other departments—for example, the open house celebrating a designated professional week (such as Physical Therapy Week or National Nurses Week)
- Participation in the organization's speakers bureau
- Hosting regional meetings of one's profession to bring attention to the organization's areas of excellence

5. The leader passes on the praise. Employees are not taken for granted; rather, their accomplishments are noted within the department and the organization. The leader takes care to nominate employees for appropriate awards such as "Employee of the Month." Departmental activities are included in the internal newsletter, with its customary "spotlight on" column. The leader submits entries for trade and professional association newsletters featuring the department. The leader finds opportunities for employees to participate in extradepartmental events, such as annual disaster or emergency preparedness drills, thereby raising the visibility and involvement of the group.

## Styles of Leadership

The manner in which a manager interacts with subordinates reflects a collection of characteristics that constitute a style of leadership. Although any manager may use several styles of leadership—choosing the style most appropriate for a given situation—one style generally emerges as that manager's predominant mode of interaction.

### Autocratic Leadership

Also referred to as authoritarian, boss-centered, or dictatorial leadership, autocratic leadership is characterized by close supervision. The manager who uses this style gives direct, clear, and precise directions to employees, telling them what is to be done and how it will be done; there is no room for employee initiative. Employees do not participate in the decision-making process. There is a high degree of centralization and a narrow span of management. The chain of command is clearly and fully understood by all. Autocratic managers use their authority as the principal, or only, method of getting work done because they believe that employees could not properly or efficiently carry out work assignments without detailed instruction.

There are two general types of autocratic leadership, exploitative and benevolent. In the exploitative type, the followers are literally exploited for the benefit of the leader. In the benevolent type, the "father-knows-best" approach to leadership is used; the leader treats followers kindly while sincerely believing he or she must make all the decisions and call all the shots. Both the exploitative autocrat, fortunately a seldom-encountered sort of leader, and the benevolent autocrat, a much more common sort than the other, are dictators; they lay down the law and the followers have no choice other than to comply or leave.

Although autocratic leadership appears to get results much of the time, it can be fatal in the long run. Employees can lose interest in their assignments and stop thinking for themselves, because there is no room for independent thought. Under certain conditions and with specific employees, however, a degree of close supervision may be necessary. Some employees prefer to receive clear and precise orders because close supervision reassures them that they are doing a good job. Even so, it can generally be assumed that an autocratic, close leadership style is the least effective and least desirable method for motivating employees to perform. This remains so whether the leader is the harsh exploitative autocrat or the kindly benevolent autocrat; in either case, the leader dictates and the followers are expected to comply.

### Bureaucratic Leadership

Like the autocratic leader, the bureaucratic leader tells employees what to do and how to do it. The basis for this leadership style is almost exclusively the organization's rules and regulations. For the bureaucrat, the rules are the law. The bureaucratic manager is often afraid to take chances and manages "by the book." Rules are strictly enforced, and no departures or exceptions are permitted. The bureaucrat, like the autocrat, allows employees little or no freedom. Some bureaucrats become so entrenched in their reliance on rules and regulations that they are essentially paralyzed when encountering a situation for which there is no applicable rule or regulation.

### Participative Leadership

In participative leadership, the contribution of the group to the organizational effort is emphasized. This style is the opposite of autocratic, close supervision. The manager who uses the participative method involves the employees in the decision-making process and in the maintenance of cohesive group interaction. The manager involves employees in determining goals, objectives, and work assignments, and similarly he or she involves them in defining the nature and extent of a problem before making a final decision and issuing directives or orders. This approach endeavors to make full use of the talents and abilities of the group members. If approached honestly and with fair consideration of employees' input, the employees who have participated in the process are likely to experience a sense of ownership in the resulting decision.

Participative management does not weaken a manager's formal authority because the manager remains responsible for the final decision whether it is made independently or by the group. The obvious advantage of the participative style of leadership revolves around the meaningful involvement of the employees, which greatly enhances the implementation of the decisions that have been made.

### Consultative Leadership

Some managers use a pseudo-participative method of leadership to give employees the feeling that they have participated in decision making. The consultative leader routinely solicits employee input, then just as routinely ignores that input and independently makes the decision. This sort of leader is often self-deluded into believing that he or she is being openly participative by soliciting employee input. However, when the employee input is ignored, employees quickly sense that the manager is manipulating people and that their participation in the decision-making process is not real.

### Laissez-Faire Leadership

Laissez-faire or "free rein" or essentially "hands-off" leadership is based on the assumption that individuals are self-motivated and generally self-directed. In this approach, employees receive little or no supervision. Employees, as individuals or as a group, determine their own goals and make their own decisions. The manager, whose contribution is minimal, acts primarily as a consultant and does so only when asked. The manager does not lead but allows the employees to lead themselves. Some managers consider this approach to be true democratic leadership, but the usual end result is disorganization and chaos. The lack of leadership permits different employees to proceed in different directions.

### Paternalistic Leadership

This is quite similar to benevolent autocracy, the "father-knows-best" approach to leadership. The paternalistic manager treats employees like children, telling them in a kindly manner what to do and how to do it. It is the paternalistic manager's belief that employees do not really know what is good for them or how to make decisions for themselves. In this approach, everyone is watched over by the benevolent manager—the benign dictator—and the employees eventually become extremely dependent on their "paternalistic boss." The paternalistic leader genuinely believes that the followers are incapable and must therefore be told every move to make. In contrast, the benevolent autocrat does not care whether the followers are capable or not, but firmly believes that he or she must think and decide for the entire group.

## Continuum of Leadership Styles

Another way to view leadership behavior is on a continuum ranging from highly boss-centered to highly group-centered. The relationship between the manager and the employee in the continuum ranges from completely autocratic, in which there is no employee participation in the decision-making process, to completely democratic, in which the employee participates in all phases of the decision-making process. The following briefly describes the gradations along the continuum:

1. *The manager makes the decision and announces it.* The manager identifies a problem, considers alternative solutions, selects a course of action, and tells employees what to do. Employees do not participate in the decision-making process; they do not provide input in any form.

2. *The manager "sells" the decision.* The manager again makes the decision without consulting the employees. Instead of simply dictating the decision, however, the manager attempts to persuade the employees to accept it largely through explaining how the decision serves both the goals of the department and the interests of group members.

3. *The manager presents ideas and invites questions.* The manager has already made the decision but asks the employees to express their ideas. Thus, the manager allows for the possibility that the initial decision may be modified.

4. *The manager presents a tentative decision subject to change.* The manager allows the employees the opportunity to exert some influence before the decision is finalized. The manager meets with the employees and presents the problem and a tentative decision. Before the decision is finalized, the manager obtains the reactions of employees who will be affected by it.

5. *The manager presents the problem, obtains suggestions, and makes the decision.* Up to this point on the continuum, the manager has always come before the employees with at least a tentative solution to the problem. At this point, however, the employees get the first opportunity to suggest solutions. Consultation with the employees increases the number of possible solutions to the problem. The manager then selects the solution that he or she regards as most appropriate in solving the problem.

6. *The manager defines limits and asks the group to make the decision.* For the first time, the employees make the decision. The manager now becomes a member of the group. Before doing so, however, the manager defines the problem and the limits and boundaries within which the decision must be made.

7. *The manager permits subordinates to function within the limits defined by the superior.* For the maximum degree of employee participation, the manager defines the problem and lists the guidelines and boundaries within which a solution must be achieved. The limitations imposed on the employees come directly from the manager, who participates as a group member in the decision-making process and is committed in advance to implementing whatever decision the employees make.

In summary, the manager's relationship with the employees influences morale, job satisfaction, and work output. Employee satisfaction is positively associated with the degree to which employees are permitted to participate in the decision-making process. In contrast, poor supervision causes employee dissatisfaction, high turnover rates, and low morale.

## Factors That Influence Leadership Style

No one style of leadership fits all situations. A successful manager is one who has learned how to apply the most appropriate method for a given situation. Before selecting a style of leadership or deciding to blend several styles, the manager must consider a number of factors:

1. *Work assignment.* If the work assignment is repetitious, properly trained employees do not need constant or close supervision. If the assignment is new or complex, however, close supervision may be required.

2. *Personality and ability of employees.* Employees who are not self-starters function best under close supervision. Others, by reason of personality and work background, can take on new and important responsibilities on their own; these individuals react best to participative leadership. The occupational makeup of a department may also influence the leadership style used by the manager. For professional practitioners (e.g., physical therapists, occupational therapists, health information specialists) or other highly skilled employees, the employee-centered participative leadership style is often most effective. When employees are unskilled or unable to act independently, the boss-centered or autocratic style of leadership may produce better results.

3. *Attitude of employees toward the manager.* The manager cannot begin to lead or influence behavior unless he or she is accepted by the group. Employees fully accept the manager's authority only when they believe that the goals and objectives of the manager are consistent with their own personal and professional interests.

4. *Personality and ability of the manager.* The manager's personality has a definite effect on the behavior and performance of employees. The manager must treat employees' opinions and suggestions with respect and must sincerely encourage employee participation.

When faced with different work group encounters and situational factors, the effective manager shifts from one style of leadership to another, often without conscious recognition of a shift in style. **Table 4-1** provides examples of the adjustments in leadership style that a manager makes to stimulate maximum effort from employees.

## Communicating Your Own Managerial Style

A manager may deliberately go out of his or her way to communicate to employees the style of leadership or management he or she practices. It is not particularly uncommon for a manager who is relatively new to an organization or department to make statements such as these: "I believe in employee participation, and I always welcome your input"; "I practice management by wandering around, so you'll see me a lot in the departments"; or, one of the most oft-heard, "my door is always open."

There are some significant hazards in introducing yourself as a manager in such a manner. In the words of a wise, anonymous observer of management practices, "It's Management 101—using the buzzwords, saying what you think you should be saying, telling people that you're what the 'management experts' say

**Table 4–1** Variables in Leadership Style

| Work Group | Key Activities | Leadership Style |
|---|---|---|
| Hospital transporters | Transport of patient<br>    Safety considerations Schedule considerations<br>    Mode of transport | Bureaucratic—policies and procedures must be followed |
| Staff physical therapist with experience | Patient evaluation "Need evaluation today"<br>    Neurological case Conference at 10:00 A.M. | Laissez-faire—manager does not need to tell physical therapist such typical evaluation elements as motor, sensory, and cognitive tests |
| Total physical therapy professional staff (five physical therapists) | Vacation schedules<br>    Consideration of patients, students, and overall coverage<br>    One staff resignation in July | Participative—manager consults with employees concerning vacation schedule and the need for proper coverage during the summer months |
| Staff physical therapist | Call from physician to staff therapist; wishes to see therapist at patient's bedside promptly at 9:15 A.M. or "Sorry to interrupt but just had a call from Dr. Jones and he requests you be at the patient's room #343 in 5 minutes" (Note: Even, nice tone) | Autocratic, nonnegotiable |

you should be." The hazards inherent in such pronouncements are found in the risk of being trapped by employee perception.

It takes only a few perceived contradictions of your self-described style to create dissonance. As soon as you are seen unilaterally making decisions without soliciting participation or input, you have created a perceived conflict between your words and your actions. And when a few employees have found you unavailable, although you have said "My door is always open," more such conflicts are created and employee perceptions begin to turn unfavorably against you, whether deservedly or not. Any given perception may not be entirely accurate, but to the perceiver perception is reality.

It is best to say as little as necessary about your own style of leadership and allow your actions to convey your true style. In other words, instead of telling employees what kind of leader you are, let your actions show them. You may not come across as the sort of leader idealized in "Management 101," but, even more importantly, you are more likely to come across as honest.

## Situational Leadership and Adjustment

What style of leadership should a manager adopt? It depends on the situation. For the experienced conscientious manager and insightful leader of people, adjusting one's style should be automatic, adapted to the particular situation at hand or to the unique needs of the moment.

Not every problem submits to the same logical process of analysis and solution. Not every need that arises in the workday can be addressed in an identical manner. And, most important to the manager, not every employee is able to respond as desired to the same management approach. Within the same group you may have individuals who must be led and who indeed often prefer to be led and have others do their thinking for them, along with people who are self-motivated and capable of significant self-direction. This is especially likely in department employing both professionals and nonprofessionals. Although the same overall "rules"—that is, the same personnel policies—apply uniformly to all employees, the manager will have to deal differently with individuals in other ways. Some you may consult and invite their participation or input; others you will simply direct.

Avoid making assumptions about people; never assume that what works with one will work with all others. Know your employees and try to understand each one as both a producer and a person. By working with people over a period of time, and especially by working at the business of getting to know them, you can learn a great deal about individual likes and dislikes and capabilities. Learn about your people as individuals and when necessary lead accordingly. If you are convinced that a certain employee genuinely prefers orders and instructions and this attitude is not inconsistent with job requirements, then use orders and instructions. Although many employees of healthcare organizations seem to prefer participative leadership, not everyone will desire this same consideration. Maintain sufficient flexibility to accommodate the employee who wants or requires authoritarian supervision. It is fully as unfair to expect people to become what they do not want to be as it is to allow a rigid structure to stifle those other employees who feel they have something more to contribute.

There is no single style of leadership that is appropriate to all people and situations at all times. Let the situation and the needs of those involved dictate your managerial style.

## ▶ Some Final Thoughts About Authentic Personal Leadership

In the preceding discussion, the manager has been identified as an agent of change. The functions of the manager have been noted, and leadership traits and foundations have been explored. All of this leads up to some final thoughts about the manager–leader as a person.

One who would aspire to leadership and become successful in its pursuit must perform some serious self-examination by asking: *why should anyone be led by me?* This can be a startling question. A person's initial reaction might be one of defensiveness or even irritation: "Shouldn't it be obvious? I am up-to-date in my field; I come in every year at or under budget; no accreditation citations arise from my department; there are few, if any, grievances from my staff; and my employee turnover is minimal. What more do *they* want?"

Now ask the latter question another way: "What more do *you* want? What kind of person are you striving to be?" Some people view the idea of self-development as trendy: dress for success, or six steps to persuading and negotiating, or similar topics suggesting artificial methods for getting ahead in the organization. Such practices even become the fodder for sit-coms and cartoons, not to be taken seriously. But for others, this focus on self is embarrassing and perhaps discouraging. Who can be the perfect person?

Such reactions could cause us to neglect this important aspect of leadership. Notice the emphasis that major business and management schools place on the cultural, spiritual, and psychological development of the manager–leader. They devote significant curriculum time and resources to these topics. Major business and management journals include regular features on these aspects of leadership. When we observe successful peers, higher-level managers, and leaders both within the organization and external to it, we notice some common traits. Specifically, they possess a set of *value-added* characteristics.

## Value-Added Characteristics

The value-added characteristics flow from a deep respect for the dignity of the human person. This genuinely high regard for oneself and for others is reflected in the presentation of self in everyday life. It is manifested through an attitude of engaged, conscious living; gracious interpersonal relationships; and calm, orderly work habits. It is embodied in the values of integrity, trustworthiness, and respect.

### Engaged, Conscious Living

Individuals who display the characteristic of engaged, conscious living have an awareness of and an enthusiasm for life. They bring positive energy to the work setting that is rooted in a balanced life—they like their life! Their approach to life keeps them from overreacting. They are not the caricature characters who are always having a bad day and give off the negative vibration: "don't even ask; you don't want to know; wait until I have had my coffee." No, these are the people who are steady; they are pleasant to associate with; they easily and routinely show graciousness.

### Gracious Interpersonal Relationships

In an age of depersonalization, coupled with overly casual ways of relating, a person can inadvertently fail at fundamental politeness. The antidote is gracious interpersonal relationships. The gracious person truly sees you and acknowledges you; a simple "good morning" is extended to coworkers, and a cordial "hello" is given to the attendees at a meeting. This person knows how to make an introduction, both informal and formal, and can offer an appropriate blessing, a toast, or a congratulatory message at a celebratory occasion. He or she sends the timely handwritten note and does not fall into the casual practice of cute, humorous, or even sarcastic commercial cards. He or she can make conversation with ease and does not rely on the latest sports headline as the only topic.

### Calm, Orderly Work Habits

The workplace is accepted for what it is—a place of business. The attentive manager–leader maintains an orderly work space, free of distracting items (e.g., mementos, knickknacks, highly personal possessions). The office is not the person's second home. The work at hand is laid out for attention and then returned to its proper holding place. A member of the organization who comes to this person's office can literally sit down without having to step over or move "files and piles." If a high-level manager brings a visitor to the office space, it should not result in embarrassment on anyone's part. There is an attitude of dignity and respect toward one's physical environment; this person is a good steward of the material goods entrusted to him or her.

### Embodiment of Values

Others can easily make positive remarks about these manager–leaders. They have integrity; they promote ethical behavior that is reflected in routine practice. There is no bootleg software in use. Their expense reports are truthful and straightforward. When given the opportunity to attend conferences and training sessions, they actively participate, take the opportunity to obtain information from vendors, and make useful contacts through networking. They are trustworthy; such a person can keep a confidence, and he or she is a thoughtful sounding board and a safe haven for letting off steam. The person confiding in this manager–leader knows that the conversation will be safeguarded.

Finally, these manager–leaders are respectful of others. People know that they are psychologically safe in such a person's presence. People know they will not be recorded, photographed, or "uploaded" onto the various social media. The respectful manager–leader truly listens to the individual in one-on-one situations and at meetings; he or she is not doodling, knitting, clock watching, surreptitiously checking for messages, or multitasking. Attentiveness, being fully present, is the hallmark behavior of such a person.

Recall the probing question: Why should anyone be led by you? The answer becomes easy and obvious when one attends to purposeful self-development.

## ▶ Growing in the Leadership Role; Enhancing One's Career Path

Several concepts coalesce when a manager reflects on the interplay of his or her leadership role, career path, and day-to-day management functions. Aligning one's career path and enhancing one's leadership activities are properly interwoven into the organization's short- and long-range plans. This integration of personal and organizational plans benefit the individual and the organization by advancing the goals of both.

Some managers might find this introspective practice awkward and embarrassing. Is it not egotistical and artificial to set out "to be a leader"? No, it is not. A manager is expected to be fully engaged in organizational life as a member of the leadership team.

## A Data-Driven Review

Just as the processes used in healthcare reviews and decision making emphasize an evidence-based, data-driven approach, so should the process of examining one's personal leadership and career-path decisions be anchored in facts. The first cluster of reflections focuses primarily on career-path decisions. In this private process of review, the manager inventories the particular circumstances of his or her personal life, role sets, and non-work-related obligations. As a general rule, an employer may not inquire into personal circumstances. However, the honest assessment of these factors, made privately by the employee, helps him or her—whether new to the management role or well into a career—avoid two pitfalls: (1) accepting a managerial position and subsequently finding themselves unable to meet the demands of the position; and (2) failure to engage with the organization's mission and plans because of personal plans. One runs the risk of being perceived as a liminal participant at best—merely a place holder, one who is just passing through, with minimal involvement in organizational life beyond what is minimally required by the job specifications. Additional examples and considerations are given in the final chapter of this book in the section about choosing to be a manager.

Here are some typical observations made by group participants at a workshop on career and leadership development in answering the question: What factors in your personal life (including other key members of your household or extended family) potentially impact your decisions? These examples represent a wide variety of factors:

- Having an agreement to participate in a student loan forgiveness program; must work in this designated geographic region with an underserved population. Requires 5-year commitment.
- Enrolled in a master's degree program (part time); 2 more years to go until completed; program also requires a 2-month continuous full-time capstone practicum.
- Spouse is active duty military, assigned to duty station in this city; we cannot relocate until the 3-year rotation is finished; 2 more years to go before we relocate.
- Developing specialty practice in industrial health and rehabilitation; need to stay in this geographic location, with its availability of potential

clients from local industries. Start-up business plan includes a projection of 2 years needed to implement a solid independent practice.

- Planning to develop specialty practice providing home care services for postacute-care clients. Need to gain experience in acute care facility's home care department.

- Cannot accept a position requiring overnight and/or out-of-area travel: family obligations—regarding care of aged parents and young children requires a regular day schedule at one central location.

A second cluster of factors reflects personal preferences:

- Prefer large, multispecialty urban healthcare center with research component; plan to immerse myself in research projects; eventually seek a full-time faculty position at university level.

- Desire to travel; have limited financial resources; will sign on with a national agency specializing in "prn" and other short-term placements; travel/relocation stipend included.

- Desire to stay in small town, quasi-rural location near extended family. Local hospital and 2 long-term care facilities are the only healthcare employers.

- Prefer nondirect care setting; plan to seek employment in a healthcare agency (city, county, or state/government); try to specialize in innovative outreach programs.

- Aware that, while I am committed to excellence in my work, I have other interests and commitments outside the organization. Thus, I am choosing to limit my involvement in the organization's voluntary activities (e.g., helping with a health fair or fund-raising activities).

A third cluster of fact-finding elements focuses on the manager's leadership accomplishments. Such information is readily available from several sources. One can compare one's actual leadership initiatives to identifiable outcomes. Sources include the department and organization's annual reports; accrediting agency reviews; critical incident reviews; and one's annual self-evaluation as a manager. These reports and reviews reflect the departmental accomplishments, challenges, and goals fully or partially achieved. A manager assesses these facts by asking two questions. What leadership actions stand out? Where were there failures of leadership or missed opportunities? In addition to the reviews and reports noted, the manager uses an additional source of detailed information, the manager's wheel book.

## ▶ Using the Manager's Wheel Book

As noted in the section on the functions of a manager in Chapter 1, the concept and uses of the manager's wheel book were described. Because this log reflects details of the manager's daily activity, a current manager could use this log as a retrospective review for the purposes of identifying distinctive leadership actions. **Appendix 4–A** contains an excerpt from a manager's wheel book. In this example, the manager has culled leadership actions accomplished during the past year. Distinctive leadership actions included:

- Actively promoting department visibility by participating in interdepartmental projects (e.g., the reimbursement issues relating to the behavioral care unit; providing consultative services to newly affiliated program; participating in mass casualty response training).

- Actively representing employee concerns and accomplishments (e.g., resolve questions about safety and security for night-shift employees; clarify telecommuting hours of work during inclement weather; nominate workers for employee-of-the-month awards).

- Actively supporting educational efforts for the organization's employees and for students from affiliated educational institutions (e.g., directed practice preceptor; in-service training for supervisors).

- Continuing professional development (e.g., STEM-H project and subsequent formal presentation of findings; enrolled in formal study program regarding project management certification).

The manager made additional observations based on the wheel book entries. There was almost no distinct training or motivational interactions regarding evening and night shifts. There was almost no attention given to the worker's environment (e.g., upgrading the lighting or improving work-flow layout). A new leadership plan of action will include actions to overcome these short comings.

The capstone chapter, Day-to-Day Management, includes additional discussion pertaining to developing one's career path.

# Appendix 4-A

## Wheel Book—Examples Relating to Leadership Role

- Participated in interdepartmental project: identify reimbursement denial trends and patterns; developed process for prebilling edits and error reviews for behavioral care center.
- Prepared readiness plan for department coverage during upcoming transit strike.
- Enrolled in formal study program to attain project management certification.
- Finalized peer exchange/reading group meeting dates, topics, and presenters.
- Presented employee concerns to human resources, re: safety and security for evening and night shift employees required to use remote parking lot.
- Submitted department nominee for employee of the month.
- Provided consultant services (initial review) to newly affiliated behavioral care center.
- Met with clinical practice coordinators from 2 baccalaureate programs, re: special projects for the 1-month practicum.

- Attended continuing education and practice center for STEM-H (science, technology, engineering, math, and health) quarterly program; round-table presenter on high-tech applications in selected health informatics jobs.
- Attended in-house emergency training: mass casualty response update; accepted position of coordinator, re: intake and registration.
- Gave presentation to Woman's Auxiliary: Your Personal Health Record.
- Briefed assistant directors and unit supervisors on educational benefits available to them for job-related study.
- Clarified with human resources: weather-related closing and questions raised by employees with prior-approved telecommute options.
- Agreed to be listed in the organization's speakers bureau website.
- Volunteered for the 100th anniversary committee of hospital's founding.

### Notes

1. Chester Barnard, *The Functions of the Executive* (Cambridge, MA: Harvard University Press, 1968), 167–169.
2. Herbert Simon, *Administrative Behavior* (New York: Macmillan, 1965), 12.
3. Ibid., 129.
4. Robert Presthus, "Authority in Organizations," in *Concepts and Issues in Administrative Behavior*, ed. Sidney Mailick and Edward H. Van Ness (Englewood Cliffs, NJ: Prentice-Hall, 1962), 122.
5. Edgar H. Schein, *Organizational Psychology* (Englewood Cliffs, NJ: Prentice-Hall, 1965), 11.
6. Hans Heinrich Gerth and Mills C. Wright, *From Max Weber: Essays in Sociology* (New York: Oxford University Press, 1946), 196–204.
7. Ibid.
8. Henry C. Metcalf and L. Urwick Harper, eds., *Dynamic Administration: The Collected Papers of Mary Parker Follett* (New York: Harper, 1942).
9. Ibid.
10. Ibid.

## CHAPTER 5

# Planning and Decision Making

## CHAPTER OBJECTIVES

- Define the management functions of planning and decision making.
- Identify the characteristics of plans and specifically address those characteristics or features that make plans effective.
- Identify participants and their responsibilities in the planning process.
- Delineate the constraints placed on planning and identify the boundaries to be observed in the planning process.
- Define and differentiate among the terms philosophy, goal, objective, functional objective, policy, procedure, method, and rule.
- Delineate aspects of project management and 500-day plans.
- Evaluate plans and decisions using after-action reviews, OODA loop feedback, and analyses of unanticipated consequences.
- Determine how to evaluate a decision's importance.
- Describe some of the tools and techniques available to aid decision making.

Planning is the process of deciding in the present what to do to bring about a desired outcome in the future. We might further qualify this description by referring to planning as the process of *tentatively* deciding what to do because we have no assurance of exactly what the future will bring.

Planning involves determining appropriate goals and deciding on the means to achieve them, making assumptions, developing premises, and reviewing alternative courses of action. It is the what, who, when, and how of alternative courses of action and of possible future actions. In planning, the manager contemplates the state of affairs desired for the future in light of what is known or can be inferred about the future. Any time people are looking ahead considering what to do in the future—whether that future is years or only minutes away—they are planning.

In the planning process, the step involving the choice among alternatives is the decision-making phase.

## ▶ Characteristics of Planning

Planning is the most fundamental management function and logically precedes all other functions. Unplanned action cannot be properly controlled because there is no basis on which to measure progress, and organizing becomes meaningless and ineffective because there is no specific goal around which to mobilize resources. Decisions may be made without planning, but they will lack effectiveness unless they are related to specific goals.

Planning goes beyond mere judgments, because judgments involve the assessment of a situation but do not stipulate actions to be taken. Planning concerns actions to be taken with reference to specific goals.

In planning, the ideal state is first identified. The initial approach to achieving that ideal is then modified, refined, and brought to a practical level through a variety of derived elements, such as intermediate target statements, functional objectives, and operational goals. Planning includes the decision-making process, particularly in the commitment phase. Logical planning includes commitment in terms of time and actions to be taken. There is a hierarchy in the process that includes the relationship of derived plans to the master course, the linkage of short-range and long-range plans, and the coordination of division and department or unit plans with those of the organization as a whole. Finally, planning is characterized by a cyclic process in which some or many goals and specific objectives are recycled.

In a sense, some plans are never achieved completely; they are continuous. For example, the goal of healthcare institutions to provide quality patient care is a continuing one that invests the many derived plans with a fundamental purpose. This goal is recycled during each planning period.

## ▶ Participants in Planning

Top management sets the basic tone for planning, determines overall goals for the organization, and provides direction on the content of policies and similar planning documents. This is not done in isolation but is based on information provided through the feedback cycle, through reports and special studies, and through the direct participation of personnel in each department or division. The manager consults the major superusers, both in the direct patient care divisions and the administrative units.

Department heads are normally responsible for the planning process in their areas of jurisdiction. They identify overall goals and policies for their departments, and they develop immediate objectives, taking into account their departments' particular work constraints. In some organizations, a special planning department is created, such as a program and development division or a research and development unit.

Occasionally, clients participate in the planning process; such participation is required in some externally funded programs. In healthcare planning, for example, members of the provider, consumer, and business community are included at each level of the review process. Professional associations frequently involve their members in the planning process at local, regional, state, and national levels. Employee involvement is yet another aspect of participation. Organizations whose members belong to collective bargaining units involve employee representatives in formulating certain aspects of planning, such as plans to downsize or to change major patterns of staffing. Because the final responsibility for planning, with the attendant legal considerations, rests with management, the input of employees and the public is advisory in nature. Their roles should be well delineated at the outset, and their input is encouraged.

## ▶ The Planning Process

Because planning is intended to focus attention on objectives and to reduce uncertainty, there must be a clear statement of goals. Once the goals to be attained have been established, premising must be developed—that is, the assumptions must be identified, stated, and used consistently. Premising includes an analysis of planning constraints and a statement of the anticipated environment within which the plans will unfold. In a healthcare organization, the premises reflect the level of care, the specific setting (e.g., outpatient clinic, inpatient unit, or home care), the specific number of beds per service, the anticipated number and kinds of specialty services or clinics, morbidity and mortality data for the outreach territory, and the availability of related services.

The department head states the premises on which departmental plans are based—for example, the number of inpatient beds, the readmission rate, the projected length of stay, and the interrelationship of the workflow. The following is an example of specific planning premises or assumptions based on the operation of a physical therapy service:

1. Anticipated hours of operation
   a. 6 days per week
   b. 8-hour day; evening coverage for selected patients and clinics
2. Anticipated caseload
   a. Inpatients—100 per day
   b. Outpatients—120 per day
3. Diagnostic categories
   a. Hemiplegics
   b. Arthritis
   c. Amputees
   d. Fractures
   e. Sports injuries

4. Patient characteristics
   a. Adults: general adult population; workers' compensation/industrial health referrals; frail, elderly people; juveniles, especially those with sports-related injuries
   b. Children
5. Level of care
   a. Acute
   b. Subacute
   c. Convalescent
   d. Chronic

Alternative approaches to reaching the desired state are developed, and the choices to be made are stated. Commitment to one of these choices constitutes the decision-making phase. Derivative plans then are formulated, and details of sequence and timing are identified. Planning includes periodic checking and review, which leads to the control process. Review and necessary revisions of plans, based on feedback, are the final steps in the cycle of planning.

# ▶ Planning Constraints or Boundaries

To constrain means to limit, to bind, to delineate freedom of action. Constraints in planning are factors that managers must take into account to make their plans feasible and realistic. Constraints, which are both internal and external, take a variety of forms. Analysis of the organizational environment by means of the clientele network, specifically the category of controller, leads to ready identification of planning constraints. The use of the input–output model also yields practical information about the constraints specific to an organization. The cost of data gathering and analysis is another constraint; if committees or special review groups are involved, the cost of their time must be considered.

General resistance to change impedes the planning process so that standing plans take on the force of habit. Without a program for regular review of plans, they become static and rooted in tradition. Precedent becomes the rule, and the bureaucratic processes become entrenched. The phase in the life cycle of the organization also affects planning, as the degree of innovation that is appropriate varies with each phase.

The nature of the organization also shapes the planning process. The extent to which the organization's members participate in planning correlates with the predominant mode of authority. Highly normative organizations tend to include more member participation in their planning than do coercive ones. Ethics and values of the larger society, of the individual members, and, in health care, of the many professional organizations help shape the goal formulation and subsequent policies and practices. There may be a greater openness to innovation and a demand for outreach programs and flexible patterns of delivery of service when professional associations or government programs highlight new areas of emphasis.

Within the organization, interdepartmental relationships may be constraints. In highly specialized organizations with many services or departments, each unit manager must consider how other departments' needs and processes are interwoven with those of the manager's own department. Effective planning includes an assessment of such factors. The manager sometimes must accept as inputs or constraints the procedures and policies of another department.

Capital investments must also be considered. When a major commitment that involves the physical layout of the facility or some major equipment purchase has been made, the degree of flexibility in changing the process is necessarily limited.

External factors to be considered in planning include the political climate, which varies in its openness to extensive programs in health care. The general state of labor relations and the degree to which unionization is allowed or perhaps even mandated in an industry may be imposed on the organization. The many regulations, laws, and directives constitute another set of constraints.

In healthcare organizations, the many legal and accrediting requirements are specific, pervasive constraints that affect every aspect of planning. Such requirements can be developed into a reference grid for the use of the manager, as compliance with these mandates is a binding element in the overall constraint on departmental functioning.

An alternative approach to the identification of constraints in any healthcare planning situation is the systematic recognition of the following major factors. (Also recall the earlier discussions on the settings and trends, and on response to change, for additional examples.)

1. *General setting.* The level and particular emphasis of care must be determined. For example, the goal of one institution may be acute care in specialized diagnostic categories; the goal of another may be long-term care of frail, elderly people. The organizational relationships that stem from the general setting should be identified (e.g., the institution's

degree of independence versus its adherence to corporate and affiliation agreements and contractual arrangements). Physical location may also be a constraining factor, although an earlier decision to develop the facility in a specific location may be part of the ideal plan. For example, the decision to develop a pattern of decentralized care so as to enhance the outreach program of a community behavioral health center will serve as a constraint on many derived plans, such as workflow and staffing patterns. Information about the general setting is readily available in long-range planning documents, licensure and accreditation surveys, annual reports, and public relations materials.

2. *Legal and accrediting agency mandates.* Each healthcare institution is regulated by a federal or state agency that imposes specific requirements for the level of care and nature of services offered. For example, a hospital is licensed by the state only after it meets certain requirements; it is approved for participation in the Medicare and Medicaid programs only after it fulfills certain conditions. In addition, a hospital must comply with special regulations for medical care evaluation. It also must comply, at a minimum, with malpractice insurance regulations and related risk management programs as well as fire, safety, and zoning codes.

3. *Characteristics of the clients.* The general patterns of mortality and morbidity for a given population must be considered, as well as related factors such as length of inpatient stay, frequency of outpatient services, emergency unit usage, and readmission rate. Patients' sources of payment relate to the stability and predictability of cash flow. Specific eligibility for treatment may be another factor, as in certain services for veterans or programs for other specific groups. Demographic profiles for the area served and the organization's internal database are the usual sources of such information.

4. *Practitioners and employees.* The licensure laws for healthcare practitioners and physicians, as well as the many federal and state laws pertaining to most classes of employees, govern the utilization of staff. These include the Labor Management Relations Act (Taft-Hartley Act), the Civil Rights Act, the Age Discrimination in Employment Act, the Unemployment Compensation and Workers' Compensation Acts, the Occupational Safety and Health Act, and the Americans with Disabilities Act. The personnel practices mandated in the accrediting agency standards and guidelines of health agencies and professional associations also

must be followed. Any contractual agreement resulting from the collective bargaining process must be taken into account. The specific bylaws and related rules and regulations for medical staff and allied healthcare practitioners are yet another constraint on plans involving employees and professional practitioners in any role.

5. *Corporate culture.* The overall vision, mission, and corporate culture invest planning and decision making with an underlying approach. It provides a framework within which these activities are developed, and reflects a level of openness to new modes of care, alternate settings, expanded roles of professional practitioners, and outreach to clients.

## Strategic or Limiting Factors as Constraints

Chester Barnard, in his classic work on the functions of managers, stressed the importance of identifying those limiting factors that constrain the development of plans.[1] Legal and accreditation requirements and contractual agreements are major examples of binding constraints. Systems interoperability is an example of an internal limiting factor. The planning team identifies these factors to prevent a waste of time and energy in the planning process; they concentrate on developing plans that are feasible. Alternative solutions are narrowed to include only those that fit the organizational goals and the availability of resources, and that satisfy the binding requirements. In exceptional situations, managers might seek exemptions from the existing regulations so as to undertake a pilot program or demonstration project focusing on innovative practices, but this is rare.

## ▶ Characteristics of Effective Plans

Effective plans are flexible. Plans should have a built-in capacity to change; they should be adaptable. A plan could include a timetable sequence, for example, that allows extra time for unexpected events before the plan goes off-schedule.

The manager seeks to balance plans so that they are neither too idealistic nor too practical or limited. On the one hand, plans that are too idealistic tend to produce frustration because they cannot be attained; they may become mere mottoes. On the other hand, plans that are too modest lack motivational value, and it may be difficult to muster support for them. Clarity and vagueness must also be balanced in formulating plans. These factors help make the goals realistic. A precise goal may be a motivational tool because it provides immediate satisfaction, but there is also merit in a degree of vagueness because with some plans, especially long-range ones, it may not be possible or desirable to state goals in precise terms. Vagueness can contribute to motivation by permitting the development of detailed plans by those more directly involved in the work. Finally, vagueness can provide the necessary latitude to compromise when this is required or is a general strategy in the development of plans throughout the organization.

Effectiveness in planning and decision making is enhanced by thoroughness of fact finding. Using these elements (the setting and the characteristics of the clients), a manager would note these in detail. This process yields both expected and unexpected results, particularly when the manager is dealing with an unfamiliar setting.

For example, consider the elements associated with correction care. These include the graying of the prison population; incarceration of the severely handicapped; healthcare needs of pregnant prisoners; withdrawal symptoms and detox care, with subsequent education and behavioral change programs relating to drug or alcohol addiction; comprehensive care for people with HIV-AIDS; infection control and infectious diseases (e.g., TB, hepatitis); living with cancer; diabetic care; medical risks for adolescent boys in correctional boot camp; suicide risk assessment and prevention.

Here is another example from a different setting, that of truck-stop dispensaries. The clients are short- and long-distance drivers; their schedules do not permit easy access to routine or episodic care or first aid. They are "on the clock" and "on the road" with strict time limits on their work time. Major (usually interstate) truck stops sometimes include limited access to first aid, some routine monitoring (e.g., blood pressure), and, with the increasing use of telemedicine, there is greater access to routine and more urgent care.

In a similar setting, that of industrial manufacturing, a full-time dispensary or clinic is usually available, owned (or on contract) and operated by the owners. Its primary focus is rapid intervention when there is an industrial accident (e.g., chemical burn, crushing wound, toxic fumes, falls). In addition, routine monitoring of hearing, eyesight, balance, blood pressure, effects of medication, and general physical fitness is part of employees' benefit packages as well as management's safety and risk prevention program. Employee physical exams (at hire and subsequently

throughout tenure as an employee) are usually the responsibility of dispensaries. Worker compensation monitoring is another major responsibility of industrial clinics. Telemedicine support is now a common feature.

A fourth example reflects a less traditional setting and client group, namely the homeless. In assessing these programs, a manager would differentiate the categories of homeless people and their healthcare needs. One segment of this population is the temporarily displaced individual or family unit, perhaps due to a fire or flood. These clients are relatively short-stay and have an available medical history and health insurance, and their health needs are relatively routine (e.g., diabetic care; first aid and respite care related to the cause of their displacement; ordinary health screening, as for a child entering school). Another category of homeless people includes a relatively stable and known group who tend to frequent the same support stations for meals and overnight lodging. It is possible to provide some level of care to these individuals, such as flu shots, basic health monitoring, and first aid. Through social service outreach, some members of this population can be brought into a supportive system (e.g., veterans' care, programs for individuals with black lung disease and similar initiatives). A third group within this population are more transient and their healthcare needs are often at the level of first aid or, when their condition massively worsens, hospitalization.

Clearly the aspects of care patterns and systems are quite different within these settings and for these groups of people than what many of us may be accustomed to. However, effective planners take note of these factors.

## Anticipating Changes and Updates in Existing Plans

The effective manager monitors the planning process as an ongoing activity so that existing plans may be modified and new plans developed to meet changes in one or several planning constraints. The manager is not caught unaware but instead has an active plan to monitor potential change. Federal and state agencies as well as accrediting agencies issue their intended changes well in advance of their required implementation. Some agencies issue annual or semiannual agendas of changes under consideration. The various inspectors general regularly make known the targeted review focus for the upcoming year.

Plans needing modification are similarly assessed. As a manager identifies a trend or issue, he or she checks existing objectives, policies, and procedures to adjust them accordingly. An equipment recycling program may have worked well in the past, but now more particular attention is required when computers are recycled or destroyed; privacy considerations as well as environmental protection requirements need to be added as factors in such a recycling or disposal process.

## Planning for the Unknown

In addition to planning based on well-known planning premises (e.g., expected number of patients per year, usual length of stay), planning for unknown events must be accomplished. The management team typically assesses the relative unknowns and seeks to make them progressively tangible. Although complete certainty is not possible, plans for rare but probable events are not only prudent but often mandated by external agencies. The strike plan is one such example. As the contract period for a given labor union agreement concludes, it is possible that a new contract may not have been agreed to yet. The workers may strike, thereby causing work disruption. Because patient care is of primary importance, management must have a contingency plan in place well before the strike deadline. Weather-related disruptions are another instance of possible-to-probable events. Managers in hurricane-prone locations or in regions with winter storms of a crippling variety have plans in place to cover those circumstances. Although managers do not know precisely how many or when such disruptions will occur, they have anticipated them well in advance and only need to fine-tune the plan when the emergency conditions escalate.

Disaster preparedness is a prime example of planning for the unknown. The types of possible disasters (e.g., epidemic, mass casualty, bioterrorism) are identified and the plans rehearsed in great detail precisely because their incidences are so unpredictable. Continuity of operations and plans for succession are essential aspects of disaster planning. These plans include such topics as alternative care sites, triage, changes in staffing patterns, and remote work site/telecommuting arrangements.

Each major function of patient care and administrative support (e.g., food, electricity, water, medications, supplies) is assessed to determine the quantities of inputs needed and the vendors and suppliers available to meet those needs. An authority–responsibility pattern is developed for each critical function so that a clear chain of command is established, including succession plans indicating who will take over the tasks should the usual job holder become unable to function. The job descriptions and the training programs

**Exhibit 5–1** Relationship of Types of Plans

I. Underlying Purpose/Overall Mission/ Philosophy/Goal
II. Objectives
III. Functional Objectives
IV. Policies
V. Procedures
  V.1 Methods
  V.2 Rules
VI. Work Standards
VII. Performance Standards
VIII. Training Objectives
IX. Management by Objectives
X. Operational Goals

for the succession team members reflects these succession considerations. Plans should also include family well-being considerations (e.g., child care, elder care) so that workers with disrupted schedules may work without distraction and concern.

## Types of Plans

The planning process involves a variety of plans that develop logically from the highly abstract, as in a statement of philosophy or ideal goals, to the progressively concrete, as in operational goals and procedures. Management literature on planning consistently includes the concepts of goals and objectives as central to the planning process. The terms *goal* and *objective* are frequently used interchangeably, except in discussions of management by objectives (MBO). The MBO concept refers to specific, measurable, attainable plans for the unit, department, or organization. For the purposes of this discussion of plans, the concept of goals will be discussed in terms of overall purpose. The concept of objectives will be discussed in terms of more measurable attainable plans, including unit or departmental objectives and functional objectives. **Exhibit 5–1** lists the sequence of planning documents from planning state through controlling by means of operational goals.

## ▶ Core Values, Philosophy, Heritage Statement, and Mission

Individuals who share a common vision and set of values come together to create a formal organization for purposes that are consistent with and derived from

---

**Exhibit 5-2  Mission, Vision, and Values of Community Hospital**

Community Hospital and Health Center exists to serve the community by providing expert, affordable, and readily available evaluation and treatment of the health needs of the residents. Educational and research activities to meet community needs and improve the quality of life of the communities we serve are part of our commitment.

**Vision**

Our vision is to offer health services ranging from primary to specialty care, with coordination among all units, thus encouraging patient care across the continuum of care. We seek to offer cost-efficient, customized care at our facility and to coordinate care with facilities in adjacent geographic areas. We seek partnership with the business, educational, and research communities for the mutual benefit of all.

**Values**

Our organizations govern our actions by the following values:

- Service: excellence and compassion in all aspects of care
- Unity: team approach among the direct care providers and support staff
- Innovation: continuous learning and searching for best practices
- Adaptability: proactive toward change and supportive of others who initiate change
- Communication: openness to receive information and feedback in a nonjudgmental atmosphere

---

their common values. The statement of core values, philosophy, or mission provides an overall frame of reference for organizational practice; it is the basis of the overall goals, objectives, policies, and derived plans. It is the groundwork for the corporate culture ethos. (See **Exhibit 5-2** for a sample of a mission, vision, and values statement of a nonprofit, community-based healthcare center.) Actual practice, as delineated in policies and procedures, should not violate the organization's underlying philosophy. As new members and clients are attracted to the organization and as the organization grows from the gestational to the youthful stage of the life cycle, the statement of principles may be made more explicit. A statement of core values may take one of several forms, such as a creed, a pledge, or a statement of principle. A heritage statement sometimes forms a sort of preamble to the core values statement, providing a context for the values and principles. This provides a context for the values to the historical development and long traditions of the founding/sponsoring organization. Here is an example of wording in a heritage statement:

> Project Caring exists because the citizens of this county recognize their responsibility to care for those in need. From 1914 to 1965, services were largely organized around the institutionalized care of the aged, orphaned, and destitute. Since 1965, the project has expanded its programs to include social and community-based services. It relies primarily on charitable funding and depends on volunteers to help the professional staff.

In addition to reflecting the values of the immediate, specific group that formed the organization, a statement of philosophy may reflect, implicitly or explicitly, the values of the larger society. To one degree or another, for example, society as a whole now accepts the burden of providing for those who need medical care. The concept of health care as a right, regardless of ability to pay, gradually emerged as an explicit value in the 1960s. Emphasis on the rights of consumers and patients emerged in a similar evolutionary pattern in the 1970s. Because free enterprise is a benchmark of the democratic way of life, a trend toward marketing and competition in health care became a feature of the 1980s and 1990s. The early 21st century is characterized by a combination of all of these considerations.

Department managers in a healthcare organization are guided by several philosophical premises. These may differ from, and even be in opposition to, the managers' personal values. However, as members of the executive team, the managers are expected to accept these premises. One of the goals of providing orientation and motivation is to foster acceptance of the underlying purpose of the organization. Typical philosophical premises in health care include the following:

- The basic philosophy of the group that sponsors or controls the healthcare institution (e.g., federal or state government agency, religious or fraternal organization, business concern)
- The guidelines promulgated by national associations regarding patient rights, safety and privacy, and similar issues

- Guidelines of accrediting agencies, such as The Joint Commission, that emphasize continuity of care, patient rights, and other topics
- Guidelines, codes of ethics, and position statements of professional associations (e.g., American Physical Therapy Association, American Health Information Management Association [AHIMA], American Occupational Therapy Association)
- Values of society in general, such as concern for privacy, equal access, employee safety, and consumer/client participation in decision making
- Contemporary trends in the delivery of health care, such as the shift from inpatient acute care to outpatient care and community-based outreach centers; the establishment of independent practices by health professionals (e.g., physical therapists) who formerly provided care only under the direct supervision of physicians; and the emergence of technical levels in several health professions and the acceptance of the care given by technicians; the expanding use of telemedicine.

Mission statements usually remain stable over the life of the organization because the fundamental purpose of the organization remains unchanged. Note that there is another concept of mission, usually associated with military or emergency operations: the mission is specific and limited, and when completed, a new mission is undertaken. The concept of mission in this discussion refers to the relatively unchanging, underlying mission of the healthcare facility.

Medical centers devoted to acute care as well as teaching carry out an ongoing mission consisting of three elements:

- Educating superior physicians
- Enhancing research and knowledge
- Improving health care in the community and region

A specialty assisted living facility defines itself through its mission statement: to provide an assisted living residence for individuals in the early to middle stages of Alzheimer's disease and other related memory impairments, in an environment of warmth, caring, safety, with the comforts and routines of home.

The following are excerpts from statements of philosophy. One health information department has its philosophy stated in a preamble:

Given the basic right of patients to comprehensive, quality health care, health information management, as a service department, provides support and assistance within its jurisdiction to the staff and programs of this institution. A major function of this department is to facilitate continuity of patient care through the development and maintenance of the appropriate health information systems, which shall reflect all episodes of care given by the professional and technical staff in any of the components of this institution.

An educational institution adheres to the following statement of philosophy:

One of the critical elements in an effective approach to health care is the establishment of the spirit and practice of cooperative endeavor among practitioners. Recognizing this need, the Consortium for Interdisciplinary Health Studies seeks to foster the team approach to the delivery of health care.

The following is from the statement of philosophy of a physical therapy department:

The physical therapy department as a component of the healthcare system is committed to providing quality patient care and community services in the most responsive and cost-effective manner possible. In addition, the department will participate in research and investigative studies and provide educational programs for hospital personnel and affiliating students from the various medical and health professions.

The philosophy of an occupational therapy private practice group is stated in these terms:

The Occupational Therapy Consultants, Inc. believe that humans are open systems that both influence and are influenced by the environment. Therefore, individuals are motivated to pursue goal-directed activities that reflect their values, roles, and interest. We use activities and environmental adaptations to provide positive reinforcement and a sense of mastery to our clients. We make "doing" possible.

The mission of this private practice group is as follows:

Occupational Therapy Consultants, Inc. will seek referrals from medical and nonmedical sources and offer high-quality, cost-effective services to clients and their caregivers whose roles, habits, and interests are limited by pathological, congenital, or traumatic incidents. Services, direct and consultative, will be offered in schools, homes, industrial settings, and outpatient facilities.

The mission of a nonprofit organization offering programs for older adults is:

> We affirm the value of older adults in our society. We seek to provide healthcare programs to assist them in maintaining and then enhancing their quality of life. We therefore seek to offer education, information, and services to this end. We offer point-of-entry and subsequent coordination of care.
>
> Our purpose is this, and flows from our original founding in 1990, to provide services to the older adult population (aged 62 and older) in the three contiguous counties of this region. Our three-fold goals are these: to provide coordination of services, both in-home and at community center sites, through social service and nurse case managers; to reduce the need for institutional care through the provision of extensive homecare programs, including transportation, shopping assistance, housekeeping, and meal preparation; to foster and promote research relating to the social, psychological, and physical well-being of older adults, and to advocate on their behalf in legislative and funding initiatives.

The values of the organization are stated explicitly in mission and vision statements. They are embodied in subsequent management practices and documents. Policies and practices for risk management, infection control, and in-service training are additional examples of vision and values informing day-to-day practice. For example, in a sample labor union contract, the shared values of fostering patient care and providing good working conditions are amplified.

## ▶ Overall Goals

The goals of the organization originate in the common vision and sense of mission embodied in the statement of purpose or the underlying philosophy. They reflect the general purpose of the organization and provide the basis for subsequent management action. As statements of long-range organizational intent and purpose, goals are the ends toward which activity is directed. In a sense, a goal is never completely achieved but rather continues to exist as an ideal state to be attained.

Goals serve as a basis for grouping organizations—for example, educational organizations, healthcare institutions, and philanthropic or fraternal associations. Goals, like statements of philosophy, may be found in an organization's charter, articles of incorporation, statement of mission, or introduction to the official bylaws. Again, like the statement of philosophy, the overall goals may not bear a specific label and may be identified only through common understanding. The planning process is facilitated when the philosophy and the goals are formally stated. Derivative plans may then be developed in a consistent manner and with less risk of implementing policies and procedures that violate fundamental values.

This overall goal statement for a publicly sponsored rural health agency is an example of the language and style used in stating these plans. This agency has three primary goals:

- To provide services that will enable older adults to maintain a relatively independent lifestyle in both home and community, rather than becoming dependent on institutional care
- To advocate for older adults in the three-county rural area
- To give priority services to those older persons with the greatest social and economic needs

## ▶ Objectives

In the planning process, the manager makes the plans progressively more explicit. The move from ideal, relatively intangible statements of mission and purpose or overall goal to the "real" plans is accomplished through the development of specific objectives that bring the goals to a practical, working level. Objectives are relatively tangible, concrete plans and are usually stated in terms of results to be achieved. The manager reviews the underlying purpose and basically answers the question: what is my unit or department to accomplish specifically in light of these overall goals?

Achieving specific objectives tends to be a continuous process; the work of the department must satisfy these objectives over and over again. An overall goal such as "to promote the health and well-being of the community" can be accomplished only through a series of specific objectives that are met on a continuing basis. Objectives add the dimensions of quality, time, accuracy, and priorities to goals. The objectives are specific to each unit or department, whereas the overall goals for an organization remain the same for all units.

Objectives may be stated in a variety of ways, and different levels of detail may be used. For example, objectives may be expressed as follows:

- *Quantitatively:* to maintain the profit margin of 6% during each fiscal year by an increase in sales volume sufficient to offset increased cost
- *Qualitatively:* to make effective use of community involvement by the establishment of an advisory committee with a majority of members drawn

from the active clients who live in the immediate geographical community

- *As services to be offered:* to provide comprehensive personal patient care services with full consideration for the elements of good medical care (e.g., accessibility, quality, continuity, efficiency)
- *As values to be supported:* to ensure privacy and confidentiality in all phases of patient care interaction and documentation

Objectives for the department as a whole may include elements essential for proper delineation of all other objectives. These may be stated as objectives for the organization and need not, therefore, be repeated in the subsequent departmental statement of objectives:

- Compliance with legal, regulatory, and accrediting standards and with institutional bylaws
- Risk management factors, including accuracy of assessment and documentation of patient safety protocols
- Privacy and confidentiality in patient care transactions and documentation
- Reference to inpatient as well as outpatient/ambulatory care and other programs sponsored by the organization, such as home care or satellite clinics

Because they are intended to give specificity to overall goals, objectives are the key to management planning. Therefore, objectives must be measurable whenever possible. They must provide for formal accountability in terms of achieving the results. Furthermore, they must be flexible so that they can be adapted to changing circumstances over time.

Two additional planning concepts must be used with the statements of objectives to make them meaningful: the statement of functional objectives and the development of policies. These related plans are both important in fleshing out departmental objectives.

## ▶ Functional Objectives

A functional objective is a statement that refines a general objective in terms of:

- The specific service to be provided
- The type of output
- The quantity and/or specificity of output
- The frequency and/or specificity of output
- Accuracy
- Priorities

Some elements, such as accuracy indicators, may be defined for the department or unit as a whole. A general objective's priority may be implied by its delineation in a related functional objective.

Planning data for organizing and staffing functions may be obtained by inference from statements of objectives. For example, the functional objective statement may include the stipulation that all documentation of patient encounters (e.g., discharge summaries) shall be entered into the electronic health record system. The workload (number of discharge summaries) may be calculated based on the number of discharges per year. A priority system for processing such summaries or a designated turnaround time for such processing provides the necessary parameters for calculating the number of workers needed to meet the objective on a continuing basis. The staffing patterns for day, evening, and night shifts may be developed, again, in a way to satisfy the priority designation and turnaround time contained in the functional objective.

The relationship of the general objective and the functional objectives that support it is illustrated in the following example, drawn from the plans for a transcription/word processing unit of a health information management service.

*General Objective:* Health information management will provide a system for dictation of selected medical reports by specified healthcare practitioners and for the timely and accurate transcription of these reports on a regular basis.

*Functional Objectives:* More specifically, this system will provide for:

1. Dictation services for attending medical staff, house officers, and associated professional staff as defined by the medical staff bylaws
2. Transcription/editing of reports will be done within the following time frame:
    a. Discharge summaries within 8 hours of receipt of dictation
    b. Operative reports within 4 hours of receipt of dictation
    c. Consultation reports within 4 hours of receipt of dictation
    d. Emergency and priority requests on a "stat" basis
3. Coordination of in-service training for using the system:
    a. New employees—at hiring and semi-annually thereafter
    b. Healthcare practitioners—at hiring and as requested thereafter
4. Maintain quality controls through monthly reviews focusing on accuracy and timeliness of report processing

This example specifies the quantity of output and the time frame and implies the priority of the objective through the designation of the time frame. A statement of accuracy is not included, because it is included in the objectives for the department as a whole. This accuracy statement, which may fall under the overall objective of risk management and quality control, may be expressed as follows:

> Health information management strives to carry out its responsibilities and activities with 100% accuracy; therefore, we strive for this level of accuracy.

The following is an example of a general objective and functional objectives from a direct patient care service:

> *General Objective:* The physical therapy department will provide evaluation and assessment procedures appropriate to the patient's condition as requested by the referring physician.
> *Functional Objectives:* More specifically, this system will provide for:

1. Evaluations within (*n*) hours following receipt of the referral.
2. A verbal summary of findings submitted to the physician following the completion of the evaluation.
3. A formal summary of the evaluation entered in the patient's health record within 8 hours following the verbal report.

## ▶ Policies

Policies are the guides to thought and action by which managers seek to delineate the areas within which decisions will be made and subsequent actions taken. Policies spell out the required, prohibited, or suggested courses of action. The limitations on actions are stated, defined, or, at least, clearly implied. Policies *predecide* issues and limit actions so that situations that occur repeatedly are handled in the same way. Because policies are intended to be overall guides, their language is customarily broad.

A balance must be achieved when policies are formulated. These comprehensive guides should be sufficiently specific to provide the user with information about the actions to take, the actions to be avoided, and when and how to respond. At the same time, they should be flexible enough to accommodate changing conditions. They should reinforce and be consistent with the overall goals and objectives. In addition, they should conform to legal and accrediting mandates as well as to any other requirement imposed by internal or external authorities. Policies and related procedures have importance in legal proceedings; they constitute the practices identified as those carried out in the normal course of business. For example, in a challenge to the legal chain of custody of evidence, the usual or customary practices, spelled out in policy and procedure, would involve a review of these documents.

Policies are relatively permanent plans, a kind of cornerstone of other, more detailed plans. Yet they must be sufficiently flexible in intent to permit change in the derived plans without necessitating a change in the policy. For example, a commitment to a centralized dictation–transcription/editing system might be made through a policy statement on health information functions. However, no specification is made as to brand of equipment, exclusive use in in-house staffing, or external agency contract. All remain options as long as the equipment selected and the staffing pattern determined meet the policy considerations of an adequate dictation–word processing function. In the dictation–word processing policy, the essential features of the word processing system are delineated. It is easy to derive from this a decision-making matrix for the comparison and selection of one or another commercial transcription–word processing service. In this sense, a policy statement serves to preform or shape detailed decision making because the overall parameters are stated within the policy or are easily derived from it.

## Sources of Policy

Department or unit managers develop the policies specific to their assigned areas, but these policies must be consistent with those originated by top management. Policies are sometimes implied, as in a tacit agreement to permit an afternoon coffee break. An implied policy may make it difficult to enforce some other course of action, however, if the implied policy has become standard—in spite of its lack of official approval. Policies are shaped in some instances by the effect of exceptions granted; a series of exceptions may become the basis of a new policy, or at least a revision of an existing one. Certain policies may be imposed by outside groups, such as an accrediting agency or a labor union, through a negotiated contract.

A rich trove of policy and related guidelines is available through national associations of the various health professionals. These associations publish practice briefs and best practice guidelines. These sources reflect state-of-the-art practices, and the wording of these documents is carefully crafted to provide clear guidance. These suggested practices and guidelines are supported by research and field testing.

Another source of wording for policy content is the official publication of a law, regulation, or standard. When these are added to a policy, appropriate citation is made and the excerpt is incorporated with the exact wording of the published law, regulation, or standard.

## Wording of Policies

Policies permit and require interpretation. Language indicators, such as "whenever possible" or "as circumstances permit," are expressions typically used to give policies the flexibility needed. Policy statements in a healthcare institution may concern such items as definitions of categories of patients and designations of responsibility. In a health information service, policy statements may specify, for example, a standardized patient record core content, the use of abbreviations, and the processing of urgent requests.

To decrease the sheer volume of policy statements, a glossary may be developed that includes the institutional definition of "patient" as well as definitions of terms and acronyms referring to members of the medical and professional staff and legal and accrediting bodies. Occasionally, a statement of rationale is included in a policy statement, but the manager should avoid excessive explanations; in general, the manager needs to couch policy directives in wording that predecides issues and permits actions. Another useful adjunct to the complete policy statement is the "Policy in Brief"—a short summary of major points for quick reference.

Policies are somewhat futuristic in that they are meant to remain in force, with little change, for extended periods. In an age of rapid social and technical change, it is helpful to think in broad terms, anticipating change. It also helps to set aside the normal biases that stem from describing the way things are now: increasing use of technology (e.g., telemedicine); expanding scope of practice by physician assistants, nurse practitioners, and technical assistants; and changing levels of care.

Departmental policies typically include these topics:

- Scope of service: list the major functions (e.g., coordination of release of information; maintaining a statistical database)
- Hours of operation and provision for access when department is closed
- Staffing: include a statement that there is a mix of full-time and part-time employees, supplemented by contractual services

- Continuity of operations and succession planning
- Confidentiality, privacy, and data security provisions
- Provision of in-service training
- Participation in education and research
- Risk management and continuous quality improvement
- Interdepartmental coordination

The wording in the following examples, drawn from a variety of settings, tends to be broad and elastic yet gives sufficient information to guide the user. The first example is a policy for the waiver of tuition for senior citizens:

> In recognition of their efforts over the years in support of education, the college will waive tuition for academic and continuing education courses for senior citizens who reside in the tricounty area. All residents who are at least 62 years of age and who are not engaged in full-time gainful employment are eligible under this tuition waiver policy. This policy will be subject to annual budgeted funds.

This example provides a general sense of why the college is granting this waiver: in recognition of senior citizen support over the years. The outer limits of its applicability are noted; both academic and continuing education programs are included. A definition of senior citizen is included, and the additional eligibility factors are stated. A final parameter is included to provide flexibility should circumstances change—namely, the limitation determined by the availability of budgeted funds. With this short policy, the necessary procedures can be developed for determining eligibility, and a relatively untrained worker can make the necessary determination.

The following are typical policies for healthcare institutions.

For employee promotion:

> It is the policy of this hospital to promote from within the organization whenever qualified employees are available for vacancies. The following factors shall be considered in the selection of individual employees for promotion: length of service with the organization, above-average performance in present position, and special preparation for promotion. Employees on their present job for a reasonable length of time, excluding probationary period, may request promotion during the customary period in which a job is open and posted as being available.

For admission of patients to a research unit:

Because the primary purpose of this unit is research in specialized areas of medicine, the primary consideration in selecting elective patients for admission to the research unit accommodations is given to the teaching and research value of the clinical findings. The research unit offers two types of service: inpatient and outpatient. The research unit reserves the right to assign patients to either service category, depending on the characteristics of the case and facilities available at the time.

For a physical therapy department:

The Physical Therapy Department shall be open from 8:30 A.M. to 4:30 P.M. Monday through Friday and on weekends and holidays as required to meet patient care needs.

For professional credentials requirements:

All occupational therapy personnel will be licensed and registered.

Each applicant will submit the names of two references, and the human resources officer will contact these individuals and check on the applicant's ability to problem solve and communicate with others and his or her work habits and commitment to patient service delivery.

The director of the occupational therapy department will check to see if the applicant has passed the national certification examination and has a current state license.

Recent graduates or therapists from foreign countries may treat patients but they must be supervised by a licensed and certified occupational therapist who reviews their patient care plans and progress notes.

Occupational therapists may not work more than 6 months under these conditions. If not registered and licensed within 6 months after hire, employment must be terminated.

For Institutional Review Board Policy:

Parental Permission and Child Assent (excerpt) Parents or legal guardians shall be informed that the study involves research whose outcomes cannot be guaranteed. They should be assured that identifiable information about them or their child will be removed from any data or biospecimen. They should be informed that biospecimens could be used for further research without additional consent. They should be assured that these specimens will not be used for commercial purposes. The parents or guardians, and the researcher will explain to the child the details of research protocols to the extent that the child can comprehend this information. Although not legally required, assent/consent will be sought from teenagers below the age of eighteen (or age of consent in the given state).

# ▶ Procedures

A procedure is a guide to action. It is a series of related tasks, listed in chronological order, that constitute the prescribed manner of performing the work. Essential information in any procedure includes the specific tasks that must be done, at what time or under what circumstances they must be done, and who (job title, not name of employee) is to do them. Procedures are developed for repetitive work to ensure uniformity of practice, to facilitate personnel training, and to permit the development of controls and checks in the workflow. Unlike policies, which are more general, procedures are highly specific and need little, if any, interpretation.

Procedures for a specific organizational unit are developed by the manager of that unit. As with other plans, departmental procedures must be coordinated with those of related departments as well as with those developed by higher management levels for all departments. For example, the procedures for patient transport to various specialized service units, such as nuclear medicine, physical therapy, or occupational therapy, are developed jointly by the nursing service and these related departments or services. In contrast, procedures relating to employee matters may well be dictated by top-level management for the organization as a whole with little, if any, procedural development done at the departmental or unit level.

## Procedure Manual Format

There are two common format types used in procedure manuals: narrative and abbreviated narrative. The narrative format contains a series of statements in paragraph form, with special notes or explanations in subparagraphs or in footnotes. This format has the disadvantage of being difficult to refer to quickly and easily. The abbreviated narrative format illustrates procedures through the use of key steps and key points (**Exhibits 5–3, 5–4**, and **5–5**). When a procedure involves several workers or departments, it is useful to identify each participant by job title. The step is

**Exhibit 5–3** Abbreviated Narrative Procedure Formal: Procedure for Terminal Digit Filing

| Key Step | Key Points | |
|---|---|---|
| Terminal digit filing system | Read from right to left, two digits at a time. Explanation: Records are filed in sections by the last two digits to the right, then the middle two digits, then the last two digits to the left. Example: if the history number is 06-52-18, find it this way: | |
| Look here last within the 18 section 06 | Look here second within the 18 section 52 | Look here first 18 18 |
| The last two digits (terminals) are color coded. The colors for each digit always remain the same, and once they are learned they can be used in many combinations of numbers. They help a person file more accurately and quickly. | | |

**Exhibit 5–4** Abbreviated Narrative Procedure Format: Procedure for Interdepartmental Coordination

| Key Step | Key Points |
|---|---|
| Determine patient care need | Review medical care record. Perform appropriate evaluation procedures. Complete related medical documentation, including information needed for consultation. |
| **Key Step** | **Key Points** |
| Contact appropriate department | Make verbal contact via telephone. Confirm through interdepartmental request form for joint conference. |

**Exhibit 5–5** Examples of Key Steps and Detailed Steps

| Key Steps | Sequence | Responsibility | Detailed Steps |
|---|---|---|---|
| Receive the incoming mail: 1. U.S. mail 2. Interdepartmental mail | Step 1 | Release of information clerk | ■ Pick up the mail from the central mail room located in room [___]. ■ The mail is ready for pickup at [___] A.M. ■ The department mailbox is number [___]. |
| Perform the initial processing | Step 2 | Release of information clerk | ■ Sort the mail by general categories: 1. Loose reports received via interoffice mail: Direct these immediately to the Storage and Retrieval unit 2. Mail marked "Confidential": Direct immediately to the department director's assistant 3. U.S. mail not marked "Confidential" ■ Open all mail except that marked "Confidential." ■ Staple the envelope to the back of each letter. ■ Date-stamp each letter in the lower right-hand area. ■ Do not obscure any information, such as the signature or date. |

| Distribute the mail and redirect nondepartmental mail | Step 3 | Release of information clerk | <ul><li>Direct loose reports to the Storage and Retrieval unit.</li><li>Direct "Confidential" mail to the department director's assistant.</li><li>Direct nondepartmental mail for<ol><li>A staff physician to the physician's office (see the telephone directory for office room numbers)</li><li>The outpatient clinic to the clinic coordinator (see the telephone directory for the office room number)</li></ol></li><li>If there is an obvious error by the sender, return the mail immediately to the sender (e.g., if the request for information is for another area hospital).</li></ul> |
| --- | --- | --- | --- |

given a sequence number, key action words are stated, and action sentences are developed for the step (see Exhibit 5–5).

The physical format of the procedure manual is important. A procedure manual should be convenient in size, easy to read, and arranged logically. If the manual is too large or too heavy for everyday use or is difficult to read because of too many unbroken pages of type, workers tend to develop their own procedures rather than referring to the manual for the prescribed steps. The choice of a format that makes it easy to update the manual (e.g., loose-leaf binder) removes a major disadvantage or limitation regarding the manual's use—pages of obsolete procedures. The use of electronic media is, of course, a convenient option.

## Development of the Procedure Manual

The manager who is developing a procedure manual must first determine its purpose and audience (e.g., to train new employees or to bring about uniformity of practice among current employees). The level of detail and the number and kinds of examples depend on the purpose and the audience. Clarity, brevity, and the use of simple commands or direct language improve comprehension. Action verbs that specify actions the worker must take help to clarify the instructions. Keeping the focus of the procedure specific and its scope limited permits the manager to develop a highly detailed description of the steps to be followed. The steps are listed in logical sequence, with definitions, examples, and illustrations.

Methods improvement is a prerequisite for efficient, effective procedure development. Flow charts and flow process charts are useful adjuncts to the procedure manual because they require logical sequencing and make it possible to reduce the backtracking and bottlenecks in the workflow.

## ▶ Methods

The way in which each step of a procedure is to be performed is a method. Methods focus on such elements as the arrangement of the work area, the use of certain forms, or the operation of specific equipment. A method describes the preferred way of performing a task. The manager may develop methods detail as part of the training package for employee development, leaving the procedure manual free of such detail.

## ▶ Rules

One of the simplest and most direct types of plan is a rule. A continuing or repeat-use plan, a rule delineates a required or prohibited course of action. The purpose of rules is to predecide issues and specify the required course of action authoritatively and officially.

Like policies, rules guide thinking and channel behavior. Rules, however, are more precise and specific than policies and, technically, allow no discretion in their application. As a result, management must direct careful attention to the number of rules and their intent. If the management intent is to guide and direct behavior rather than require or prohibit certain actions, the rule in effect becomes a policy and should be issued as such.

Like procedures, rules guide action; unlike procedures, however, rules have no time sequence or chronology. Some rules are contained in procedures (e.g., "Extinguish all smoking material before entering this facility"). Other rules are independent of any procedure and stand alone (e.g., "No smoking"). The wording of rules is direct and specific, such as:

- Food removed from the cafeteria must be in covered containers.

- Books returned to the library after 4:00 P.M. will be considered as returned the following day, and a late fine will be charged.
- Children younger than the age of 12 must be accompanied at all times by an adult who is responsible for their conduct.

# ▶ Project Planning

In addition to developing the operational plans for day-to-day functioning, managers sometimes undertake intensive project planning for major initiatives. Examples include:

- Implement an organization-wide electronic health record over a 4-year period.
- Develop a regional poststroke rehabilitation center over a 2-year period.
- Enhance the revenue cycle processes to maximize reimbursement by collecting all the revenues to which the organization is entitled. To accomplish this in a timely manner, systems and workflow changes are to be implemented during the first 3 months of the new fiscal year.
- Develop a leadership succession plan for the next 3 years in anticipation of planned retirement of (*n*) executive-level managers.

Extensive projects, such as planning and opening a new service, developing an educational division, or expanding an existing program to include satellite facilities, generally fall under the rubric of major project planning.

A major project reflects the elements of general planning (e.g., assumptions, constraints, goals and objectives, timeline). Project planning is sometimes expressed primarily in terms of time frame, as in a 500-day plan to gain momentum and to demonstrate major achievements. In the 500-day plan, a rolling cycle of designated periods is delineated (e.g., 90 days, 100 days, 13 weeks), with adjustments to the plan made at the conclusion of each phase. The designated periods are not necessarily the same for each activity. As one phase is completed, an additional phase is added until the rollout of the project has occurred. Planning for the next phase is fine-tuned in light of the outcomes in the preceding period. The goals for such initiatives reflect actions that have the potential to yield the most results. For example, a fetal alcohol syndrome disorders clinic might focus on early intervention through emphasis on prenatal care. Other aspects of the program simultaneously unfold, but the major focus is this aspect of care.

## The Project Manager

The project manager is the designated coordinator of the planning and execution of the project. For large, organization-wide projects, this manager may hold an executive level position. For projects within a division or department, the middle manager might take on that role, or he or she might delegate it to an assistant who has authority and responsibility over the system that is the focus of the project. Sometimes an outside consultant is hired as the project manager as in the case of new products, systems, and equipment. This individual would have knowledge of the new system, along with expertise in implementation. Colleges and universities, along with private organizations, offer training and certification in project management. Professional organizations offer similar programs, tailored to the interests and needs of the particular profession.

# ▶ Elements and Examples of Major Projects

At the outset of developing a major project, the project manager and team decide on the desired level of detail of the plan. In general, a major project includes the customary elements, described here, with some examples of wording. **Exhibit 5-6** provides a more detailed example of the project elements, timelines, and wording of a major project plan with a 500-day timetable. This type of plan is the framework for many derivative plans. It is essential that no shortcuts be taken; in terms of its nature, such a plan is very detailed. Some elements may seem obvious or excessively plodding, but a manager must resist the temptation to gloss over seemingly small details.

## Name of Project

This should be precise but informative, as in *Developing and Implementing a Neighborhood Health Center in the Northeast Catchment Area of the City of Clarion*.

## Focus and Scope of the Project

This section provides an overview of the project. Specify whether the project is a new one or an extension of an existing project. Provide brief background information. Has funding been obtained? Have feasibility studies completed? Sample wording of focus and scope might be:

> This new project has as its focus the development and implementation of a comprehensive neighborhood health center in catchment area 25 of Clarion City's master health plan. The projected time line is augmented by a detailed timeline and milestone event listing included in the body of this proposal. The overall timeline is:
>
> - January 1, year one: Development phase
> - July 1, year one: Phase One—limited opening of clinic for maternal and infant care as well as school-age youth care
> - October 1, year one: Phase Two—opening of all the remaining clinics; programs fully operational
> - July 1, year two: Transition from grant funding to freestanding, community-sponsored clinic, with 6-month transition funding (July–December)
> - January 1, year three: Transition funding ends; clinic is self-supporting

## Scope of Service

The clinic is a primary care facility, with as-needed referrals to a tertiary care hospital and specialty clinics. It deals with ambulatory care—scheduled, walk-in, or urgent.

The target population includes mothers and infants, preschool and school-age children and youth, and adults. There is a special emphasis on homeless youths and adults. (The target population figures/planned numbers would be given here.)

## Project Manager and Project Team

Key personnel are identified, with a listing of name, title, and organizational authority/responsibility. For example:

> The Project Manager is Dr. Leslie H. Deal, Associate Vice President for Community Outreach, Clarion Health Systems. Project Manager Associates are the designated representatives from the direct patient care and support services staff. (A list of names and titles would be given here.) These associates report directly to the project manager, who, in turn, reports to the Vice President for Community Outreach, Clarion Health Systems.

## Time Frame and Milestone Events

The time frame provided in the opening section on the focus and scope of the project is repeated and amplified in this section. Managers develop a level of detail best suited to the project and their management style. If time is critical, with little or no leeway, and/or if there are multiple contingent activities, the timeline is detailed and precise. For example, time specifications could include three estimated time calculations: the probable, most likely (realistic considerations noted); the pessimistic (if everything or many things go wrong); and the optimistic (everything goes as scheduled, no equipment breakdowns, no staff turnover, no delay in obtaining material). The beginning and ending time frame for each activity is specified.

Milestone events are listed. These are the markers for major accomplishments, such as completion of equipment selection, completion of site renovations, and accomplishment of an immunization and physical examination program for preschool children.

Activities are carried out to lead to the completion of a milestone or landmark event. For example, developing a job analysis, job descriptions, and a wage and salary scale for clerical and technical support staff leads to the milestone of completion of foundational analysis and description of clerical and technical support staff documents. *Note:* Activities and events are not solely sequential; some activities, and therefore the accomplishment of events, may occur simultaneously.

## Cost Factors

Project managers develop a related tracking process for budgeting; the monitoring timeline is associated closely with the step-by-step implementation. This financial monitoring and auditing can be built into the evaluation process.

## The Evaluation Process

Both public and private organizations require sound evaluation processes. The federal government's Program Evaluation for Effectiveness Review is one example of detailed evaluation requirements. Program evaluation focuses on the systematic collecting, evaluating, and using information to answer the basic question. Did the program accomplish what it set out to do? Did the program meet its proposed goals?

There are two categories of evaluation: process and outcome. Process evaluation focuses on the start-up activities that need to be in place before direct services can be offered (e.g., site location secured, physical

**Exhibit 5–6** Project Plan for Neighborhood Health Center with 500-Day Timeline

(*Note:* This exhibit shows excerpts from the project plan to illustrate the usual content and wording. There would be several supplementary attachments, such as budget and audit protocols.)

### Name of Project

Development and Implementation of a Neighborhood Health Center in the Northeast Catchment Area of the City of Clarion

### Focus and Scope of the Project

This new project has its focus on the development and implementation of a neighborhood health center (NHC) in catchment area 25 of Clarion City's master health plan. The health center's services will be coordinated with the city health department clinic and the outpatient clinics of the University Hospital's tertiary care center. A combination of a federal grant and private funding has been secured by the University Hospital for the first 2 years of operation. A plan for transition to freestanding status has been developed. The grant application, including feasibility study and related background information, is attached.

   A full range of services will be offered. There will be primary care, with as-needed referrals to the University Hospital tertiary care hospital and its clinics. Ambulatory care will include both scheduled and walk-in routine and urgent care services. The target population is a mix of adult and children. Initial emphasis will be given to maternal and infant care and young child care (preschool children and children in primary grades). Then the scope of service will be expanded to older children and adults. Special emphasis will be given to homeless youth and adult populations.

### Overall Time Frame

| | |
|---|---|
| January 1, 20x1–June 30, 20x1 | Preliminary development phase |
| July 1, 20x1–September 30, 20x1 | Phase One of clinic service: maternal and infant care, young child care (preschool children and children in primary grades) |
| October 1, 20x1–November 30, 20x1 | Phase Two of clinic service: general population (youths and adults); clinic fully operational |
| December 1, 20x1–December 31, 20x1 | Phase Three: outreach program begun for homeless (both youth and adult) |
| July 1, 20x2–December 31, 20x2 | Transition phase from University Hospital sponsorship to freestanding neighborhood center, under sponsorship and control of community agency |
| January 2, 20x3 | Independent, freestanding neighborhood center fully operational, with 2-month transitional funding from grant obtained by community agency |
| March 1, 20x3 | Fully self-sustaining clinic |

   (A detailed timeline, with key events, is attached.) The 500-day pattern of planning cycles reflects 100-day cycles, with the rolling addition of 100-day cycles as each planned cycle is completed.

### Project Manager and Project Team

The Project Manager is Dr. Leslie H. Deal, Associate Vice President for Community Outreach, University Hospital. Project Manager Associates are the designated representatives from the direct patient care staff and administrative support services of the hospital. (A complete list of names, titles, and responsibilities is attached.) The associate project managers report directly to the project manager who, in turn, reports to the Vice President for Community Outreach, University Hospital.

### Cost Factors and Tracking

The generally accepted financial practices will be followed. This includes a monthly internal audit by the finance department of University Hospital; special oversight review and audit by the Vice President for Community Outreach to conform to grant funding requirements. A quarterly audit by an independent auditing firm augment the internal audits. (Sample audit protocols are attached.)

## Evaluation

Both internal and external evaluation processes have been developed. Evaluations will be done throughout each phase of the project. Their frequency varies from 1 month to 6 weeks to quarterly, depending on the focus of the review. Process evaluation methods will be used for administrative activities. Outcome evaluation methods will be used to reflect patient care and client and community-at-large satisfaction with clinic services. (A detailed listing of the timeline and evaluation methods is attached.)

Evaluators include internal review committees and teams and external, independent reviews, including peer teams from the sponsoring hospital and its related university, as well as peer professionals from clinics in the region. An independent review will be carried out by a designated accrediting agency that provides preliminary coaching reviews for outpatient services.

## Detailed Timeline of Activities: 500-day plan (excerpts)

**Cycle One**: 100 days (January 1, 20n1–April 10, 20n1)

### January

- Incorporation filed; state agency approval to operate received
- Physical site secured; renovations begun
- Administrative processes developed
- Mission; goals and objectives; policies; procedures
- Staffing patterns developed
- Monthly budget review and reconciliation completed by NHC staff

(This review will be done every month and would be listed as an activity and related event for each month using this same wording.)

### February

- Neighborhood community board configured and members selected and oriented
- Collaborative arrangements completed for mutual referrals (University Hospital, city health department clinics, local schools—prekindergarten and primary grades)
- Monthly budget review of previous month completed
- Process evaluation completed by peer review team from University Hospital and NHC staff
- Process evaluation completed regarding legal, regulatory, corporate compliance (carried out by Vice President for Corporate Compliance and Chief Development Officer of University Hospital)
- Patient care practitioners and administrative support staff recruited for Phase One: program opening (for July 1)

### March

- Equipment selected, received, and debugged
- Quarterly external financial audit and budget review completed
- Pilot run completed (intake and registration; flow of patient care through care site)
- Peer group review of administrative and patient care processes completed by NHC staff and University Hospital clinic counterparts

### April

- Direct patient care staff and administrative support staff recruited for Phase Two of clinic operations (scheduled for late October)
- Quarterly financial audit completed by external auditors
- Process evaluation of administrative functions completed by NHC staff

**Cycle Two:** 100 days (April 11, 20n1–July 19, 20n1)

### April

- Outreach to community completed (detailed outreach plan is attached)

### May

- All hiring and orientation completed
- All requirements met regarding billing Medicare, Medicaid, and city health agency

*(continues)*

**Exhibit 5–6** Project Plan for Neighborhood Health Center with 500-Day Timeline    *(continued)*

*June*
- Pilot run completed: sampling of patient population recruited and treated (200 maternal and infant care patients, 50 prekindergarten children)
- Final review of administrative and patient care processes completed

*July 1*
- NHC officially opened

**Cycle Three:** 100 days (July 20, 20n1–October 28, 20n1)

*July*
- Evaluation of outreach program completed by NHC staff

*August*
- Outreach program completed (youth and adults for Phase Two)
- Outreach program evaluation completed (NHC staff, community board, representatives from local schools)

*September*
- Outcome evaluations completed for maternal and infant care and prekindergarten care
- Additional staff for Phase Three hired and oriented (social worker and nurse practitioner)
- Outreach program for Phase Two completed (general population)
- Process review of intake and care flow completed (maternal and infant care and prekindergarten care)
- Patient satisfaction information captured and compiled (maternal and infant care)

*October*
- Phase Two programs opened (general population)
- Agreements with nonprofit Host Home Program for at-risk youths completed
- Agreements with local homeless shelters (referrals) completed
- Quarterly external financial audit completed

**Cycle Four:** 100 days (October 29, 20n1–February 5, 20n2)

*November*
- Transportation needs survey completed and analyzed
- Community Board input and review of transportation needs completed
- Action plan developed:
  - Donation of van obtained
  - Schedule of transportation to and from University Hospital specialty clinics developed
  - Van driver hired ($10.00/hour for 8-hour day Monday through Friday)
  - Budget allocations reassigned to cover driver's wages and fringe benefits; money taken from training budget and from refurbishing funds for 20x2; arrangements made for free training by University faculty as an in-kind donation

*December*
- Homeless and at-risk youths outreach extended to youths not attending school (street outreach, soup kitchen, emergency winter shelters in catchment area [four overnight shelters, two day shelters])
- Coordination of shelter services with partnering agencies completed (focus on homeless adults)
- Coordination of services, and referral processes completed (community mental health agencies for adults; clean and sober programs for adults)
- Process survey completed (focus on patient/client satisfaction with transportation and with intake-care flow)
- Peer review completed
  - Focus on administrative processes: regional peers
  - Focus on direct care provision: regional peers

*January*
- Quarterly external financial audit completed
- Internal review completed: billing compliance (review team coordinated by Vice President for Compliance and Chief Financial Officer of University Hospital)
- Patient care outcomes review completed (focus on wellness and immunizations; medication compliance; patterns of care: chronic conditions of diabetes, obesity, and blood pressure)

*February*

■ Process evaluation: review of transportation services completed

**Cycle Five:** 100 days (February 6–May 17, 20n2)

*February*

■ Repeat patient care outcomes evaluations completed; comparison study completed

*March*

■ External regional peer review completed (focus on administrative processes and outcomes, with emphasis on data from comparison studies)

*April*

■ Quarterly external financial audit completed
■ Community agency, nonprofit corporation formed
■ Preliminary plans for transition in 20n3 begun
■ Outcomes review completed: community-at-large survey

*May*

■ Transitional funding request for 20n3 completed and submitted to city's Community Development Fund

　　May 17, 20n2 END OF FIRST 500-DAY CYCLE

**Cycle Six:** 100 days (May 18, 20n2–August 26, 20n2)
(activities and events reflecting ongoing operations)

**Cycle Seven:** 100 days (August 27, 20n2–December 5, 20n2)
August (activities and events reflecting ongoing operations)

*September*

■ External funding for transition received
　October

■ Quarterly external financial audit completed
■ Billing compliance internal review completed
■ Additional administrative processes implemented regarding incomplete and late billing
■ Preliminary close out for line items in budget completed
■ Revenue projections for 20n3 completed

*November*

■ Transition plan completed

*December 5*

■ Transition plan implemented

**Cycle Eight:** 100 days (December 6, 20n2–March 16, 20n3)

*December*

■ Process review of all administrative systems completed
■ Outcomes review of patient care (all categories) completed
■ Due Diligence Review completed
■ December 31, 20n2:
　● Official end of University Hospital sponsorship
　● End of 2-year funding grant

*January 1*

■ New funding cycle (transitional funds) begun

*February*

■ Detailed plan for self-sufficiency funding developed and implemented
■ Final audit of 2-year University Hospital funding completed (reflecting late charges and final billing as well as closeout of budget line items)

*March 16*

■ Transitional funding completed; clinic is fully self-sustaining renovations completed, license to operate obtained). In addition to a major process review at the end of the development phase of the project, ongoing process review occurs throughout the life of the project to ensure smooth operations. For example, in a project with limited service offerings, followed by full-scale service offerings, particular attention would be given to the functionality of the systems when the program is expanded. Evaluation methods could include sampling of workflow, equipment, error rates, turnaround times, flow of intake, and registration process.

Outcome evaluation focuses on the results in terms of effect on target population. Did the project reach the intended numbers and categories of patients? Factual data are presented. For example, data for a social service project might show:

| | Goal (# of persons) | # of Cases | # of Persons |
|---|---|---|---|
| Planned | 1500 clients | 300 | 5 per case (average) |
| Actual | 1200 clients | 240 | 5 Per case (average) |

A short narrative explanation of reasons for overprojection or underprojection would be included.

If the project focus includes behavior changes in patients, these would be reported (e.g., successful smoking cessation rates, wellness behaviors). Client satisfaction with services is another indicator of program success. (Interviews and surveys are the source of this information.)

The sources of information about patient care outcomes include studies drawn from documented care, patient satisfaction surveys, aggregate data about infection rates, patterns of "no-show" appointments or noncompliance, and number of return visits. If there are unexpected results, these are explained in detail. For example, the need for coordination of transportation from clinic to tertiary hospital's clinics might surface. Or the planned focus on school-age at-risk youth might have changed to a wider focus to include at-risk youth who no longer attend school.

The evaluation process properly includes both internal and external review, along with appropriate intervals of review. One final review is insufficient to make course adjustment. The internal review and its time frames are developed to correspond with milestone events (e.g., frequent reviews during development phase to ensure on-time opening of a clinic). These reviews are internal for the most part. An outside peer review, perhaps from the affiliated health system, would usually be invited because the systems of the two organizations need coordination. External review teams include the peer review, as noted, along with coaching reviews by accrediting agencies, external financial audit, or community boards.

Exhibit 5–6 provides excerpts from a major project, coupled with the 500-day planning approach. See also Chapter 12 of this text on strategic planning and related examples.

# ▸ The Plan and the Process

Referring back to the beginning of the chapter, it is perhaps pertinent to offer a reminder that planning always involves tentatively deciding what might be done in a time period that is not yet here—that is, at some point anywhere from the very near to the far distant future. People plan because they do not know for certain what changes will occur in the environment; they plan because every decision carries with it some elements of risk and uncertainty.

Of course, the environment will change between the time people make their tentative decisions and the time the future becomes the present, and of course they enter the overall process with less-than-perfect information about not only what the future will bring but often also what the present contains. Because change is continual and only partially predictable, people know at the outset that rarely will their plans be fulfilled exactly as planned. This does not, however, mean that planning is a futile activity. On the contrary, it means all the more than might be suspected that planning is essential.

In and of themselves, plans—those collections of stated targets with dates and desired results attached—are not especially valuable. What is of inestimable value is the planning *process*, that cycle of activities in which people gather information, tentatively decide what is to be done and do it, monitor progress, alter methods as the environment changes and the unforeseen occurs, modify targets as necessary, and go through it all over again but differently. Even if the stated target remains fixed and valid but not attained, the simple presence of the target provides information people would not have had without it—they know by how much they missed, and thus they know how much they must correct their approach for the next attempt.

Giving special attention to the decision-making phase may be a useful adjunct to this phase of planning.

# ▸ Decision Making

## Evaluating a Decision's Importance

By its nature, decision making means commitment. The importance of a decision may be measured in terms of both the resources and the time being committed. Some decisions affect only small segments of the organization, whereas others involve the entire organization. Some decisions are irrevocable because they create new situations. The degree of flexibility that remains after the commitment has been made may also be used when evaluating the significance of a decision. Are the resulting conditions tightly circumscribed, with little flexibility permitted, or are several options still available in developing subsequent plans? Decisions regarding capital expenditures, major procedural systems, and the cost of the equipment that must be prorated over the projected life of the equipment are examples.

The degree of uncertainty—and therefore the degree of risk—associated with a decision is another dimension that must be evaluated in weighing its impact. The greater the impact in terms of time, resources, and degree of risk, the more time, money, and effort that must be directed toward making such decisions. Uncertainty is caused, in part, by a lack of necessary information or the impossibility obtaining comprehensive, reliable data. The consequence of some events may not be known until an action or a project has been undertaken and sufficient information is generated to make additional plans.

The management team must proceed in some instances without full certainty. There are costs associated with inaction and indecision. For example, the opportunity to expand a program, to increase client base, or to obtain special funding may be lost if timely action is not taken. Other aspects of inability to make decisions, which have associated costs and impacts, include:

- Failure or delay in making necessary capital improvements, resulting in (1) increased safety hazards for clients and workers and (2) greater costs due to deterioration of physical plant
- Loss of licensure or accreditation because of failure to meet standards
- Decrease in client perception of the organization's quality, causing clients to seek service elsewhere

Therefore, the management team attends to decision making, even in the face of uncertainty. The team uses such strategies as incremental implementation, taking advantage of the unfolding dynamic in which unknowns become knowns; thus, uncertainties become clearer, and plans can be revised.

The degree of impact and probability could be assessed through certain terms, including:

*High impact with low probability*: For example, a young client chooses to obtain disability and long-term care insurance; he is in his early twenties and has no history of major illness, no disability, and no family history of genetic disorders. Should he develop some such condition, there would be high impact (e.g., job loss/income loss, high cost of long-term care); the probability, given his history, is low.

*High impact with high probability*: For example, serious weather-related disruption to a healthcare facility located in a region of annual hurricanes. The storm-related destruction results in high impact; the regional location indicates high probability.

*Short- or long-term impact*: For example, the short-term impact of a temporary relocation of a clinic during major renovations is projected as 4 months; contrast that to the physical relocation of the entire agency to another geographic area. The decisions relating to a major relocation have long-term impact because such decisions are relatively permanent.

*Degree of reversibility of decision*: For example, ending an affiliation with a medical school training program for an academic cycle. The decision to reaffiliate could be made during the next academic cycle. Much more difficulty arises in ending a relationship with an umbrella corporation, thus becoming an independent healthcare entity. Re-establishing complex corporate arrangements involves root decision making by both parties and is subject to stringent review.

Finally, in any organization, effects of a decision on humans are a major factor. The environmental impact and social costs must be assessed. Decisions have a cascading impact—sometimes positive, sometimes negative. In the planning–decision phase, managers anticipate second- and third-order effects: the desired outcome is the first cause–effect dyad. This, in turn, causes a second-order effect, which leads to a third-order effect. By way of example: consider the decision by a healthcare team to open an outreach, walk-in clinic in a busy, congested neighborhood. This is done with the positive result of easier access by clients to the care they desire. As the client usage rises, so does the traffic and related parking congestion; this second-order effect is a negative one, with both merchants and residents becoming disaffected with the clinic. They, in turn, begin to boycott the clinic and call for increasing inspection and regulation of the facility; this is a third-order event.

Managers try to anticipate second- and third-order effects in order to prevent or mitigate them. Managers seek to avoid unanticipated consequences, as for example, the efficient regrouping of transportation for frail, elderly people in a continuing care facility. In one instance, instead of picking up one person at a time, designated pick-up stations were set up. This resulted in more falls and accidents in inclement weather, causing obvious harm to the clients, and an increase in lawsuits for negligence. Originally, the cost-savings idea had seemed like a good one, but the reality reflected a different result. Both positive and negative factors influence the process by which alternatives are evaluated.

## Evaluation of Alternatives

To evaluate alternatives, a manager must adopt an underlying philosophical stance and make a preliminary decision about the approach to decision making that will be taken. Depending on this philosophical stance, certain alternatives will be considered acceptable, and others will be excluded automatically. Root and branch decision making, satisficing, maximizing, and the use of Paretian optimality are among the fundamental types of (or approaches to) decision making that partially determine the decisions that are actually reached.

## Root and Branch Decision Making

Certain decisions are so basic to the organization's nature that their effects are pervasive and far-reaching in terms of organizational values, philosophy, goals, and overall policies. Such decisions—termed *root decisions*—invest the organization with its fundamental nature at its inception and carry it through periodic, comprehensive reviews of its fundamental purpose, often resulting in massive innovation. Thus, in the life cycle of an organization, root decisions may be associated with gestation, when the fundamental form and purpose of the organization are crystallized. They may also occur in middle age, when new goals are developed and new organizational patterns are adopted. Finally, during old age and decline, a fundamental decision to dissolve the organization may be made.

The pervasive effect of root decisions may be seen in the decision of a board of trustees to change a 2-year college into a baccalaureate degree–granting institution or to convert a hospital into a multicomponent healthcare center. Consider the decision made by a health information administrator who chooses to use off-site commercial storage for hard copy records. When this change is implemented, the existing space for hard copy records will be eliminated and will not easily be recovered. Policies and procedures, budget considerations, and changes in staffing patterns also result. Such a decision has long-lasting implications. For these reasons, it ranks as a root decision.

Other examples of root decisions can be found in the major changes made by some professional associations, such as the AHIMA's decision to open active membership to all who are interested in the primary work of this organization. Another example of such change is the American Physical Therapy Association's decision to emphasize doctoral-level preparation as the norm for its practitioners.

Management theorist Charles Lindblom described root decisions and their opposite, *branch* or *incremental decisions*.[2] According to Lindblom, these incremental, limited, successive decisions do not involve a reevaluation of goals, policies, or underlying philosophy. Rather, objectives and goals are recycled and policies are accepted without massive review and revision. Change occurs by degree, and only a small segment of the organization is affected.

Branch decision making is more conservative in its approach than is root decision making, with innovation being inhibited during the former. The stability of organizational life is enhanced, in many cases, when decision making is of the successive, incremental type, because the manager does not have the option of completely reviewing the organizational structure, functions, staffing patterns, equipment selection, and similar capital expenditures. Incrementalism also simplifies decision making because it tends to limit conflicts that might occur if the patterns of compromise, consensus, organizational territory, and subtle internal politics are disturbed. Moreover, incrementalism may be the simple outcome of previous root decisions. However, the manager may overlook some excellent alternatives because they are not readily apparent in the chain of successive decisions. Incrementalism lacks the built-in safeguard of explicit, programmed review of values and philosophy.

## Satisficing and Maximizing

"It might easily happen that what is second best is best, actually, because that which is actually best may be out of the question." This quotation, attributed to the philosopher–educator Cardinal Newman, expresses the idea contained in the concepts of satisficing and maximizing. In decision making, the one best solution may be determined by developing a set of criteria against which all alternatives are compared until one solution emerges as clearly preeminent. In the form of decision making known as *maximizing*, this one best solution is the only acceptable one.

In the form of decision making known as *satisficing* (a term used by Simon[3]), a set of minimal criteria is developed, and any alternative that fulfills those criteria is considered acceptable. A course of action that is "good enough" is selected, with the conscious recognition that better solutions may exist. When the manager seeks several options, satisficing may be employed. Like incrementalism, satisficing obstructs absolute, rational, optimal decision making, yet it simplifies the process. In satisficing, the manager accepts the fact that not every decision need be made with the same degree of intensity.

## The Pareto Principle (Paretian Optimality)

Vilfredo Pareto (1848–1923) was an Italian economist and sociologist who postulated a criterion for decision making that is referred to as the *Pareto principle* or *Paretian optimality*.[4] He suggested that each person's needs be met as much as possible without any loss to another person. In this mode of decision making, certain alternatives are rejected because they would produce a decrease in benefits for one or several groups. Decisions that result in a major gain for one individual with a concomitant major loss for another are avoided. This approach involves compromise and consensus, with each manager accepting the needs of other units of the organization as legitimate and the needs of the organization as a whole as paramount. The concessions and trade-offs in the budget process or in the labor negotiation process illustrate the balance required to satisfy the needs of many departments or groups without penalizing any one of them (or by penalizing all departments or groups in equal measure if penalties are unavoidable).

## Continuing Assessment of Decisions

Two major tools for evaluating the outcome of decisions are the after-action review (AAR) along with the OODA loop analysis. The second useful method is the analysis of unintended consequences.

The decision-making process includes continuous analysis of decisions. Through the feedback process, a new agenda is generated and new alternatives are revealed. The steps in the control process provide a link back to the planning and decision-making functions. This feedback process necessarily pervades organizational life. Planned, formal review is built into operational plans and decisions such as budget preparation, accrediting self-study processes, and labor union contract review. In addition, there is need for continuous real-time assessment of decisions that require rapid response to changing situations. An example of such a condition is an outbreak of an epidemic; disruption of service because of a protracted and polarizing labor strike is another such circumstance.

In this type of situation, the AAR and the classic OODA loop, or Boyd cycle, provide methods of rapid assessment and real-time adjustments to the pressing situation. This strategy was developed by Colonel John Boyd of the U.S. Air Force (retired) and has been widely used in military operations.[5] Businesses have adopted the general schematics of the OODA loop in responding to rapid change in their own and their competitors' environment. OODA is the acronym for:

- *Observe:* the fact-gathering stage, which emphasizes the immediate situation and its changed reality
- *Orient:* an assessment of one's own position in relation to the changed situation
- *Decide:* a rapid decision to commit to a new course of action in light of the changed circumstances
- *Action:* implementation of the new course of action immediately, without delay

The use of the OODA loop is predicated on managerial flexibility and a high degree of delegation of authority. This decision-making process is intended for use in the field by highly skilled professionals who need to act without continual reference back to some other authority. Rapid adjustment to the plans is a key characteristic.

The AAR, or "hotwash" review, is a method used in emergency response–disaster management. As soon as possible after the crisis has been dealt with, but before the response team leaves, a rapid review is completed—what worked, what did not, and what situations need further review; lessons learned. For example, on the "plus" side, there may have been rapid and coordinated response of two or more local service units with a coordinated disaster response. When surge capacities at the treatment sites were reached, adequate supplies and personnel were available. On the "minus" side, there also may have been portable lighting on scene that was insufficient, traffic diversion that needed to be accomplished earlier, and radio frequencies that required recalibration. Using AARs, a lessons-learned session may be held at a later date to consolidate the findings and make recommendations. Some other situations in which the AAR is used include an immediate review after surveyors have finished their site visit; a review of a strike plan immediately at the conclusion of the strike; immediately after a misadventure such as live TB vaccine exposure in a research unit. A detailed example of an AAR is provided in Chapter 7 in the scenario reflecting group deliberation.

## Analysis of Unanticipated Consequences

The following examples reveal the results of decisions that, at one level, lead to successful outcomes, but with a less-than-positive overall outcome. A national professional association, for example, begins extensive webinar offerings for continuing education, with great success. However, local and regional associations and local community colleges experience a drastic drop in attendance at their continuing education offering. One example from an emergency department illustrates a helpful process, but one that violates patient privacy. A nurse assistant moves through the busy ER, asking patients about their situation, and groups them by common need. In a similar attempt to improve patient safety and reduce risk, a patient is asked repeatedly, in earshot of others, what is their name and date of birth. With medical identity theft being a growing problem, this practice needs rethinking. One final example involves a pleasant outreach to new parents. A photo wall of newborns includes names and dates of birth along with the photos; again, this is an opportunity for identity theft. See also the section on "When Plans Fail" in Chapter 13.

## ▶ Decision-Making Tools and Techniques

Managers have available a variety of historical records, information about past performance, and summaries of their own and other managers' experience. In addition, managers may test alternatives through the use of decision-making tools and techniques.

## Considered Opinion and Devil's Advocate

A manager may obtain the considered opinion of experts and use the technique of the "devil's advocate" to sharpen the arguments for and against an alternative. In the first instance, the manager asks staff experts or other members of the management team to assess the several alternatives and develop arguments for and against each. The resulting comparative assessment helps the decision maker to select a course of action.

When the devil's advocate technique is used, the decision maker assigns an individual or group the duty of developing statements of all the negative aspects or weaknesses of each alternative. Each alternative is then tested through frank discussion of weaknesses and errors before the final decision is made. The underlying theory is that it is better to subject alternatives to strict, internal, organized criticism than to run the risk of having a hidden weakness or error exposed after a decision has been implemented. The devil's advocate does not make the decision but simply develops arguments to ensure that all aspects are considered.

## The Factor Analysis Matrix

For the decision maker who must overcome personal preference to make an impartial decision, the matrix of comparative factors is an effective tool of analysis. As a first step, the decision maker develops the criteria under two major categories: essential elements (musts) and desired elements (wants). The manager begins this process by listing key factors relating to the topic. For example, in weighing alternatives to select an outsourcing service for dictation–transcription functions, the manager would consider the following points:

- Health Insurance Portability and Accountability Act (HIPAA)-compliant encryption
- Accepts dictation from landline phone systems and personal digital assistant devices
- Document distribution system by secure e-mail and remote print
- Electronic edit and authentication
- One-screen tracking of documentation from beginning of recording through the finished document received at the client site
- Temporary or total outsourcing services for seasonal peak loads
- Customized formatting
- STAT capability
- 24-hour/365-day support center
- Turnaround time of 12 hours for routine reports
- Conformity with standardized billing method principles
- Zero capital investment on site: use of standard Internet connections

The choices available are compared by developing a table or matrix. The factors can be assigned relative weights, as in a point scale, with the alternative with the highest point value becoming the best option. Even without the weighting factors, the matrix remains useful as a technique of factual comparison. **Table 5–1** illustrates the use of the "must" and "want" categories to compare equipment for departmental use. A similar process could be used to evaluate applicants for a job; personal bias can be set aside more easily and candidates compared on the basis of their qualifications for the position (**Table 5–2**).

## The Decision Tree

A managerial tool used to depict the possible directions that actions might take from various decision points, the decision tree forces the manager to ask the "what then" questions (i.e., to anticipate outcomes). Possible events are included, with a notation about the probabilities associated with each. The basic decisions are stated, with all the unfolding, probable events branching out from them. Decision trees enable managers to undertake disciplined speculation about the consequences, including the unpleasant or negative ones, of actions. Through the use of decision trees, managers are forced to delineate their reasoning, and the constraints imposed by probable future events on subsequent decisions become evident. Each decision tree reveals the probable new situation that results from a decision.

**Table 5–1** Matrix of Comparison for Equipment Purchase

|  | Brand A | Brand B | Brand C |
|---|---|---|---|
| ■ Maximum cost | Acceptable | Acceptable | $14,000 |
| ■ Compatibility with related equipment | Yes | Yes | No |
| ■ Expected years of service<br>■ 5 year minimum | 5 years | 5 years | 3 years |
| ■ Availability of service | Yes | Yes | Yes |
| ■ Renovation of existing space needed | No | Yes | No |
| • Safety features | Yes | Yes | Yes |
| • Trade-in value for present equipment | No | No | Yes |
| • Available delivery date | Yes | No | Yes |
| • Special training for use | No | Yes | Yes |
| • Lease option | No | No | Yes |

■ = must (required); • = want (desirable)

**Table 5–2** Matrix for Evaluation of Job Applicants

|  | Applicant A | Applicant B | Applicant C |
|---|---|---|---|
| Meets productivity standard at Level 1 | Level 2 | Level 2 | Level 1 |
| Previous experience in this type job | 0 | 1 year | 1 year |
| Previous experience in related clerical job | Unit Clerk | Unit Clerk | None |
| Years in organization (policy: preference internal applicants) | 3 years | 1 year | 0 |
| Willing to accept salary of $29,000 | Yes | Yes | Prefers higher; wants raise within 6 months |
| Full-time | Yes | Yes | Yes |
| 3:00–10:00 P.M. shift acceptable | Yes | Yes | Prefers day; plans to switch as soon as opening is available |

It is possible to use a decision tree without including mathematical calculations of probability, although computers are commonly used to calculate the probability of events when such detailed information is available. Managers in business corporations with sufficient market data about profit, loss, patterns of consumer response, and national economic fluctuations include these data in the construction of a decision tree for the marketing of a new product, for example.

Managers who lack detailed information of this type can still use decision trees to advantage. In developing decision trees, these managers use symbols to designate points of certainty and uncertainty. For example, events of certainty may be placed in rectangles; events of uncertainty in ovals. This technique emphasizes the relative risk in each decision track. The goal to be reached is the continual reference point. The sequence of decisions that leads to the goal with the least uncertainty emerges as a distinct track, thereby facilitating the manager's decision. For decisions in which the manager has intense personal involvement, this approach is a valuable aid in overcoming emotional barriers to objective choice.

When managers devote time and effort to sound decision making, the planning process is enhanced, leading to consistent achievement of organizational goals.

## Notes

1. Chester Barnard, *The Functions of the Executive* (Cambridge, MA: Harvard University Press, 1968), 202.
2. Charles Lindblom, "The Science of Muddling Through," *Public Administration Review* (Spring 1959): 79–88.
3. Herbert Simon, *Models of Man* (New York: John Wiley & Sons, 1957), 207.
4. Vilfredo Pareto, *Mind and Society* (New York: Harcourt, Brace, 1935).
5. Grant Hammond. *The Mind of War: John Boyd and American Security* (Washington, DC: Smithsonian Institution Press, 2001).

## CHAPTER 6

# Organizing and Staffing

## CHAPTER OBJECTIVES

- Define the basic management function of organizing and identify the steps in the organizing process.
- Define the key concepts of hierarchy, chain of command, succession plan, splintered authority, and concurring authority.
- Identify the factors that shape the span of management.
- Differentiate between line and staff relationships, and identify basic line and staff relationships.
- Describe the dual pyramid organization arrangement found in healthcare authority patterns.
- Identify the basic patterns of departmentation.
- Introduce the concept of the matrix organization and define the applicability of this apparently contradictory concept.
- Identify patterns of organizational flexibility: temporary agency, contractual outsourcing, the use of independent contractors and consultants, flexible time scheduling, and remote work options.
- Identify the principles involved in developing an organizational chart.
- Describe the elements of a job analysis.
- Introduce job descriptions, including their uses and the elements necessary in their development.
- Describe the job rating and classification system.
- Identify the content and uses of the management inventory.
- Describe the role and activities of the professional practitioner as consultant.

Organizing is the process of grouping necessary responsibilities and activities into workable units, determining the lines of authority and communication, and developing patterns of coordination. It is the conscious development of the role structures of superior and subordinate, line and staff. The organizing process stems from several underlying premises:

- There is a common goal toward which work effort is directed.
- The goal is articulated in detailed plans.
- There is a need for clear authority–responsibility relationships.
- Power and authority elements must be reconciled so that individual interactions within the organization are productive and goal directed.
- Conflict is inevitable but may be reduced through clarity of organizational relationships.

- Individual needs must be reconciled with and subordinated to organizational needs.
- Unity of command must prevail.
- Authority must be delegated.

## ▶ The Process of Organizing

The immediately identifiable aspects of the organizing process include clear delineation of the goal in terms of scope, function, and priorities. For example, will a healthcare institution focus on acute care for inpatients or comprehensive care, including outpatient care and home care? Will the organization expand its services through decentralized locations and active outreach programs?

The development of a specific organizational structure must be considered. What degree of specialization will be sought? Specialization is a major feature of healthcare organizations; it is dictated and shaped in part by the specific licensure mandates for each health profession. The manager must assess the question of line and staff officers and units. A major organizational question concerns the division of work. What will be the pattern of departmentation? The development of the organizational chart, the job descriptions, and the statements of interdepartmental and intradepartmental workflow systems must be assessed and implemented as part of the management function of organizing. Finally, the changes in the internal and external organizational environment must be monitored so that the organizational structure can be adjusted accordingly.

The degree of centralization/decentralization is a fundamental decision, one having an effect on hierarchical pattern, levels of supervision, and amount and type of interdepartmental coordination required. A highly centralized hierarchy, with successive levels of middle managers, results in a "tall" organization. The pattern is sometimes referred to as the silo arrangement, with distinct organizational units and precise authority designations. The opposite arrangement, namely a highly decentralized hierarchy, with emphasis on teams and participative management style, fewer middle managers, and wide span of management, results in a "flat" organization. The following example reflects some of the consequences of a highly centralized pattern.

A social service agency, part of a state-wide umbrella organization, had, in its origin, a philosophy of decentralization, with several smaller offices and service sites. The benefits of this approach included a close relationship with the local community. Volunteers, because they were familiar with the agency and aware of its value to the community, readily and easily became involved with the agency's work. Local civic and social groups readily contributed to the agency's financial and logistical needs. Local merchants and area businesses routinely donated money, goods, and services as part of their own outreach, commitment to the community, and basic public relations initiatives. Local law enforcement and the social service agency had well-established relationships. All in all, the agency was a stable one, with a regular client base and reliable resource suppliers.

In a state-wide reorganization initiative, top-level management at the state level decided to centralize the smaller organizational units into regional entities, each covering approximately a 75 mile (120 km) radius. While some cost savings were immediately gained (e.g., fewer physical sites to maintain), other less positive outcomes resulted. The number of clients dropped approximately 35% as clients did not wish to, or could not, travel to the centralized location. They also postponed seeking assistance because of necessity to travel to a large, unknown location, resulting in a greater need for care of more advanced clinical or social service intervention. The number of volunteers dropped by 40%. They cited reasons for dropping out; these reasons included the fact that they would be expected to go to locations and events out of their immediate locale. Travel conditions, especially in harsh weather-related events, were a burden, as was the simple requirement of additional travel time to an unfamiliar location. Trying to adapt to assisting "strangers" versus dealing with a well-known local population was another factor, although one that was only reluctantly discussed.

The availability of physicians and other professional care givers was impacted by the centralization decision. In the decentralized arrangement, the local hospital could easily release caregivers for a short period of time in an emergency or for practice drills, but this was no longer practicable when the additional travel time was factored in. Local resource suppliers, such as merchants and service groups, continued to be willing to support locally based agencies, but were unwilling to go beyond their customary marketing and service areas.

This example provides insight into the factors relating to centralized versus decentralized decision making. In summary, the basic steps of organizing are these:

1. Goal recognition and statement
2. Review of organizational environment
3. Determination of structure needed to reach the goal (e.g., degree of centralization, basis of departmentation, committee use, line and staff relationships)
4. Determination of authority relationships and development of the organizational chart, job descriptions, and related support documents

# ▸ Fundamental Concepts and Principles

Relationships in formal organizations are highly structured in terms of authority and responsibility. The resulting hierarchy—that is, the arrangement of individuals into a graded series of superiors and

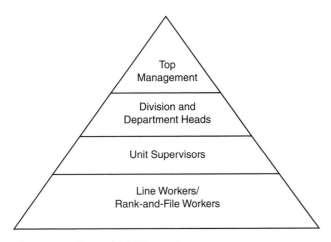

**Figure 6–1** Pyramidal Hierarchy.

subordinates, authority holders, and rank-and-file members—constitutes one of the most obvious characteristics of formal organizations. A pyramid-shaped organization tends to result from the development of a hierarchy (**Figure 6–1**).

The authority and responsibility that can be observed in the hierarchy constitutes a distinct chain of command, also referred to as the scalar principle: the chain of direct authority from superior to subordinate. It was long maintained that strict unity of command—the uninterrupted line of authority from superior to subordinate so that each individual reports to one, and only one, superior—was fundamental to hierarchical relationships in organizations. It was seen as essential to have a clear chain of command showing who reports to whom, who is responsible for each individual's actions, and who has authority over each worker. In situations of mandatory reporting, critical events, and similar matters, it is important that this set of relationships (i.e., who has the responsibility to report—and to whom) be well established and stated with clarity. In the organizational succession plan, there needs to be clear designation, by job title, of the officer who will act in place of the primary office holder. This plan reflects ordinary coverage, as in vacation time, leave of absence, and educational conference attendance. It also reflects the chain of command in emergency situations such as a disaster. The section on planning and decision making includes further discussion of succession plans.

Although unity of command is the usual practice, an alternative is reflected in split-reporting relationships in which a single subordinate reports to two or more superiors. Split-reporting relationships are proliferating as healthcare organizations merge into larger organizations or join together in health systems. It is not at all uncommon to find, for example, a single manager over the same functions at two sites who is therefore answerable to two different site administrators. Such combinations have occurred out of economic necessity, and many of them make sense in terms of operating efficiency and optimal utilization of management capability. This efficiency can be put at risk, however, as the absence of unity of command can create a new set of problems.

The individual who reports to two superiors is put in the position of having to balance the two reporting relationships. If either superior is inflexible or overly demanding, the stage is set for subordinate burnout as the individual attempts to reconcile conflicting demands. Much of the determination of whether a split-reporting relationship works lies beyond the reach of the individual. Even the most highly capable subordinate can be rendered frustrated and ineffective by two superiors who have not coordinated their demands and expectations or who have tried to have their way with the subordinate at the expense of the other superior.

Also, a split-reporting relationship more than doubles the communication demands on the subordinate manager. Not only does the manager have to communicate regularly with two superiors, but he or she must do so in a manner that attempts to provide coordination between the needs of the two superiors.

Split reporting may generate potential conflict when managers differ in their interpretation or application of policy. For example, one manager may readily give liberal leave in bad weather or allow early closing before a holiday, whereas another manager may have a stricter interpretation of such practices. The employee in this situation is caught in the middle of an ambiguous situation.

Split-reporting relationships may be necessary under certain circumstances, but they should always be entered into with full awareness and consideration of the problems that may be encountered. The concept of unity of command should not be abandoned without good reason and without planning to meet the increased communication needs of the alternative arrangement.

The authority delegated to any individual must be equal to the responsibility assigned. This principle of parity—that responsibility cannot be greater than the authority given—ensures that individuals can carry out their assigned duties without provoking conflict over their right to do so. In developing policies and documents that support the organizational chart, managers must avoid contradicting this principle. At the same time, managers cannot so completely delegate authority that they become free of responsibility. This is reflected in the principle of the absoluteness of responsibility; authority may (and must) be delegated, but ultimate responsibility is retained by the manager. This, in turn, is the basis of the manager's right to exercise the necessary controls and require accountability.

Normally, managers have adequate authority to carry out the required activities of their divisions or units without recourse to the authority possessed by other managers. Two situations occur, however, in which the authority of a single manager is not sufficient for unilateral decision making or action. Occasionally, because the work must be coordinated and because there are necessary limits on each manager's authority, a problem cannot be solved or a decision made without pooling the authority of two or more managers. These problems of splintered authority are overcome in three ways: (1) the managers may simply pool their authority and make the decision or solve the problem, (2) the problem may be referred to a higher level of authority until it reaches a single manager with sufficient authority, or (3) reorganization may be done so that recurring situations of splintered authority are eliminated. Such recurring situations sometimes require adjustment in the delegation of authority.

Concurring authority is sometimes given to related departments to ensure uniformity of practice. For example, the packaging department of a manufacturing company may not change specifications without the agreement of the production division. A computer systems manager in a healthcare setting may be given concurring authority on any data element changes, although this is the primary responsibility of the health information practitioner, to foster compatibility throughout the information processing function. Concurring authority, as a control and coordinating measure, can be a normal part of the routine checks-and-balances system. Splintered authority and concurring authority are the natural consequences of the division of labor and specialization that make it necessary to coordinate the authority delegated to different managers.

Maintaining unity of command in disasters and emergency situations has received particular attention over the past several years. The National Incident Management System (NIMS) was implemented as part of a nationwide Homeland Security initiative in 2001–2002. One feature of this system is the concept of unified command, a mechanism wherein a command team, which consists of representatives from various response agencies, develops a collective set of strategies. This process takes into account that different responding groups (e.g., police, fire companies, emergency medical response personnel) have differing jurisdictions and responsibilities. Within the structure of unified command, incident commanders from each agency coordinate their efforts. A lead agency or team will have primary authority and responsibility, with the other groups deferring to them. The lead agency or team could change as the situation changes and a different skill set or jurisdictional authority becomes the preferred one (e.g., a fire company hands off a situation to police; an emergency first responder team hands off the care of injured patients to an advanced field triage team). Healthcare organizations are adopting similar organizational patterns in their disaster planning, both internal and external.

## ▶ The Span of Management

If authority is to be delegated appropriately, consideration must be given to the number of subordinates a manager may supervise effectively. Four terms are used to refer to this concept: *span of management, span of control, span of supervision,* and *span of authority*. Stated another way, the span of management is the number of immediate subordinates who report to any one manager. It is essential to recognize that the number of individuals whose activities can be properly coordinated and controlled by one manager is limited.

There is no ideal span of management. A span of 4 or 5 subordinates at higher levels and a span of 8–12 at the lower levels have sometimes been suggested. Many modifying factors shape the appropriate span of management for any authority holder, however. These factors include the following:

- *Type of work.* Routine, repetitive, and homogeneous work allows a larger span of management.
- *Degree of training of the worker.* Those workers who are well trained and well motivated do not need as much supervision as a trainee group; the more highly trained the group, the larger the span of management may be.
- *Organizational stability.* When the organization as a whole, as well as the specific department, is stable, the span of control can be broader; when there are rapid changes, high turnover, and general organizational instability, a narrower span of control may be needed.
- *Geographical location.* When the work units are dispersed over a scattered physical layout, sometimes even involving separate geographical

locations, closer supervision is necessary to control and coordinate the work.

- *Flow of work.* If much coordination of workflow is needed, there is a corresponding need for greater supervision and a narrow span of control.
- *Supervisor's qualifications.* As the amount of training and experience of the supervisor increases, the span of control for that supervisor may increase as well.
- *Availability of staff specialists.* When staff specialists and selected support services, such as a training, human resources, or development department, are available, a supervisor's span of management may be increased.
- *Value system of the organization.* In highly coercive organizations, a supervisor may have a large span of management, because there is a pervasive system to help ensure conformity, even to the extent of severe punishment for deviation from the rules. In contrast, in a highly normative organization, there may be an emphasis on participation in planning and decision making and a resultant complexity in the communication process; thus a smaller span of management may be appropriate. In healthcare organizations (traditionally normative settings with respect to the professional worker), the span of management may be large because the healthcare professional is a specialist within an area and does not always require close supervision.

As an example, the span of management in a laboratory department is shown in the partial organizational chart in **Figure 6–2**. In this figure, one can trace the chain of command from each supervisor in the department back up to the chief executive officer.

## ▶ **Line and Staff Relationships**

The terms *line* and *staff* are key words in any discussion of organizing. In common usage, staff refers to the groups of employees who perform the work of a given department or unit. The director of nursing speaks of the nursing staff, the chief dietitian discusses the dietary/food service staff, and the physicians who practice in a hospital are referred to as the medical staff.

In management literature, a differentiation is made between line and staff departments or officers. Line refers to those workers who have direct responsibility for accomplishing the objectives of the organization, and staff refers to those employees who help the line units achieve the objectives. In a healthcare organization, direct patient care units are considered to perform line functions, and all other units are listed as staff services. The problem with this distinction becomes apparent when it must be applied to such units as the dietary, supply chain division, or housekeeping and environmental services. Are these functions any less essential to the operation of a healthcare organization than a direct patient care unit? Some organizational specialists prefer to list such units as service or support departments, reserving the term "staff" for a specific authority relationship.

The concept of line and staff was inherited by management theorists from the military of the 1700s and 1800s. An examination of a typical military encounter during this era makes it easier to conceptualize the notions of line and staff. The soldiers literally formed a line; the immediate commanding officers were those who commanded the line—that

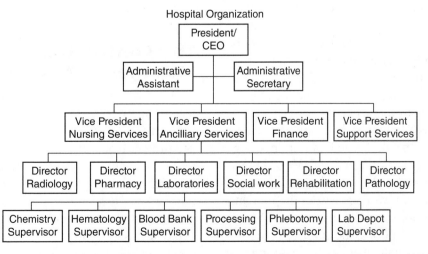

**Figure 6–2** Partial Organization Chart Illustrating Span of Management (Tracing from President/CEO through Vice President/Ancillary Services and Director, Laboratories)

is, line officers. The actual fighting of the battle was the duty of these troops and officers. In turn, these troops and officers were assisted by staff officers and other units that provided logistical support, supplies, and information. The idea carried over as formal bureaucratic organizational theory developed in the 1800s.

## The Relationship of Line and Staff Authority

The term staff also connotes a certain kind of authority relationship. Again, the original usage of the term was derived from the military, in which the staff assistant pattern was developed as a means of relieving commanders of details that could be handled by others. The staff officer was an "assistant to" the commander, and this assistant's authority was an extension of line authority.

Line authority is based on a direct chain of command from the top level of authority through each successive level of the organization. A manager with line authority has direct authority and responsibility for the work of a unit; the line manager alone has the right to command others to act. A staff assistant provides advice, counsel, or technical support that may be accepted, altered, or rejected by the line officer.

Functional authority is the right of individuals to exercise a limited form of authority over the specialized functions for which they are responsible, regardless of who exercises line authority over the employees performing the activities. For example, the information services staff is responsible for developing and implementing a specific computerized data collection system. The unit manager has functional authority over processing input documents, although these documents may be originated and completed by workers in other units, such as the admission office, business office, nursing service, or health information management. A human resources officer may be charged with monitoring organizational compliance with affirmative action programs or labor union contracts; the advice of such an officer cannot be rejected or altered arbitrarily by a line officer.

A manager may hold a staff position. Such an individual may be the designated officer in charge of a support department, such as the legal or human resources department. Yet this manager may also have charge of one or several workers within the unit and would exercise line authority within that unit. Organization charts, job descriptions, and similar documents should contain clear statements as to the nature of each position: whether it is a line or staff position, what kind of authority it possesses, and what its area of responsibility includes.

## Line and Staff Interaction

Various types of staff arrangements may be developed to channel line and staff interaction. As noted earlier, one basic mode of interaction is to designate a staff member as the personal assistant to an individual holding office in the upper levels of the organization. This position should not be confused with that of an assistant department head or assistant manager, who generally shares in direct line authority. Managers in the upper levels of the organization may have several assistants, each carrying out highly specialized tasks. When there is only one position of assistant, this individual's work may be general, varied, and determined by the needs of the superior officer. The style of interaction may be highly personal, as when the staff assistant is seen as an alter ego of the line officer. When such a staff member indicates a point of view, a desired action, or a preferred decision, other members of the organization recognize that this individual is reflecting the opinion and wishes of the line officer.

A full department that gives specialized assistance and support frequently has a general staff. The relationship between staff and line personnel is less intimate than the assistant relationship. The work tends to be technical and highly specialized (e.g., the work of logistical staff in the military).

A third aspect of line and staff relationship is the organizational arrangement of the specialized staff. Specialized staff members (or departments in a large institution) give highly specialized counsel, such as that provided by engineers, architects, accountants, lawyers, and auditors. Finally, as noted, departments can be arranged in terms of direct line entities, assisted by support or service units.

## The Contractual Management Team

There is a growing practice of using a contractual management team in place of the direct-hire chief executive and/or chief operating officer and some key department manager positions (e.g., director of nursing). The board of trustees hires, on contract, an outside individual or team to take over, for some period, the executive functions in the organization. The board has directly given this individual or team authority to make necessary changes and maintain regular operations. The reasons for using an outside group include necessary restructuring due to downsizing or mergers, need for turnaround measures, and preparation for a merger or for disinvesting by the original sponsoring organization. These expert outsiders identify and implement necessary changes, absorb any hostility from workers and clients, and deal with overcoming the resulting demoralization. They may be in residence for several months or years, depending on the reasons for using them. More than consultants whose role is limited to making recommendations, these individuals are empowered to implement.

# ▸ The Dual Pyramid Form of Organization in Health Care

Healthcare institutions are characterized by a dual pyramid form of organization because of the traditional relationship of the medical staff to the administrative staff. The ultimate authority and responsibility for the management of the institution is vested in the governing board. In accordance with the stipulations of licensure and accrediting agencies, the board appoints a chief executive officer and a chief of medical staff, resulting in two lines of authority. The chief executive officer is responsible for effectively managing the administrative components of the institution and delegating authority to each department head. Within the administrative units, there is a typical pyramidal organization with a unified chain of command.

Physicians and dentists are organized under a specific set of bylaws for the governance of the medical and dental staff. With governing board approval, the chief of the medical staff appoints the chief of each clinical service. Physicians and dentists apply for clinical privileges through the medical staff credentials process and receive appointment from the governing board. A second pyramid results from this organization of the medical staff into clinical services, with each having a chief of service who reports to the chief of the medical staff.

In an effort to consolidate authority and clarify responsibility, the top administrative levels of a healthcare organization may be expanded to include a central officer to whom both the administrator and the chief of the medical staff report. In some institutions, however, there may be no permanent medical staff position that corresponds to the position of chief executive officer on the organizational chart. The elected president of the medical staff may fill this role when there is no organizational slot for a medical director per se.

It is important to determine the precise meaning of titles as they are used in a specific healthcare setting. The following titles are commonly used:

- *Chief of staff.* This is the officer of the medical staff to whom the chiefs of medical and clinical services report. The chief of staff is appointed by the governing board.
- *Chief of service.* Each chief of service is the physician–director of a specific clinical service (e.g., chief of surgery) and is the line officer for physicians who are appointed to that specific service.
- *Department chairperson.* The chairperson of a department is the director of a specific clinical service in an academic institution, such as a teaching hospital. (This title may be used as an alternative to "chief of service" in this type of setting.)
- *Medical director.* This is a position in a line authority structure. It is sometimes seen as the counterpart of the chief executive officer for the medical staff.
- *President of the medical staff.* The president is the presiding officer for the medical staff and is usually elected for a year. In the absence of a full-time medical director, this individual serves as coordinating officer for the medical staff.

Although all authority flows from the governing board, there are two distinct chains of command—one in the administrative structure and one in the medical sector. Furthermore, in matters of direct patient care, the attending physician exercises professional authority; thus, a single employee not only may be subject to more than one line of authority but also may have professional authority. Line officers in the administrative unit may find that their authority is limited in some areas because of the specific jurisdiction of medical staff committees, such as the pharmacy and therapeutics committees. The director of the physical therapy department, for example, may report to a committee of physicians of the active medical staff, which limits the authority mandate of this line manager. Because of the dual pyramid structure, much coordination is needed.

# ▸ Basic Departmentation

The development of departments is a natural adjunct to the specialization and division of labor that are characteristic of formal organizations. Departmentation overcomes the limitation imposed by the span of management. The organization, through its departments and similar subdivisions, can expand almost indefinitely in size. Departmentation facilitates the coordination process, as there is a logical grouping of closely related activities.

Basic departmentation may be developed according to any one of several patterns:

1. *By function*. Because it is logical, efficient, and natural, the most widely used form of departmentation groups all related activities or jobs together. This permits managers to take advantage of specialization and to concern themselves with only one major focus of activity. Hospital departments are usually developed according to function (e.g., the finance office and the health information management, human resources, environmental services, maintenance, and dietary departments).

2. *By product*. All activities needed in the development, production, and marketing of a product may be grouped for purposes of coordination and control. This pattern of departmentation is used in business and industry where one or a few closely related products are grouped. It facilitates the use of research funds, the use of specialized skills and knowledge, and the development of cost control data for each product line. Functional departmentation may be an adjunct of product departmentation.

3. *By territory*. In business, the marketing process may be developed according to geographical boundaries. In service organizations, a decentralized pattern based on customer or client groupings may be appropriate. In some healthcare organizations, territorial departmentation is used because funding stipulations designate specific catchment areas or require coverage of certain population centers. Local needs, such as participation of clients and prompt settlement of difficulties, may be accommodated more easily through departmentation by territory. Grouping by geographical territory is a common element in outreach programs and home care services because it fosters efficient movement of personnel to client locations.

4. *By customer*. Departmentation may be based on client needs. Specialty clinics in health care tend to follow this pattern. Government programs frequently focus on a specific client need, partly in response to the lobbying of interest groups. Specific examples of customer departmentation include special maternal and infant care programs, memory care units in long-term care facilities, and programs for migrant workers. A university may have components such as day, evening, and weekend divisions, as well as continuing education programs, to accommodate the needs and interests of differing student populations.

5. *By time*. Activities may be grouped according to the time of day they are performed. This pattern, which is usually based on the use of shifts, is common in manufacturing and similar organizations in which the activities of a relatively large group of semiskilled or technical workers are repetitive and continue around the clock. Organizations that provide essential services throughout the day and night use this pattern, usually in conjunction with functional departmentation.

6. *By process*. Technological considerations and specialized equipment usage may lead to departmentation by process. This is similar to functional departmentation in that all the activities involving one major process or some set of specialized equipment are grouped. In healthcare organizations, the formation of radiology and clinical laboratory departments is an example of departmentation by process as well as by function.

7. *By number*. Departmentation may be accomplished by assigning certain duties to undifferentiated workers under specific supervision. This form of departmentation is used when many workers are needed to carry out an activity. Its use is relatively limited in modern organizations, but it was traditional in early societies, such as tribes, clans, and armies. Organizing by sheer number may be used in such activities as house-to-house soliciting campaigns and membership drives. Unskilled labor crews may be organized in this pattern.

## Orphan Activities

Certain activities may not merit grouping into separate departments, and there may be no compelling reason to place them in any specific location in the organization. Yet these orphan activities must be coordinated and interlocked with all others. The "most use" criterion is followed to resolve the question of organizational placement. The major department that most often uses or needs the service absorbs it. Other units that need the service obtain it from the major department to which it has been assigned.

Patient transportation in a hospital involves such a set of activities. These services are used by the physical therapy, occupational therapy, and radiology departments, among others, but overall coordination is assigned to the inpatient nursing units because one central placement is needed for these groups of workers. As another example, in small nursing homes one worker often performs several activities on a limited basis, such as general maintenance activities, running errands, and transporting patients to appointments with private physicians. The individual with these responsibilities may report to a central manager, such as the director of nursing, because the director or a delegate is present on all shifts. This arrangement provides coordination and control of the activities.

## Deadly Parallel Arrangements

In an alternative organizational pattern, the higher levels of management establish dual organizational units for the purposes of control or competition. As a control device, the parallel arrangement permits comparison of costs, productivity, and similar parameters.

Competition may be enhanced, if this is desired as a means of motivation, because productivity and performance can be compared.

## ▶ Specific Scheduling

The determination of specific coverage of key functions through specific scheduling, usually by shift, is an essential aspect of organizing. **Exhibit 6-1** provides

---

### Exhibit 6-1 Specific Scheduling by Shift: Health Information Services

**Planning Premises**

1. Clinic days and hours
   Monday through Friday 8:00 A.M. to 7:00 P.M.
   Scheduled appointments and walk-ins
   Saturday and Sunday 8:00 A.M. to 4:00 P.M.
   Primarily walk-ins; occasional scheduled appointments
2. Tasks and deadlines (based on operational goals for department; hybrid system with active use of hard copy records)
   Pull and deliver charts for appointments for chart availability 1 hour before clinic opening.
   Pull and deliver charts for walk-ins within 15 minutes of call for chart.
   Refile charts within 2 hours of return by clinic (pick up and return of charts scheduled every 2 hours).
   File (or data entry) late and continuing care reports within 2 hours of receipt.
3. Full-time equivalents (FTEs) needed
   Eight (to be full-time employees)
4. Number of floaters needed to provide vacation, holiday, and sick-time coverage
   Two FTEs, to consist of four part-time positions assigned as needed based on vacation, holiday, and sick-time experience.

**Monday Through Friday**

7:00 A.M. to 3:00 P.M. Shift: Two FTEs
   Search for charts missing or not found on initial attempt.
   Pull and deliver charts for walk-ins throughout shift.
   Pick up and return charts to file, 2-hour rotation.
   Pull charts for next day's clinic appointments.
9:00 A.M. to 5:00 P.M. Shift: Two FTEs
   Pick up and return charts to file, 2-hour rotation.
   Pull charts for next day's clinic appointments.
   Process late and continuing care reports. (hard copy file, or data entry)
   Search for charts missing or not found on initial attempt (for late afternoon and early evening clinic appointments).
   Pull and deliver charts for walk-ins 3:00 P.M. to 5:00 P.M.
3:00 P.M. to 11:00 P.M. Shift: Two FTEs
   Pull and deliver charts for evening clinic walk-ins.
   Pick up and return charts to file, 2-hour rotation.
   Process late and continuing care reports. (hard copy file, or data entry)
   Carry out quality control audit of files.

**Saturday and Sunday**

8:00 A.M. to 4:00 P.M. Shift: One FTE per day
   Pull and deliver charts for walk-ins.
   Pick up and return charts to file, 2-hour rotation.
   Process late and continuing care reports. (hard copy file or data entry)
   Carry out quality control audit of files.

an example of the development of coverage based on workflow. A mix of full-time and part-time workers and overlapping shifts at times of high-volume demand in the workflow are essential considerations in developing this particular plan, which reflects the needs of a large group practice with a hard copy record system in use while it gradually implements an electronic health record system.

# ▶ Flexibility in Organizational Structure

Managers, in their role as change agents, continually seek ways to respond to change in the external and internal organizational environment. It may be necessary to adjust traditional organizational patterns because of advances in modern technology, increases in workers' technical and professional training, the need to offset employee alienation, and the need to overcome the problems inherent in decentralized, widely dispersed units. In addition, managers must take into account certain characteristics of today's workforce: the two-wage earner family, the single parent, and the worker who is also caretaker of an elderly family member. These workers need a modicum of flexibility such as that provided in flexible hours, telecommuting, and similar remote work sites as alternatives to on-site work.

In general, functional departmentation has been predominant, and there has been a strong emphasis on unity of command. When technical advice or assistance was needed, staff roles were developed to assist the line managers. When intraorganizational communication and cooperation among several units were needed, the committee structure was used. Three alternative temporary or permanent organizational patterns allow managers to retain the benefits of these traditional practices and to reduce some of their disadvantages: (1) the matrix approach, (2) temporary departmentation, and (3) the task force. These approaches may supplement the traditional organizational structure or, in the case of the matrix approach, supplant it.

## Matrix Organization

Matrix organization, a design that involves both functional and product departmentation, is used predominantly to provide a flexible and adaptable organizational structure for specific projects in, for example, research, engineering, or product development. This pattern is also called grid or latticework organization and project or product management. The matrix of organizational relationships involves a chief for the technical aspects, an administrative officer for the managerial aspects, and a project coordinator as the final authority. This dual authority structure is a predominant characteristic of the matrix organization and stands in distinct contrast to the unity of command in the traditional organizational pattern.

Workers are essentially borrowed from functional units and temporarily assigned to the project unit. Rather than designating line and staff interactions, the developers of the matrix pattern seek to create a web of relationships among technical and managerial workers. Multiple reporting systems are developed and communication lines are interwoven throughout the matrix.

Participants in the matrix organizational pattern tend to be highly trained, self-motivated individuals with a relatively independent mode of working. These functional personnel are grouped together according to the needs dictated by the phase of the project that has been undertaken. In the matrix arrangement, workers receive direction from the technical or the administrative chief as appropriate, but it is assumed that they have the ability to develop the necessary communication and work patterns without specific direction in every aspect. The project coordinator has the traditional responsibilities of guiding the technical and administrative groups and of developing the basic channels of communication and lines of coordination; however, there may be none of the detailed stipulations that are commonly associated with the highly bureaucratic traditional organizational pattern. In the healthcare organization, a matrix organization frees nurses, physical therapists, occupational therapists, and other direct patient care professionals from some of the relatively rigid elements of formal organization.

## Temporary Departmentation

The temporary department or unit reflects a management decision to create an organizational division with a predetermined lifetime to meet some temporary need. This lifetime may be imposed by an inherent, self-limiting element, such as funding through a defense contract or private research grant. Although the predominant organizational structure may be modified periodically, there is an implicit assumption that the basic unit will remain substantially unchanged for the life of the organization. The use of the term "temporary" may be somewhat misleading; temporary departmentation usually reflects an organizational pattern that will exist for more than a few months, as an activity limited to only a few months' duration would be placed under the category of special project or task force rather than temporary departmentation. The temporary department may exist for several years (i.e., for the life of a research grant), although there is no set rule.

The development of a new product (i.e., the calculation of comparative cost data, product development, and marketing) may be placed under a temporary department assigned to carry out the necessary research development and marketing within a specific period. A team of workers with the necessary specialized knowledge may be assembled under the jurisdiction of the temporary department, deadlines set, necessary accounting processes developed, and related functions delineated.

In businesses and institutions with defense contracts or research grants, temporary departmentation provides the necessary organizational structure without interfering with the establishment's normal efforts. Equipment is purchased and workers hired with special funds designated for that purpose. These workers are not necessarily subject to the same pay scale, fringe benefits, union contracts, and similar regulations as are regular employees. The manager must make it clear to these workers that their jobs are temporary, limited to the life of the contract or grant. There should also be a clear understanding about worker movement into the main organizational unit: is this employee eligible for such movement with or without having accrued seniority and similar benefits? Patients who receive full or partial subsidy for their care in a healthcare institution under a special research grant or project should be informed about the limited scope of the project, and their options for continuity of care about the life of the project should be explained.

## Temporary Agency Services

Staffing flexibility may also be achieved or enhanced through the use of temporary help from agencies that specialize in supplying trained personnel to cover short-term needs. "Short-term" in this sense is ordinarily construed as a period not exceeding 6 months. The workers engaged under an arrangement with a temporary help agency are employees of the agency, not the utilizing organization.

There are several advantages to the use of agency "temps." The organization is spared the effort and expense of recruiting, hiring, training, and separating employees who will be in the workforce for

perhaps only a few weeks. Also, in many instances, these temporary employees come trained in the basics of the job and require only specific departmental orientation. Although the organization pays something of a premium in that the rate for a temp includes the person's pay and benefits and the agency's profit, the temp alternative is often more economical than paying overtime premium to regular staff to cover the need. There are in health care, however, some marked exceptions to this claim of economy in health care. Professional staff such as registered nurses, physical therapists, and a number of others are always more costly as temporaries than regular staff. Presently the reasons for engaging professional temps have little or nothing to do with "short-term needs"; the key reasons for today's use of professional temps are the shortage of adequate staff and the attendant difficulties experienced in recruiting critically needed personnel.

It should be stressed that temporary help arrangements need to be limited to a period of less than 6 months. Federal law requires that anyone working for an organization for a period exceeding 6 months must be considered an employee for purposes of earning credit toward retirement. Some nonhealthcare organizations' past practices—often involving laying off employees and hiring them back as "temporaries" at lower rates of pay and with fewer benefits and the inability to accrue retirement credit—were seen as a deliberate strategy to avoid certain costs.

In any event, a temporary engagement that has extended beyond the 6-month guideline should be examined closely for alternative ways of meeting the need. The key criterion for the appropriate use of temporary staff is the short-term nature of the need. In the healthcare setting especially, the prolonged use of temps to meet a continuing need is never as economical as engaging permanent staff.

## Outsourcing

Outsourcing is the process of having certain services that could be provided internally performed by agencies or individuals external to the organization. As with the temporary agency arrangement, these workers are employees of their agency, not of the contracting organization. Outsourcing has been an actively used alternative in manufacturing industries for many years. It is common in manufacturing for a company to rely on external suppliers to provide it with various components made to the company's specifications. In fact, what we now know as outsourcing probably began in manufacturing in the manner just described, although the label "outsourcing" is considerably newer than the activity itself.

Many of the decisions favoring outsourcing are made for economic reasons. Quite simply, if a service can be obtained externally for less than the cost of providing it internally, outsourcing may be considered a preferred alternative (providing, of course, that the external source meets all of the organization's quality requirements).

Often the economic decision favoring outsourcing is driven by volume considerations. Should there not be enough of a particular activity required to justify hiring and staffing to perform it (e.g., some specialized task requiring just a few hours each week), outsourcing may be the logical alternative.

Outsourcing decisions may also hinge on the presence or absence of particular skills or capabilities. For example, a large healthcare organization may have its own in-house legal counsel, whereas a smaller organization will outsource all of its legal work to an external law firm. Or perhaps a group practice that is having difficulty keeping up with medical transcription because of position vacancies or abnormally high volume of dictation will farm out some of its transcription work to an external service.

In recent years, outsourcing has become a "hot-button" issue with many Americans. More and more activities have been farmed out not just to suppliers external to an organization but to suppliers outside the country. Some businesses have taken this approach in an effort to reduce their operating costs or improve their competitive positions; in tough economic times, some have seen outsourcing as enhancing their chances of survival. Regardless of why outsourcing is undertaken, however, it frequently leads to the loss of jobs. Foreign outsourcing invariably means lower costs for various products and services and fewer jobs in the domestic economy.

Nevertheless, for the modern healthcare organization, outsourcing has its legitimate uses. Outsourcing is often essential for acquiring services that cannot be provided on an in-house basis, and it is sometimes the most economical means of addressing a temporary need.

## Contracted Services

The general heading of outsourcing includes the use of contract management services and the use of independent contractors. Under contract management, the entirety of a particular service associated with the organization is managed by or perhaps provided in full by an external organization that specializes in that service. Probably the two most common hospital and nursing home services provided under contract management are food service and housekeeping, although in one setting or another essentially every conceivable service has been contracted out by some healthcare organizations. Contract management may involve management alone or the complete provision of the service. At one particular hospital, for example, an external firm supplies the management of food service while the rank-and-file food service workers remain hospital employees; at the same hospital, housekeeping is provided by an external firm using its own staff with no involvement of hospital employees.

The use of independent contractors has received considerable government attention over the past couple of decades. Generally, to qualify under Internal Revenue Service (IRS) guidelines as an independent contractor and thus be paid as a supplier rather than as an employee, a worker is required to demonstrate a level of independence not commonly found in an employer–employee relationship, as evidenced by the following principal factors:

- The worker personally invests in facilities and equipment that are used in performing the services.
- The worker can expect to either make a profit or experience a loss from the activity (other than because of simple nonpayment for services provided).
- The worker provides services for two or more unrelated clients or customers within the same period of time.
- The worker makes services available to any or all potential clients or customers on a regular and consistent basis.

It is the presence of the foregoing conditions that the IRS will look for in assessing the nature of the relationship in which an external service is provided. Using an independent medical transcriptionist as an example, if this individual acquired his or her own equipment and offers transcription services to a number of organizations including Hospital A, chances are he or she will be considered an independent contractor. If, however, the individual is performing transcription for Hospital A only and working in his or her home using equipment largely or completely provided by Hospital A, he or she will be considered an employee of Hospital A. As an employee he or she must be on the payroll of Hospital A with all that such a status implies (various personnel expenses for the hospital, and withholding taxes).

---

**Exhibit 6–2** Guidelines for the Use of Contractual Services (Transcription Services)

---

Contracts with incorporated contractual services should be approved by the Human Resources Division and should include the following elements as a minimum:

- HIPAA-compliant confidentiality and security measures
- Accept dictation from land-line phone systems, PC microphones, handheld digital recorders
- Document distribution by secure line fax, secure e-mail, remote print
- Electronic editing and signature
- Tracking system for each document, from beginning of recording through document received
- Customized format
- Ninety-nine percent error-free guarantee
- STAT capability
- Access to listen or view transcriptions 24/7 (365 days/year)
- 24/7 support center (365 days/year)
- Turnaround time of (n) hours
- Conform with nationally accepted billing method principles

---

The use of independent contractors may generate cost savings because of the elimination of personnel expenses associated with training, physical space requirements, unemployment compensation, and other aspects of direct employment. However, the healthcare organization department that makes use of independent contractors must have consistently applied guidelines governing such working relationships. **Exhibit 6–2** provides a set of sample guidelines for contract specifications for independent contractors using, for illustrative purposes, guidelines applied in arrangements with an outsourced dictation–transcription service.

## Flexible Options for Worker Scheduling

Flexible options for worker scheduling may be offered as part of recruitment, retention, and motivation. Two commonly used options are flextime arrangements and remote work site/telecommuting. These options provide workers with more control over their schedules as well as requiring them to be more independently responsible for meeting their work assignments. Official lateness is usually reduced because these options include leeway for start time.

## Flextime

Flextime is an arrangement wherein employees choose their own schedule within parameters set by management. The work week is defined, for example, 40 hours, Monday through Friday. The work day includes extended opening and closing hours, for example, start time as early as 7:00 A.M. and end time no later than 7:00 P.M. Core time is defined; this is the large portion of time during which all employees are expected and required to be at the workplace so that coordination and communication is assured. The core time might start at 10:00 A.M. and conclude at 3:00 P.M. Thus, a worker could start the work day at 7:00 A.M. and leave at 3:00 P.M., or start at 10:00 A.M. and leave at 7:00 P.M. A worker might, on occasion, choose to work a short day (10:00 A.M.–3:00 P.M.) offsetting this with a longer day during the specific week (assuming no overtime or other rules prohibit this). With the flextime option, there is the underlying assumption that the worker is self-motivated, does not require a high degree of supervision, and is engaged in work that permits this variation in schedule. A manager must be mindful that not all workers can use flexible options because of the nature of their job duties. The potential for conflict and/or demotivation could result.

## Telecommuting

If an individual does all or most of his or her work at home, serving only Hospital A and using some Hospital A's hardware and software, he or she may be considered a telecommuting employee. This ambiguity should be cleared up so that his or her status is properly categorized.

Telecommuting is an employment arrangement in which a person who is on the organization's payroll works an agreed-on or perhaps regularly scheduled amount of time each week at home or some other external location with the support of the appropriate equipment and services. As a flexible workstyle option, telecommuting is a significant step beyond what is often called "flextime." A telecommuter works in a setting other than the traditional office or shop and is supervised by means other than management provided by an immediately present supervisor.

Whether they work full-time or part-time, telecommuters are regular employees on the payroll of the organization. They are decidedly not independent contractors or freelancers who are paid per piece or per job and excluded from employee benefits, and they do not conform to the criteria by which the IRS defines independent contractors.

Telecommuting is never appropriate for employees whose primary duties involve direct interaction with clients or customers, and it is inappropriate for people who work on team undertakings that require regular employee interaction. And even if a particular job's duties would seem to lend themselves to telecommuting, such an arrangement should never be considered for employees who have yet to prove themselves as reliable self-starters.

Telecommuting cannot be a hit-or-miss proposition. It requires a consistent policy delineating the rules for its use, specifying:

- Where the telecommuter can work: whether just at home or at other sites as well
- Work status: whether full-time or part-time
- When one can work: whether the employee sets the hours, the organization sets the hours, or the employee is allowed to flex around required "core" hours
- Technology required: whether what is needed is determined by the telecommuter or designated by the business
- Work space: compliant with the Health Insurance Portability and Accountability Act (HIPAA), with security of confidential data

In developing a telecommuting policy, it is best to secure the input of not only affected managers but also some of the likely telecommuters. The telecommuting policy should require that any such arrangement be described by specific objectives, detailed results expected, and methods for measuring accomplishments.

For certain kinds of activities, telecommuting has been practiced for years. For example, traditional telecommuting arrangements have included data entry, customer billing, and medical transcription. However, possibilities for telecommuting include most jobs that are performed independent of other people and those that do not require high-cost specialized equipment. Many jobs can lend themselves to telecommuting as long as the arrangement can satisfactorily serve the needs of all concerned.

The individual in a telecommuting situation stands to benefit from reduced travel time and fewer transportation concerns, comfort of work environment and dress, freedom from interruptions, possibly flexible hours, and in some instances, relief from child care concerns. Some professional and technical employees find that on telecommuting days they are more available for telephone consultation than when they are in a busy office environment. The organization frequently gains productive efficiency and is often able to reduce expenses and save energy and in general reduce the strain on facilities and services. In fact, some organizations have adopted telecommuting as a means of avoiding the addition of more space. Telecommuting can also aid in recruiting and retaining employees.

Telecommuting is not likely to succeed with the occasional employee who is unable to cope well with isolation from coworkers and the absence of traditional supervision. And the manager who is constantly— or, at the other extreme, never—checking up on the unseen employee will not do well with telecommuting employees. Managers inexperienced with telecommuting often fear they will not be able to monitor employee activities sufficiently, perhaps feeling they cannot effectively manage people who are not under their full-time direct supervision. Thus the manager of telecommuters must necessarily manage by results, using goals, objectives, and quotas.

Before going forward with any telecommuting arrangement:

- Check with counterparts at other organizations of comparable size and complexity about their experiences with telecommuting.
- Be certain the desired arrangement is consistent with the organization's personnel and business systems (e.g., time reporting, payroll).
- If unionized employees are potentially involved, sound out the union concerning its stand on telecommuting and bring union officials into the process early.

Needless to say, a great many employees would likely jump at the opportunity to work at home. However, telecommuting should never be adopted simply because some employees want to do it. Telecommuting should be seriously considered only if doing so would seem to make good business sense.

# ▶ The Organizational Chart

The management tool used for depicting organizational relationships is the organizational chart. It is a diagrammatic form, a visual arrangement that depicts the following aspects of an institution:

1. Major functions, usually by department
2. Relationships of functions or departments
3. Channels of supervision
4. Lines of authority and of communication
5. Positions (by job title) within departments or units

There are numerous reasons for using organizational charts:

- An organizational chart maps major lines of decision making and authority, so managers can review it to identify any inconsistencies and complexities in the organizational structure. The diagrammatic representation makes it easier to determine and correct these inconsistencies and complexities.
- An organizational chart may be used to orient employees, because it shows where each job fits in relation to supervisors and to other jobs in the department. It shows the relationship of the department to the organization as a whole.
- The chart is a useful tool in managerial audits. Managers can review such factors as the span of management, mixed lines of authority, and splintered authority; they can also check that individual job titles are on the chart so it is clear to whom each employee reports. In addition, managers can compare current practice with the original plan of job assignments to determine if any discrepancies exist.

Certain limitations are inherent in the rather static structure presented by organizational charts, and these limitations can offset some of the advantages of using the charts:

- Only formal lines of authority and communication are shown; important lines of informal communication and significant informal relationships cannot be shown.
- The chart may become obsolete if not updated at least once a year (or whenever there is a major change in the organizational pattern).
- Individuals without proper training in interpretation may confuse authority relationship with status. Managers whose positions are placed physically higher in the graphic representation may be perceived as having authority over those whose positions are lower on the chart. The emphasis must be placed on the direct authority relationships and the chain of command.

- The chart cannot be properly interpreted without reference to support information, such as that usually contained in the organizational manual and related job descriptions.

## Types of Charts

There are two major kinds of organizational charts: master and supplementary. The master chart depicts the entire organization, although not in great detail, and normally shows all departments and major positions of authority. A detailed listing of formal positions or job titles is not given in the master chart, however. Each supplementary chart depicts a section, department, or unit, including the specific details of its organizational pattern. An organization has as many supplementary charts as it has departments or units.

The supplementary chart of a department usually reflects the master chart and shows the direct chain of command from highest authority to that derived by the department head. The master chart usually shows the major functions, whereas the supplementary chart depicts each individual job title and the number of positions in each section, as well as full-time or part-time status. Additional information, such as cost centers, major codes, or similar identifying information, sometimes appears on the charts.

## General Arrangements and Conventions

The conventional organizational chart is a line or scalar chart showing each layer of the organization in sequence (**Figure 6–3**). In another arrangement, the flow of authority may be depicted from left to right, starting with major officials on the extreme left and with each successive division to the right of the preceding unit. The advantage of this form stems from its similarity to normal reading patterns. A circular arrangement, in which the authority flows from the center outward, is sometimes used; its advantage is that it shows the authority flow reaching out and permeating all levels, not just flowing from top to bottom.

Certain general conventions are followed when an organizational chart is drawn. Ordinarily, line authority and line relationships are indicated by solid lines, and staff positions are indicated by broken or dotted lines. In **Figure 6–4**, the position of health information consultant has a staff relationship to the administrator, which is, accordingly, shown by a broken line. Sometimes the staff relationship is indicated by a small "s" with a slash mark setting it off from the job title.

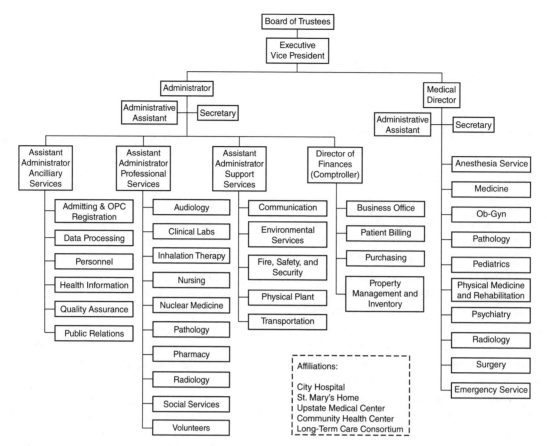

**Figure 6–3** Organizational Chart of a Hospital

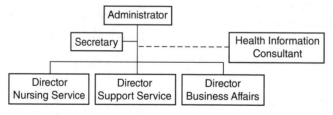

**Figure 6–4** Staff Relationships: Consultant in Advisory Role

Occasionally, an affiliated relationship is indicated by surrounding an entire unit or even another organization with broken lines and leaving it unconnected to any line or staff unit. Such a unit is included in the organizational chart to call attention to the existence of a related, auxiliary, or affiliated organization. This technique is used in Figure 6–3 to indicate the relationship of the teaching institutions affiliated with the hospital.

## Preparing the Organizational Chart

If the chart is prepared during a planning or reorganization stage, the first step is to list all the major functions and the jobs associated with them. The major groupings by function then are brought together as specific units—for example, all jobs dealing with health information services or with patient identification systems, all jobs dealing with physical medicine and rehabilitation, or all jobs dealing with information processing and computer activities. If there is a question about the proper placement of one or several functions, managers can derive significant information by asking the following questions:

- If there is a problem, who must be involved to effect a solution?
- Do the supervisors at each level have the necessary authority to carry out their functions?
- If a change in systems and procedures is needed, who must agree to the changes?

- If critical information must be channeled through the organization, who is responsible for its transmission throughout each unit of the organization?

As an aid in developing the organizational chart, it is useful to prepare a simple tabulation showing the following information:

1. Job title
2. Reporting line: supervised by whom (title)
3. Full-time or part-time
4. Day, evening, or night shift; Monday through Friday; weekend coverage (Friday evening, Saturday, and Sunday)
5. Hours of work, including flextime option; requirements concerning availability: on call, availability through phone, messaging, e-mail; mandatory overtime
6. Designation as essential versus nonessential worker for response to work schedule modification (such as weather or emergencies)
7. Residency requirements: that worker must reside in a specific region (e.g., township, city, county)
8. Line or staff position

The inclusion of the incumbent's name is optional for this worksheet preparation, although names may be useful in a subsequent managerial audit of the department in which the manager is comparing present practice with the original plan. The use of names as the basic means of developing the chart could be misleading, however, as it may block managers' thinking, causing them to describe organizational relationships as they are rather than as they should be. It may be best to show names only on a staffing chart that is prepared after the organizational chart has been developed.

After obtaining the necessary information about work relationships, shifts, supervisory needs, and span of management factors, managers develop the final chart, using the general conventions for depicting organizational relationships. A support narrative or a section of the organization's manual can be developed to give additional information.

## ▶ The Job Description

The duties associated with each job should be determined by the needs of the department. Frequently, jobs evolve as duties are assigned to an employee. These jobs are accumulations of tasks rather than products of prior planning. Some form of control is necessary to keep assignments within intended limits.

To provide this control of the various work assignments, the duties and responsibilities of each job should be set forth in written form. This helps ensure that employees' concepts of their duties will be consistent with those of the manager and with the needs of the department.

In every formal organization, there are job descriptions/position profiles to cover all jobs. To fill the various positions with the appropriate employees, it is necessary to match the jobs available in the department with the individuals. This can be done only with the help of job descriptions, which are written objective statements defining duties and functions. Each job description includes responsibilities, experience, organizational relationships, working conditions, and other essential factors of the position.

If a specific position is part of the continuity of operations plan, or if team participation is an essential component of the position, these expectations should be clearly stated.

## Job Analysis

Preceding the development of a job description, there should be a thorough job analysis that serves as a single source for the various uses to be made of information concerning a specific job. In addition to providing all of the information necessary for the development of the job description, the job analysis serves a variety of other uses, including performing a job evaluation (establishing an appropriate pay grade for the job), developing recruiting specifications, conducting employee orientation and education, and planning for staffing requirements. Reminder: not every element will apply to every job; the job analysis pattern is, however, applied to every job so that comparison and classification of jobs is possible. Typical content includes the following:

- Job responsibilities: details of work, frequency of action (e.g., routine, periodic, emergency), any other distinguishing features (e.g., on-call duties) (note percentage of time spent on each duty)
- Level of supervision: working under direct supervision or independently, with only periodic review of work by second-level supervisor or department manager
- Supervisory responsibilities: providing direct supervision (indicate job titles and numbers of employees supervised); providing direct training and supervision of students on affiliation rotation (indicate if duties include employee evaluation, discipline, and/or hire-or-fire decisions as well as if duties include orienting, training,

coaching, scheduling, developing, counseling, and measuring performance of [n] employees)

- Consequences of errors:
  - Are errors easily detected and remedied?
  - Are errors difficult to detect, with long-range consequences?
  - Is the work performed independently?
  - Could a serious error occur in direct patient care?
- Confidential data: having limited access or full access to patient records, financial information, or review committee proceedings (e.g., infection control reports, safety reviews, audits, credentialing reviews, employee evaluations, labor contract background information)
- Mental and physical demands and effort: having various physical abilities, such as (1) lifting and supporting patients (n pounds) and (2) lifting and pushing equipment (n pounds; indicate type of equipment); ability to walk and stand throughout the work day, to tolerate prolonged sitting throughout the work day, to maintain calm demeanor when faced with agitated or demanding clients, and to drive an automobile; having visual and aural acuity
- Environment/working conditions: routine office environment; indoors; no major exposure to noise, infections, or hazards (identify these [e.g., exposure to infections, high noise levels, outdoor work in extreme weather conditions]); telecommuting option; travel requirements; shift work (permanent or rotating); site rotation (regular or occasional)
- Preparation and training: entry level requirements only (e.g., high school diploma or equivalent), advanced training (e.g., master's degree in a specific field of study), certification as specialist in a specific area, graduation from an approved/accredited training or educational program, computer skills, language and degree of fluency in specific language

A specific advantage of the use of a job analysis is that a single job analysis can sometimes serve as a template for a family of jobs. Consider, for example, a job analysis of perhaps six pages in length for *registered nurse* (RN). This thorough job analysis would be written to be descriptive of all RN positions in the organization, with all duties or groupings of duties described in general terms. Related to this master job analysis, there may be any number of one- or two-page job descriptions addressing the specific variations of RN, such as RN, Emergency Department; RN, Medical/Surgical; RN, Operating Room.

# Job Description Content and Format

The job description provides essential information about duties, responsibilities, and qualifications for specific positions. Because of the continual adaptations to change, including technological factors and certain laws and regulations, job descriptions are usually reviewed on a periodic basis, at least once a year. A cluster of jobs might have common characteristics and fall under broad categorization with more specific details added to the common-core descriptors. The position of registered nurse is an example of common-core descriptors, with specialty information supplementing these basic descriptors. As nursing roles and functions change, new categories emerge, for example: nurse navigator for the cancer unit; nurse information technology coordinator; registered nurse case manager and coach—stroke rehab unit.

The format of a job description should present the information in an orderly manner. Because there is no standard format, job descriptions vary with the type of facility and with the size and scope of the department. The following format, along with some sample wording, is suggested as a guide:

- *Job title.* The job should be identified by a title that clarifies the position. The inclusion in the job title of such words as "director," "supervisor," "senior," "staff," or "clerk" can help to indicate the duties and skill level of the job. Examples of job titles that indicate such specificity are Medical Safety Clinical Pharmacist; Operations Manager—Health Information Service; Human Resources—Training Specialist; Regulatory Standards Manager; Certified Health Data Analyst; Electronic Health Record Data Extractor; Physical Therapist—Vestibular and Balance Program Coordinator; and Health Information—Coding and Reimbursement Clinical Specialist; Certified Documentation Improvement Practitioner; and Voice Recognition Editor. Professional associations provide guidelines about job titles and descriptions.
- *Immediate supervisor.* The position and title of the immediate supervisor should be clearly identified. This information reflects the organization chart. For managerial positions, include information about succession plan responsibility.
- *Job summary.* A short statement of the major activities of the job should indicate the purpose and scope of the job in specific terms. This section serves principally to identify the job and

differentiate the duties that are performed from those of other jobs. Sample wording might be:

> This is a clerical position in the health information service of an acute care facility affiliated with a medical school and a research institution. This full-time, day-shift position is under the direct supervision of the Assistant Health Information Administrator. The work is performed with relative independence and any exceptions to policy should be referred to the unit supervisor.

- *Job duties.* The major part of the job description should state what the employee does and how the duties are accomplished. The description of duties should also indicate the degree of supervision received or given.
- *Job specifications.* A written record of minimum hiring requirements for a particular job comes from the job analysis procedure. The items covered in the specifications may be divided into two groups:
  1. The skill requirements include mental and manual skills, plus personal traits and qualities, needed to perform the job effectively:
     - Minimum educational requirements
     - Licensure or registration requirements
     - Experience expressed in objective and quantitative terms, such as years
     - Specific knowledge requirements or advanced educational requirements including cyber skills
     - Manual skills required in terms of the quality, quantity, or nature of the work to be performed
     - Communication skills, both oral and written; specific language fluency
  2. The physical demands of a job may include the following:
     - Physical effort required to perform the job and the length of time involved in performing a given activity
     - Working conditions and general physical environment in which the job is to be performed; external travel requirements; several or multiple settings (as in a decentralized organization)
     - Mental demands, including ability to work with frequent interruptions; ability to remain courteous, tactful, and cooperative throughout the work day
     - Job hazards and their probability of occurrence

The date of latest revision is provided at the end of the description.

**Exhibit 6–3** is a sample job description. Human resources manuals and professional association publications are excellent sources of job description content and wording.

In some institutions, job specifications are organized as a separate record because the information is not used for the same purpose as the information

---

**Exhibit 6–3** Excerpts from a Typical Job Description: Clerical Position

**Job Summary**

This is a clerical position in the health information service of an acute care facility affiliated with a medical school and a research institution. This full-time, day-shift position is under the direct supervision of the Assistant Health Information Administrator. The work is performed with relative independence and any exceptions to policy should be referred to the unit supervisor.

**Job Duties**

1. Receives visitors to the department, processes their requests by routing them to appropriate supervisors, assists requestor as needed, and schedules appointments
2. Processes reports from dictated media and/or from rough draft and transcribes according to prescribed format

**Job Specifications**

1. Fluency in English language, both oral and written expression
2. Ability to create final copy, from both dictation and handwritten copy, error-free minimum of 70 words per minute
3. Minimum of high school diploma or its equivalent and at least 1 year of secretarial experience or successful completion of postsecondary secretarial school

Note flexibility in requirement 3; this fosters a nondiscriminatory approach to hiring, giving flexibility to the manner in which an individual may qualify for the position.

contained in the job description. The specifications receive the most usage in connection with the recruitment and selection of employees, as this part of the job description defines the qualifications that are needed to perform the job. Job evaluations and the establishment of different wage and salary schedules are other functions that depend on the data contained in the job specifications (**Exhibit 6–4**).

## Job Rating and Classification

Before employees are selected and hired, the organization develops a job classification. This classification is based on the results of the job rating process. In job rating, each set of functions within each unit of the organization is analyzed using some set of common denominators. In health care, these variables include complexity of duties; error impact; contacts with patients, families, and other individuals both within and outside of the organization; degree of supervision received; and nature of duties, ranging from unskilled to highly technical and professional. Mental and physical demands as well as working conditions may also be assessed because these variables may make a job different from seemingly similar positions in the organization.

When developing a job description, it is useful to compare the draft of the description with the job rating scale specific to the organization. From this dry run, changes in actual wording may result so that the final expression of job duties and related conditions matches the categories or factors to be assessed. Without such correlation between the job rating scale and the job description's wording, inequities could be

---

**Exhibit 6–4** Job Description—Administrative Assistant (an alternate example of job description format and content)

| | |
|---|---|
| Job Title: | Administrative Assistant to Director of Dietary and Food Service |
| Department: | Food Service |
| Manager: | Incumbent reports to Director of Dietary and Food Service |
| Job Titles reporting to Administrative Assistant: | None |
| Exempt/nonexempt | Nonexempt |
| Line/staff: | Staff |
| Full time/part time: | Full time; Monday through Friday, 7:00 A.M. to 3:00 P.M. |
| Essential/nonessential: | Essential |
| Location/work setting: | Central dietary-food service department |
| External travel: | None |

Job Duties: this is a staff/support position; work is carried out according to established policies, procedures, and systems. Primary responsibility is the provision of administrative support to the Director of Dietary and Food Service. Specific duties include, but are not limited to:

1. Timely and accurate completion of data entry and documentation of department records
2. Timely and accurate processing of correspondence and inquiries
3. Maintenance of department records according to organization's record keeping and retention policies
4. Coordination with IT department regarding office equipment and systems
5. Processing vendor specifications and proposals; scheduling vendor interviews
6. Scheduling and coordinating food safety inspections
7. Requisitioning food service supplies and equipment
8. Track purchasing requisitions; carry out inventory control
9. Prepare payroll information
10. Monitor budget and account for variations
11. Maintain appointment schedule for Director of Dietary and Food Services
12. Maintain confidentiality of patient, employee, and organization's information

### Job Requirements

1. Ability to communicate effectively
2. Proven administrative experience
3. Knowledge of office management duties
4. Ability to maintain positive interpersonal skills throughout the work day
5. Ability to maintain productivity and prioritize work throughout the work day with its frequent interruptions
6. Ability to use standard office equipment and systems, including proficiency in computer skills
7. General knowledge of budgeting and accounting practices

fostered. Similar jobs could receive different ratings based on a lack of proper wording in a particular job description.

Ideally, the overall job rating process contains safeguards against discrepancies; ideally, the human resources manager makes such job rating information available to unit managers. It is still the duty and prerogative of line managers to take active steps in these matters and anticipate the job rating process.

In addition to the overall job classification, the wage and salary and fringe benefit package may be predicated on information gained in the job description or job rating process. Another key to success in developing useful job descriptions is to assess the written document for its adequacy in conveying information about the factors used in job rating and wage and salary considerations.

Two additional outcomes of the job classification that concern the manager are the determinations made for exempt and nonexempt positions under the Fair Labor Standards Act (FLSA) and the applicability of a union contract in terms of jobs included in a particular bargaining union. In both of these cases, information about supervisory activity is critical. Thus, there is another benchmark against which to measure the adequacy of the job description. Does it contain sufficient information to justify inclusion—or exclusion—of a job in terms of overtime pay and related FLSA provisions? Is the nature of the job clearly delineated in terms of rating as skilled or unskilled, technical or professional, for purposes of union contract applicability?

## Recruitment

Certain steps in the recruitment process involve information derived from the job description. Internal job posting may involve the placement of the complete job description in a specified location, such as on an employee bulletin board and website. Potential transfer employees essentially participate in a self-selection or rejection process as they read this job description. They can take the opportunity to assess such practical aspects of a job as shift work or weekend coverage requirements in terms of their availability to work such hours.

The physical, mental, or technical demands of the job also may sway the potential transfer employee to reconsider applying for a position. Then, too, the job description may have the effect of encouraging applicants. Does the job description contain enough information to help prospective employees make such a preliminary determination?

Those involved in the preliminary selection interviews, usually members of the human resources department, need sufficient information about all the jobs in the institution to carry out initial screening. The unit managers must convey, through the job description, key points of information about duties, responsibilities, and qualifications. It is important to note that the unit manager is the individual most familiar with the work of the unit. This information must be conveyed in a way that it can be understood by persons who are not involved in the unit or department on a daily basis.

Awareness of the wide audience who will use the job descriptions will help the manager write them in understandable form. The unit manager may find it useful to try out the wording of a job description on another manager. Does the wording convey enough information for this person, familiar with the healthcare setting but not necessarily familiar with the details of the specific department, to form a basic idea of the job?

## The Final Selection Process

A major use of the job description occurs during the selection process as the candidate is matched to the job. During the selection interview, information about the duties, responsibilities, and qualifications is conveyed. One sensitive overlay to the selection process, which includes all aspects of the interview, testing, and physical examination, is strict avoidance of discriminatory practices, even inadvertent discrimination.

When the job, as summarized in the job description, is the focus of the interview, it is easier to avoid the pitfalls of interviewing that could suggest discriminatory practices. Thus, with a job description that spells out such expectations as weekend coverage, shift work availability, and similar requirements, the manager and prospective employee can deal with that set of expectations without the manager probing in any way into such questions as days of religious observance, arrangements for child care, and other topics that are off-limits for direct inquiry. The emphasis is on the job as it is described.

Job qualifications and mental, physical, and technical demands become the objective measures of candidate suitability when they are derived from job duties. These in turn foster a positive climate of compliance with nondiscriminatory practices.

For example, if the job duties include frequent routine interaction with patients in need of emergency care and the patient population involved is non-English speaking, a qualification of fluency in a specific language is not discriminatory. If the unit manager can tie each qualification to one or more job duties, the likelihood of discriminatory practices in the employment selection process is diminished. Sometimes it may seem that one is stating the obvious, such as ability to read, write, speak English (or some other language) with ease, hear, see, and lift—so why spell these out? These elements are specified in detail when they are true requirements. The purpose of the job description, with its explicit requirements, is to provide all parties with necessary information about the job so that there is no misunderstanding later.

Another method to use in making a dry run of the job description that helps the manager determine the level of detail needed under the foregoing conditions is working with human resources management using a sample of applications that have been received over some period of time. How does the manager's job description hold up? On what basis would the manager hire, or not hire, a particular individual in light of the job description as it is written?

## Employee Development and Retention

At each point of employee development, activities focus on the work to be done within each job. Orientation and training programs take on greater meaning as they are tailored to specific job duties and qualifications. Training outcomes can be stated in terms of the trainee's ability to perform the duties. This is another step toward objective evaluation of candidates.

Job descriptions also provide a focus for performance evaluations. Has the worker accomplished the duties and responsibilities made known in the job description? Error correction, retraining, and, if necessary, disciplinary action are carried out in the context of the job for which the individual was hired. In cases of grievance, emphasis is given to the worker's accomplishment of the job duties, with the presumption that these have been made known to the worker. A comprehensive, up-to-date job description is a valuable management document in such cases.

Finally, in cases of illness or injury under review by workers' compensation groups or agencies such as the Occupational Safety and Health Administration (OSHA), the basic determination of job relatedness is made using the job description.

Following is a summary of uses of the job description. How would the manager's current descriptions hold up when scrutinized in relation to each of these applications?

## Summary of Uses of the Job Description

The job description does the following:

- Fosters or contributes to overall compliance with legal, regulatory, contractual, and accrediting mandates
- Serves as a basis for job rating, job classification, and wage and salary administration
- Serves as a basis for determining exemption or inclusion under provisions of the FLSA and collective bargaining agreements
- Provides information to prospective employees and to employer representatives during the recruitment and selection process
- Serves as a basis for orientation and training programs at the time of initial selection, transfer, or promotion
- Serves as a basis for performance evaluation, error correction, retraining requirements, and grievance determinations
- Provides information to determine eligibility for claims under workers' compensation groups, OSHA, and similar programs

Jobs, like the organizational structure of a hospital, are dynamic in nature. Changes in the size and nature of the organization, the introduction of new equipment, or the employment of new treatment techniques—to mention only a few factors—have a definite influence on the duties and requirements of jobs. Thus, the manager and the employees of a department must review the description of each job on a periodic, regular schedule (at least once a year). The document should be dated when it is first prepared, re-dated when it is reviewed, and again re-dated when it is revised. An up-to-date accurate job description is essential when the human resources department recruits applicants for a job or when the manager hires new employees, appraises the performance of existing employees, and attempts to establish an equitable wage and salary pattern within the department.

## ▶ The Management Inventory

Part of planning and organizing involves the assessment of current and projected staffing needs. One tool for gathering such information is the management inventory, a simple, factual listing of each specific job; name of the incumbent; and any relevant notation. Notation would include such known factors as: (1) an employee who has given 3-month notice of intent to retire; a summer intern leaves in late August; an employee who has requested and has been granted family leave time starting on September 1, with a planned return date of December 15; and an employee who has provided manager with military reserve duty dates, including a 2-week span in mid-July. Managers also include training level accomplished or needed, cross-training indications, changes upcoming because of system change, and phasing out of certain functions. The management inventory is, of course, a highly confidential document used for planning purposes. It is compiled from information given to the manager; managers may not inquire into personal matters, especially those that might infer race or sex discrimination.

## The Credentialed Practitioner as Consultant

Because the contemporary healthcare organization is frequently involved in new patterns of organization, the credentialed practitioner is sometimes called on to be an external consultant or independent contractor. Consultants offer advice and counsel and carry out professional activities within the scope of their competence and licensure. Consultative arrangements generally fall into three categories:

- One-time-only arrangements wherein the consultant carries out an in-depth assessment of current practices or assists in development of a major project. For example, an occupational therapist might assist the management team of a long-term care facility with its plan to open an adult day care service. The occupational therapist would typically identify and describe the range of activities for the occupational therapy unit's services; calculate and determine the pattern of staffing needs for the unit; and identify equipment and space needs, along with layout considerations.
- Initial survey with implementation. In this instance the consultant and the healthcare organization's representatives agree that the professional practitioner will remain under contract to implement the initial findings. Using the example given previously, the occupational therapist would be given the mandate to contact vendors; compare vendor bids; and, with the organization's approval, select the equipment and oversee its placement.

- Ongoing maintenance of project or program. In this arrangement, the professional practitioner agrees to provide continuous service over some specific, and usually prolonged, period of time. For example, a physical therapist is hired to upgrade the in-service training program at an industrial health clinic. Having developed an overall training plan, based on the facility's needs, the physical therapist commits to a plan to provide the in-service training on a regular basis—for example, 1 day per month for the upcoming year.

## The Independent Contractor

When the professional practitioner is hired to provide regular, ongoing services for a protracted period of time (as in the third example in the previous section), the relationship of the practitioner to the contracting organization may fall into the category of independent contractor. Both parties to such an arrangement need to review pertinent federal and state laws and regulations regarding independent contractor status. Particular attention should be given to the Internal Revenue Code's definitions of independent contractors. Regulations set forth in HIPAA contain specific provisions concerning privacy and confidentiality requirements for business partners and independent contractors. Professional liability insurance provisions, workers' compensation laws, collective bargaining agreements, and similar labor-related mandates need review as to their applicability to the particular arrangements.

## Guidelines for Contracts and Reports

Whether fulfilling the role of consultant or independent contractor, the professional practitioner works under written contract and provides formal reports to the administrative coordinators of the facility. Following are guidelines for the content of contracts and reports.

### The Contract

The professional practitioner, working with a properly qualified attorney, would develop a contract specific to the given situation. The contract typically includes at least the elements of a clear statement of parties to the contract, the period covered, services to be provided, fees and payment schedule, ownership of materials, privacy and confidentiality of patient and business information, and provisions for termination of the contract. An attorney would provide the appropriate level of detail and additional provisions necessary for a sound agreement.

## The Written Report

The consultant provides the administrative coordinators with periodic written reports, formal and detailed in their content. Following are guidelines for such reports:

1. Consultant reports are formal business records and, as such, must be retained by both the consultant and the organization for the required retention period for such business records. See the specific state laws and federal tax laws governing the retention period.
2. Consultant reports are subject to inspection and review by licensing and accrediting agencies and by third-party payment auditors. The report, therefore, should be complete, formal, and accurate.
3. Keep the report focused on compliance with required licensure, accreditation, and professional practice standards. Include both positive and negative findings. A useful practice, and one that also motivates the recipients to continue to strive for excellence, is to list the positive findings first, followed by the heading "Areas Needing Improvement."
4. Provide specific recommendations for each topical area needing improvement. For example, suggest the content of an in-service training program on the topic or provide sample forms or procedures.
5. Prioritize the findings in order of importance. To prioritize findings:
   - Priority Class One: Address any practice that has potential for direct harm to the patient. An example in health information documentation would be contradictory physician orders concerning medications. This finding would be reported orally to the nursing staff as soon as it is identified by the consultant. The written report, as follow-up, would contain the formal recommendation for corrective practices, with the notation that an oral report was made to the nursing staff in a timely manner.
   - Priority Class Two: Address any practice for which the facility received a citation in the last external survey or auditor review, with particular attention to the practices for which a plan of correction was filed with state or federal agencies. Also, address any practice having repeat citations over the past several years, even if the current survey showed full compliance for the immediate year.
   - Priority Class Three: Address any practice that is out of compliance with:
     - State licensure requirements. For example, mention record retention practices that do not meet the state's required retention period.
     - Federal conditions of Medicare. For example, cite any failure to update the patient plan of care according to the required time frames.
     - HIPAA regulations. For example, note any failure regarding the disclosure of patient information without appropriate consent.
     - Accrediting standards (if the facility participates in an accreditation program). For example, address the failure to document interdisciplinary progress notes according to suggested standards.
     - Generally accepted principles of professional practice. For example, mention failure to put complete patient identification on each page of the hard copy record or on each data entry for an electronic record.

An example of a cover letter, a formal report with priority indications, and a project timetable is included here.

## ▶ Sample Contract for a Health Information Consultant

*Note:* The following example is not intended as legal advice. The professional practitioner who plans to enter into consultant activity should consult an attorney for the development of a contract appropriate to the specific situation.

## ▶ Consultant Agreement for Health Information Services

**Parties to the Agreement**: The parties to this agreement are Morgan Dean, MS, RHIA, Consultant (referred to as Consultant), and The Gabriels Continuing Care Center (referred to as Gabriels Center), Anywhere, Anystate. As a licensed continuing care facility in this state, Gabriels Center is governed by the applicable state and federal laws and regulations.

**Effective Date**: February 1, 20n1. This agreement continues in effect until one of the parties chooses to terminate it by providing a written notice to that effect 1 month prior to the termination date.

**Independent Contractor**: Consultant's status is that of an independent contractor. Consultant is not an employee or agent of Gabriels Center. Consultant is not a participant in any benefits program, labor contract agreement, or any other program offered by this facility. Consultant is not a designated officer in the continuity of operations or succession plan of the facility.

**Professional Competence**: Consultant agrees to provide formal, written evidence of professional competence as defined by the national credentialing body for health information practice. This documentation shall be provided at the inception of this contract and on an annual basis (on the anniversary date of this contract) thereafter.

**Scope of Service**: Consultant's activities are limited to the skilled care, assisted living, and personal care components of Gabriels Center as currently configured.

**Terms of Payment**: The fee for services is ($_____) per quarter. A 5% increase shall be made at the beginning of each new year of the contractual relationship if this contract remains in effect. This increase shall be effective on the anniversary date of the initial contract. Consultant, as an independent contractor, is responsible for Social Security contributions and any applicable withholding tax or contribution as required by federal, state, and local taxing authorities. Consultant will present a written bill for services rendered for each quarter. This bill must be filed within five working days of the conclusion of the quarter. A quarterly written report must be filed at the same time. Gabriels Center agrees to pay Consultant within five working days of the receipt of the quarterly bill and report. This is the whole and entire reimbursement.

**Confidentiality**: Consultant agrees to keep confidential any and all information about Gabriels Center's operations and practices and to follow HIPAA-compliant practices. Reports shall be filed with the designated official contact of the center.

**Ownership of Materials**: Consultant agrees to develop materials such as, but not limited to, policies, procedures, forms, job descriptions, and training programs for use by Gabriels Center in its skilled and assisted living and personal care components. These materials become the property of Gabriels Center. Gabriels Center agrees to limit their use solely to these levels of care as currently configured. Gabriels Center agrees not to sell or distribute the materials to any other component or entity. Gabriels Center agrees to obtain Consultant's permission to use the materials in any other manner. The consultant retains the right to use the same or similar materials without facility identification.

**Responsibilities**: Consultant will review the health information services and the healthcare documentation practices of the skilled care, assisted living, and personal care components of Gabriels Center.

Consultant will make at least quarterly site visits and remain available by telephone and/or electronic messaging.

The specific duties are listed in the attached *Key Activities of the Health Information Consultant*. Consultant will make formal, oral reports to the chief executive officer or designate at the conclusion of each quarter at a mutually agreed-on time and date. A formal, written report shall be filed within five working days of the conclusion of the quarter. One interim written report per quarter shall be made at a mutually agreed-on date.

**Entire Agreement**: This is the full and entire agreement as stated in these terms and signed by both parties on the date listed below. This agreement may be amended in writing with both parties signing and dating the acceptance of the changes.

| Chief Executive Officer | Morgan Dean, MS, RHIA |
|---|---|
| The Gabriels Continuing Care Center | Health Information Consultant |
| Date: February 1, 20n1 | Date: February 1, 20n1 |

# ▶ Key Activities of Health Information Consultant (Addendum to February 1, 20N1, Contract)

Consultant shall oversee the health information system (HIS) and documentation practices for the skilled and assisted living and personal care components as follows:

1. Identify applicable federal and state laws and regulations and generally accepted principles of health information practice. Assess the degree of compliance with these regulations and recommend

improved practices associated with areas needing upgrading. Assist the management team in preparing for periodic federal and state reviews and related plan of correction development.

2. Monitor proposed changes in applicable federal and state laws and regulations; monitor trends in health information practices and provide the management team with this information.

3. Prepare and periodically update the following documents:
   - Policy and procedure manuals
   - Forms design for hard copy and electronic data capture

4. Analyze and review each component of the health information system and the documentation practices of the facility:
   - Patient identification
   - Creation and maintenance of official health record
   - Data entry and dictation–transcription/voice recognition editing
   - Record retention, storage, and retrieval
   - Coding and reimbursement support
   - Support data and studies for patient care reviews, quality improvement studies, and management use
   - Release of information

5. Participate in staff development and in-service training:
   - Annual presentation of documentation standards to professional staff
   - Training program for new HIS employees
   - Annual training program for each HIS employee

6. Assist management in the development of:
   - Staffing pattern
   - Job descriptions
   - Space allocation and equipment acquisition
   - Budget preparation

7. Participate in the patient care review committee and the emergency preparedness committee:
   - Recommend items for consideration
   - Provide support materials for items under consideration
   - Attend regularly scheduled meetings

End of listing of key activities as of February 1, 20n1.

# ▶ Sample Cover Letter and Report

*Background information for this fictitious setting:*

1. State-licensed as a continuing care facility; last licensure survey was last year on December 20

2. Privately owned and sponsored by a nonprofit corporation

3. Medicare certified under applicable provisions

4. Fiscal year: July through June

5. Components:
   - Independent Living: 100 units; average length of stay: 8 years
     - Eighty percent of residents move to the assisted-living or skilled unit when one of these levels of care is needed
   - Assisted Living: 50 units; average length of stay: 3 years
     - Ninety-five percent of residents move to the skilled care unit when this level of care is needed
   - Skilled Care: 90 units; average length of stay: 1.5 years
   - Personal Care: 30 units; average length of stay: 3 years
   - Annual discharges average 45, including 25 discharges to acute care; 10 discharges from skilled care, returning to the assisted living unit; 10 deaths (natural causes)

6. Health Information Services (HIS): There is no full- or part-time credentialed practitioner. The consultant was hired on February 1, 20n1, and remains under contract.

7. Expansion plans: The facility is considering the addition of an adult day care unit, a memory-care/dementia care unit, and a home care service for the independent living unit.

# ▶ Cover Letter

July 5, 20n1
Bernard Downey, Chief Executive Officer
The Gabriels Continuing Care Center
253 Main Street
Anywhere, Anystate 00999

Dear Mr. Downey:

I have enclosed the written report and bill for the April–June 20n1 quarter. The report reflects my findings and recommendations about the health information services (HIS) of the skilled and assisted living and personal care components of your center.

As we discussed at our June 30 meeting, I will continue the regularly scheduled duties and responsibilities as outlined in the current contractual agreement. As we agreed, we will meet on July 12 to update and expand this contract to reflect my involvement in the plans for the adult day care program, the home care project, and the development of the personal health record for the independent living unit. We also agreed to give additional efforts to the following topics:

- Review and update of all HIS job descriptions and titles
- Participation in a focused study of pattern of care and related documentation for short-term, postacute care and respite care admissions versus balance-of-life admissions
- Special review of documentation and reporting of suspected elder abuse, including involuntary seclusion in the personal care unit
- Focus on efforts to regain Five-Star Medicare rating
- Focused review of pattern of admission from, and readmission to, acute care facility for same diagnosis within (*n*) days
- Focused review of pattern of care for patients with advance directives who are, nevertheless, transferred to acute care
- Thorough review of record retention policy and practice, with particular attention to legacy hard copy records from the 2007 merger of three facilities, along with planned destruction of all hard copy records for which the mandatory retention period has been met

If you have any further question about these findings, please do not hesitate to contact me.

Sincerely,
Morgan Dean, MS, RHIA
Health Information Consultant

Enclosures: quarterly report and bill for period ending June 30, 20n1

## ▶ Quarterly Report: Health Information Services

April 1, 20n1–June 30, 20n1
Report filed on July 5, 20n1

### Dates of Site Visits and Primary Activities

April 13: Continuing review of systems and documentation

Attended Emergency Preparedness committee; presented updated version of the portable emergency file for individual residents

May 10: Continuing review of systems and documentation

Training program for new coder

May 16: Continuing review of systems and documentation

In-service training program on documentation requirements; presented to professional staff

June 28: Attended Emergency Preparedness committee; finalized updated version of portable emergency file

June 28: Completed suggested response to Plan of Correction

Met with chief executive officer to review quarterly report and discuss additional activities regarding the Center's expansion

### Persons Interviewed During Site Visits

Chief executive officer, director of finances, director of nursing, director of social services, consultant occupational therapist, consultant physical therapist, staff activities therapist, health information staff

### Key Activities

1. Licensure review preparation: assisted with preparation for annual licensure review, completed report sections relating to HIS, developed suggested Plan of Correction responses for the deficiencies noted at the December 20 (last year) site visit by state agency.
2. Monitoring of proposed changes in legislation and regulation and trends: assisted in the development of an in-service training program concerning medical identity theft prevention, assisted risk management and nursing service in development of a procedure for providing photo identification for residents who are admitted to the local hospital or who receive care at the local hospital's clinic. I reviewed compliance with the licensure agreements associated with computer software in the HIS; no breaches were identified. I proposed the development of a project for the implementation of the personal health record for the independent living unit. This project will be discussed during the next quarter; the consultant's agreement will be amended to reflect this involvement.
3. Policy and procedure manual development: the section of release of information was updated to reflect the changes associated with the newly implemented computerized system.
4. Participation in staff development and in-service training: annual presentation to professional staff on core data/documentation requirements was given on May 16. The preliminary information on

the photo identification issues was also presented at this session. On-the-job training of the HIS coder was given during the week of May 12–16.

5. Committee participation: attended meetings of Emergency Preparedness Committee on April 13 and June 8 to develop an updated version of the portable emergency file for residents.

6. Review of HIS: Each component of the HIS was reviewed.

    *Patient identification:* The comprehensive system is in place; 100% accuracy noted; each patient has full identification, documented at admission and updated at least quarterly.

    Practice needing improvement: some frail, elderly patients have used, and continue to use, a familiar name ("nickname") and that is the name to which they most readily respond. (Examples: Sarah Smith uses Sally as her familiar name; Jonathan Michael Lake uses Mike.) This familiar name should be added to the identification information, noting that it is the familiar and preferred name as used by the resident. The full legal name should, of course, be listed. Discussion of these issues is appropriately included at admission and in the patient care plan conference. Suggestion: confer with legal counsel and risk management to develop an appropriate policy and procedure.

    Priority Class One: residents could become confused and/or agitated when they are addressed using only a formal name.

    *Creation and maintenance of an official health record:* A formal health record was readily located for each resident. In all but two cases, there were no data entry errors within the records. In two cases, residents with the same first and last name (but different middle names and dates of birth) were mixed. The contents of these two records were promptly corrected under the supervision of the director of nursing.

    Practice needing improvement: proper data entry; attention to accuracy of identification and data entry

    Priority Class One: potential harm to resident

    A second issue was noted: the creation of "shadow charts." The physical therapy, occupational therapy, and social services departments have created their own full-scale health record; the content of these records duplicate some portions of the official health record, and some information in the "shadow chart" is not included in the official record.

    Practice needing improvement: elimination of "shadow charts"

Priority Class Three: the applicable laws and regulations indicate that there is one official health record.

    *Coding and reimbursement:* A 10% sample of coding was carried out, giving attention to completeness, accuracy, and timeliness. Completeness and accuracy met the required standard, but there is a delay in timely coding due to staff absence associated with illness and vacation. This affects the reimbursement process, causing delay in that system.

    Practice needing improvement: timely coding through provision of alternate staff to carry out this function when regular staff is absent

    Priority Class Three: reimbursement schedules require timely submission of billing information.

    *Storage and retrieval:* During the month of May, the closed (inactive) files from 14 years were moved to another location because of renovations to the former storage area. The new location is a temporary one—the storage shed on the upper campus. This storage area does not meet the privacy, security, and protection requirements. The records are in boxes in the same space as items for the craft and yard sale fund-raising events, there is only a padlock on the door, there is no sprinkler system, and access is not restricted. Before similar actions are taken in the future, and before remedial action is taken now, it is necessary to check with the HIS consultant to ensure compliance with laws, regulations, and best practice.

    Practice needing improvement: relocation of records to secure environment; recommended removal to a commercial storage facility that meets record storage requirements or cull these records for destruction if the retention period has been satisfied.

    Priority Class Three: applicable laws and regulations require secure storage.

    A second issue was noted: The records from last year's discharges due to death were not found in the central storage and retrieval unit. These records had been inadvertently kept with the patient care review committee files. They were subsequently retrieved and placed in their proper location.

    Practice needing improvement: review and enforce the procedure for the return of records after committee review.

    Priority Class Three: applicable laws and regulations require secure storage.

7. Review of health information documentation: These findings are based on the results of the routine reviews done at time of admission, patient

care plan conference, transfers within levels of care, and discharge. An additional 10% sampling was carried out. Overall, there is continuing improvement in documentation practices. However, the following areas need attention:

*Patient care plan:* The initial care plan and the first two updates are adequate; there is only limited update of the plan reflecting changes in care when a major episode occurs (e.g., bed rest or other restrictions due to a fall). Activities therapy plans are not updated to reflect the circumstances of a resident's increased impairment due to physical or cognitive diminishment. The plan of care for final weeks of care when a patient is close to death is not fully reflective of palliative care, review of healthcare directives, and family conference.

*Physical examination:* Approximately 20% of residents do not have their annual physical examinations completed within the mandated time frames.

*Transfer support documents:* Approximately 10% of residents do not have up-to-date transfer support data entries available at the time of transfer. The average delay in providing these documents was 2 days.

In addition to the routine review of documentation, five special studies were carried out. The findings were presented to the Patient Care Review committee and were made part of the minutes of that committee:

- Restraint-free protocol compliance
- Adequacy of consent for treatment and for release of information
- Adequacy of data entries/documentation at time of transfer into the Center and at discharge to another facility
- Patterns of care: comparison of length of stay between short-stay respite care and short-stay postacute care
- Indicators and patterns of social isolation of semi-bedridden residents and memory care residents.

In addition to these topics, the patient care committee discussed whether or not a detailed spiritual history should be obtained and included in the residents' social history that is recorded during intake. This concept has been brought up in some externally sponsored training programs by some who view this comprehensive documentation as part of a holistic approach to care. The committee unanimously rejected the concept for these reasons:

1. There is a standard entry to show a resident's religious affiliation, should they wish to do so.
2. There is follow-up to this entry to determine if there are dietary needs, medical interventions prohibited (e.g., blood transfusion), and any particular accommodation needed for religious reasons.
3. The services of a chaplain of choice is available to residents. Chaplaincy notes are made according to standard documentation protocols. These are brief and do not include confidential information.
4. Residents, their families, and some volunteers might not be aware that, should more detailed information be incorporated into the formal medical record, it is discoverable.

## CHAPTER 7

# Committees and Teams

## CHAPTER OBJECTIVES

- Provide a generalized definition of a committee.
- Provide examples of committees and task forces commonly used in healthcare settings.
- Differentiate among committees, standing as well as ad hoc, and plural executives and task forces.
- Describe the generally accepted purposes and uses of committees.
- Enumerate the advantages as well as the limitations and disadvantages of committees.
- Provide guidelines for ensuring committee effectiveness.
- Identify the role and functions of the committee chairperson.
- Provide guidance for creating and preserving documentation of a committee's formal proceedings.
- Examine the modern management phenomenon of the employee team (in a number of possible forms) as a special case of the committee.
- Provide guidelines for group deliberations, with application to a multidisciplinary review process.

Committees have become a fact of life in modern organizations. The democratic tradition in American society, the committee system's history of success in organizations, and the legal and accrediting authority mandates for such activity contribute to the widespread use of committees in healthcare organizations. Consider the variety of committees, task forces, and teams in healthcare organizations, noting that their development tends to flow from one of four sources:

1. *The corporate culture*: the mission and vision statements of the organization set the tone; committee and task force structures are set up to implement routine actions to carry out these value statements, for example:
   - Commitment to excellence: continuous quality improvement committee and its adoption of benchmark/best practices standards
   - A culture of cooperation and coordination: multidisciplinary review committee of disaster response; clinical care review committee
   - A culture of safety and security: safety and security committee; risk management review committee
   - A culture of outreach: patient and family advisory committee; community relations task force
2. *The organizational structure*: there is a need for coordination among units, for example, the joint operations committee for cancer treatment, the medical executive committee, and joint conference committee.
3. *Response to a specific need*: for example, pandemic preparedness coordinating committee, 100th anniversary commemoration planning.
4. *Mandates contained in licensure laws and accreditation standards*: these mandates may be stated broadly, allowing the organization considerable leeway in structuring its committees. A state law for an outpatient adult care center might simply indicate that an oversight process be developed to assure compliance with administrative,

organizational, and client care directives of the state's healthcare agency. The mandate might include a general directive that written policies, procedures, and recommendations for improvement be reviewed on an annual basis.

Conversely, a mandate might contain highly specific, detailed requirements. For example, utilization review committee directives include required committee composition, specific topics for review (e.g., over- and under-utilization; review of extended stay cases; appropriateness of care setting/level of care, medical necessity for admission, and timely discharge planning). The dates of committee meetings and the names of members in attendance are required. Practices to ensure confidentiality of reports and patient review forms are required.

The bylaws of the organization usually set out the composition of the board of trustees/governing board along with specific duties, usually carried out by committees, for example, an audit and compliance committee, contractual review group, fiscal soundness, investments, and budgetary issues.

Having noted these typical examples, we turn our attention to a detailed discussion of important aspects of committees and task forces.

The committee structure complements the overall organizational structure because it can be used to overcome problems stemming from specialization and departmentation. The weakness of specialization is the potential loss of broad organizational vision on the part of the individual manager; however, coordination of action and assessment of the overall organizational impact of a decision may be facilitated when a committee brings together a number of specialists for organized deliberation.

Healthcare organizations need committees to help consolidate the dual authority tracks within the medical authority structure and the administrative/support structure. The joint conference committee, consisting of representatives from the medical staff, the board of trustees, and the administration, is commonly used for this purpose. Functions of healthcare organizations typically monitored and assessed by committees include pharmacy and therapeutics, infection control, patient care evaluation, surgical case review, health records/clinical documentation, quality assurance, and patterns of care review.

Committee participation, development of support data, and development of policies and procedures are expected parts of the daily routine of the chief of service, department head, or manager. A review

of the manager's daily wheel book entries provides insight into the nature and extent of managers' committee involvement. See **Appendix 7–A**, Wheel Book Excerpts Reflecting Committee and Team Activity.

A starting point for understanding the importance and scope of committee activity in healthcare organizations is found in legal and accrediting mandates that require such a framework. The executive—leadership officers of the organization develop the framework for compliance with mandated reviews and oversight processes. This framework is incorporated into the official bylaws, rules, and regulations of the organization. Usually, this framework consists of a mix of committees and review boards, developed to meet the specific needs of the organization. This framework also incorporates the required reviews and oversight activities stemming from state licensure and regulation, federal laws and regulations, and accrediting agency standards. Matters relating to the medical staff (e.g., selection, credentials review, appointment, peer review) are usually grouped under the purview of the Medical Executive Committee.

Each committee and review board is important, but some activities move into prominence because of new or intensified interest in the topics related to such groups. Historical examples include the increased role of the ethics committee in response to the Patient Self Determination Act of 1990 or the Institutional Review Board mandates for research on human subjects (1974). Both continue to deal with recurring as well as emerging topics. The Quality Committee or the Performance Improvement Program is an example of current and continuing emphasis. This committee, usually headed by the senior medical officer and the quality improvement officer, focuses on developing and implementing organization-wide performance improvement plan. Benchmark data, proven practice protocols, and institutional data and trends provide the basis of the plan and its ongoing review. Membership on the committee includes both direct patient care staff as well as managerial and support staff/department representatives so that all aspects of care are coordinated and reviewed.

Some organizations place all externally and internally mandated reviews in one comprehensive committee: the healthcare compliance (corporate compliance) committee of the board of trustees. A chief compliance officer oversees the corporate compliance program. As a relatively independent and objective position within the organization, the compliance officer develops, maintains, and communicates the system-wide plan. The work entails a high degree of collaboration with each department/service as well as with the organization's committees and review boards. Examples of mutual collaboration involve risk management, Health Insurance Portability and Accountability Act (HIPAA) review for data security, coding and reimbursement, claims review and processing, and standards of conduct.

Because middle managers interact with these key committees, an understanding of the nature of committees, their function, and their composition helps managers foster committee effectiveness.

# ▶ The Nature of Committees

A committee may be defined as a group of persons in an organization who function collectively on an organized basis to perform some administrative activity. A committee is more than an informal group that meets to discuss an issue and share ideas, even if such a group meets regularly. The manager who informally calls together a team of subordinates or other managers to talk over an idea or problem is not dealing with a committee. The emphasis in the committee concept is the creation of a structure that has an organized basis for its activity and interaction and that is accountable for its function. The predominant characteristic of the committee is group deliberation on a recurring basis done in the context of a specific grant of authority.

Committees may be temporary or permanent. The temporary, or ad hoc, committee is created to deal with one issue, such as cost-containment compliance initiatives, and its work is limited to that issue. If the problem assigned to an ad hoc committee becomes a recurring one, it may be handled by an existing committee, it may be referred to an existing department, or a new standing committee may be created to deal with it.

Standing committees, which are relatively permanent, focus on recurring matters. The individual members change, but the committee is continuing with respect to the number of members, the distribution of representatives, and its basic charge. Typical standing committees in healthcare organizations include those responsible for dealing with credentials, infection control, patient care policies, patient care documentation, and quality assurance. A department may have specific standing committees, such as departmental quality assurance, safety control, or professional development committees.

A committee may have either line or staff authority. If the committee has authority to bind subordinates who are responsible to it, it is part of the line unit structure. For example, a governing board may have an executive committee that gives directives to the chief executive officer of the institution and thus exercises line authority. A grievance committee, whose decision is binding because of a policy or union contract, exercises line authority in producing its determinations; managers are not free to act contrary to such decisions. In contrast, if the committee has an advisory relationship to line managers, it is a staff unit.

In actual practice, the distinction between line and staff authority of a committee is sometimes blurred. A credentials committee of the medical staff may have limited line authority in that, except for unusual cases, the next levels of authority are bound by the recommendations it makes. A union contract governing faculty at a medical school or university may require that a faculty committee review each case of promotion and tenure and make a recommendation to the line officer, the dean, who in turn must add a recommendation, with the final decision made by the board of trustees. Participation in the decision process by several layers in the hierarchy is mandatory in such cases. In that sense, the credentials committee of the medical staff, as well as the promotion and tenure committee of a college, may be viewed as a line committee with limited but explicit input into decisions concerning professional colleagues. Their decisions are not final, but their recommendations are well protected by custom and, in some cases, by law.

## The Plural Executive

Although most committees are nonmanagerial in nature, there is a structural variation in which a committee is created that has line authority and undertakes some or all of the traditional functions of a manager. These committees are created as a result of policy decisions. A familiar example in the healthcare setting is the executive board of a national professional association. Established through the bylaws of the organization, the executive board typically consists of the elected officers and has the authority to act on behalf of the membership in prescribed areas. The board of trustees in a hospital is also a plural executive, although it is almost universal practice to appoint a chief executive officer and assign management functions to that officer.

The plural executive may be established by law, as in federal regulatory agencies (e.g., the Federal Communications Commission and the Securities and Exchange Commission). The law creating such agencies stipulates that there be a regulatory board which has line authority as a board. The board varies greatly in the amount of power held and authority exercised.

Although the board has formal authority, the center of true power in the organization may shift from the executive board to the appointed chief executive officer, who reports to the executive board.

The individual officeholders who constitute the plural executive must rely greatly on an appointed officer, such as the executive director, and on the staff chosen by that officer. Although the executive officer is in a continuing position, the plural executive group may meet infrequently, and its membership may change as frequently as every year. Furthermore, the members of the plural executive unit tend to remain less visible, as they give directives to the executive, who issues these under the office's title. This common practice often obscures the authority constellation proper to the plural executive and may even reduce it to one of symbolic rather than actual authority and power.

## The Task Force

A temporary organizational unit, the task force is created to carry out a specific project or assignment and present its findings to some person or committee that has line authority. It has as its focus highly specific work that requires technical expertise. The task force analyzes the question, completes the research, and makes its recommendations, which may take the form of a complete plan of action. Unlike committees, which remain in existence until specifically dissolved, the task force automatically ceases functioning when its assigned task is completed.

Members of a task force are chosen on the basis of technical competence and specialized training to form a composite, interdisciplinary team. They are not selected to represent a special group interest, and not every department or organizational unit is represented. A task force rarely, if ever, has line authority. Its findings sometimes are referred to a committee that deliberates issues of a basic policy nature; the work of the task force complements that of committees by providing technical research and preparing background information. The group may be created as a result of committee deliberations; for example, the executive committee or the board of trustees of a healthcare institution may wish to expand its services or to develop an entirely new physical complex. These technical problems could be referred to a task force for study; when the work of the task force is done, the executive committee or board takes appropriate action.

Examples of these types of task forces include those concerned with the pandemic response preparation.

In this case, technical experts from several disciplines were needed to study the issues and make recommendations. Representatives from external agencies concerned with public health and safety (e.g., police, county emergency management) were included to make certain that these essential services were integrated into the planning.

Another example of the appropriate use of a task force is to focus on the trend toward a renewal of short-stay, respite care, along with the reduction of long-term care beds. A skilled care facility would benefit from setting up a task force to study this issue, monitor the pending state regulations, and review its marketing and outreach plans.

A task force sometimes is created for its symbolic value—a common political use. The various presidential commissions of the past decades are examples of the use of task forces to call attention to an important issue (e.g., civil rights, space technology, and care of the aged). To ensure that recommendations are made in an arena that is relatively free from vested interests and particular biases, a task force—rather than an administrative agency, or department personnel—may be assigned the responsibility of studying an issue.

## ▶ The Purposes and Uses of Committees

Committees are created to fulfill various specific needs. The following purposes and uses of committees include the advantages that accrue to an organization as a result of effective committee structure development.

## To Gain the Advantage of Group Deliberation

Many management problems are so complex that their impact on the organization as a whole is best assessed through group deliberation and decision making. Decisions may have a long-range effect, and no single manager likely has the knowledge necessary to see all possible ramifications of a problem. In a committee structure, no one manager bears the burden of a decision that will have far-reaching consequences. Probing of the facts and their implications is likely to be more thorough if the knowledge, experience, and judgment of several individuals are brought to bear on the problem in a coordinated manner. The stimulation of shared thinking may lead to a better decision than could be reached by an individual. Finally, group deliberations may be mandatory in some organizations because of the stipulations in a union contract, an accrediting agency, or a regulatory body.

## To Offset Decentralization and Consolidate Authority

In the process of organizing, each manager is given only a portion of the organization's authority. Normally, each manager receives sufficient authority to carry out the responsibilities of the branch or unit of the organization over which that individual has charge. When the organizational structure is consolidated, efforts are made to avoid splintered authority. Yet, because of the limits placed on the manager's authority, every problem a manager faces cannot be solved, and every plan cannot be implemented unilaterally. It is necessary to consolidate organizational authority through specific coordinating efforts; committees provide an additional organizational structure that can be used for this purpose.

The creation of a special-purpose committee to deal with a project or problem involving several units of an institution is an acceptable means of augmenting the normal organizational structure. If the problem is a recurring one, the structure itself should be adjusted to consolidate authority in a formal manner. For nonrecurring special problems, however, special-purpose committees are appropriate.

Coordination among units in a highly decentralized organization may be fostered through committees. The focus under these circumstances is on the need for consistency of action and coordination of detailed plans among several units, which are often separated geographically. A statewide health coordinating committee in healthcare planning is an example of a committee created specifically for the purpose of coordinating activity among units with wide geographical distribution and multiple categories of membership.

## To Counterbalance Authority

The checks-and-balances system in an organization is subject to many pressures. When individuals in decentralized locations surrender authority to higher levels in the hierarchy, there is an attendant desire to monitor those higher levels. For example, to avoid a concentration of power in an executive director, a professional organization or a union with nationwide membership may create an executive committee with power to finalize all decisions, to approve the budget and authorize payments over a stated amount, and to act as sole decision-making body in many areas.

In a situation in which there has been significant fraud or deception or extreme authoritarianism, an officer may be retained temporarily to avoid a public scandal that would have negative effects for the organization. To limit the actions of such an individual during the transition period, the authority of the office is stripped away and placed in a special group that acts as a line committee in place of the official, who retains only the title and selected symbols of office. This committee functions until the officer is safely removed in a politically acceptable manner and a successor is chosen. The committee structure can be costly in economic terms, but an organization may be willing to pay the price to offset concentrated power and to obtain a diffused authority pattern in certain circumstances.

## To Provide Representation of Interest Groups

Occasionally, certain groups have a vested interest in an organization and seek representation in its decision-making arenas, including committee participation. Wanting to protect the value of their degrees, alumni of a college seek positions on the board of trustees or on advisory committees to specific programs. Community members concerned with both long- and short-range plans of a healthcare organization seek input into patient care policies and community health programs through committee participation.

The organization, in turn, is interested in obtaining the support of specific groups and extends to them an opportunity to participate in its deliberations, often through the committee structure. A college may seek alumni representation to consolidate financial support from that group. A hospital or health center may seek community representatives for its advisory committee so that it can better determine local sentiment, assess probable responses to changes in the pattern of services offered, gain tangible financial support, and create goodwill toward the institution.

## To Protect Due Process

In disciplinary matters, an organization may seek to reflect the larger societal value of due process, even when there is no legal or contractual requirement to do so. For instance, in recent years, an increase in litigation has added an almost legal flavor to processes in which an individual's performance is evaluated. A committee of the individual's peers, even if the peer group does not have line authority, may be constituted to make a recommendation to the line officer or governing board. Examples of this approach include the promotion and tenure committee of a university, the ethics committee of a professional association, or the credentials committee of a medical staff. A union contract may specify the composition and function of a grievance committee to ensure that it includes line workers as well as management officials.

## To Promote Coordination and Cooperation

When individuals affected by a decision have participated in making that decision, they are more likely to accept it and abide by it. Participants in group deliberations develop a fuller understanding of each unit's role. The communication process is facilitated because the managers affected by the decision have had an opportunity to present their positions, the constraints under which their departments function, and their special needs, as well as to express disagreements. All members can evaluate the overall plan, review their own functions, and become familiar with the tasks assigned to other units that depend on their unit's output or, in turn, constrain the work assigned to their unit. In its final decision or recommendation, the committee states the assignments for each unit, and these are known to all. This approach is especially valuable when the success of the work depends on the full understanding and acceptance of the decision and plan of execution.

## To Avoid Action

A manager who wishes to avoid or postpone an action indefinitely may create a committee to study the question or may refer it to a panel that has a long agenda and sends its findings to yet another committee for action. If members are selected carefully or if the assignment to an existing committee is made strategically, action will be slow. The issue may die owing to a lack of interest or may become moot because of a decision made in some other arena or because of the departure from the organization of the individuals concerned. Although this intentional delaying tactic can be misused by a manager, it may also be a positive strategy; for example, delay through committee deliberation may be a form of "buying" time for issues to become less emotionally charged.

## To Train Members

Committee participation may be used as part of the executive training process. Exposure to multiple facets of a decision, the defense of various positions, and the development of insight into the problems and considerations of other managers' decisions are part

of this training experience. The potential manager is assessed by other members of the executive team during this interaction, and appropriate coaching and counseling may be given to the management trainee.

## ▶ Limitations and Disadvantages of Committees

Humorous and disparaging comments sometimes reflect the limitations and disadvantages of committee use: "a camel is a horse that was designed by a committee," or "there are no great individuals in this organization, only great committees."

Committee interaction, with its emphasis on deliberation and group participation, is slow. The committee structure, therefore, is not the proper arena when decisions must be made quickly. The time consumed, including the hours spent in formal meetings, is also costly. In highly decentralized organizations or professional associations, travel and lodging costs alone may run well into the thousands of dollars for a meeting of only a few members. The cost of an individual member's attendance (separate from travel and related costs) is calculated by establishing an average hourly rate per member and multiplying the meeting time by this rate. Additionally, there are costs associated with preparation, follow-up time, or the cost of staff support and services. The results of committee action should offset the costs in time, money, and overall effort.

Because of time pressures, committee deliberations may be cut short, thereby eliminating the major advantages of the committee structure (i.e., group participation and presentation of multiple viewpoints). The committee may be indecisive because there is insufficient time to deliberate, or the discussion may become vague and tangential, leading to adjournment without action. Members' lack of preparation prevents full discussion of issues. Being present and on time is only part of a committee member's responsibility; member preparation is a critical factor.

There are several pitfalls to be avoided in regard to preparation. Material may be prepared and distributed in a timely manner, but the committee members may fail to brief themselves prior to the meeting. A member of a subcommittee may fail to carry out an assignment that is critical for the panel's further action. Staff aides or the chairperson may be late in preparing items so that committee members arrive to find large quantities of critical material at their places and are expected to reach decisions even though they have not had enough time to develop an informed opinion.

Absenteeism or tardiness may obstruct the committee's work. If a quorum is required, absence or lateness (or early departure) of several members may upset the critical balance. When the discussion of an agenda item is dependent on a particular member's presence, this part of the meeting must be delayed or postponed if that member is absent or late. Furthermore, time spent waiting for members to arrive to provide a quorum or to discuss a particular agenda item generates cost with no offsetting productivity.

Obstructionist behavior in committee meetings can limit debate. On the one hand, a member who continually declines to give an opinion and who continually votes "abstain" muddies the outcome. Such a committee may be seen as lacking in decisiveness, and its recommendations may be set aside more easily. On the other hand, an individual or a few members may try to dominate the committee. When unanimity or at least major consensus is required, such members may refuse to give in or may insist that the committee endorse their own suggestions for compromise. If it is to act, the committee must accept this dominance by a few. A ready solution to this problem is the encouragement of minority reports. Some open discussion of group dynamics may also foster solutions to this type of roadblock.

Even with much goodwill and a high degree of commitment on the part of members, certain aspects of committee dynamics tend to limit the group's effectiveness. In seeking common ground for agreement and in dealing with small-group pressures to be polite and maintain mutual respect, diluted decisions or compromise to the point of the least common denominator may characterize committee outcomes.

Furthermore, a committee never can take the place of individual managers who accept specific responsibilities and exhibit leadership. Managers must accept the responsibility for certain decisions, even when they are unpopular. It may be especially important to have a specific individual held responsible for decisions in conflict situations. The proverbial buck stops at the highest level of officers, and one manager must be the first among equals when it is a decision in that manager's area of jurisdiction.

## ▶ Enhancement of Committee Effectiveness

Committees, in spite of their limitations, are valuable for organizational deliberations. Their effectiveness may be enhanced by the following actions:

- Viewing committee activity as important and legitimate
- Providing the necessary logistical support
- Assigning clear-cut responsibilities and specific functions to the committee
- Considering committee size, composition, and selection of members carefully
- Selecting the committee chairperson carefully
- Maintaining adequate documentation and follow-up activity
- Creating task forces as an alternative to the proliferation of committees
- Ensuring that members are sensitive to group dynamics and organizational conflict

## Legitimization of Committee Activity

The top management of an organization must create a climate in which the work of committee members is valued. The evaluation system for merit raises and promotions should include the assessment of individuals' work on committee assignments. Committee membership should be viewed positively by members rather than merely tolerated as a duty. Job descriptions should include committee assignment as a necessary component of the work. When staffing patterns are established, work hours should be allotted for essential committee participation. Committee structure should be streamlined so that action is purposeful and members can see the results of their work. Training specifically for effective committee involvement should be part of the overall training program for members rather than left to chance.

## Logistical Support

All necessary staff assistance should be given to the committee chairperson and members. Staff assistants may prepare specific material, devise research questions, gather necessary support data, and carry out follow-up activities. Clerical support should be provided for recording and transcribing minutes and related documents. Adequate space should be made available for meetings. Top management may enhance committee workings by requiring that committee meetings be scheduled regularly and that membership be drawn from several organizational components. Setting aside a certain block of time for interdepartmental meetings and proscribing intradepartmental sessions during that period facilitates the coordination of schedules. If it is deemed preferable, committee meetings may be scheduled for longer periods of time at less frequent intervals.

# Scope, Function, and Authority

When a committee is created, its purpose and function, as well as its scope of activity, must be presented clearly. Will its purpose be merely to deliberate? Will it deliberate and make a recommendation, or will its decision be a binding one? What subjects will it consider? For example, will the medical care evaluation committee concern itself only with assessments of the topics of quality assurance that are mandated by outside review agencies, or will it expand its function to organization-wide quality assurance and education? Will patterns of care review remain a separate function? Will the clinical documentation committee focus only on the documentation requirements for inpatients or on the records of all patients who receive care in the institution regardless of patient category (e.g., inpatient, outpatient, group practice)?

The scope of the committee's work is shaped by its authority. If the credentials committee of the medical staff only makes recommendations to the governing board, while the board retains final authority to make staff appointments, this division of duties should be stated in the bylaws creating the panel and setting forth its mandates. The committee's accountability also needs delineation. To whom does it make its reports? How frequently? Is coordination required with certain administrative components or with other committees?

# Committee Size and Composition

No absolute figure can be given as the optimal size of a committee. Given that open, free deliberation is a major reason for a committee, the size of the group should be small enough to permit discussion. At the same time, it should be large enough to represent various interests. The organization's bylaws and charter may stipulate required committee composition, which in turn will affect a committee's size. Some hospital policies, for example, state that all chiefs of service are members of the executive committee; therefore, the size of the committee is determined by the organization's department structure.

The need for a quorum to undertake official committee action presents special problems if members' schedules simply do not allow them to attend meetings on a predictable basis. Committee size may be increased in order to ensure a quorum so that business may be conducted.

Committee composition is one of the most important factors in the success of a group's work.

Whether they volunteer, are appointed, or are elected, members should possess certain personal qualities. Specifically, they should be able to meet the following criteria:

- Express themselves in a group.
- Keep to the point.
- Discuss issues in a practical rather than theoretical way.
- Give information that advances the thinking of the group about the topic rather than about themselves.
- Assess a topic in an orderly yet flexible way.
- Suppress the natural desire to speak for the sake of being heard or of saying what they think the leader or some powerful member wants to hear.

The members also should have sufficient authority to commit the units or groups they represent to the course of action adopted by the committee. If an individual is appointed to a committee to represent a busy executive, that person should have the power to cast a vote that binds the executive who deputized the member. Deputizing is not without its hazards, but these potential problems may be avoided by careful review and discussion between the executive and the representative before the meeting.

Generally, committee members should be of approximately equal rank and status in the organization to permit the free exchange of ideas. The presence of ex officio members, who may be viewed as more powerful than the elected members, may deter free discussion. Individuals who attend meetings as staff assistants should respect the limits placed on their participation. There should be a clear understanding that the duties of secretary of the committee are those of the individual appointed or elected from within the group; other persons present to carry out the clerical aspects of secretarial work, such as taking down the raw proceedings from which minutes will be extracted, should not be asked to participate in the discussion and should not volunteer information or opinions as they are not official members. If a parliamentarian who is not a member of the committee attends the meetings, this individual should confine any interaction with the committee to points of parliamentary procedure and should withhold all opinions, agreements, and disagreements concerning the issues under discussion. A group that appoints or elects a committee should have confidence that only those individuals duly appointed or elected will make decisions and recommendations on its behalf.

Although diverse points of view should be represented in deliberations, not every participant must be a full-time committee member. Individuals can be invited to attend a meeting or a portion of one to answer questions from the committee, share information, or present a point of view. Like staff assistants, individuals who attend meetings as guests should respect the limits of their participation.

In summary, committee size and composition are matters of individual organizational determination. Committees should be large enough to represent various interest groups and ensure adequate group deliberation but small enough to ensure that the deliberation will be effective.

## Periodic Review of Committee Purpose and Function

There is an occasionally encountered phenomenon experienced by some committees, primarily standing committees, although even ad hoc committees are not totally immune. That phenomenon is the tendency of some committees to remain in place, meeting regularly and cranking out meeting minutes, when the essential reasons for their existence have either changed or vanished. By way of example, consider the common and well-intentioned practice of resident or client or customer representation committees or councils. Student representation groups in higher education are another such structure, and employee representation groups are yet another example. At an early stage in the life cycle of the organization, there might have been many issues to resolve, with input from the client group being useful in this regard. As practices became routinized, and as other structures were put in place (e.g., a grievance process, an appeal process, an open forum with management sessions, special focus committees), however, the original purposes of the client representation group became diminished. What to do now? If there is still a need for such a group, examine its mandate and its composition. Perhaps less frequent meetings might be in order, with the capacity for scheduling more meetings if a need arises. In this way, the representative structure is maintained but meetings with virtually no agenda are avoided.

Some have likened a committee to a physical structure that, once built, tends to remain in place in its original form even though it becomes empty or perhaps is just partially occupied. In other words, committees are often seen as self-perpetuating or even self-propagating, regardless of whether the reasons for their formation have vanished or changed.

Any committee should be subjected to periodic review of its purpose and function. This purpose and function might be referred to as a "mission," perhaps a "charter," maybe simply a "charge," or some other label to describe the reason for its existence. Certainly some standing committees will not often require such review. Consider, for example, the executive committee or the finance committee of an institution's board of directors, which will likely remain in place as long as the organization's basic mission remains unchanged. But even those supposedly stable committees might benefit from periodic review. For instance, certain conditions in the environment or perhaps in the organization itself might suggest some appropriate change in committee membership or composition.

The review of a committee's purpose and function should not be left solely to the committee itself. Depending on how some committee members view membership on the committee, members could conceivably vote to continue a useless committee or to disband a committee that has valid reasons to continue. Some committee members, and certainly the committee's current chairperson, can legitimately be involved in the review. These individuals, as the participants closest to committee activity, will be in a position to provide information to others involved in the review. It is most appropriate that the review be led by persons placed at the level of management to which the committee reports. In other words, a committee of the board of directors would be evaluated by the full board; a medical staff committee would be evaluated by the medical staff leadership; an institution's safety committee would be evaluated by a member or two of administration, including the executive to whom the committee answers.

Some of the principal questions to be addressed by those evaluating a committee's purpose and function are these:

- Has the mission, charter, or charge of the committee changed somewhat, significantly, or not at all?
- What would appear to be the net effect on the organization if this committee were eliminated?
- If this committee is to be retained, what changes, if any, should be made to its mission, charter, or charge?
- If this committee is to be retained, should the frequency of meetings be altered in any way?
- Can the functions of this committee be constructively combined with the functions of another committee?
- What changes, if any, should be made in committee structure and composition?
- Should there be any changes made to the committee's reporting requirements?

It is true that many committees tend to take on a life of their own. It is also true that many in management feel they are "committeed to death" and could make good use of the time that could be freed if they had fewer meetings to attend. It follows, therefore, that regular, systematic review of committee purpose and function—at least once per year for the majority of committees—can help weed out ineffective or unneeded committees. In brief, periodically make each and every committee justify its continued existence.

## ▶ The Committee Chairperson

### Selection and Duties

The position of chairperson of a committee may be filled in several ways. One is direct appointment by the individual with the mandate and the authority to do so. For example, the bylaws of an organization may direct the president of the medical staff to appoint a committee chairperson. The manager of a department may be the chairperson of a related committee as a matter of course, the director of the patterns of patient care review program may be the appointed chairperson of the utilization review committee, and the individual who holds the line position responsible for safety will probably automatically become the chairperson of the safety committee.

Managers may appoint themselves chairpersons of committees that they constitute and over which they wish to exercise control, or they may offset powerful members by appointing as chairperson an individual sympathetic to their position. Selection of committee chairpersons may or may not be left to the group's membership. In committees where members are elected from the panel as a whole and where there is an accepted egalitarianism in the group, this is a common practice. The group conveys the idea that all those selected for membership have equal ability and that equal confidence is placed in all of them. Conversely, the group could also convey the idea that the committee is not very important so it does not matter who is chairperson. A group that elects the members of a committee may select the chairperson as a separate action by a special vote or may direct that the individual who receives the highest number of votes automatically assumes the chair.

Occasionally, the office is simply rotated among members of the committee to avoid a power struggle.

When a specific activity of a standing committee requires extensive and recurring follow-up work and staff assistance is limited, the work of the chairperson is divided by rotation; because the burden of staff support must be shared by the chairperson's department or unit, this approach spreads the support work over several organizational units. When the committee's work is viewed as mere compliance with bureaucratic red tape and the work is valued neither by its members nor by the group as a whole, the position of chairperson is sometimes downplayed by this rotation process. Finally, individual members may volunteer to accept the assignment as chairperson because of a sense of duty, because of a desire to advance themselves or protect some potentially threatened interest, or because the committee deals with an issue within their field of expertise.

An able, well-qualified individual sometimes refuses to accept the position of chairperson because it would limit his or her ability to participate in deliberations. Eligibility factors sometimes determine the choice of a chairperson. Prerequisites might include prior membership on the committee, tenure as a faculty member, a specific number of years of service as a full-time employee, or a certain technical or professional degree.

A committee chairperson's duties include arranging for logistical support, chairing meetings, and monitoring follow-up assignments. The logistical duties include the following tasks:

- Coordinating the schedules of committee members
- Correlating committee activities with the work of related committees or departments
- Checking for compliance with mandated deadlines and actions
- Obtaining meeting space
- Issuing meeting notices as to time, date, place, and agenda
- Coordinating and distributing support information before meetings
- Preparing the agenda, including sequencing items according to priority

### Chairing the Meeting

The chairperson sets the tone of meetings, controls the agenda to a major extent, guides deliberation on the issues, and provides or denies opportunities for committee members to express themselves. The degree of formality or informality is indicated not only by the manner in which the chairperson conducts the business of the meeting but also by an explicit statement. At the outset, the chairperson makes known the rules of debate—for example, whether there will be general discussion followed by a formal vote and whether strict adherence to parliamentary procedures will be required throughout the meeting.

It is the duty of the chairperson to conduct the meeting efficiently by starting the session on time, following the agenda, and providing sufficient time for deliberation. Subtle leadership skills must be brought to bear as the chairperson referees the members' deliberations. The process of group deliberation and participation must be protected and promoted. The chairperson must artfully provide time for individuals to be heard, which involves far more than merely letting each person have a turn to speak. Group cohesion must be fostered even when there are differences of opinion.

The agenda is usually prepared by the chairperson, who invites members to provide timely input. Although the agenda is intended to guide the proceedings, the chairperson may take an item out of sequence if the course of discussion creates a natural opening for the deliberation of related agenda items. The chairperson keeps the meeting flowing by moving from one agenda item to another at appropriate times, calling the group's attention to work accomplished and work yet to be done.

The chairperson must seek to prevent polarization, overhasty decisions, or the eruption of blatant conflict. It is the chairperson's duty to prevent the group from moving into discussion of unrelated topics or returning to issues that have already been settled. The chairperson periodically integrates the discussion by summarizing major points, calling for motions, and appointing subcommittees or individuals to carry out special assignments.

To summarize the primary duties of the chairperson, in chairing a meeting this individual should follow these guidelines:

- Except in the face of highly unusual circumstances, always begin the meeting at the stated time, and do not repeat information for late arrivals.
- State the purpose of the meeting at the start and determine that everyone knows why they are present.
- Ensure the privacy and confidentiality of the proceedings by reminding participants that use of recording devices (including cellphones) of any kind are prohibited.

- Ensure that someone (a "recorder") is assigned to record the proceedings for the purpose of minutes and assignments, and that someone (a "scribe") will capture (via computer display, or some other means) points and ideas that arise for discussion. (At a small meeting, these two activities could probably be handled by a single person.)
- Encourage discussion. Ask direct questions, especially of participants who otherwise tend to remain silent. Consciously attempt to secure everyone's participation.
- Remain in control of the proceedings. Do not lecture or dominate, do not tell others what to say, do not argue with participants, and do not try to be funny.
- Remain in control of the group itself. Do not permit tangential digressions, and do not allow monopolizers or ego-trippers to take over or to intimidate less-vocal participants.
- End with some specific plan. Allow no one to depart without full understanding of the decisions made, actions to be taken, individuals responsible for implementation, and when things will be done. Every meeting must end with a statement of who will do what by when.
- Follow up after the meeting to ensure, as necessary, that what was decided and assigned has been accomplished.

## Follow-Up Activity

The final duty of the chairperson is follow-up. The chairperson participates in the preparation of minutes either directly by formulating them or indirectly by reviewing and approving them as prepared by the committee secretary. Periodic reports must be made to administrative officials. In addition, the chairperson issues invitations to special guests, consult technical staff, hold informal sessions with members between meetings, and attend subcommittee meetings or those of related committees; all these duties fall within the category of follow-up.

The chairperson must periodically review the work of the committee. Is the work satisfactory given the committee's basic charge? Is the committee fulfilling its designated function? The minutes of several recent months may be examined and specific follow-up inquiries made to individuals and subcommittees concerning the progress of work assigned; agenda items that were set aside or those not discussed for lack of time should be brought to the committee's attention again. All unfinished business should be

---

**Exhibit 7–1** Sample Format for Minutes

| The committee directed its attention to new guidelines concerning the content of discharge summaries. A random sample of discharge summaries from medical and surgical discharges from the past 4 months was compared to mandated content from federal and state regulations to determine areas of noncompliance and areas of strength. | Discharge summaries<br>February 8, 20n1<br>June 9, 20n0 |
| --- | --- |

---

monitored and active follow-up initiated. **Exhibit 7–1** is an excerpt from a form that may be helpful in following up on committee action.

# Committee Member Orientation

Members often come to committees with varying degrees of knowledge about committee purpose, function, and procedures. In most instances, therefore, some orientation to a new committee assignment is recommended. This may amount to little or nothing for a professional appointed to a committee involving a specific function. For example, a nurse functioning as a quality assurance specialist may need very little orientation to membership on the institution's quality assurance committee. By comparison, someone appointed to a committee that cuts across a number of functional lines may require more orientation and familiarization. For example, an individual from the admitting department who is appointed to the institution's safety committee may require more extensive orientation.

To cite some examples of committee member orientation:

- In a particular small hospital, a new member of the safety committee meets with the committee chairperson one on one before the new member's initial meeting.
- In a midsize not-for-profit human services agency, a newly appointed member of the finance committee of the board receives a 2-hour orientation with the agency's chief executive officer, finance director, and finance committee chairperson.
- In a midsize hospital, a new member of the board of directors receives a half-day orientation with the hospital's chief executive officer, the compliance officer, and the executive committee of the board.

Before ever agreeing to committee service, the person who is invited to serve should be fully advised of the purpose and function of the committee, the time commitment necessary, and the meeting schedule. Once this information has been conveyed and an individual's agreement to serve is secured, the committee chairperson can proceed with arrangements for a customized orientation depending on the needs of the individual. It should, of course, go without saying that a significant part of this orientation should involve answering the questions of the new member.

# Minutes and Proceedings

Sound practice requires that an organization maintain official documentation of business transacted. Minutes serve as the permanent factual record of committee proceedings. An explicit statement in bylaws or policies may state that the minutes shall be maintained, including a record of attendance; that they shall reflect the transactions, conclusions, and recommendations of each meeting adequately; and that they shall be kept in a permanent file. Some other time frame for retention that reflects the legal and statutory requirements for the organization may be stated. Committee manuals should contain such information.

When properly formulated, minutes summarize business transacted, including matters that require follow-up action, matters on which there is substantial agreement or disagreement, and issues that remain open for committee deliberation. Minutes are sometimes transmitted to individuals who are not currently members, as determined by the policies on distribution and by legal and accrediting requirements. The historical record provided in the minutes gives new members an overall sense of committee activity. A surveyor checking for compliance with patterns of patient care review requirements, for example, might request the minutes of the utilization review committee over the past year. Representatives of The Joint Commission may call for minutes and proceedings of the medical staff committees to help in determining whether the staff is fulfilling its medico-administrative responsibilities.

In legal proceedings, the admissibility of committee minutes and proceedings as evidence rests on the premise that these records were made in the normal course of business at the time of the actions or events, or within a reasonable time thereafter. Thus, minutes of the official business of the organization's committees must be prepared, reviewed, and distributed in a timely manner (i.e., close to the time of the actual proceedings). This preliminary set of minutes is marked "DRAFT" to indicate that it has not yet been approved. The minutes are reviewed formally at the next meeting to obtain general agreement that their content reflects the business transacted. Should a lawsuit be instituted regarding the possible negligence, malpractice, denial of privileges, or discipline of a practitioner, the minutes of such proceedings might, in some instances, be admissible as legal evidence; the laws on this point vary from state to state.

It could be argued that minutes do not reflect all the business transacted by the committee. The counterargument is a question: why not? The effort spent on proper documentation in the normal course of business is a legitimate use of organizational time and staff. It has also been argued that minutes could be altered to reflect business that, in fact, was not transacted, but this is true of any form of documentation. Review of minutes by all members is one way to safeguard accuracy. Managers can only go forward guided by their own ethical code as well as by the organizational and societal presumption that the work was carried out "in good faith."

## Preparation of Minutes

Minutes are prepared in two stages. First, either the proceedings are transcribed in their entirety by clerical staff or a summary of key points is compiled by a staff assistant. Then, the official secretary to the committee (if there is such an officer) or the committee chairperson formulates the official minutes from the transcript or summary. If there is no clerical assistant or staff aide, the chairperson (or member—secretary) uses self-compiled notes to formulate the minutes. Any required approval is obtained, and the minutes are sent out according to a prescribed distribution list. The distribution process may be simplified by developing a standing list of the names and titles of members, administrative officers to whom certain minutes are sent because of their organizational jurisdiction, or the chairpersons of related committees. The chairperson then needs only to check the names of those who are to receive a particular set of minutes. It is useful to include the phrase "Standard Distribution" and to list any additional individuals to whom minutes were sent as a point of information. The inclusion of a list of support material or enclosures makes the minutes more complete.

Exhibit 7–1 illustrates a format that makes it possible to scan the pages of a volume of minutes and focus on specific topics. The topic key is placed in the right-hand margin; if the left-hand margin is used for the topic key, it may be placed too deeply in a bound or semi-bound margin for ready reference. Inclusion of the dates on which there was previous discussion gives the user an easy means of reference to related information. This format generates an index of committee topics, and members have the benefit of ready reference to past deliberations of a related nature.

## Content of Minutes

Minutes are more than a mere listing of committee actions in chronological order. The topics discussed are normally grouped—a process facilitated by adherence to a formal agenda. In relatively informal meetings, however, the discussion may be diffuse and less focused on discrete topics than is a discussion in a meeting conducted under strict parliamentary procedure.

The minutes should reflect what is done, not what is said. Adequate minutes as a matter of course contain such information as the following items:

- The name of the committee
- The date, time, and place of the meeting
- Whether it is a regular or special meeting
- The names of members present (specify ex officio if appropriate)
- The names of members absent (include a notation of excused absence if appropriate)
- The names of guests, including title or department as an additional indicator of reason for attending

The opening paragraph of the minutes, which is relatively standardized, normally includes the following information:

- The name of the presiding officer
- The establishment of quorum, if this is done routinely or at the request of a member
- A routine review of the minutes of the previous meeting, noting whether they were reviewed as read or only as distributed and whether any corrections were made

The proceedings are summarized. The names of those who made formal motions are given, but the names of those who seconded the motions need not be recorded. All main motions, whether adopted or rejected, are included.

The bulk of the business may be reflected in general discussion only. There are five basic dispositions of agenda items, and each item should be listed with its disposition:

1. Item is discussed and a formal motion is made; formal wording of motion is given. Votes for and against, as well as abstentions, are recorded. Notation is made whether motion is adopted or rejected.

2. Item is discussed and there is general consensus. No formal motion is made. Summary statement of general discussion is entered with notation that there was general agreement with action taken.

3. Item is discussed and tabled informally or set aside for discussion at another time because members need more information. Reasons for setting it aside may be stated; indeed, it is useful to give this information for later reference.

4. Item is discussed, with subsequent formal motion to table it permanently.

5. Item is not discussed. This is not stated directly; item is simply carried as old business.

A precaution is in order relative to outcomes three, four, and five, concerning items that are "tabled informally," "set aside for discussion at another time," "tabled permanently," or "simply carried as old business." These particular actions—representing largely more inaction than action—are often taken for truly legitimate reasons. Perhaps study is required, more information is needed, or the individuals most appropriate to a particular item are not present. Often, however, items of business that represent thorny, emotional, or generally controversial issues are repeatedly put off via one or another of the means cited. Certain items of business seem to be put off, then brought up again only to be put off again.

Some unresolved and recurring agenda items can languish without action forever, such that they simply accumulate and nothing happens to them except postponement after postponement. It is suggested that any accumulation of such agenda items be reassessed regularly, with the intention, if possible, of either moving them onto an active schedule—for example, "To be addressed at the February meeting"—or dropping them altogether. Often committee participants and other decision makers behave as though they believe that an issue ignored long enough might just go away of its own accord. It is true that occasionally some issues, even those involving seemingly difficult or insoluble problems, simply vanish as a topic of review; however, the issue per se remains and continues to need attention.

Whether a particular issue is thorny or controversial or not, and whether the issue in question seems to defy rational solution, it falls to every committee member to be aware that postponing a problem is, in fact, "deciding not to decide." There may often be completely valid reasons for doing so, but there can be a price associated with this practice. The exercise of this "no-decision option" is itself a decision, and frequently it turns out to be the decision of the greatest potential consequences. Therefore, recurring or unresolved agenda items should not be allowed to coast in open-ended fashion for a prolonged period of time. Either place them on a reasonable track toward resolution, or get rid of them altogether.

A useful practice for providing background information for new members of a committee or for review of past committee action is to include a rationale statement for each motion that is made. Although this is not required, such a statement provides a succinct summary of the underlying reasons for an action:

> It was moved and seconded that documentation review will be carried out by health information department personnel for all patients in the long-term care/rehabilitation unit whose length of stay exceeds 14 days. This review will be made on a weekly basis for each patient.
>
> Rationale: Because of the extended length of stay for this category of patients (an average of 47 days in this facility), the detection and subsequent correction of patient care documentation deficiencies should be carried out during the patients' stay.

Both the positive and negative discussions of each topic may be summarized. If there is a specific follow-up action to be taken and a committee member is assigned this task, the name of the individual should be included in the minutes. If a subcommittee is created, the names of its members are given. In the minutes of a formal meeting, points of order and appeals, whether sustained or lost, are noted.

At the conclusion of the minutes, the name of the individual who compiled them is given. The legend "minutes compiled by" may be used instead of the somewhat archaic phrase "respectfully submitted." If minutes are approved or reviewed by the chairperson before distribution, this fact is stated. The minutes should be signed by the person who compiled them (e.g., the committee secretary) and the person who approved them for distribution. If the committee does not have an official secretary, the chairperson's name and signature are entered.

Minutes and proceedings reflecting patient care often are summarized in tabular form. See **Exhibit 7–2**, which reflects a documentation review of geriatric clients in the Adult Daily Living Center.

# ▶ Where Do Teams Fit In?

With the continuing expansion of employee involvement, it is increasingly likely for problem solving to be approached through the use of employee teams.

Teams have been at the forefront of the implementation of total quality management (TQM) programs, as they were in previous undertakings under various other names, such as quality circles, in which an individual "circle" was neither more nor less than an employee problem-solving team.

Today's team essentially fits within the broader definition of committee dealt with earlier in this chapter. There are, however, some points of difference between teams and the more traditional forms

---

**Exhibit 7–2** Documentation Review: Geriatric Clients in Adult Daily Living Center

**Focus of Review: Documentation of Discharge Process—Planned Discharges**

Number of client records reviewed for proper documentation: 40
Standard of compliance: 100%
Actual compliance: 88%

Elements of documentation to be noted:

- Age 60 or older
- Reason for initial admission
- Listing of initial and subsequent structured programs (date, specific program)
- Discharge Planning Conference—Staff
  - reason for planned discharge
  - timeline: minimum of 30-day notice to client and family/caregiver and planned discharge date
    - Family Conference—Staff and family/caregiver representatives
    - plan of care for post-discharge
    - family/caregiver needs
    - referrals to community agencies
    - referrals to support groups
    - specific information and training for certain needs (e.g., self-medication, lifting, moving client)
    - preparation Special Needs Assessment Information (SNAP) form for use in emergencies (such as disasters, first responders)
    - date and time of planned discharge
- Date and time of final discharge, to whom discharged, and destination.
- The discharge summary:
  - reflects initial screening and placement
  - reflects the initial plan of care and its subsequent revisions
  - medical status
  - Activities of Daily Living competencies
  - medications
  - diet
  - socialization activities
  - final destination (e.g., home, inpatient care center)
  - discharged to the care of (family member, caregiver)
    - Cardiovascular medication
    - Psychotropic medication
    - Use of four or more medications
    - Cognitive impairment
    - Decrease in hip strength
    - Poor balance when walking
    - Prior falls in the home
    - Chronic pain/pain status
    - Environmental factors (e.g., rugs, stair rails)
    - Compliance by client with safety instructions
    - Compliance by family/caregivers with safety instructions

of committees. Like other committees, a team may be "standing," with a continuing life beyond its initial concern, such as a departmental team that exists to continually scrutinize the department's procedures. By contrast, a team may also exist temporarily to address a specific problem or situation.

Generally, a team is seen as less formal or less structured than a committee. People often see committees as existing by virtue of some higher authority, such as the committees of the medical staff or the board of directors, or at least as deliberative bodies established by higher management. By comparison, teams, although perhaps standing in the sense of having open-ended assignments, are generally perceived as nonpermanent.

The term *committee* is more likely to be associated with more formal processes such as parliamentary procedure and the requirement for thorough minutes of proceedings. Also, as compared with a team, a committee is more likely to be associated with voting, which may or may not be a feature of a given team's activities.

Therefore, given the foregoing few points of variation, a team may be referred to as a committee. There is, however, one unique dimension of an employee team that deserves special attention, and that is the questionable legality of some teams relative to their missions.

## ▶ As Employee Involvement Increases

Participative management and employee involvement have been talked about for several decades and have been practiced in an increasing number of work organizations since the human relations approach to management began to make inroads into the authoritarian management of the past. Thanks to TQM and other initiatives, more and more is being done with the involvement of employees by way of teams. There are some good reasons for wanting to include employees in some team activities and deliberations. In most instances, nobody knows a given job better than people who do it every day. Also, it only makes sense to try to account for employees' needs and desires when designing a benefits program.

However, there are areas of employee involvement in which teams are seen as intruding on the territory of labor unions. There is a constant risk that a given employee team could be judged an illegal labor organization under the National Labor Relations Act (NLRA). Suggestions for employee participation, although well intended, readily lead to groups that could be considered as infringing on the rights of collective bargaining organizations.

The problem has actually existed since the NLRA became law in 1935, but it was brought into sharp focus by the Electromation decision of December 1992. In 1989, Electromation, a manufacturer of electrical equipment, established several employee committees. One was created to investigate bonuses, one to look at premium pay, one to study absenteeism, one to examine employer–employee communications, and one to deal with a no-smoking policy. Management defined the subjects, set the number of members for each committee, appointed managers to all of the committees, and paid workers to participate. When Electromation's five employee committees were challenged, the National Labor Relations Board (NLRB) agreed with the challenge. (The NLRB is an independent federal agency created to enforce the NLRA.) According to the NLRB, these employee representation committees were essentially employer-dominated labor organizations that discussed wages and other terms of employment. The NLRB concluded that the company was not simply dealing with quality, productivity, or efficiency but was creating the impression among employees that their differences with management were being resolved bilaterally. The NLRB's reason for the ruling suggested that in establishing the NLRA years earlier, Congress prohibited employer interference with labor organizations to ensure that such groups were free to act independently of employers in representing the interests of employees.

Following the Electromation case, there was a similar case in which the DuPont Company was ordered to disband seven labor-management committees, six created for safety issues and one for recreation. In addition, there was a similar case in which the Polaroid Corporation was forced to disband its long-standing employees committee after the U.S. Department of Labor determined that it was actually a "labor organization."

Generalizing from the experiences of Electromation, DuPont, Polaroid, and others, an employee team or committee might be considered to be an employer-dominated illegal labor organization for any of a number of reasons. First, and probably foremost, is if the group is dealing with wages, hours, benefits, grievances, or other terms and conditions of employment. These are, of course, among the issues most frequently subject to collective bargaining and are seen (at least by the NLRB) as the exclusive province of unions. Second is if team suggestions or recommendations result in management decisions but the group itself does not have the power to make the decisions and if employees are elected to the group as representatives of larger bodies of employees. Third is if (1) employees see the group as a means of resolving their concerns with management and (2) meetings appear to involve "negotiation" between employees and members of management.

Many in business consider the NLRB's decision in the Electromation case an unfortunate occurrence—an expression of Depression-era assumptions that relationships between employees and employers must always be adversarial. The strongly pro-labor position of the NLRB often seems to work against the establishment of a healthy employee relations climate in an organization. Experiences stemming from the cases cited above seem to suggest that a violation will most likely be found if an employee team is actually set up during a union campaign, participation is made mandatory, and the employer picks the members or controls the method of their selection.

Because of what happened with Electromation and other companies, there may be a tendency for some organizations to shy away altogether from teams or committees that include rank-and-file employees. Some justify a diminished emphasis on teams by pointing out that attacking employee committees has become an active tactic of unions that are either in place or seeking acceptance.

However, the Electromation case did not open up any truly new issues; it simply brought some that had existed for years to the surface. Long before this case, it was recognized that the more effective an employee team is, the more likely the NLRB is to find it an illegally dominated and supported company union in violation of existing labor law. However, potential difficulties should not be allowed to completely deter the use of such a team. The active use of employee participation and input via teams or committees lies at or near the heart of every initiative intended to improve quality or productivity. If management believes what is said to employees about the value of their input, "empowerment," and "owning your job," then management had best make maximum use of participative processes, including teams.

## ▶ Employee Teams and Their Future

### Avoiding "Committee Paralysis"

Rather than paralyze employee teams because of legal risk, it makes more sense to look for ways in which management may make the fullest possible use of

employee input while avoiding legal entanglements. The value of including employees in problem solving is undeniable; surely it makes sense to account for employees' needs and desires in making changes within the organization. The active use of employee participation and input, largely via teams or committees, actually lies at or near the heart of every TQM initiative.

## Occasional Shortcomings of Teams

Some team members, especially managers serving on teams with nonmanagers or others of perceived lesser rank, are unwilling to set aside position and power for the sake of the team. Also, unequal levels of knowledge and ability among team members can lead some team members to dominate the others, some to anticipate their contributions will be diminished or overruled by the "authority" present, and still others to become overwhelmed or lost in the crowd.

Some extremely important and highly disruptive effects on teams are found in reward and compensation systems that continue to focus on individual effort rather than on team performance. This has been a frequently encountered barrier to successful TQM implementations as organizations have tried to alter how they do business without changing the systems or processes by which they do business. Indeed, some reward systems support individual performance to such an extent that they can discourage teamwork.

Performance appraisals that do not account for team performance also present barriers. An organization's performance appraisal process is usually one major business support system that has to change dramatically to appropriately support the activities and accomplishments of teams. In evaluating employees, most present appraisal processes tend to identify "stars"—that is, the exceptional individual performers. In reality, a team will not long remain a productive body if some members feel they work in the shadow of a few people who are regarded as better performers and receive higher individual appraisal scores. Therefore, it is necessary to change some employees' concept of evaluation from a focus on the individual to emphasis on the team. Moreover, because not all of the organization's employees will be serving on teams, the performance appraisal process must offer a variation by which to evaluate group efforts as well as continue to accommodate individuals as usual.

There is another sort of shortcoming that now and then arises to frustrate the well-intended efforts of some team members. This shortcoming comes in the form of the "coaster" or "free rider," who contributes only minimally to the team's work, if at all, but stands to share the credit when the team, carried forward by its productive members, registers successes. This apparent footdragger becomes a concern of the other team members and especially of the team leader. Ordinarily a team's leader will be a working leader who both serves as a contributing member and provides some direction to the group as a whole. This leader must sometimes lean on a nonproductive member to "shape up or ship out." Indeed, if the leader does not do so, discontent is likely to spread among the other team members. Thus, individual team members will often directly address the slacker in their midst. The well-run team that discovers one of these nonproductive members in its ranks will be self-policing; that is, the team will either help to get the footdragger up to speed or, failing that, have the individual removed or replaced.

Whether for TQM projects or any other undertaking that involves committees or teams, lack of top management commitment to the process is a sure means of undermining effectiveness. It should go without saying that top management that fails to "walk the talk" will be perceived as insincere.

Some problems with teams are inherent in the labels used to describe these bodies—labels such as "self-directed," "autonomous," and the like. These names are misleading in that they convey the belief that these groups are independent and free to act as they choose. No effective teams in business really provide their own total direction. Instead, each team should be directed by its specific charge or mission or assignment and by the goals of the organization. As such, all teams should actually be interdependent with other organizational elements. Effective teams require clear direction, comprehensive guidelines, and open, nonthreatening leadership.

## What to Avoid in Using Employee Teams

It is possible to empower teams that include rank-and-file employees and use them—legally—to maximum effect by observing a few simple limitations:

1. Never allow an employee team to deal with terms and conditions of employment, such as wages, hours, benefits, and grievances. Even consideration of working conditions in general should be avoided. As a member of management who might be part of a team, do not deal with other team members, and specifically nonmanagers, concerning terms and conditions of employment. If a

team's activities take it from a legitimate topic into the realm of terms and conditions of employment, its direction should be altered or it may be seen as being an illegal, employer-dominated labor organization.

2. Do not solicit from team complaints, grievances, or suggestions about terms and conditions of employment. If such issues arise on their own, refer them to the proper points in the organization, usually either administration or human resources.

3. Do not let team meetings degenerate into gripe sessions in which members simply complain about aspects of their employment.

4. Do not mandate employee participation, ask employees to represent other employees, or sanction employee elections to choose representatives. Ask for volunteers, and appoint all members.

5. Do not allow an employee team or committee to exist and function without a clear, understandable mission or charge and without fully and plainly delineated limits on its authority and responsibility.

## Proper Focus of Effective Employee Teams

Short of actually establishing teams or committees to wrestle with certain issues, a number of steps can be taken to encourage employee participation. It is possible, and frequently desirable, to consider bringing together loosely defined groups of managers and employees simply to brainstorm ideas, gather information, and help define problems, as long as no proposals are offered or recommendations made. It is also proper to assemble an employee group to share information and observations with management, again, as long as no proposals or recommendations are made.

Beyond one-time or limited informal gatherings and in the realm of actual teams or committees, use the following points of focus:

1. When establishing a team or committee, identify it up front as not intended as an employees' channel to management. Define a clear mission or charge before soliciting team membership, and have the team's functions and limits identified before any team activity begins.

2. Keep the team focused on productivity or quality improvements only. This pursuit requires clear guidelines and plenty of continued vigilance. It is difficult to talk about quality, efficiency, productivity, and such without conditions of employment becoming involved, so be constantly aware of the

potential need to redefine the team's boundaries periodically. Also, be mindful that in such a gathering of employees it is sometimes all too easy for a complaint or two to trigger a full-blown gripe session.

3. Staff teams with volunteers, or use rotating membership selected by some means that is not management dominated.

4. If a team is empowered to make a final management decision—that is, the team decides in place of management, not just makes recommendations to management—it can be seen as acting as management. This is acceptable. In fact, it has been suggested that the ultimate protection against being ruled an illegal labor organization exists when the team can make final decisions in its own right.

5. If an issue is sufficiently narrowly defined that all persons affected by it can be included in a single group, a "committee of the whole" including everyone, is usually legally safe. In such an instance nobody can be seen as "representing" anyone else.

6. For standing committees or long-lived teams, maintain a majority membership of managers. A committee or team composed of a majority of managers stands less chance of being adjudged illegal under the NLRA. Such teams do present a significant drawback, however; a team composed mostly of managers is far less likely to be seen as a legitimate vehicle for employee participation.

7. Rather than always creating teams or committees that tend to develop a continuing existence, consider establishing specific problem-solving or work-improvement ad hoc groups, each with a specific, well-defined charge and a specific problem to solve, and disband each group after its goal has been attained. Such ad hoc groups can much more safely consist of a majority of non-managers than can permanent teams or committees. For teams composed largely of rank-and-file employees, however, it is legally safest to have management representatives serve as observers or facilitators, without the power to vote on proposals or dominate or control the group.

For collaborative group problem solving and participative decision making in general, it is always appropriate to bring into the group those people who have the skills needed for dealing with the group's charge. It is necessary, however, to recognize that those persons who have skills pertinent to the problem at hand will likely have greater influence on group decisions.

Recognize also that teams or committees become unwieldy as they increase in size. Small groups are generally better; active participation in tasks seems to decrease with increases in group size. In fact, team participants tend to rate small groups as more satisfactory, positive, and effective than larger groups.

Employee participation may well be the key to continuing increases in quality, efficiency, and productivity. Employee participation is essential. As noted earlier, no one knows the inner workings of a job better than the person who does it day in and day out. Also, there are few, if any, problems whose solutions are not enhanced by multiple viewpoints and inputs. A team brings to the problem the power of the group.

# ▶ Guidelines for Group Deliberations

Committees, task forces, and teams generally have a small number of participants who are usually well known to each other. Their deliberations are structured, relatively frequent, and routine. By way of contrast, consider the characteristics of large-group deliberations. The number of participants tends to be high, 30 to 40 or more. Although participants share a common interest, they do not necessarily know one another. The group is less cohesive than a committee or team because it meets only once, or a few times, and disbands at the conclusion of deliberations.

A manager's challenge in guiding group deliberations involves efforts to achieve effectiveness. Most of the guidelines for enhancing committee and team effectiveness, noted in earlier sections, apply to group deliberations (e.g., adequate space, staff support). In addition, a manager attends to other considerations when conducting large group deliberations. The brief scenario described below reflects aspects of group discussion, dynamics, and guidelines. A similar after-action review (AAR) is commonly used for assessing response to workplace disruptions, including active threat/shooter, bomb threat, protests, pandemics, internal systems failures (e.g., heating, water supply), regional disruptions (e.g., transit strike), and weather-related disasters.

Group deliberation is a useful technique for gathering and processing pertinent details about such incidents. The following key points for group deliberation reflect examples from a workplace disruption due to a weather-related event.

1. Precise focus of deliberations:
   a. The June 6, 2:45 P.M. storm: unexpected, not forecast, out-of-season microburst with wind shear and hailstorm.

b. The storm's impact on medical center operations, both inpatient and outpatient.

2. Stated purpose of deliberations:
   a. Review of organizational response to this event.
   b. Assess effectiveness of the disaster plan.

3. Timeliness of the review: conduct the initial group deliberations within a couple of days of the event. Rationale: details of the experience are easily recollected.

   Schedule a follow-up review to focus on longer-term impact and to process the input from the group deliberation.

4. Selection of participants: obtaining direct feedback from individuals involved in the disaster event is the primary goal. Input from line workers, support services, and managers is essential. Department heads will select participants from their line workers and support staff, using these criteria:
   • Must have been present on campus during the event, either on duty or arriving/leaving from regularly scheduled shift.
   • Full-time line workers from security, maintenance, housekeeping/environmental services, food services, parking, admissions/intake, health information/clinical documentation, appointments and scheduling, and public relations.
   • Professional staff from inpatient and outpatient services: medical, surgical, OB, pediatrics, intensive care, behavioral care; emergency department or clinical decision-making unit.
   • Volunteers from gift shop, coffee shop and snack kiosks; information kiosk, greeters, messengers, and escorts.

   Members of the management team will attend as observers during the second half of the day's activities, but will not participate in the deliberations. Rationale: their presence during initial brain-storming sessions might unintentionally inhibit the free flow of input by line workers. Management representatives will include CEO spokesperson, disaster management coordinator, security, public relations, human resources, risk management, health information/clinical care documentation, appointments/scheduling, and billing.

5. Schedule of deliberations: a realistic plan for the day with a balance of free-flowing discussion and input with more structured, small-group sessions. As a practical matter, include break times and a lunch period. Allow sufficient time for participants to check in with their regular work stations as needed (e.g., check cellphone and e-mail messages); these offset the common tendency of splitting one's attention from the discussion while checking one's messages, as necessary as this might be.

6. Engage the participants in the process: welcome and overview of the day's proceedings; clear statement regarding their selection (as noted above); head off "monopolizers" and passive participation; include every participant.

   Strategy for engaging all participants: have each participant introduce themselves (name, department, job title) and briefly answer the questions: Where were you when the storm hit? What was the first action you took?

   A second strategy involves the use of small-group discussion and brain storming throughout the day, using structured, focus questions.

7. Summarize the deliberations: have each small group briefly present highlights of their findings; inform participants that a brief, formal summary will be compiled by the management team and made available; inform participants that a memo to file will be made, indicating their participation in the group deliberation.

8. Carry out the follow-up actions: brief summary to participants with a thank you memo; memo to each participant's file; formal summary to senior management; schedule follow-up meeting to review disaster plan in the light of group deliberation findings.

# The Manager's Wheel Book Reflecting Committee and Team Activity

As with other management concepts and applications, this reference provide a manager with reminders and insights about committees and teams. See Appendix 7–A, Wheel Book Excerpts Reflecting Committee and Team Activity.

# Appendix 7-A

## Wheel Book Excerpts Reflecting Committee and Team Activity

| | |
|---|---|
| June 24 | regular clinical documentation committee; prepared analysis of documentation of home care initial assessment |
| June 25 | 100th anniversary commemoration planning committee |
| Feb. 4 | safety committee; presented issues concerning evening and night shift—travel to and from remote parking |
| Feb. 5 | regular clinical documentation committee |
| Feb. 12 | budget committee: quarterly reviews |
| March 4 | public relations committee—plan for health information management week |
| | HR task force meeting: input merit pay section of employee handbook |
| March 19 | compliance and accrediting committee: TJC site visit preparation; the state licensure agency annual report—follow-up actions; status report |
| March 26 | 100th anniversary commemoration—subcommittee on honors and awards |
| April 9 | half-day, combined meeting: utilization review; clinical documentation, reimbursement task force |
| April 29 | Infection control review and quality assurance; prepared quality assurance review profiles—months of January through March. |
| May 1 | labor relations/management group: preliminary review of current union contract |
| May 13 | follow-up subcommittee—labor relations/current contract |
| May 16 | regular monthly meetings: clinical documentation; infection control |
| May 23 | human resources committee: briefing on holiday and vacation policies |
| June 6 | emergency meeting—safety and disaster subcommittees regarding immediate action during the storm event; evening meeting for preliminary after-action review reports |
| June 12 | follow-up meeting—safety and disaster subcommittees regarding overall review of response and continuing impact |

# Budget Planning and Implementation

## CHAPTER OBJECTIVES

- Identify the need for fiscal planning and related budgeting practices.
- Discuss budget development in the context of laws, regulations, and corporate culture.
- Identify the levels of responsibility from the board of trustees through middle management level.
- Identify in detail the middle manager's responsibilities in developing and implementing departmental budgets.
- Explain the basic revenue cycle and assert the critical need for constant attention to cash flow.
- Enumerate the requirements of successful budgeting.
- Introduce the budget as a special-purpose financial plan that is an essential part of the department manager's planning function.
- Enumerate the various types of budgets employed and identify the commonly encountered budget periods.
- Differentiate between traditional budgeting and zero-based budgeting approaches.
- Enumerate the steps in the budget cycle.
- Relate the dynamics of the budget approval process to the development of the budget.
- Identify the steps in budgetary control through analysis of budget variances.

Successful healthcare organizations adopt proven fiscal practices, including detailed budgets. These practices ensure that resources are goal-directed, prevent fraud, and foster accountability and transparency. The licensure and charter of an organization reflect state and federal laws, requiring sound fiscal planning. Development and implementation of the budget is a shared responsibility, starting with the owners and board of directors/trustees, then top level management, and then middle management/department heads. The owners and board of directors/trustees make root decisions such as for-profit or nonprofit status; educational programs (e.g., medical school) and research in addition to direct patient care; general patterns of reimbursement; a commitment to act as a "safety-net" facility for underserved and uninsured patients. They oversee the investment portfolio and set the debt limit of the organization. Related decisions flowing from these root decisions include balancing loss of, or reduction in, revenue by accepting uninsured patients with fairness to other clients; use, or nonuse, of cost shifting practices (increasing fees charged to insured groups to offset loss or reduction in payment) or debt forgiveness in hardship cases; debt collection actions (perhaps even setting up its own debt collection agency); general policies on waivers and/or reduction of charges for certain groups (e.g., first responders, military members, employees and their families).

The owners and board of directors/trustees determine the overall corporate culture of the organization. Sound fiscal management is part of a culture of excellence that is reflected in obtaining a high financial rating from external finance rating groups. This includes investment in high-yield return on investment initiatives such as owning non-health-related enterprises (e.g., real estate ventures). A commitment to staff development, training, and internal mobility is another aspect of excellence. Transparency in fiscal practice is yet another important element in corporate culture. Annual plans and reports, audit practices, and internal and external reviews are part of the processes to support the practice of transparency. A commitment to community outreach and to philanthropy is reflected in special programs and initiatives. Innovation is fostered through research and development of alternate sites of care and flexible staffing patterns.

The board selects top-level management officials to develop and implement policies and practices that flow from the root decisions. A chief executive officer, assisted by a chief financial officer, and a corporate compliance officer oversee these programs, policies, and practices. They are attentive to trends, challenges, and opportunities and take the lead in responding to these. Examples include developing a response to rationing or limits on certain aspects of care. The challenge to reduce readmissions might include expansion of the observation/clinical decision-making unit to stabilize a patient, followed by a supportive home care program. Aspects of medical tourism might be the focus of review. For example, is the organization losing clients to other facilities (including overseas locations) because of services and treatments offered, and/or pricing considerations? Conversely, the healthcare organization might be attractive for international clients who seek shorter waiting periods or the availability of treatments not covered under certain national health insurance programs.

Top-level management is tasked with responding to new legislative mandates such as the issues relating to posting/making public the cost of care. This involves clarity and explanations about the various pricing factors (e.g., group membership in special insurance plans; eligibility for waivers and discounts; inpatient stay vs. outpatient service; complexity of care due to comorbidities). Emerging technologies require adjustment to fee structure. What is the cost of telemedicine encounters? There are no facilities charges per se, as is customary in billing for onsite care. Yet, there are costs associated with this technology; therefore, an effective, reliable IT service is essential for the organization.

Committee composition and designated activities are developed by top-level management. These groups typically include a cost containment committee, an audit committee, and an employee input process.

With all of these factors and considerations noted, the middle manager develops and implements a departmental budget along with the department's annual plan on which the budget is based. Department managers coordinate and support other departments in their budget planning. For example, quality assurance studies might focus on patterns of care relating to potentially unnecessary admissions, length-of-stay variables, potentially unnecessary medications, and return rate to observation unit. Managers participate in project preparation and the identification of possible funding (e.g., through their professional associations). Managers participate in cost containment and audit review committees, and prepare support materials for these deliberative groups. An example of a detailed study is reflected in an audit of emergency/observation unit care. The comparison of costs was made to determine patterns of care, and their effectiveness. The questions, and cost assessment, included the following: Were patients using the ER as an alternative to private physician office or clinic visit? Were relatively short ER visits, followed within a week, by another ER visit or inpatient admission for the same diagnosis, resulting in extra cost when a more thorough assessment at first encounter might have been more effective? What was the pattern of ER visit, discharge home, and return to ER for the same condition? These and similar studies relating to cost and effectiveness of care are essential components of overall financial oversight.

Managers cooperate with supply chain managers, providing information about special vendor offers made through professional associations. The department manager works within this dynamic environment as a valuable, reliable participant.

# ▶ The Revenue Cycle

Described in its simplest possible form, the revenue cycle consists of comparing money coming in with money going out. However, for a given healthcare organization of any appreciable size, this cycle is far from simple and only partly predictable. Money does not always come in according to an established pattern, but much of the money that must go out is expected to move according to an established pattern (payroll and certain other expenses such as utilities) or be paid out on external demand (e.g., bills from suppliers).

## Revenue Sources

There are two broad categories of revenue: operating and nonoperating. Of primary interest here is operating revenue—income generated by providing services for patients or clients. Nonoperating revenue is that coming from other sources related to the organization's existence, such as grants or donations.

Operating revenue originates from a number of sources, including the government programs Medicare and Medicaid, insurers such as the not-for-profit Blue Cross and Blue Shield programs and commercial insurance carriers, contracts with managed care organizations, uninsured patient-care pools, and private-pay patients. Each of the different third-party payers has a somewhat different set of reimbursement rules usually resulting in different billing practices.

For the majority of healthcare organizations, the most significant sources of revenue are Medicare and Medicaid, followed by Blue Cross and Blue Shield and managed care organizations (which are often one and the same). Revenue flows in from these sources but not always at a predictable rate. The largest portion of reimbursement is related to numbers of patients served. Consider, however, some of the variations that can occur:

- Fluctuations in number of patients served, perhaps because of outbreaks or epidemics, seasonal variations due to a facility's location (e.g., resort area), weather events or disasters, competition with other providers in the area, and in general any event or circumstance that can cause activity to increase or decrease.
- Variable payment practices of the third-party payers. Payment for providers' services arrives weeks or months after the services are rendered. Sometimes this lag is predictable, but occasionally it changes. Some payers will reject a billing submission because of errors and require revision and resubmission (sometimes seen as a payer tactic used to delay payment in support of its own cash-flow circumstances).
- Fines and penalties assessed for billing errors, not unusual with governmental programs, and fines and penalties arising from changing regulations (e.g., readmission rates for certain categories of care).
- Removal of caps on certain specialties such as physical and occupational therapy services.
- Delays in collecting copays and deductibles from patients.
- Revenue never received because of treatment of uninsured, underinsured, and indigent patients.

- Changes in reimbursement systems, such as changes in coding systems, problems associated with very late billing, and the practice of bundled care, wherein a flat rate is applied (and known ahead of time) for precare, inpatient admission, and postcare.

The preceding issues are some of the more commonly encountered factors affecting the receipt of revenue by a healthcare provider organization. The point to be stressed here is that an organization's cash flow—what comes in as well as what goes out—requires careful and often aggressive management.

## Cash and the Revenue Cycle

There is an extremely simple bit of wisdom to remember in connection with the management of the revenue cycle: *cash is king.*

The organization's cash budget for any given year sets the stage for the management of the revenue cycle. This budget addresses cash needs against projections of cash to be received over the period covered by the budget (usually 1 year). The pattern of cash-in versus cash-out is extremely important because of the need to remain solvent in the short run. It does little good to appear rich "on paper"—to have impressive amounts of money owed to the organization, say in the form of extensive accounts receivable—if there is not enough cash in the bank to pay current bills or to meet payroll.

Should cash be in extremely short supply, the organization might become more aggressive in collecting accounts receivable or perhaps delay payment of a few bills to more closely match cash receipts. A lack of cash can also lead to short-term borrowing that sometimes results in difficulties in obtaining credit and creates more operating expense because of interest rates. Many an organization in today's healthcare climate has found itself in a hand-to-mouth existence in managing cash flow.

Cash is king because it is the ultimate necessity for organizational solvency. Organizations of all sizes and in all lines of business are subject to the same ultimate financial constraint: revenue must be sufficient to cover expenditures within a reasonable period. Many businesses that once looked good on the balance sheet—with a fortune in accounts receivable and large amounts of nonliquid assets—have ceased to exist simply because of negative cash flow.

## ▶ The Budget

Budget preparation and administration are major duties of the department head. Before dealing with the actual budget calculations, the manager must understand the basic concepts and principles of budgeting. The budget details presented here are treated from the perspective of the department head rather than the accountant or top-level administrator. In addition, this presentation is intended for the inexperienced manager; terms are defined and examples are provided in detail to facilitate budget preparation and analysis by an inexperienced user.

The first part of the discussion treats basic concepts such as budget periods, budget types, uniform code of accounts, approaches to budgeting, and the overall budget process. The second part of the discussion focuses on the details of the budget proper: capital expenses, personnel budget, supplies, and related expenses. All dollar values and examples are fictitious and intended only to illustrate budget calculation processes.

Sound budgetary procedures are based on six requisites:

1. Sound organizational structure so that the responsibility for budget preparation and administration is clear
2. A consistent, defined budget period
3. The development of adequate statistical data
4. A reporting system that reflects the organizational structure
5. A uniform system or code of accounts so that data are meaningful and consistent
6. A regular audit system so that variances are explained in a timely manner

## ▶ Uses of the Budget

Budgeting is both a planning and controlling tool. As a plan, the budget is a specific statement of the anticipated results, such as expected revenue to be earned and probable expenses to be incurred in an operation for a future defined period. This plan is expressed in numerical terms, usually dollars. A statement of objectives in fiscal terms, the budget is a single-use plan that covers a specific period of time; it becomes the basis of future or continuing plans when the incremental approach to budgeting is used, whereby the next budget is formulated through the addition of specific increments to the existing budget. It is a statement of what the organization intends to accomplish, not merely a forecast or a guess.

When the budget is properly administered, it becomes a tool of control and accountability in that it reflects the organizational structure, with each unit or department given a specific allocation of funds based on departmental goals and functions. The budget is an essential companion to the delegation of authority; the line manager who has the responsibility for developing the plans for the department or unit must be given the necessary resources to accomplish the approved plans. In turn, this manager accepts responsibility for assigning specific budget amounts to the personnel and material categories and monitoring the use of these resources. Because the budget permits a comparison of planned with actual performance, control is enhanced. The department head is responsible for those costs that are controllable, such as overtime authorization, supplies, and equipment purchases, but not for those that are arbitrarily assigned to the departmental budget, such as fringe benefits calculated as a flat percentage of personnel budget or administrative overhead calculated as a flat percentage of operating costs.

## ▶ Budget Periods

A budget specifies the amount to be spent in a predetermined period. This budget period varies according to the purpose of the budget. The capital equipment or improvement budget may be developed for a long period, such as a 3-, 5-, or 10-year period; the budget for supplies, expenses, and personnel costs may be developed for the immediate fiscal year. Given the various regulatory requirements for long-range planning and budgeting for capital improvements in healthcare organizations, these organizations commonly have such a combination of long- and short-term budget periods.

The accounting period encompassed by the overall budget framework is the fiscal year. The fiscal year may or may not coincide with the calendar year. In the past, many hospitals—especially teaching institutions—used the July through June cycle, which reflected changes in staff (e.g., medical and nursing staff in training programs and residencies) at the end of the teaching year. In recent years, however, a number of government entities have encouraged—and in some instances have essentially required—the adoption of the calendar year as the fiscal year.

Within the accounting year, there are a number of accounting periods. It is common practice to keep track of payroll and certain other expenses on the basis of 1, 2, or 4 weeks and to accumulate this information for 13, 4-week accounting periods in the year; however, other important financial information is accumulated by calendar month either because it is necessary to do so or because this is clearly the most sensible data collection period.

Because of the inevitable presence in the budget of some information in 2- and 4-week increments and some in full-month increments, it is usually necessary to manipulate some of the figures by adding in or backing out certain amounts at either end of a period to have complete financial information for the period of interest.

## Periodic Moving Budget

Another approach to the definition of budget period is the periodic moving budget. In the moving budget, the basic forecast for the year is adjusted as specific periods are completed. As each period is completed, an equal time period is added:

| Year One | Jan. | Feb. | Mar. | |
|----------|------|------|------|--|
| | Apr. | May | June | |
| | July | Aug. | Sept. | |
| | Oct. | Nov. | Dec. | |
| Year Two | Jan. | Feb. | Mar. | (Added when the Jan.–Feb.–Mar. of Year One period is completed) |

The periodic moving budget allows the manager to make use of the more up-to-date information that becomes available as each period closes and, therefore, to make a more accurate prediction. In organizations using the 500-day plan or similar long-range plans with periodic (e.g., 200-day moving update) review points, this type of budgeting is the natural process.

## Milestone Budgeting

In milestone budgeting, the budget periods are tied to subsidiary plans or projects. As these milestone events are accomplished, costs can be determined and budget allocations for the next segments of the project can be established. The budget periods are not uniform but rather depend on the projected time frame for the subsidiary plan. During the implementation of the electronic health record, for example, several milestone events would be noted, with budgeting forecasts associated with each segment. Milestone budgeting usually covers more than 1 year. Recall the discussion of project management and the 500-day plan in Chapter 5 (Planning and Decision making) as an example of periodic and milestone budgeting.

# ▶ Types of Budgets

The budget may be developed to give emphasis to one of several aspects of the overall plan. The revenue and expense budget is the most common type of budget. It reflects anticipated revenues, such as those from sales, payment for services rendered, endowments, grants, and special funds, and it includes expenses, such as costs associated with personnel, capital equipment, or supplies. In the personnel or labor budget, projections are based on the number of personnel hours needed or the types and kinds of skills needed rather than on wages and salaries, as in the personnel costs of the revenue and expense budget. A production budget expresses the information in terms of units of production, such as economic quantities to be produced or types and capacities of machines to be used.

The fixed budget presumes stable conditions; it is prepared on the basis of the best information available, such as past experience and forecasting. The plans, including cost and expense calculations, are made on the basis of this expected level of activity. The variable budget concept was developed because operating costs, and level of activity may fluctuate. For example, a university may calculate its unit budgets according to credit hours generated, but student enrollment may be lower than anticipated; a hospital may use dollars per patient-day or average census as its basis, but the daily census in the hospital may drop and remain low. Thus, costs and expenses are established for varying rates. As actual income and operating costs become known, the budget is adjusted. The periodic moving budget is used with variable budgeting, as is the step budget.

The step budget is a form of variable budgeting in which a certain level of activity is assumed and the impact of deviations from this level of activity calculated. If the manager wishes to show several possibilities predicated on various factors, such as level of production or number of clients served, the step budget is used. These other levels may be greater or less than the basic estimate. For example, a step budget showing probable estimates plus pessimistic and optimistic allowances might be developed. The advantage of using the step budget is that it permits (or even forces) the manager to examine the actions required in the event of a variation from the estimated revenue and expense. When a step budget is prepared, the fixed costs and revenues—that is, those that are not tied to volume of service, production levels, or other factors related to operational costs—are stated. Then the variable revenues and costs are calculated according to the volume of service, operating costs, anticipated revenues, and similar factors.

The master budget is the central, composite budget for the total organization; all the major activities of the organization are coordinated in this central budget. The department budgets are the working, detailed budgets for each unit; they are highly specific so as to permit identification of each item as well as close coordination and monitoring of revenue and expense. To coordinate the several department or unit budgets into a master budget and to make budget processes consistent, a uniform code of accounts and specific cost centers must be developed.

## The Uniform System or Code of Accounts

The standard classification of expenditures and other transactions made by an organization is the uniform system or code of accounts (also referred to as the uniform chart of accounts). Such a uniform code of accounts contains master codes and subdivisions to reflect such information as the specific transaction (e.g., personnel expense, travel expense, capital improvement) and the organizational unit within which the transaction occurred (e.g., food service, human resources, public relations). The delineation of the specific organizational unit facilitates responsibility reporting, because it becomes possible to relate specific expenditures to the manager in charge of that organizational unit.

The chief financial officer of the organization develops the necessary guidelines for a uniform chart of accounts. These guidelines typically reflect those of national associations of healthcare financial management professionals. These account codes are used in the budget to group line items, such as a purchase requisition or a position authorization request. Account codes for a particular institution might include:

- 200 Furniture
- 210 Capital Equipment
- 520 Equipment Rental
- 530 Equipment Maintenance and Service Contracts
- 580 Purchased Services (e.g., an outside contract with a coding and abstracting service)
- 600 Education and Travel
- 610 Dues and Subscriptions

Budget worksheets are coordinated with these account codes, with specific items listed, line by line, under each account code. Line item is a term commonly used to refer to such specifications. For example, the worksheet for budget preparation and, subsequently, the line items of the budget for the category of Dues and Subscriptions reflect the item in detail and the unit with which it is associated:

| 610.1 | Hospital association (regional) dues | $1000.00 |
| 610.2 | Professional dues paid for Chief of Service | $300.00 |
| 610.7 | Accrediting agency regulations annual update subscription | $700.00 |
| 610.8 | Attendance at annual meeting of professional association | |
| | 50% cost for Chief of Service | $700.00 |
| | 25% cost for each staff assistant | $350.00 |
| 610.9 | In-service workshop for support staff (2-day seminar, in-house) | $480.00 |

The code of accounts varies from one institution to another; the items and costs given here are for illustrative purposes only.

## Cost Centers

An activity or group of activities for which costs are specified, such as food service, maintenance and repairs, telephone service, and similar functions, is a cost center. Usually predetermined, cost centers generally parallel the department or service structure of the organization. For example, direct patient care cost centers, with their associated codes, may include:

| 45 | Physical Therapy |
| 46 | Occupational Therapy |
| 47 | Home Care Program |
| 48 | Social Services |
| 49 | Medical Imaging and Radiology |

Administrative cost centers may include:

| 50 | Computer and Information Service |
| 51 | Health Information Service |
| 52 | Admissions Unit |
| 53 | Food Service |

Additional cost centers reflect costs associated with the overall expense of operation:

| 1 | Employee Health and Welfare Benefits |
|---|---|
| 2 | Depreciation: Buildings and Fixtures |
| 3 | Depreciation: Equipment |
| 4 | Payroll Processing |

## Responsibility Center

A unit of the organization headed by an individual who has authority over and who accepts responsibility for the unit is a responsibility center. These centers parallel the organizational structure as outlined in the organizational chart. The departments or services are responsibility centers, each with its detailed budget. The cost center codes and responsibility centers normally parallel one another.

## ▶ Approaches to Budgeting

The two major approaches to the budgeting process are incremental budgeting and the zero-based system (historically referred to as the planning–programming–budgeting system [PPBS]; currently referred to as planning—programming—budgeting—execution, or PPBE).

In incremental budgeting, the financial database of the past is increased by some given percentage. For example, the personnel portion of the budget may be increased by a flat 5% over the last budget period allotment, capital expenses by 7%, and supplies by 4%. There is some efficiency in this approach because the projected calculations are relatively straightforward. There is also a danger, however; significant changes, shifting priorities, or pressing needs within some unit of the organization may be overlooked. As with incremental decision making, there is an implicit assumption that the original money and resource allocation was appropriately calculated and distributed among organizational units. Incremental budgets are object-oriented—that is, they are developed in terms of personnel, materials, maintenance, and supplies. Traditional budgeting is control-oriented, whereas PPBS, or PPBE, is planning-oriented.

The PPBS approach became popular when it was mandated in the Department of Defense in the early 1960s. PPBS (or a similar performance-based approach), as the name implies, emphasizes the budgeting process in systems terms. The outputs for specific programs are assessed, and resource allocation and funding are related directly to the program goals. It is also referred to as "zero-based" budgeting because past dollar allocations are not the basis of projection.

A major feature of this approach is its departure from the traditional 1-year budget cycle. Funding is projected for the period of time (frequently 3 or more years) needed to achieve the goals of the program. In the planning phase, the general objectives are stated and refined, the projected schedule of activities is established, and the outputs are specified. These refined objectives are grouped into programs, resulting in a hierarchy within the plans.

The alternate means of achieving the plans are assessed through cost-effectiveness analysis. Units of measure for the outputs are developed (e.g., number of clients to be served, length of hospital stay, geographical area to be covered). Costs and resulting benefits for each approach are calculated, and the best alternative in terms of cost–benefit ratio is selected. With this approach, managers seek to increase the number of factors that can be used to provide top-level decision makers with sufficient information to make the final resource allocation. An adequate information system is, therefore, required; this is consistent with the classic systems approach, which includes an information feedback cycle.

The PPBS approach has several disadvantages. First, it is a time-consuming process, involving long-range planning, development and comparison of alternatives in terms of cost-effectiveness, and final budgeting. Second, not all goals can be stated precisely; not all worthy objectives can be quantified in specific measures, with a specific dollar cost attached. Third, there is the presumption that all alternatives are known and attainable. Fourth, the value, the legitimacy, and the actual survival of the program or organization are questioned. This, in turn, reopens conflict and exposes the accumulation of internal and external politics—the power plays, the bargaining, and the trade-offs that have developed over time. The concern for program survival may intensify to the point that line managers may seek to withhold negative information, and the feedback cycle may become distorted.

Although the zero-based budgeting approach is probably not used in preparing the routine budget for the ongoing operations of the organization, it is the approach underlying the cost justification for special projects of great magnitude. For example, the managers of a healthcare facility might commit to a major change in computer applications or support systems. Millions of dollars may be involved in the conversion to the new system. Detailed analysis of the project will typically include cost comparisons of several vendor options, with specifics provided for each. Cost breakouts for such a project are presented by category, such as illustrated in the following example:

| *Financial services module:* | |
| --- | --- |
| Application software | $700,000 |
| Software maintenance/yearly | $150,000 |
| Implementation services | $600,000 |
| (one-time cost in year one) | |
| *Training:* | |
| No cost in year one; included in implementation | |
| Annual cost for consultant training staff | $90,000 |
| *Licensing fees—annual* | $50,000 |
| (subject to review at the end of 3 years) | |

In both approaches, the budgeted funds are used during the designated period, with any unspent funds being turned in at the end of the fiscal year. However, some organizations follow a revenue retention rule to reward efficiency: a department keeps a portion of unspent funds at the end of the year to augment the upcoming year's funds.

## ▶ The Budgetary Process

### Initial Preparation

The budgetary process is cyclic; the feedback obtained during one budget period becomes the basis of budget development for the next period. The budget process usually begins with the setting of overall limits by top management. The supply chain manager is a key participant throughout the budgeting process, overseeing procurement, vendor compliance, and contracts. The specific guidelines for budget preparation reflect the mandatory federal, state, and accrediting requirements as well as union contract provisions and the financial assets of the organization. The timetable and particular forms to be used in budget preparation are issued along with these guidelines.

Development of the unit budget is the specific responsibility of the department manager. In some instances, a department manager may wish to use the "grassroots" approach to budgeting, in which unit managers or supervisors prepare their budgets and submit them to the department manager for coordination into the overall department budget. The supervisors or unit managers must, of course, be given

sufficient information and guidance to carry out this function. An alternative way of involving supervisors and subordinates is to ask for suggestions about equipment needs, special resources, or supplies. In highly normative organizations, such as a university, there may be an advisory or review committee composed of selected employees who make recommendations to line officials regarding budget allocations. In any event, the department head bears the responsibility for final preparation, justification, and control of the budget.

## The Budget Reference Portfolio

A manager will find it useful to develop a budget reference portfolio, gathering in one file all the working material relating to the budget. There is an exactitude to budgeting that warrants such precise attention. Current managers and those who come after them will benefit from notations, explanations, sources of information, and pertinent directives that shaped specific budgets over the years. Some of the useful items to include are:

- Current budget, with notations, detailed justifications, audit reviews, budget freezes or cuts; notations about items that cannot be cut.
- Past 2 or 3 years for historical reference and reuse of standard explanation calculations and justifications; carry-over information about such actions as an agreement to postpone certain expenditures for the fiscal year, with the expectation that these expenditures will be restored in the next budget.
- Directives and timeline for preparing the upcoming budget.
- Directives about wage/salary and benefit increases (or decreases); current minimum wage requirements.
- Directives from supply chain manager regarding leases, bulk purchases; equipment amortization schedules.
- Management inventory regarding personnel (confidential listing of known information, e.g., pending leave of absence; continuing sick leave); patterns of turnover by unit and/or job title.
- Calculations regarding vacation, personal days, holidays, and projected sick day usage, and plan of coverage.
- Excerpts from employee handbook and union contract regarding vacation, holidays, etc.
- Training needs and training plan.
- List of all equipment contracts and leases, with due dates.

- Area wage rates and/or national wage and salary listings.
- Resources for purchasing specialty items associated with particular functions (e.g., coding guidelines issued by an authoritative source such as a national professional association).
- Review of the manager's wheel book for entries relating to budget matters (e.g., contract renewal made; meeting about merit raise guidelines; budget freeze begun)

During the budget preparation phase, the manager reviews, challenges, and updates the working assumptions. Trends are noted, priority needs are identified, and initiatives for the upcoming year are stated. Effective managers rely on a continuous process of gathering facts throughout the year. Information includes changes in workload quantity and patterns (e.g., an increase in the number of industrial health-related cases, the opening of a satellite clinic for school health). Equipment and maintenance logs reflect the useful life estimates or depreciation values of all major items, including the cost of maintenance and repair. Delayed maintenance of the physical structures is noted. The department history log (similar in concept to the classic wheel log of a ship's captain) is reviewed; this log shows the ongoing history of departmental changes in systems and in departmental capital improvements (e.g., rewiring, painting) as well as major systems changes (e.g., introduction of off-site storage, ongoing conversion from hard copy to electronic health records).

The availability of previously unavailable external resources is identified, as in ensuring the availability of a reliable transcription service for outsourcing this function in health information services. The increased availability of specialists in an area of occupational therapy opens up the possibility of introducing new service in that unit of patient care.

Major trends in the field of professional practice, along with emerging department issues, are noted and appropriate initiatives stated. A department manager's initiatives might include increasing retention through in-service education programs and bonus or incentive plans, developing more specialist coverage, upgrading work stations, introducing new treatment modules, or developing outreach programs in community-based locations.

An essential part of budget preparation is the justification statement. Suggested wording is given later in this chapter for the major budget categories of capital expenses, supplies, maintenance and repair, specialty references, staff development, and personnel costs.

# The Review and Approval Process

Competition, bargaining, and compromise in the allocation of scarce resources—personnel, money, and space—occur in the review-and-approval phase of the budget process. It is important for the manager to have the necessary facts to support budget requests; control records to demonstrate fluctuations in the workload, staffing needs, equipment usage, and goal attainment are essential sources of such information.

The internal approval process begins with a review of the department's budget by the department head's immediate budget officer. Compliance with guidelines is checked, and justifications for requests for exceptions are reviewed. The organization's designated financial officer may assist the chief executive officer in coordinating the department budgets into the master budget for the organization, but the chief executive officer is the final arbiter of resource allocation in many instances.

There is continuing emphasis, both within the organization and from external pressures, on cost containment, and a cost-containment committee may be involved in the budget review process. Current voluntary efforts contribute to the routinization of this aspect of budget review. Cost-containment committees vary in structure and mandate, but their tasks typically include advising, investigating, and even participating in the implementation of cost-containment measures. Such a committee should have a questioning attitude as its primary philosophical stance; data are scrutinized and compared in an effort to identify areas where costs can be contained.

The budget hearing or review provides the department manager with an opportunity to make the case for his or her unit. Forthrightness and thorough preparation should characterize the manager's presentation. As the individual closest to the special issues of the particular unit, the manager should use this occasion to brief higher-level managers on critical issues. The manager should indicate willingness to trade off certain costs so that another department, with a more pressing need, may be accommodated; in turn, the manager should be able to make the argument for why such a trade-off is not possible. A manager might be willing to defer major improvements as well as routine maintenance (such as annual painting of the department) until another year, thereby freeing money for use by another department needing new equipment or increased staffing. This deferred maintenance might be tied to planned changes for the coming year, such as implementation of a major upgrade in equipment because of a technological change not yet available this coming budget year but definitely available in 2 more years. Instead of viewing the budget process as a win–lose proposition, a manager could partner with other department heads to preview mutual needs and trade-offs, thus fostering a win–win approach.

The customary planning approach of overaim or contingency planning is the usual principle followed in budget development. During the budget review, the manager would be prepared to give an optimistic, best-case scenario estimate (e.g., revenue increased, turnover decreased); a worst-case scenario, with definite indicators of expenditures that can be reduced or cut should this become necessary at a later time in the budget year; and a middle-ground estimate. During the review process, the values of open communication and integrity are paramount so that prudent, cost-effective decisions can be mutually agreed on.

The final approval for the total budget is given by the governing board. In practice, a subcommittee on budget works with the chief executive officer, and final, formal approval is then given by the full governing board, as mandated in the organizational bylaws or charter of incorporation.

The budgets of organizations that receive some or all of their funds from state or federal sources may be subject to an external approval process—for example, by the state legislature or the federal budget bureau. A certain predictable drama in the budget process becomes more evident in the external review process. There is a tacit notion that budgets are padded because budget requests are likely to be cut. The manager attempts to achieve a modicum of flexibility in budget maneuvering through overaim. There is also a necessary aspect of accountability, however. The public more or less demands that federal or state officials take proper care of the public purse. Even as clients (the public) seek greater services, they want cost containment, especially through tax relief. Public officials, then, must dramatize their concern for cost containment, partly by a highly specific review of budget requests and a refusal to approve budgets as submitted.

Conversely, should an agency request a budget allocation that is the same as, or less than, that of a previous year, it might be seriously questioned whether the agency is doing its job. At best, the manager must recognize the subtle and overt political maneuvers that affect the budget process.

## Implementation Phase

The final phase of budgeting is the implementation stage, when the approved budget allocation is spent.

During this phase, revenues and expenses are regularly compared—for example, through periodic budget reconciliation. Should revenues fall short of the anticipated amount or should unexpected expenses arise, there may be a budget freeze or certain items may be cut. For example, overtime may be prohibited; personnel vacancies may not be filled, except for emergency situations; and supplies or travel money may be eliminated.

Specific internal procedures must be followed to activate budgeted funds in the normal course of business. For example, the budget may contain an appropriation for certain supplies, but a companion requisition system must be used to effect the actual purchase of such supplies. When an individual worker is to be hired, a position authorization request may be used to activate that position as approved in the budget. Finally, during the budget year, preparation for the following budget period is made, bringing the manager full circle in the budget process (**Exhibit 8–1**).

Budget variance review and the periodic audit are discussed later in this chapter.

## ▶ Capital Expenses

An organization owns and operates capital facilities of a permanent or semipermanent nature, such as land, buildings, machinery, and equipment. Capital budget items are those revenues and costs related to the capital facilities. These expenses may be centralized as a single administrative cost for the entire organization, or they may be specified for each budgetary unit. The manager at the departmental level is normally concerned primarily with capital improvements for the department, such as acquisition of additional space, renovation and repairs, special electrical wiring, and painting.

The second capital expense in the departmental budget is major equipment. The equipment budget usually includes fixed equipment that is not subject to removal or transfer and that has a relatively long life. Major equipment that is movable is also included. The distinction between major and minor equipment is usually made on the basis of the cost and life expectancy of the item; major equipment commonly includes any item over a specific cost (e.g., $1000) that has a life expectancy of more than 5 years. As with other aspects of budgeting, however, a specific organization may use some other cost or life expectancy factor to define major equipment/capital equipment expense. Major fixed equipment includes the heating fixtures, built-in

**Exhibit 8-1** Annual Budget Plan: Based on Fiscal Year July 1–June 30

| Activity | Current Year | | | | | | | | | | | | Projected Year | | | | | | | |
|---|---|---|---|---|---|---|---|---|---|---|---|---|---|---|---|---|---|---|---|---|
| | Jul. | Aug. | Sep. | Oct. | Nov. | Dec. | Jan. | Feb. | Mar. | Apr. | May | Jun. | Jul. | Aug. | Sep. | Oct. | Nov. | Dec. | Jan. | Feb. |
| 1. Current budget executed; monthly reconciliation and adjustments made | | | | | | | | | | | | | | | | | | | | |
| 2. CEO and Controller develop forecasts; issue budget guidelines to departments | | | | | | | | | | | | | | | | | | | | |
| 3. Department heads formulate budgets and submit | | | | | | | | | | | | | | | | | | | | |
| 4. CEO and Controller develop master budget | | | | | | | | | | | | | | | | | | | | |
| 5. Department revisions made and submitted | | | | | | | | | | | | | | | | | | | | |
| 6. CEO and Controller finalize budget | | | | | | | | | | | | | | | | | | | | |
| 7. Board of Trustee subcommittee review; further adjustments made and final approval given | | | | | | | | | | | | | | | | | | | | |
| 8. TRANSITION: close out current year accounts | | | | | | | | | | | | | | | | | | | | |
| 9. New fiscal year budget in effect OR tentative budget in effect, pending full approval and/or further revisions | | | | | | | | | | | | | | | | | | | | |

cabinets or shelves, and appliances. Major movable equipment includes file cabinets, patient beds, computer stations, and a variety of treatment modular equipment.

When budgeting for major equipment expenses, the manager may calculate the acquisition cost and prorate this cost over the expected life of the equipment. Depreciation costs are a factor in equipment selection. The budget guidelines developed by the chief financial officer's staff includes reference tables for estimating the useful life of major equipment and a formula to calculate composite depreciation rates for each unit of equipment. Vendors for major equipment generally provide depreciation data as part of the support information relating to their products. An item that is more costly to acquire may be less expensive in the long run because of a lower operating cost, longer life expectancy, or slower rate of depreciation. This information should be included on the supplemental information forms used to justify equipment selection. When a lease agreement is considered, justification notes would reflect considerations such as: allows for purchase of equipment at end of lease; includes standard service at no additional cost; allows for upgrades during life of the lease to meet changing technological advances; delivery and set-up free of charge.

The worksheet for capital expenses includes the account code number from the uniform code of accounts, item description, unit cost, quantity, and total cost (**Exhibits 8-2** and **8-3**).

## ▶ Supplies and Other Expenses

The many consumable items that are needed for the day-to-day work of the department are listed under the category of supplies. It may be tempting at first to group all these items under "Miscellaneous," but the clear delineation and listing of such items in the appropriate budget category alerts the manager to the magnitude of these costs and facilitates control. A useful designation for these items is *consumable supplies*. Items considered consumable supplies typically include routine items such as pens, pencils, notepads, letterhead stationery, staples, scissors, rubber bands, and paper clips. Such detailed calculations for these kinds of supplies may seem tedious, but the dollar value of these items is, in fact, significant. The manager's working notes include the support calculations about consumables, and only the final total is listed under the broad term of consumable supplies. Careful assessment of needs prevents excessive inventory and problems associated with stockpiling. Stockpiling of unnecessary quantities takes up space, invites petty theft, and may lead to excess inventories of items that become outdated (e.g., forms, specialty supplies for equipment no longer

**Exhibit 8-2** Sample Worksheet for Capital Expenses: Health Information Services

Department: Health Information Services
Fiscal Year: July 1–June 30

| Account Code | Account Title: Item Description | Item Quantity | Item Cost | Total |
|---|---|---|---|---|
| 210.6 | Secretarial Desk | 1 | $760.00 | $760.00 |
| 210.7 | Side Chairs | 3 | $150.00 | $450.00 |

**Exhibit 8-3** Sample Worksheet for Capital Expenses: Physical Therapy

Department: Physical Therapy
Fiscal Year: July 1–June 30

| Account Code | Account Title: Item Description | Item Quantity | Item Cost | Total |
|---|---|---|---|---|
| 210.3 | Parallel Bars—10 foot | 1 | $2800 | $2800 |
| 210.4 | Shoulder Wheel—Deluxe Heavy Duty | 1 | $620 | $620 |

in use). Common-sense practices of regular inventory control and good recordkeeping by an office manager provide a department head with both the planning and the control appropriate to a seemingly incidental cost. Postage is included in this category unless it is absorbed as a central administrative line item.

A given department may have special consumable supplies that are essential to its operation. The direct patient care units incur expenses related to medical and surgical supplies, for example. The clinical laboratory has a major expense in reagents. A health information department may have continuing expenses associated with the transition from hard copy records to electronic media. Thus, there may still be a need for color-coded, preprinted folders used for patient records. Special forms approved and mandated for medical record documentation (e.g., the fact sheet/identification sheet used in the admission unit, the preoperative anesthesia report form used in the surgical unit, the laboratory requisition/report form for laboratory studies) may be charged to each department as they are requisitioned and used. An alternative practice is to charge the health information department or central forms design unit with the cost of all preprinted forms. When the emphasis in the budgeting process is on control, however, it is preferable to charge the unit using such supplies so that administrative control may be fixed.

Special expenses commonly incurred at the department level include the lease and rental of equipment; the purchase of technical reference books, software, and periodicals; training and education costs; and travel and meeting expenses. Contractual services for a special activity (e.g., transcription, statistical abstracting, special laboratory studies) are included under the expense category. Justification notes would include, by way of example, the cost of work station shredders as these are needed as part of the department's "Shred-as-You-Go" project. This is based on our continuing efforts to enhance HIPAA compliance. Efforts to prevent unauthorized access to confidential data include the use of relatively small shredders at each work station, thus eliminating information exposure. This method would replace the current practice whereby material is placed in a central bin in the department, but not collected until end of work day or, in some situations, not until after closing hours. Each shredder costs approximately $100.00. The total cost for shredders is $800.00 (8 shredders at $100.00 each = $800.00).

The promotional items associated with the celebration of Health Information Management week are available through the national association for a total cost of $285.00. This amount does not exceed the general budget guidelines limiting such expenses to $500.00. The materials will be used as part of outreach and client education about HIM activities such as release of information.

The worksheet for budget requests for supplies and expenses typically includes the required account number from the organization's uniform code of accounts, the item description, the item cost, and the total requested (**Exhibit 8-4**).

Notice that the budget worksheets reflect the totals for each line item. The manager retains the detailed calculations in a working file for reference during budget presentation and then for use during budget implementation. These working files contain levels of detail about specifications such as brand names, software details, discounts, and usual vendors. Examples of such details include the following working file notations:

| | |
|---|---|
| Books, Subscriptions, and Training Materials | $600.00 |
| Webinars and DVD Seminars for Training | $800.00 |
| Coding Update for Emergency Department Services | $161.00 |
| Hospital Outpatient Reporting Module | $242.00 |
| Nonphysician Practitioner Services: Coding and Reporting | $190.00 |

Notes to file: Obtain from AHIMA as authoritative source; also use discount by purchasing four at one time. These references are needed for coding and reimbursement update for the coming year. All will need annual replacement.

## Maintenance and Repair

Cost allocations are made under this category to reflect both routine maintenance and occasional repairs. Two approaches to these arrangements are:

1. *The fee-for-service plan*: Payment is made for time and materials per service. The price may vary, usually by way of an increase, but this method may be cost-effective for equipment that is new and still under warranty. Newer equipment generally needs few repairs, if any, early in its "life."
2. *The service agreement*: A contract, with fixed cost, is made with a service company. This agreement typically includes preventive maintenance as well as rapid on-call service. For departments having a mix of new and older equipment, such plans are cost-effective.

**Exhibit 8–4** Sample Worksheet for Supplies and Other Expenses: Health Information Services

Department: Health Information Services
Fiscal Year: July 1–June 30

| Account Code | Account Title: Item Description | Item Quantity | Item Cost | Total |
|---|---|---|---|---|
| 610.2 | Annual Professional Dues Paid for Department Head | — | $600 | $600 |
| 610.7 | Accrediting Agency Regulations Annual Update Subscription | 4 | $121 | $484 |
| 610.4 | Drug Usage Manual, Current Edition | 1 | $85 | $85 |

A mix of the two approaches is a third possibility. Cost comparisons of these approaches would provide the manager with a basis for decisions in this matter.

## Specialty References and Licensure Software

A required line item is associated with the legal requirement to pay licensure fees for software packages. Specialty software is needed in most departments, and the associated licensing fees are generally charged to the department. This is a line item that must be calculated in detail and may not be cut even when other expenditures must be reallocated. The budget justification document is the licensure software agreement, which specifies this obligation to pay a periodic fee for usage.

Specialty references (books, periodicals, and software) constitute another consideration for resource allocation. Certain references change from year to year, reflecting external agency requirements and practices. Examples include the latest interpretations of coding and reimbursement guidelines, accrediting standards, prescription drug references and compendia, and guidelines on certain aspects of clinical practice. These references are needed for the proper processing of mandated reimbursement practices. As with software licensure agreements, some of these costs cannot be omitted or reduced. These items are, of course, differentiated from other journal subscriptions, software, or references that, although highly desirable and convenient, are not absolutely necessary and could be cut should a financial emergency occur.

## Staff Development

This set of line items reflects costs associated with staff development, including travel and training opportunities and material. Costs associated with travel are

among the most vulnerable of line items. The manager should have a well-developed rationale for such expenditures; these costs should be linked to specific departmental and organizational goals, with their related projects. For example, attendance by the manager at a national meeting of a professional association provides the manager with opportunities to preview systems and equipment on a scale not available locally. Such a meeting may also provide critical updates concerning new mandates, as well as methods of complying with existing requirements such as accreditation, risk management, or reimbursement requirements. Specialty-oriented tutorials may be available at such events, providing the manager with updated skills that he or she can then teach to department staff. For example, a hospital may be planning to increase its observation unit capacity; health information services must, therefore, be up-to-date in the coding and billing strategies under outpatient payment systems. Attendance at a training session at a national meeting would pay dividends because of the resulting upgrade in coding and billing quality.

In developing travel budget estimates, the general policies of the organization are followed; for example, travel should be conducted by the most cost-effective means, with lodging and per diem limits specified. As part of recruitment and retention of specialty staff, managers (with appropriate approval) sometimes offer a guaranteed amount of time and money for such travel. A related benefit is that of payment (up to a set amount) of continuing education costs for job-related programs (e.g. conference fees). When such agreements have been entered into, that part of the travel cost is a given and may not be cut. These benefits may not be cut, once offered and accepted.

In-service training is a cost-effective method for keeping staff up to date in technical and specialty areas, no travel cost is incurred, and materials are used by more than one worker. Examples of topics include web-based coding courses, clinical data analysis, clinical documentation improvement.

Examples of cost calculation associated with training, along with ideas for cost justification, are included in the section on training (Chapter 9).

# ▶ The Personnel Budget

The cost of personnel is typically the largest category of expense in the budget of a healthcare organization, accounting for as much as 85% of the total budget in many cases. Personnel costs include the wage and salary calculation for each position and for each worker, including anticipated raises (e.g., cost of living increases, merit increases) and adjustments resulting from a change in status (e.g., from probationary employee to full-time, regular employee). The department manager normally calculates these costs. Special justification for an increase in the number of positions or for adjustments to individual salaries or wages is also included.

Also calculated and justified by the department manager are those costs associated with vacation relief, overtime pay, temporary or seasonal help, and sign-on bonuses. Specific support information may be required for these budget requests, such as a calculation of the personnel hours required to give proper departmental coverage and a calculation of the hours not available to the organization because of vacation time and holidays. If there is a high employee turnover rate or a distinct pattern of absenteeism, historical information, such as the average time lost over the past year or several years as a result of these circumstances, may be cited as support information.

In calculating the costs for personnel needs, the manager deals with impersonal costs—that is, those costs associated with the position, regardless of the incumbent. Such costs include the wage or salary range for the position and the number of full-time equivalent (FTE) positions. In addition, there are other costs that are associated with the incumbent and change with the holder of the position; these costs include those associated with the number of hours scheduled for work each week, the number of years in the job category, the eligibility for merit increases, and the anniversary date for a scheduled increase in pay. The following factors must be considered in any budget calculation:

1. Minimum wage. Federal and state laws mandate a base pay rate for certain jobs. Some categories of temporary help may be exempt from this wage; the manager must seek the guidance of the human resources specialist for details of this provision.

2. Union contract stipulations. Each class of job and each incumbent must be reviewed in light of contractual mandates for basic wage as well as mandatory increases. Where there is more than one contract in effect, the provisions of each contract must be reviewed and applied as appropriate. Wage and salary increases on a straight percentage basis may be mandated. In some cases, the contract may state that either a given percentage or a flat dollar amount, whichever gives the greater increase, is to be awarded. A hiring rate may be indicated for employees on "new-hire" status; a related job rate may be indicated, with the employee moving to the job rate at the end of the probationary period (**Table 8–1**).

3. Organizational wage and salary scale. Except for the specific provisions of union contracts, the organizational wage and salary scale applies. Positions are listed by job category or class, and the individual employee's rate is calculated from this scale. Increases may be in terms of a percentage or in terms of step increases dependent on the number of years in the position.

4. Cost of living increase. The organizational guidelines or contract provisions establish cost of living increases. Frequently, this amount is given as a flat percentage increase added to the base rate of pay, although it may be given as a flat dollar amount added to the base rate of pay.

5. Area wage and salary considerations. Periodically, benchmark data are made available within a geographic region. Such data are generally developed by a chamber of commerce group, regional healthcare organizations, or labor unions, to reflect the market-basket costs of the region. Similar to overall cost of living calculations reflecting nationwide factors, these area wage and salary surveys drive the costs associated with hiring and retention of workers. These data are usually refined to reflect

**Table 8–1** Sample Salary Structure (Clerical)

| Pay Grade | Hiring Rate (Weekly) | Job Rate (90 Calendar Days) |
|---|---|---|
| B | $310 | $330 |
| C | $330 | $346 |
| D | $340 | $360 |

several variables: size and complexity of the healthcare organization, profit versus nonprofit enterprises, years on the job, and specialty training and credentialing.

6. Merit raise or bonus pay. These costs may be shown as an overall amount given to the department as a whole. The manager may not be able to assign dollar amounts to an individual worker at the beginning of a year, because the merit award may not be given until some time period has passed and the worker has earned the increase. Specific guidelines are given to the manager concerning the calculation of merit or bonus pay as part of the base rate of pay or as a one-time increase that does not become part of the employee's base rate of pay.

7. Special adjustments. From time to time, a special adjustment may be made to the wage or salary structure. An organization that is adjusting its wage and salary structure to satisfy Equal Employment Opportunity Commission mandates may grant a one-time adjustment to a class of workers or an individual (e.g., women and/or minority workers) to bring their rate of pay in line with other workers' pay scales. When long-term employees' rates of pay shrink as compared with those of incoming workers, a special one-time adjustment may be made to keep the comparative wages of new versus long-term employees equitable.

The budget worksheet or budget display sheet generally includes the following items, which progress logically from the factual information based on the present salary of the incumbents to the projected salary through the coming budget period:

1. Position code or grade code, obtained from the master position code sheet for the department and organization.
2. Position description: abbreviated job title or category.
3. Budgeted FTEs: the number of personnel hours per position divided by the hours per full-time workweek. Example (based on a 40-hour workweek):

| Worker A | 40 hours |
| --- | --- |
| Worker B | 27 hours |
| Worker C | 20 hours |
| Worker D | 13 hours |
| Total = 100 hours = 2.5 FTEs | |

4. Employee number, usually assigned by personnel division or payroll division for identification of payroll costs and employee records.
5. Employee name: name of incumbent. If position is vacant, this information is noted.
6. Actual FTEs: number of employed workers and number of vacancies (see **Exhibit 8–5** for an example of calculating FTEs in the health information department budget process).
7. Current rate of pay: hourly rate, biweekly rate, or job rate. The hourly rate is calculated by dividing

### Exhibit 8–5 Calculating FTE's for Health Information Services

To calculate the number of employee hours needed to process the work in a given function, the manager first establishes the basic definition of a full-time equivalent position. This calculation is based on the usual workweek as defined by the facility:

1 FTE = 40 hours / week

40 hours / week × 52 weeks = 2080 hours / year

The hours needed may be concentrated in one full-time position or distributed between two or more part-time workers to total 2080 hours/year. The latter method provides flexibility.

The second part of the staffing calculation consists of estimating the volume of work to be done.

Work standard: 24 minutes to process one request

Volume per day: 30 requests

30 requests × 24 minutes = 720 minutes needed

1 FTE = 480 minutes per work day

1.5 FTE needed to process 30 requests per day 480 / 720.0

Needed: 1.5 FTE to process 30 requests per day.

the total salary by the number of work hours per budget period, and the biweekly rate by dividing the total salary by 26. The job rate is usually specified in the wage scale, especially as given in a union contract.

8. Projected annual base salary, calculated by multiplying the rate by the appropriate unit of time. This projected salary is specific to the incumbent. Should the incumbent separate from the organization with the replacement worker hired at entry-level pay, the annual base salary would be lower.
9. Incumbent's anniversary date, used to calculate cost of living or other raise associated with date of employment.
10. Projected annual increase because of cost of living increase, merit or bonus pay, or special adjustments.
11. Projected total salary: present salary plus projected annual increase.

*Example*

| Grade Code | 4 |
| --- | --- |
| Position Title | Compliance Specialist |
| Shift | Full-time, day |
| Incumbent | M. Caretto |
| Current Biweekly Pay | $1,575 |
| Projected Annual Base | $40,950 |
| Anniversary Date | Dec. 20 of current year |
| Projected Annual Increase | $1,250 |
| Projected Total Salary | $42,200 |
| Hours per Pay Period (biweekly) | 80 hours |

Sign-on bonuses and other recruitment/retention offers are listed, noting the specific costs and the fact that they are promised benefits.

Special pay adjustments, often a one-time allotment, are sometimes made to offset the disparity of wages when long-term employees' wages fall behind that of newer hires.

Coverage for paid time-off is calculated in one of two ways. (1) A generalized method simply uses an average, for example, all workers receive 10 paid sick days per fiscal year, but not every worker takes all 10 days; therefore, an average based on actual use could be calculated. All workers receive 2 paid personal days. In addition, there is a paid vacation allotment based on period of service. This varies by employee

hiring date and length of service. Again, a simple average might be used.

Note: all workers receive holiday pay, but if the department is not open on holidays, obviously no coverage is needed.

(2) A more exact method of calculation of coverage is to refine the calculations by identifying the exact benefit for the vacation days. Sick days would still be based on an average, and the paid personal days remain as stated. Here is an example reflecting one worker who will, in the next year's fiscal year, complete 7 years of employment, thus accruing 14 working days (as stipulated in the employee handbook or labor union contract), plus the 2 personal days, plus the 10 sick day allotment. Twenty-six days of coverage would (potentially) be needed to cover this worker's time off. The only variable is the actual number of sick days used; this figure would not be available at the time of budget preparation; thus, the full 10 days is built in.

Each worker's total days of coverage calculation is prepared using this method.

# Direct and Indirect Expenses

A department budget also reflects costs under the categories of direct and indirect expenses. Direct expenses typically include salaries, services and contracts, dues and subscriptions, and equipment. Indirect expenses are charged to the departmental budget on a formula basis or some process of assessment. These indirect costs are associated with the organization as a whole and are prorated per department. Examples of indirect costs and their units of assessment are shown in **Table 8–2**.

# Budget Justification

As mentioned earlier, support or explanatory documentation may be required for budget requests. If a particular type of equipment is requested, the manager is expected to explain why that particular model or brand is needed. The reasons may include compatibility with existing equipment, guaranteed service contracts, availability, or durability. Projected patient usage is another element of support data; the acquisition of a particular item may enhance patient care because of its safety features.

Sometimes the facility may need an item simply to remain competitive and thereby retain a given patient

**Table 8–2** Indirect Expenses Charged to Health Information Services

| Item | Amount | Basis of Calculation |
|------|--------|----------------------|
| Fringe benefits/health and welfare | $156,000 | Percentage of salaries |
| Equipment depreciation | $30,000 | Depreciation schedule |
| Telephone costs (equipment) | $8,000 | Number of telephones |
| Maintenance and repairs | $2,300 | Number of work orders |
| Physical plant operation (e.g., heat, air conditioning) | $42,000 | Number of square feet |
| Building depreciation | $6,000 | Number of square feet |

population. The budget justification may take the form of a cost comparison, such as that between rental or long-term lease of equipment and outright purchase plus maintenance costs. For a health information department, a cost comparison between an in-house word processing–transcription unit and a contractual service might be included. A careful review of the proposed change includes the challenging question: Is there a true cost saving? Some contractual services require a stipend to cover office, internet, and phone expenses for work-at-home businesses. A related observation is: Can the physical space truly be used for some other activity in the department? If not, the indirect cost calculated on square footage remains. If contracted work is done onsite, there is a potential cost saving because fringe benefits are not paid. However, such contractual work often costs more per hour than the regular wage for a traditional employee.

## The Budget Cut

When financial exigencies warrant a budget adjustment, either in the form of a partial reduction in a line item or category or the elimination of an entire expenditure, the manager uses the budget justification details to guide this process. Certain items cannot be cut (e.g., software licensure agreements, sign-on bonuses promised to specific employees). The manager looks to those categories of planned overage to determine which items to reduce or cut. For example, desired staff training programs may be best accomplished by sending workers off-site, but adequate programs could be developed by the management staff and offered at substantial savings.

Similarly, bulk purchases (e.g., a 3-year supply of custom-designed forms) could be cut back to the purchase of 1-year supply. The discount for the bulk rate might be lost, but in a tight budget situation of a given year, this more limited expenditure might be necessary to meet the "bottom line." Another option might be available from wage and salary lines: a manager could delay hiring a replacement when a vacancy occurs. The wage and fringe benefit amount could be used to pay for a temporary or contract worker. By delaying the hire of the new full-time worker until the next fiscal year, the pay increase is also saved. Alternatively, the manager could fill the position immediately but at an entry-level pay grade.

## Cost Comparison

Budget justification also includes cost comparison. One example would be that of comparing costs of in-house or outsourced medical transcription/editing. This type of information would also be the basis for requests for proposals when the selection process is implemented. See the earlier example included in the section on budget justification.

## ▶ Budget Variances

During the fiscal year, the manager receives periodic reports showing budgeted amounts versus amounts spent. This report may categorize such information under the headings of "overbudget" or "underbudget" for the period and for the year. The manager uses this information as a monitoring and control device. A particular unit's budget may include money for overtime that is assigned arbitrarily to budget quarters. A periodic report may show that the manager was overbudget in that category for the quarter but not for the year. Such a report is an internal warning system that alerts the manager to that line item. Filed with higher-level management, the variance report reflects the manager's awareness of the expenditure for the quarter and its relationship to the yearly amount as a whole. Should there be some unexpected cause for using these overtime funds, such as high absenteeism because of employee illness or injury, this information is noted in the variance report.

Underbudget indicators require similar explanations as part of the control process in budgeting. Explanations for underbudget items are not required in every instance, but particular attention must be given to large sums that have not been spent because of delay factors in the outside environment. For example, the purchase of a large, expensive piece of equipment may be included in the budget for the fiscal year. If it is not available until the next fiscal year, the delay could throw a carefully planned budget out of balance; that is, funds are not expended in the year, and no funds are allotted for this purchase in the upcoming budget. The manager should anticipate such a situation and make arrangements for the transfer of funds in a timely way.

Direct patient care service budgets include projections of care to be rendered. Actual revenue generated per patient visit is compared with projected revenue. The explanations—overprojections or underprojections of care to be rendered—are made by the budget officer for the service. If patient care services are

below those projected, plans for increasing services may be included with the explanation.

## Example of Variance Analysis

**Exhibit 8–6** displays a year-to-date summary of expenditures. The fiscal year in this example runs from July through June. This report reflects year-to-date costs as posted through April 30, the close of the third quarter. The department manager reviews these figures for the following purposes:

Verify the accuracy of posting (making sure costs are posted and none are omitted due to error). The department daily ledgers are compared to this official listing prepared by the finance office.

1. Review specific object codes where the actual costs exceed the approved budgeted amounts. An item may be over budget for the period but not for the year. The manager would note these and prepare explanations.
2. Review specific object codes where actual costs are below the approved budgeted amounts. If the allotted money is not going to be spent in the

### Exhibit 8–6 Summary of Expenditures, Year-to-Date

#### Cost Center 234

| Object Code | Supplies | Budgeted | Actual | Over/Under |
|---|---|---|---|---|
| 021 | Printed forms, stationery, office supplies—vendors | 51,999.00 | 50,000.00 | 1,999.00 |
| 026 | Books | 400.00 | 304.00 | 96.00 |
| 027 | Journals and software subscriptions | 620.00 | 754.00 | (134.00–) |
| 028 | General stores, supplies—internal | 2,400.00 | 1,987.00 | 413.00 |
| 035 | Parking | -0- | 30.00 | (30.00–) |
| 044 | Travel | 1,700.00 | 1,917.00 | (217.00–) |
| 051 | Film rental | -0- | 42.00 | (42.00–) |
|  | Supplies—subtotal | 57,119.00 | 55,034.00 | 2,085.00 |
| **Object Code** | **Services** |  |  |  |
| 122 | Contractual temps | 850.00 | 600.00 | 250.00 |
| 131 | Equipment rental | 2,000.00 | 1,811.00 | 189.00 |
| 134 | Outside contractual service | 5,000.00 | 3,750.00 | 1,250.00 |
| 136 | Equipment repair contracts | 380.00 | 31.60 | 348.40 |
| 138 | Computer license agreement | 32,000.00 | 9,000.00 | 23,000.00 |
|  | Services—subtotal | 40,230.00 | 15,192.60 | 25,037.40 |

approved category, the manager may seek approval to use these funds for some other need. Particular attention is given to an underbudget category in which a major expense has been, or soon will be, incurred but that has not yet been posted. Object code 138, Computer License Agreement, reflects a major cost yet to be posted—namely, the fourth-quarter payment.

# The General Audit

Through the related processes of posting entries to the proper line items, monitoring variances and explaining their causes, and tracking each item from its budgeted approval entry through its actual expenditure, the manager has developed an audit trail. The required forms, documentation, and approvals for actual expenditures all dovetail with these practices to provide sound control over the financial resources. The department manager will usually carry out periodic partial audits during the fiscal year, and both internal and external auditors will carry out a full audit at least once during the year.

Examples of such audit practices include the prevention of "ghost employees" or "ghost patients"—every employee will be clearly identified as to job title, hours worked (payroll data), and paycheck issued and processed. In some organizations, all employees must sign in person for paychecks on a random or regular basis to prevent such potential fraud. The audit trail of a given patient is easily tracked: (1) the master patient index provides name and other identifying information, (2) a complete and accurate patient care document should match this information, (3) names of care providers are matched against provider rosters, and (4) billing records are matched against the documentation of the care.

Similarly, expenses relating to purchases of equipment can be tracked by noting the purchase requisition, the installation date, the actual location of the equipment at the time of the audit, and the appropriate entries in the equipment inventory. Some examples of audit findings, results of the audit trail, and the follow-up action are:

- *Item*: Sign-on bonus for coder not activated

*Results of audit trail*: Coder sign-on bonus was conditional on coder having remained in this job for 6 months. Coder transferred to physician practice division after 4.5 months.

*Follow-up action*: Sign-on bonus cancelled.

- *Item*: Equipment lease ended 3 months before originally contracted date but payment was made for the full 11 months

*Results of audit trail*: Refund needed for the 3 months; contract has a no-penalty clause and a refund clause

*Follow-up action*: Referred to purchasing/contract coordinator. Because of lateness of the refund claim (June 24, 20n2), the refund will not clear until early July of the upcoming fiscal year.

- *Item*: Former employee (Name) received payment as employee while, at the same time, receiving payment as a contractual worker; dates of dual listing are March 4 through March 22.

*Results of audit trail*: This individual was carried as an employee during these days. These were the unused vacation and personal days; organizational policy does not provide for cashing out such days. Official termination date was end of day, March 22. Worker started as contractual worker on March 4 and was paid under the payment provisions of the contract.

*Follow-up action*: Matter referred to human relations for policy clarification for future application. A waiver to the cashing-out policy was requested (and granted) for this former employee so that there was not a dual listing.

## The Audit Committee

An audit committee is formed to assist the board of trustees in fulfilling its oversight responsibilities. This committee monitors the integrity of the organization's financial statements and its compliance with legal and regulatory requirements (e.g., the Centers for Medicare and Medicaid payment/fraud controls) and works with independent outside auditors. The committee also reviews and monitors compliance with ethical codes for senior financial officers, chief executive officers, and department managers. The organizational values of integrity and stewardship are promoted through such ongoing activities, closing the loop from plan through execution, with each step properly documented.

# Sample Budget: Health Information Service

**Appendix 8–A** is a complete annual budget for a health information service.

*Note:* The figures are only examples. Actual rates will vary geographically and over time.

In preparation for developing the budget, the manager reviewed related entries in the ongoing Manager's Wheel Book. See **Appendix 8–B** Wheel Book Excerpts—Budget Issues.

# Appendix 8-A

## Sample Annual Budget—Health Information Service

*Note:* These figures are only examples. Actual costs and wage rates vary geographically and over time. Background planning notes for upcoming fiscal year:

1. Department is in final stages of migration from hard copy records to electronic health records. Planned completion is in 18 months (all 12 months of upcoming budget year plus 6 months of the following budget year).
2. Starting July 1, work order charges are $200.00 for initial response to work order request. On average, the department has had 14 requests per budget year.
3. The department plans to sponsor an on-site meeting of the regional professional association and a week-long promotion effort regarding health information management, privacy, and security. Costs associated with this plan include food, parking, printing (in house), and promotional/commemorative items.
4. Books, software, and journal subscription line items include the costs for updates of coding, billing, and accrediting resources.

Budget premises:

1. Fiscal year: July 1–June 30
2. Workweek: 40 hours/week; 2080 hours/year per FTE
3. Cost of living increase: 5% of current base rate (see **Table 8–3** for detailed cost of living calculations by position title)
4. Effective date of cost of living increase: January 1
5. Overtime rate: time and a half, based on current base for employee
6. Holiday pay: regular base rate (for employees who work on a scheduled holiday: double time, calculated on current base for each employee)
7. Temporary agency rate: average rate is $13/hour for clerical workers, no fringe benefits given
8. Sick pay: calculated on each employee's current base
9. Fringe benefits: 29% of total wages and salaries for the department; 29% for each individual employee
10. A special initiative to increase data security is included (a "Shred-As-You-Go" method); this requires small shredders at each work station.
11. Sign-on bonus and free continuing education offerings cannot be cut when they are part of employment offer, made and agreed to.
12. Wage and salary calculations are displayed to show these details:

| Factor | Example |
|---|---|
| Current annual base | $58,000 |
| July–December of current calendar year—total earnings | $29,000 |
| January 1 cost of living increase (5%) | $2,900 |
| New annual base effective January 1 | $60,900 |
| January–June of coming calendar year—total earnings | $30,450 |
| Total needed for full 12-month period of the fiscal year | $29,000 + $30,450 = $59,450 |

Table 8–3 displays the wage and salary by position and title.

**Table 8–3** Wage and Salaries by Position Title

| | Current Base | July Through December | Jan. 15 (%) Increase | New Base | January Through June | Total for Fiscal Year |
|---|---|---|---|---|---|---|
| Director | 78,000 | 39,000 | 3,900 | 81,900 | 40,950 | 79,950 |
| Compliance Specialist | 49,999 | 24,999 | 2,499 | 52,499 | 26,249 | 51,248 |
| Registries Coordinator | 45,000 | 22,500 | 2,250 | 47,250 | 23,625 | 46,125 |
| Coder A | 40,000 | 20,000 | 2,250 | 42,250 | 21,125 | 41,125 |
| Coder B | 40,000 | 20,000 | 2,250 | 42,250 | 21,125 | 41,125 |
| Evening Shift Coder | 41,000 | 20,500 | 2,050 | 43,050 | 21,525 | 42,025 |
| Billing Compliance Specialist | 38,000 | 19,000 | 1,900 | 39,900 | 19,950 | 38,950 |
| Release of Information Specialist | 36,000 | 18,000 | 1,800 | 37,800 | 18,900 | 36,900 |
| Secretary | 27,000 | 13,500 | 1,350 | 28,350 | 14,175 | 27,675 |
| Transcriptionist A | 36,000 | 18,000 | 1,800 | 37,800 | 18,900 | 36,900 |
| Transcriptionist B | 36,000 | 18,000 | 1,800 | 37,800 | 18,900 | 36,900 |
| Evening Shift Transcriptionist | 36,500 | 18,250 | 1,825 | 38,325 | 19,163 | 37,413 |
| Release of Information Support Clerk | 25,000 | 12,500 | 1,250 | 26,250 | 13,125 | 25,625 |
| Registration Specialist | 34,000 | 17,000 | 1,700 | 35,700 | 17,850 | 34,850 |
| Certified Documentation Improvement Specialist | 45,000 | 22,500 | 2,250 | 47,250 | 23,625 | 46.125 |
| Health Record Specialist grade II | 25,000 | 12,500 | 1,250 | 26,250 | 13,125 | 25,625 |
| Health Record Specialist grade I | 24,480 | 12,240 | 1,224 | 25,704 | 12,852 | 25,092 |

# Health Information Department Budget

## Personnel Costs

| Object Code | | |
|---|---|---|
| 01 | Wages and salaries | $673,653.00 |
| 02 | Fringe benefits | $195,359.00 |
| 03 | Vacation relief coverage | $4,000.00 |
| 04 | Sign-on bonuses | $9,600.00 |
| | Subtotal A | $882.612.00 |

## Equipment

| Object Code 10 | |
|---|---|
| Work station shredders (8 at $100 each) | $800.00 |
| Office chairs (6 at $128 each) | $768.00 |
| Step stools (3 at $59 each) | $177.00 |
| Multiterminal word processing system | $74,000.00 |
| Subtotal B | $75,745.00 |

## Supplies

| Object Code | | |
|---|---|---|
| 021 | Printed Forms and Folders (2-year supply; external vendor) | $51,999.00 |
| 026 | Books and Software | $3,380.00 |
| 027 | Journals Subscriptions | $1,620.00 |
| 028 | General Stores Supplies (internal supply chain) | $3,400.00 |
| 030 | Specialty Items (health information management week commemorative/promotional items; external vendor) | $610.00 |
| 035 | Parking (guest) | $500.00 |
| 044 | Travel | $2,430.00 |
| 051 | Training Materials (rental) | $600.00 |
| | Subtotal C | $64,539.00 |

## Services

| Object Code | | |
|---|---|---|
| 122 | Contractual Temporaries | $3,850.00 |
| 131 | Equipment Rental | $2,000.00 |
| 134 | Outside Contractual Service | $5,000.00 |
| 136 | Equipment Repair Contracts | $2,000.00 |
| 138 | Computer License Agreement | $32,000.00 |
| | Subtotal D | $44,850.00 |

## Cost Transfers

| Object Code | | |
|---|---|---|
| 150 | Telephone | $3840.00 |
| 151 | Work Orders | $1400.00 |
| 152 | Postage | $360.00 |
| 153 | Photocopy/Print Shop | $200.00 |
| 158 | Food Service | $560.00 |
| | Subtotal E | $6360.00 |

## Summary

| | |
|---|---|
| Personnel Costs | $882,612.00 |
| Equipment | $75,745.00 |
| Supplies | $64,539.00 |
| Services | $44,850.00 |
| Cost Transfers | $6,360.00 |
| TOTAL | $1,074,106.00 |

# Appendix 8-B

## Wheel Book Excerpts—Budget Issues

These entries reflect various budget-related actions: last quarter of fiscal year 20n1 and July 20n2, the beginning of new fiscal year.

| Date | Activity |
| --- | --- |
| Mar. 17 | Agreed to postpone capital improvement expense to next fiscal year; money needed by another department for emergency repairs |
| Apr. 20 | Calculated and submitted report regarding cost of modified operations schedule—the weather-related event of March 30; two-day coverage costs.Prepared and submitted request from supply chain coordinator regarding required brand name supplies vs. generic supplies |
| Apr. 30 | Clarified with HR department that sign-on bonus is not part of base salary |
| May 7 | Closed out third-quarter expenses |
| May 9 | Budget freeze begins |
| May 23–25 | Attended state association annual conference; obtained vendor information regarding potential purchase of equipment; arranged vendor meetings at department for June |
| Jun. 11 | Shifted money from unused wage and benefits to cover cost of temporary agency workers; resignation of (N) lead coder |
| Jun. 14 | Reviewed pattern of overtime, temporary agency, and contractual provider usage for input into labor union contract negotiations; clarified with HR department: merit raise guidelines |
| Jun. 21 | Annual report preparation done regarding absentee rate, sick day usage, and turnover rate by department unit; reviewed findings with unit supervisors |
| Jul. 1 | New fiscal year begins |
| Jul. 10 | Reassessed wages for (N), transcriptionist and (N) secretary; longevity raise requested for them due to changes in entry-level wage structure |
| Jul. 18 | Final close out: fourth quarter of fiscal year 20n1 |
| Jul. 31 | Met with development office regarding grant money for training |

## CHAPTER 9

# Training and Development: The Backbone of Motivation and Retention

## CHAPTER OBJECTIVES

- Acknowledge the importance of and necessity for employee orientation programs and ongoing training and development activities.
- Relate orientation, training, and development to the management functions of planning, organizing, directing, and controlling to employee motivation.
- Identify the components of effective employee orientation programs.
- Recommend an approach to communicating standards of conduct and behavior to new employees.
- Identify the components of employee training programs.
- Explore the availability of resources for training and development activities.
- Identify the components of the clinical affiliation/clinical practice program and contract.

## ▶ Employee Development

It is a fundamental responsibility of every manager to endeavor to shape and enhance the behavior of employees so that they possess the necessary knowledge, skills, and attitudes to fulfill their assignments according to the policies, rules, and regulations of the institution. Advances in technology necessitate continual retraining of experienced employees to perform new and altered tasks. Training and staff development are the fundamental means by which behavior can be improved to meet the immediate and long-range needs of the institution.

Training and development are ongoing activities, beginning with the orientation of a new employee and continuing throughout the employee's tenure with the organization. Participation in formal orientation and training programs must be documented for each employee, with copies of all reports provided to the employee for personal use and placed in the official personnel record of each employee.

# Relationship of Training and Development to the Basic Management Functions

The need for sound orientation and training flows from several considerations. The mission and values of the organization usually include a commitment to quality. Certain organizational policies and practices usually reflect the intent and expectation that internal development—that is, promotion from within the organization—is the norm. Training and staff development foster a culture of success and excellence. Concurrently, the organization continuously seeks to meet its external mandates which include requirements for appropriate orientation and training. The licensing and accrediting agencies include in their surveys and site visits reviews of such programs. Part of marketing and public relations initiatives often include statements about the organization's compliance with training, for example, a statement that all direct patient care providers are required to attain a certain number of contact hours for continuing education requirements, often exceeding the minimum required by state law. Also, labor contracts may contain explicit provisions for training programs and related benefits, such as compensatory time for training programs attended at off-site locations. With the increased attention being paid to succession planning and the continuity of operations, cross-training for key positions has become yet another reason for managers to develop appropriate training programs.

Quality improvement programs and risk management oversight both require proper orientation and training. Management concerns such as employee evaluation or performance review, assessment of productivity measures, and the operation of merit and bonus pay programs all require—if only out of fairness to employees—that all workers be properly oriented and trained for their jobs.

The employee who knows what is expected and how to completely perform the work is likely to be a productive employee who experiences job satisfaction. When employees are generally satisfied, complaints, grievances, and job turnover decrease accordingly. The management team further assists employees in their personal development and their growth on the job by making additional training possible—for example, through tuition reimbursement benefits, release time for educational purposes, additional stipends for incidental costs (books, fees, travel), and provision for specialty scholarships.

As a practical matter, training is necessitated by the need for workers who possess specific knowledge and skills. When the labor pool in the area does not provide a ready source of specially trained support staff, managers must engage in planned training to meet their staffing needs. Changes resulting from technology or system upgrades require ongoing training as well.

# ▶ Orientation

A sound beginning for each newly hired employee provides a positive atmosphere of mutual expectation between the employee and management. Ideally, the formal orientation will be brief, highly focused, and completed on the worker's first day of employment or as soon as possible thereafter. Orientation is a responsibility shared by the department head, the human resources department, and other designated specialists such as those in employee health and safety, information technology services, and public relations. The orientation program elements common to all employees are ordinarily developed and coordinated by the human resources department. Information and special practices associated with a specific department—that is, a departmental orientation—is the responsibility of that department's manager.

## General Orientation

The typical content of a general orientation program includes the following information:

- A brief history of the organization along with explanation of its mission and its vision
- The institution's ownership form, mode of governance, and administrative structure
- An overview of the various departments and services
- A review of specific employee policies, including:
  - Drug, alcohol, and substance abuse considerations
  - Sexual harassment
  - Nondiscrimination issues
  - Conflict of interest prohibitions and gifts
  - Dress codes
  - Use of computers, accessing the Internet, using electronic mail (e-mail)
  - Computer security and passwords
  - Privacy and confidentiality of all aspects of patient care
  - Security, fire and safety
  - Infection control
  - Review of the organization's disaster plan including modified operations schedule in emergencies

An additional portion of the general orientation ordinarily consists of a review of employee benefits, with direct assistance provided to new employees in signing up for such benefits. If workers are covered under a specific labor union agreement, the provisions of the applicable contract are explained at the general orientation.

The outline of the contents of a typical general orientation to a healthcare provider organization is given in **Exhibit 9–1**.

## Departmental Orientation

The departmental orientation aspect of the new employee orientation is customized to the individual worker. The mission and goals of the department are shared. The departmental organizational chart, including names as well as job titles, is made available. The manager pays particular attention to acquainting the new worker with the other employees who will likely share common duties and work space. Preferably the manager will have made prior arrangements with an established member of the group to act as a "buddy" to the new employee to facilitate the transition into this new work environment.

Departmental policies, procedures, work standards, and productivity monitors, if any, are highlighted, with the understanding that these will be explained in detail during the formal training period. Issues relating to patient safety and privacy are reiterated, and the confidentiality statement is again reviewed and signed by the employee (if this has not already been done at time of hire or at the general orientation). So oriented, the new employee is ready for the transition to the training phase.

**Exhibit 9–2** is an outline of one possible departmental orientation schedule. The departmental orientation

---

### Exhibit 9–1 General Orientation Contents and Checklist

The following checklist is initiated in General Orientation, following which it will be permanently retained in the employee's personnel file. It is to be completed and submitted to the Human Resources representative at the conclusion of General Orientation.

Employee Name (please print)

_____

Affiliate or Division (if applicable)

_____

Department

_____

Orientation Topics (Initial to indicate completion of each topic)
_____ Organization's mission, vision, and values
_____ Organization's history and structure
_____ Overview of operations: how all departments work together
_____ Compliance mandate: standards of conduct
_____ Confidentiality of patient-related information
_____ Cultural proficiency: diversity awareness
_____ Domestic violence and its signs
_____ Electrical safety and the Safe Medical Device Act
_____ Emergency preparedness (disaster plan) and Modified Operations Schedule
_____ Fire safety
_____ Hazardous communications and the right-to-know law
_____ Improving organizational performance
_____ Risk management
_____ Incident reporting
_____ Infection control
_____ Bloodborne pathogens/tuberculosis control
_____ No-smoking policy
_____ Patient rights
_____ Professional misconduct
_____ Security management and crime watch
_____ General age-specific competencies
_____ Use of the organization's property and systems
_____ Internet, e-mail, and social media use
_____ Introduction to personnel policy and procedure manual
_____ Received identification badge
_____ Completed and submitted confidentiality statement
_____ Received and reviewed employee handbook and submitted signed receipt

**Exhibit 9–2** Department Orientation Contents and Checklist

This form is to be initiated by the department manager or other designated individual for each new employee's department-specific orientation. Please complete the form and submit it to Human Resources following orientation; the completed form will be retained in the employee's personnel file.

Employee Name (please print)

_____

Affiliate or Division (if applicable)

_____

Department

_____

Orientation Topics (Manager, preceptor, or instructor should initial on completion of each topic)
_____ Welcome, tour of department, introduction to staff
_____ Department fire and life safety requirements
_____ General safety rules, specific hazards, personal protective equipment
_____ Infection control practices, if applicable
_____ Review of job description and performance expectations
_____ Reporting incidents and emergencies
_____ Department's role in emergency or disaster; departmental modified operations schedule
_____ Work hours, schedules, time reporting, absence reporting, modified operations schedule
_____ Dress code
_____ Parking
_____ Employee health department and annual health review requirement
_____ Pay rate, pay cycle, pay increase policy, performance appraisal process
_____ Telephone, internet, and social media use
_____ Grievance procedure and progressive discipline process
_____ Continuing education, mandatory requirements
_____ Other considerations (if any) unique to the employee's position

_____

I have reviewed the foregoing topics with my supervisor (or preceptor or instructor) during my orientation.

_____ Employee Signature

I have reviewed this employee's completed orientation form.

_____ Supervisor Signature

may vary from one department to another depending on the nature of any given department's work.

# Of Special Concern: Standards of Conduct and Behavior

An organization's code of ethics is reflected in its standards of employee conduct and behavior, which in turn are usually published in complete form in a personnel policy and procedure manual and in summary fashion in an employee handbook. Certain behavioral expectations should be emphasized with every new employee, and the new-employee orientation presents the best opportunity for doing so.

## Conflict of Interest

An organization's employees ordinarily retain the right to engage in outside business or financial activities as long as these activities do not interfere with the complete performance of their duties. It is necessary for the working healthcare professional to avoid both actual conflict of interest and any behavior that creates the appearance of conflict of interest. The issue of appearance is important; a perceived conflict may not in fact be real, but to the perceiver, perception is reality.

A conflict of interest occurs when one's loyalty becomes divided between job responsibilities and some outside interest. A conflict of interest may be perceived when an objective observer of one's actions has cause to wonder whether the actions are motivated solely by organizational concerns or by external concerns.

Conflict of interest is the area of ethical concern likely to emerge most often in the management of a department. Some of the following guidelines apply to employees at all levels, whereas some are most pertinent to specific employees (e.g., purchasing agents). Because many of these considerations affect employee behavior, they are important to every department manager. Whether you are a manager or nonmanager:

- Never place business with any firm in which you or your family or close outside associates have an interest.

- Derive no personal financial gain from transactions involving the organization unless the organization is advised of—and approves of—your potential benefit.
- Conduct all aspects of a personal business venture outside of the organizational environment and on nonwork time. This guideline is regularly violated and often implicitly condoned by management through failure to address the offending behavior. For example, soliciting orders for cosmetics, food containers, jewelry, and so on during work hours is in violation of ethical standards. Also, using the organization's equipment to make photocopies for a part-time activity or other outside interest is similarly in violation.
- In situations in which you have the authority to hire or so recommend, do not employ relatives.
- Do not solicit, offer, accept, or provide any consideration that could be construed as conflicting with the organization's business interests, such as meals, gifts, loans, entertainment, or transportation.
- Do not accept gifts exceeding the maximum value established by the organization (limits may exist in amounts up to perhaps $50 but are commonly lower). Never accept gifts of cash in any amount.
- Safeguard patient and provider information against access or use for financial gain by unauthorized interests.

If in doubt, disclose the situation and seek resolution of an actual or potential conflict of interest before taking what might later be seen as an improper action. Questions concerning potential conflicts of interest can usually be addressed with the organization's human resources department.

Finally, in many organizations managers and professionals are asked to sign a conflict-of-interest statement, indicating either the presence or absence of potential conflicts. This statement is usually the same as that executed by members of the board of directors.

## Use of Organizational Assets and Information

It is the responsibility of all employees to protect the assets of the organization against loss, theft, and misuse. Neither may the organization's property be used for personal benefit, nor may it be loaned, sold, given away, or disposed of in any manner without appropriate authorization.

The organization's assets are intended for use for business purposes only during legitimate employment. Improper use ordinarily includes unauthorized personal

appropriation or use of tangible assets such as computers and copiers and other office equipment, medical equipment, vehicles, supplies, reports and records, computer software and data, and facilities. Intangible assets such as intellectual property; trademarks and copyrights; and proprietary information, including computer programs, confidential data, business plans, and such must be protected as vigorously as tangible property.

It also is necessary to protect patient property and information in accordance with established policies requiring patient information to be shared only with those who are authorized to receive it and have a legitimate need for it.

The responsibility for protection also extends to proprietary information entrusted to the organization by vendors, referral sources, contractors, service providers, and others. This standard includes the requirement to use only legally licensed computer software, with the use of bootleg or pirated software considered illegal as well as unethical.

Concerning information, an organization's ethical standards of conduct may set forth the following principles:

- It is prohibited to disclose proprietary information to anyone external to the organization, whether during or after employment, except as specifically authorized.
- All organizational property and information in employees' possession must be surrendered on termination of employment.

## Referral Practices

The laws governing Medicare, Medicaid, and other federally sponsored programs prohibit payment in any form in return for the referral of patients. The federal antikickback statute imposes criminal penalties for knowingly and willfully seeking or receiving payment for referring patients. The kinds of payments prohibited by the statute include kickbacks, bribes, and rebates. The Self-Referral Law (known as the Stark law) prohibits physicians holding a financial interest with an entity providing any designated health service from referring Medicare and Medicaid patients to that entity. The law also prohibits billing federal healthcare programs for items or services ordered by a physician who has a financial relationship with the billing entity.

These and additional considerations may be incorporated in an organization's ethical standards of conduct in the following manner:

- No employee shall solicit, receive, offer to pay, or pay remuneration of any kind in exchange for referring or recommending referral of any individual to another person, department, or division of the organization for services or in return for the purchase of goods or services to be paid for by a federal program.

- No employee shall offer or grant benefits to a referring physician or other referral source to secure the referral of patients or patient business.
- No physician shall make referrals for designated health services to entities in which the physician has a financial interest through either ownership or a compensation arrangement.
- No physician shall bill for services rendered as a result of an illegal referral.

## Political Activity

An organization's code of conduct often includes an expectation that employees who participate in political activity will ensure that they are not doing so as representatives of the organization. There is, in fact, a legal prohibition against political activity by not-for-profit hospitals and nursing homes, and participating in political activity can jeopardize the employer's tax-exempt status.

## Employee Privacy

Personnel files are the property of the employer. The organization will have a privacy policy limiting access to these files to those persons having a legitimate need for the information. The policy will usually state that personnel information will be released externally only on employee authorization or in response to a subpoena or other legal order.

## Patient Confidentiality

Records relating to or concerning individuals to whom the organization is providing or has provided service should be held in the strictest confidence. It is a violation of the ethical code of conduct to reveal patient information to anyone outside of the organization without the express written authorization of the patient (or the patient's guardian, administrator, or executor), or a court order or other appropriate legal instrument. Within the organization, patient information is to be retained in confidence and revealed on a need-to-know basis only.

## Employee Relationships

The following is a suggested model for the portion of an organization's ethical standards of conduct addressing relationships with employees:

Every employee will be treated and judged as an individual on the basis of individual qualifications without regard to race, gender, sexual orientation, religion, national origin, age, disability, veteran status, or other characteristic protected by law. This pledge extends to all areas of the employment relationship, including hiring, promotion, benefits, training, and discipline.

[The organization] will conscientiously observe all federal, state, and local laws and regulations applicable in any way to the employment relationship.

[The organization] is committed to providing a work environment in which employees are free from harassment, sexual or otherwise. No employee will be made to feel uncomfortable in the work environment through exposure to coarse, profane, or sexual language or derogatory comments.

Employees are encouraged to express themselves freely and responsibly through established channels and procedures. Complaints will be treated as confidential information and will be revealed only to those who need to know as part of a process of investigation or resolution. Interference, retaliation, or coercion by any employee against an employee who registers a concern or complaint will not be tolerated.

We will observe the standards of our professions and exercise judgment and objectivity at all times. Significant difference of professional opinion will be referred to the appropriate management for prompt resolution.

We shall show respect and consideration for one another regardless of position, status, or relationship.

## Contemporary Concerns: E-mail, the Internet, and Social Media

The use of e-mail and the Internet by business has become widespread for a number of years, and it is clear that their use will likely continue expanding for some years to come. These technologies have also been experiencing widespread personal use. E-mail, Internet use, and social networking can, and does, intrude on business.

These technologies are subject to misuse and abuse. E-mail is even more problematic than the next most misused business technology, the photocopier. Many photocopiers, as we all know but frequently choose to ignore, handle a significant volume of non-business copying, ranging from cartoons, jokes, and recipes to announcements, schedules, and newsletters for outside organizations. E-mail not only carries a high volume of nonbusiness material, but—unlike the photocopier—also carries business information that is communicated in slapdash, generally careless fashion that frequently serves more to raise questions than to convey information.

If you have to spend one-third to one-half of your e-mail time sorting through unimportant communications and personal information before getting into pertinent messages, many of which you must then interpret or question before passing along or acting upon, then your e-mail is out of control. The discussion on communication offers specific guidelines for the business use of e-mail.

E-mail and the Internet have facilitated significant increases in efficiency in a number of activities, but they have also given life to a number of practices that are contrary to reasonable expectations of employee conduct. In other words, these modern computer-based conveniences are highly susceptible to abuse. For this reason, it is necessary to establish rules for their use.

## *Policy*

Each organization should develop a formal policy governing the use of its Internet facilities, including e-mail systems, clearly stating that these technologies are to be used for business purposes only by employees and other authorized users and they are subject to the following standards and requirements. Reminder: issues continue to arise, policies and rules are subject to challenges, and clarification (including rulings by outside agencies such as the NLRB) continues to develop about these topics (internet use, e-mail, social media). See Chapter 11 (Communication) for further discussion of these issues. As with all policies and rules, a middle manager will develop department-level directives that are consistent with the organization's overall policies. The following points reflect common elements of such policies and rules.

**Internet.** Only authorized employees are allowed Internet access and then only for valid business reasons. Assigned account numbers and access codes are personal to each user and must not be shared with others. Management reserves the right to deny or terminate access to the Internet at its own discretion.

Employees do not have an expectation of privacy with respect to their use of the organization's Internet facilities. Any and all messages, data, images, or other information received, transmitted, or archived using the Internet facilities may be accessed, copied, and used by systems administrators and management.

Also, any messages, data, or images may be disclosed to legally entitled third parties such as regulators, law enforcement agencies, and courts. The organization reserves the right to monitor, log, and filter Internet access by employees. There may be a prohibition about clearing internet search histories to avoid detection of prohibited use.

Prohibited uses of Internet facilities include, but are not limited to, the following:

- Viewing, displaying, copying, or communicating libelous, threatening, or sexually explicit material, material that fosters a hostile work environment, or material that fosters discrimination of any kind as defined in the Civil Rights Act of 1964 and subsequent antidiscrimination laws
- Supporting an outside activity, whether a commercial venture, charitable or political cause, or other private undertaking
- Developing personal home pages
- Recreational "surfing" during work hours
- Playing games, participating in online gambling and/or contests

**Electronic Mail.** All employees are advised that e-mail is available within the organization for business use only. Transmitting jokes, cartoons, recipes, personal messages, and other non-business-related information constitutes misuse of the organization's communications capacity and misuse of work time.

All users of e-mail should also be aware that in spite of individual accounts and passwords, an individual's e-mail can be readily accessed by unauthorized persons and may also be subject to monitoring internal to the organization. There is no expectation of e-mail privacy; all e-mail messages are potentially public.

**Social Networking Media.** These personal platforms of social interaction present a challenge concerning the right of an individual to free self-expression versus the organization's need to uphold its mission and its public image. A few considerations come to mind. Yes, one has a right to free speech, but at the work site, issues such as the protection of patient privacy or the maintenance of a nonhostile workplace for employees must be addressed. How far can the employer go to limit the use of off-duty action, using personally owned devices? Certainly the generally accepted standards of ethical and professional behavior continue to be the expected norm. The use of the organization's logo, badges, identification insignia, or symbols is another area where limits would be set. Orientation and training focusing on maintaining a nonhostile workplace could include a discussion of the impact of negative comments made about ethnic, religious, and similar sensitive topics on one's social networking site. When a person chooses to make these attitudes public, they are, in fact, public and could be used as examples of how he or she is potentially biased. When an employee is under consideration for advancement, the information and views posted in these forums may well be included in the assessment.

Another aspect of social networking simply falls under the heading of rude behavior. At a meeting, when one or more attendees are sending or receiving instant messages, the message to the rest of the group is simple: these individuals do not value the interaction of the group and are being disrespectful of the other attendees' time. In addition, these individuals, either inadvertently or by design, might be sending information about the proceedings to someone outside the room. As a general rule, employees should use electronic devices in such a manner that all those in their presence may feel psychologically safe.

## ▶ Training

An organized, formal training program designed to meet certain objectives is the most effective method of changing the behavior of employees. To establish such a program, the manager and those individuals involved in the organized training activities must (1) identify training needs, (2) establish training objectives, (3) select appropriate methods and techniques, (4) implement the program, and (5) evaluate the training outcomes. (See **Appendix 9–B** for excerpts from a training program designed for release of information specialists.)

### Identification of Training Needs

The manager reviews various aspects of the work, including individual employee performance, to determine training needs. Such detailed review might include the following elements:

1. Comparison of specified job requirements (as stated in the job descriptions) with current or new employee skills.
2. Analysis of performance ratings. Where are workers having difficulty meeting accuracy or productivity standards? Where are errors concentrated? Is there a pattern of difficulty in some technical aspects of the work?
3. Analysis of personnel records and reports. Is there a pattern of lateness, absenteeism, accidents, safety violations, client complaints, or equipment damage?

4. Analysis of short- and long-range plans. These often indicate the need for training in new procedures or in skills for dealing with new client groups.
5. Analysis of current trends and changes in laws, regulations, accreditation standards, and new technologies. When new regulations or standards are promulgated or new technological support becomes available (e.g., a new software program), retraining is required.
6. "Just-in-time" training. In rare circumstances, a group of workers might be pulled from their regular work and posted to a work situation where immediate, specific training is needed. Examples of these circumstances include blizzard or hurricane preparations, when patients need to have appointments canceled and rescheduled. A team of workers would receive the necessary training to make these calls, assess the patients' concerns and needs, and make the new appointment. Another example of the use of "just-in-time" training is a situation in which all visitors must be screened or rerouted, such as during a pandemic. The screening team would receive instructions appropriate to the changing situation, perhaps as often as every 2 or 3 hours.

A director of health information systems used an analysis of grievances over 5 months (**Exhibit 9–3**), a quarterly audit of the storage and retrieval function (**Exhibit 9–4**), and a 4-year long-range plan excerpt (**Exhibit 9–5**) to determine training needs. The first aspect of this overall analysis focused on the question: is this a systems problem or a training problem? Notice that six incidents in Exhibit 9–3 involved work standards and procedures, indicating a systems problem. Then notice that there are several incidents that indicate a specific training need—for example, a worker who is unable to meet work standards, the series of misfiles in the storage/retrieval area, and the supervisor and the uneven application of department policy.

The audit of the storage and retrieval system (Exhibit 9–4) leads the manager to review the system itself (dual system for historic reasons, available space and possible overcrowding, lighting, general "housekeeping"). The manager then notes that there are specific training needs—to make certain that the workers understand the two different filing systems and to review safety and ergonomics to prevent injury.

The short- and long-range plans for the organization and the department (Exhibit 9–5) provide yet another series of training needs. For example, as the healthcare organization undergoes its expansion

**Exhibit 9-3** Analysis of Grievances (May to October)

| Substance/Issue | Employee | Outcome for Management |
|---|---|---|
| 1. Harassment by supervisor: inconsistent application of late/absentee docking | File clerk | Lost |
| 2. Arbitrary and excessive work standards in file area | File clerk | Lost |
| 3. Excessive work standards in file area | File clerk | Sustained |
| 4. Firing for unauthorized release of record | File clerk | Sustained |
| 5. Arbitrary change in procedure for delivery of records to outpatient clinics | File clerk | Lost |
| 6. Excessive work standard for transcription | Word processing specialist | Lost |
| 7. Arbitrary employee evaluation | Word processing specialist | Lost |
| 8. Inconsistent merit money allocation | Release of information clerk | Sustained |
| 9. Harassment: inconsistent application of work rules re: dress code | Release of information clerk | Lost |
| 10. Arbitrary selection of candidate for job promotion | File clerk | Lost |
| 11. Firing for failure to meet work standards | File clerk | Lost |
| 12. Unequal rate of pay | Coder | Sustained |
| 13. Harassment for failing to meet work standard | Transcriber | Sustained |
| 14. Suspension for insubordination | File clerk | Sustained |

**Exhibit 9-4** Audit of Storage and Retrieval System: Legacy Files (July to September)

Percentage of misfiles—active records; terminal digit, color-coded system:

| | |
|---|---|
| Percentage of misfiles—legacy records; terminal digit, color-coded system: | 14% |
| Percentage of missing or incorrectly placed outguides: | 11% |
| Percentage of loose reports misfiled in records: | 8% |
| Percentage of "permanently lost" records: | 4% |
| Percentage of records unavailable at time of appointment: (appointment request had clear patient ID) | 33% |

*Number of Accidents/Incidents*

| | |
|---|---|
| Falls from ladder: | 3 |
| Back strain—moving/accessing boxes of emergency room reports: | 1 |
| Eye injury—hit in eye by falling outguide: | 1 |
| Bruised hip due to file cabinet drawer jammed open: | 1 |

*(continues)*

---

**Exhibit 9–4** **Audit of Storage and Retrieval System: Legacy Files (July to September)** *(continued)*

*Other Problems Noted*
20% turnover rate
All employees in unit = entry level
Poor "housekeeping" in inactive area; active storage = okay
Active storage area: terminal digit and color coded
Inactive storage area: middle digit and different color-coded record jackets

---

**Exhibit 9–5** **Five Year (20n1–20n5) Long-Range Plans (Excerpt)**

Organizational Expansion:

| | |
|---|---|
| Sports medicine outpatient clinic—juvenile sports injuries | July 20n2 |
| Expansion of regional telemedicine program | July 20n2 |
| Affiliation with local university's college of health professions | September 20n2 |
| Home care and hospice program | July 20n3 |
| Adolescent crisis day care program | January 20n4 |
| Contract with regional industry-on-site clinic | January 20n4 |

Departmental objectives (in addition to plans stemming from organizational expansion):
  Conversion to EHR: continuing development until completion in 20n4
  Move to new building—Campus #2 January 20n5

---

of specialties (home care, hospice, sports medicine), there will be a need to train the health information specialists in the related aspects of documentation, coding, and registries appropriate to those services. There is a training need that is ongoing regarding the continuing implementation of the electronic health record. The manager would revisit the long-range plan periodically as training needs become certain.

Once training needs have been identified, the manager must establish the objectives for the program. The objectives should be written in measurable terms and should state the specific outcomes to be achieved at the conclusion of the training program. For well-established, performance-related outcomes, the training objectives are specific and stated in measurable terms, because the desired results can be factually determined through recordkeeping. Written objectives serve as the fundamental guide for organizing the program and evaluating the desired outcomes.

This type of training objective is stated in stylized language. Usually each objective contains the following elements:

- The statement of the main focus (what is to be demonstrated or stated).
- The level of mastery or an acceptable performance level (e.g., "error-free" or "with 100%

accuracy"). When mastery-level performance is adopted, a realistic time limit to obtain mastery (e.g., after a certain number of practice sessions) may be stated.

- Any conditions, such as use of specific regulations or use of designated equipment.
- A time frame or performance standard, which may be presented in stages, with an initial phase of untimed performance followed by progressively increased performance levels until the work standard is met.

These training objective elements may be stated in whole or in part at the beginning of the training design for each unit and need not be repeated. For example, the various activities or processes that the trainee carries out must be in "accordance with the specified policies and procedures." Having stated this condition initially, the training specialist need not repeat it for each learning objective.

A second type of training objective focuses on affective matters—namely, values and attitudes. Their measurement is less tangible, so a performance level would not usually be stated. **Exhibit 9–6** is an example of a training program that emphasizes the underlying values of patient privacy and dignity. Workers who are not involved in direct patient care could benefit

**Exhibit 9–6** The Health Record: Mirror of Dignity, Privacy, and Patient Participation

The content of the health record reflects the important quality-of-life indicators of patient dignity, privacy, and participation in the treatment/care process. The policies and practices associated with health record systems and functions support these considerations. Review of institutional policies and practices provides both management and caregivers with a tool for assessing commitment to these values. Participants in this training session will have an opportunity to increase their understanding of the underlying values that find expression in the documentation and review processes. Specific attention will be devoted to the following topics:

1. Quality of Life: Indicators of Patient Care
2. The Health Record: Mirror of Dignity, Privacy, Choice, and Participation
   a. Patient rights documents
   b. Consent for treatment
   c. Guardianship and power of attorney
   d. Use/access of one's own financial recourses (as in a long-term care facility)
   e. Patient care plans, with specific emphasis on patient and family participation
   f. Supportive care plans in end-of-life situations
   g. Activities therapy plans, including the specific expression by the patient about declining to participate in some activities
3. Health Information Processes and Practices
   a. Relationship of these processes and practices to the protection and enhancement of privacy and dignity
   b. Specific practices:
      i. Release of information
      ii. Correlation of financial/billing information and documentation
      iii. Timely and thorough review of documentation during the inpatient stay and at time of discharge
4. Audit Topics
   a. Privacy and dignity: compliance with external directives and the organization's mission and core values
   b. Participation by patient in healthcare decisions: comparisons of patient expressions of wishes and values with elements in the plan of care
   c. Compliance with end-of-life ("living wills") directives

from such a program in that their own understanding of the importance of their behind-the-scenes work will be increased. Direct patient care providers, who sometimes feel burdened by the "paperwork" requirements, could be given this opportunity to take a fresh look at how their documentation and review efforts foster a climate of positive values.

A third type of training objective is that associated with patient and family education. Examples include program offerings to such groups as parents of autistic children, family caregivers for patients with Alzheimer's disease, and support groups for a specific clinical situation. The objectives of this type of educational offering include the following:

1. Providing information about community resources
2. Enabling participants to use support services
3. Coming to terms with the limits and the possibilities associated with the given clinical situation (e.g., stroke or breast cancer survivor)
4. Strategies for dealing with individuals (including family and neighbors as well as the general public) who are not familiar with special needs associated with a given clinical situation (e.g., an autistic child)

A measurable outcome would not be included in a general program offering, but when such training is part of the patient care plan, monitoring of progress would be included.

## Training Module Content

Detailed content is developed for each sequence of the training module when the training plan focuses on performance outcomes in job-related training. The manager takes care to use materials consistent with professional standards. Materials made available from professional associations are reliable and up-to-date. There is an advantage to using such resources: these training materials represent best practices and widely accepted methods. They have been developed and vetted by teams of experts and supported by research. They are revised on a regular basis to reflect changes in requirements. The testing materials have been developed by experts in testing design. The materials reflect the body of knowledge required for certifications at various levels.

The manager augments these standardized materials with information specific to the organization. Finally, the manager sequences the training modules in logical order. For example, a training module on the release of information would follow a training module on the Health Insurance Portability and Accountability Act (HIPAA).

The use of training modules lessens the need for detailed briefing and training when an interdisciplinary, all-day training session is planned, for example, a disaster drill. Ideally, the participants would have completed such topical modules for dealing with persons with special needs (e.g., Autism, Alzheimer's disease, intellectual disabilities), handling news media requests, safeguarding patient privacy, intake procedures, and similar topics.

# Training Methods and Techniques

The manager has many training methods available to achieve the desired outcomes. The methods most often used are profiled next.

## Job Rotation

Job rotation is a popular approach to staff training and development. Under a rotational scheme, job assignments may last anywhere from 3 to 6 months. This approach gives an employee the opportunity to acquire the broad perspective and diversified skills needed for professional and personal development. Job rotation can also be used to introduce new concepts and ideas into the various units within the department and to help individual employees to think in terms of the whole program rather than their immediate assignments.

Job rotation also supports the concept of *cross-training*. In cross-training, employees working in different jobs that are comparable in pay grade and skill level are trained in each other's jobs. This provides the manager with increased flexibility in covering positions in times of absence or fluctuating demands, and it provides employees with variety in their work and the opportunity to learn and grow. This process also supports succession planning in emergency situations and in modified operations scheduling.

## Formal Lecture Presentations

The lecture method is one of the oldest techniques used in training and development programs. The fundamental purpose of the lecture is to inform. The lecture format saves time because the speaker can present more material in a given amount of time than can be presented by any other method. The lecture should be supplemented by visual aids and variation in presentation format, for example, the use of frequently asked questions (See **Appendix 9-A**). Such methods help offset the downside of the lecture method where conventionally during the lecture, employees are passive. Outside disturbances or mental wanderings frequently distract individuals and render the lecture ineffective.

## Seminars and Conferences

The major purpose of seminars and conferences is to allow for the exchange of ideas, the discussion of problems, and the formulation of answers to questions or solutions to problems. The opportunity for employees to express their own views and to hear other opinions can be very stimulating. Employees who actively participate are more committed to decisions than they would be if the solutions were merely presented to them. Remember that true and lasting learning occurs in direct proportion to the amount of individual involvement in the discussion process.

## Role Playing

Acting out situations between two or more persons is a training method used successfully with all levels of employees. Interviewing, counseling, leadership, and human relations are a few of the content areas in which role playing has been used. By playing the roles of others, employees gain valuable insight not only from their own actions, but also from the comments of observers.

## Committee Assignments

Through committee assignments, employees can explore topics or problems to gain a broader or new perspective, experience situations involving the resolution of different ideas, learn to adjust to someone else's viewpoint, and practice reaching decisions. Committee assignments also offer opportunities for employees to assume positions of leadership that they would not otherwise have.

## Case Studies

Based on the premise that solving problems under simulated conditions enables employees to solve similar problems in actual work situations, the case study method requires employees to become actively involved in problem-solving situations, either hypothetical or real. The case studies used in developing problem-solving skills should be carefully selected and pertinent to the job so that their use meets the training and development requirements of the employees.

## Program Implementation

Throughout the implementation phase, the physical and psychological environment must be constantly monitored. For example, the time schedule, the learning environment, and the pace need to be checked periodically.

The primary consideration in any training program is the establishment of a time schedule to provide the greatest educational impact possible without reducing work output or, in healthcare institutions, patient care. The training program and the methods to be used should be announced well in advance. This approach allows everyone involved sufficient lead time to arrange individual schedules so that work assignments can be adequately covered during the employee's absence.

The arrangement of the room in which the training is to occur can either promote or handicap the process of learning. It is important to ensure that each participant can see and hear each member of the group. The traditional classroom setting in which the "teacher" sits in the front of the room and the participants are seated in neat rows should be avoided whenever possible, because it creates a stiff and formal atmosphere. One of the best arrangements for a training session is to put the tables in an open-ended rectangle, with chairs placed only on the outside perimeter. In addition, the room should be well lighted and adequately ventilated.

The pace and timing of each session are also important during the implementation phase of a training program. The function of pace is to maintain interest; therefore, the pace should be quickened when interest begins to wane, or it should be slowed if individuals are having difficulty absorbing content. A training session should not last longer than 2 hours. In fact, a 1-hour session is believed to produce better results. If a 2-hour session is necessary, a break should be allowed at the midpoint. Common sense and individual attention spans dictate how long adults accustomed to active work can be kept relatively immobile.

## Evaluation of Outcomes

Probably the most difficult aspect of a training program is evaluating the outcomes to determine whether they are or are not what was desired. This difficulty arises because there are no concrete and precise measuring tools for assessing changes in behavior and attitudes. Outcomes must be measured indirectly and conclusions based on inference. The evaluation is not just a single act or event but an entire process. Evaluation is made easier, however, if objectives have been clearly stated in measurable terms.

A before-and-after comparison may be a useful way of evaluating change. If the manager and those individuals involved in the training program assess the behavior factors they wish to change before training and examine the same factors after training has been concluded, they can determine if a change occurred.

For material of a factual nature, where precise knowledge should be demonstrated, fact tests are used. More commonly, however, trainees are evaluated through performance tests. Each trainee has activities to carry out; these are drawn from the usual work of the job. The final evaluation may be carried out in stages: practice activity, followed by real work activity under immediate supervision, followed by real work activity with diminishing levels of immediate supervision.

The evaluation brings the training process full circle. Each trainee has been given specific objectives to attain, appropriate didactic and practice materials have been explained, and practice activities with appropriate feedback and correction have been provided. The evaluation, therefore, consists of determining the trainee's capacity to perform the work outlined in the job description and specified through the detailed policies and procedures of the department.

## Resources for Training

The manager should endeavor to provide timely and thoroughly developed training materials. The cost of training materials and the time to be expended are also factors to consider. The manager can use to advantage the many programs developed by professional associations. For example, the American Health Information Management Association has developed training programs for coding, making it easier for health information department employees to enhance that particular skill set. Their webinars and training materials about privacy and confidentiality are authoritative sources on these topics, and these materials are suitable for training new employees and for reuse in a periodic review session. Distance learning is yet another option in which both technical and professional-level courses are readily available.

Some topics are common to several disciplines, thus enabling the management team to share resources and split the cost over multiple groups of employees. The training material for HIPAA implementation represents one such training program that is suitable for interdepartmental use.

Training, while desirable as well as necessary, can be costly. Budget decisions and justification for such expenditures may be systematized by reviewing training resources against a set of criteria. **Exhibit 9–7**

**Exhibit 9–7** Budget Justification for Training Resource

Title of Resource: *Confidentially Speaking: Keeping Patient Information Private*

Sponsor: Norton and Collins, Inc.

Target Population:

- New employees of Health Information Services
- Students accepted for clinical internship in Health Information Services
- Employees needing a refresher course in basic principles

Job Skill: Fostering and maintaining confidentiality of patient information

Cost:

- Two-part webinar: $104.00
- Shipping and handling: $11.00
- Total cost: $115.00

Additional notes:

1. Webinar can be reused within the department.
2. Webinar can be loaned to other departments.
3. Webinar content has been reviewed by experts in the field of HIPAA compliance.
4. Content meets continuing education approval by national association.

reflects such an assessment. Good, solid justification of necessary training activity is essential. Surely every department manager has heard executive management consistently praise the value of training when conditions are at least stable financially. Nevertheless, when a financial crunch arises and it is necessary to reduce expenditures, the education and training budget is often one of the first areas cut.

## Addressing Diversity

It is highly probable that the majority of healthcare managers will be called on to manage increasingly diverse work groups. The diversities encountered in the workforce may be rooted in ethnicity, religion, race, gender, or social differences, but in the work organization all of these areas of difference have been gathered under the term *cultural diversity* or just simply *diversity*. This term represents a broad range of differences, also implying, for example, differences in values, assumptions, expectations, and needs.

Labor projections continue to advise organizations that in the early decades of the 21st century, the majority of new entrants into the workforce are likely to be women, minorities, and immigrants. This has become true in a number of areas of health care.

It is reasonable to assume that the majority of people are most at ease around others who look,

think, and act as they do. However, these days rarely do people of a single cultural group populate an entire function, department, or organization. Rather, it is common to find most employee populations culturally mixed to some extent. Lack of understanding of the differences between and among cultures gives rise to difficulties for the manager, often indicating the need to train managers and staff in matters of diversity.

Workplace tensions can arise from failure to recognize or understand cultural differences, and these tensions can cause interpersonal conflict, reduced productivity, absenteeism, turnover, and charges of discrimination and other legal complaints. In addition, communication problems arise from language and literacy concerns related to individual background, and other issues develop from lack of cultural awareness and respect.

In the workforce in general, it is now and will become increasingly more necessary to interact with people who have different values and beliefs. Increasing diversity in the workforce is unavoidable, especially in health care. In health care, diversity is present at all working levels. Although in health care, diversity is greatest in the entry-level positions in housekeeping, nursing assistance, and food service, it is also significant in professional areas such as nursing service.

## Recognizing Differences

In the absence of knowledge of cultures other than our own, people incline toward stereotypes in their thinking about others. Although stereotypes are usually superficial or simply wrong, they nevertheless tend to influence thinking and decision making.

A manager should be able to respect each employee as an individual and hold all employees to the same standard of job performance. Yet in the one-to-one relationship between manager and employee, the manager must recognize individual differences that are culturally based. A few examples of differences one may encounter as a manager are:

- In some cultures, prolonged, direct eye contact is acceptable, whereas in others it is considered rude and improper.
- People from some cultural backgrounds believe it is disrespectful to offer opinions or suggestions to a superior (potentially quite frustrating to the manager who wants employee input).
- Workers from some cultural backgrounds are uncomfortable with being singled out in any way, even for praise.
- Workers from some cultural backgrounds will point out their own successes with pride,

whereas others will remain silent no matter how successful; to them, self-praise or self-promotion is not acceptable behavior.

- In some cultures, physical touching or entering another's close personal space is acceptable, but in some it is not.
- Some male workers from certain cultures may be extremely ill at ease reporting to a female manager.

These and other factors add up to numerous individual differences that a manager may have to account for in relating to each individual member of a work group.

### In the Manager–Employee Relationship

All employees should be expected to adapt to the reasonable requirements of the job and the workplace as necessary, but they always bring their individualism to the job as well. The effective manager always remains aware of individual differences and respects these differences in the relationship with each employee.

It is also to the manager's advantage to become familiar with applicable aspects of antidiscrimination laws. In reacting to culturally based individual differences, it is sometimes possible to unintentionally enter into discriminatory practices out of ignorance of the law.

### What About Diversity Training?

Every healthcare employee, and especially every healthcare manager, stands to benefit by attending a sound cultural diversity program and making a determined effort to learn about the cultures prevalent in a department or organization. The manager must not only successfully relate to each employee but also must deal with the interactions between and among employees to ensure that equal treatment, opportunity, and respect exist for all. It seems at times like a nearly impossible task to treat all employees alike regarding observance of policies while recognizing and adjusting for cultural differences among employees.

Along with the term *cultural diversity,* one is also likely to hear of *cultural competence* or *cultural proficiency.* Diversity itself must be prevalent and valued before one may be considered culturally competent or culturally proficient. Thus, in promoting the need to value diversity, the organization is encouraging the process of including the perspectives of underrepresented, nondominant groups to ensure they have a voice in the organization.

The shape and substance of any particular organization's diversity training will depend considerably on the cultural mix within the organization. There are, however, a few general guidelines to keep in mind when considering diversity training:

- As with all organization-wide undertakings, diversity training must have the visible participation and support of top management. Many potentially beneficial programs have withered and died because top management either did not provide visible support or provided token support at the start before backing away.
- Anecdotal evidence suggests that the most effective diversity training programs are those conducted by outside providers engaged for that purpose. When presented by insiders, there is sometimes the perception that the division or department presenting the program is advancing its own agenda.
- The presenters of the most effective programs should be seen as more or less culturally neutral. That is, no single underrepresented group should be seen as dominant such that some participants might perceive that this group is simply advancing its own agenda.
- Even highly successful diversity training should be repeated or reinforced periodically. For many participants, such training is counter to lifelong beliefs, attitudes, and prejudices that cannot be erased or altered by a one-time presentation or program.

It is clear that in the coming few decades, the more effective organizations will be those that successfully manage workforce diversity and tap the maximum potential that each employee has to offer.

## ▶ Mentoring

Professional practitioners may find themselves in the special teaching role of mentor. Mentoring is a process in which a more experienced and usually older person guides and nurtures a younger or less experienced employee. The mentoring relationship may be informal and limited—for example, in the instance of a senior practitioner encouraging a visiting student during the student's part-time job. Alternatively, the relationship may be formal and limited, as in the relationship of the clinical supervisor during training rotation or in assisting with thesis supervision. The relationship may then become informal and ongoing, as in a partnership of interest, leading to shared projects, co-presenting at workshops, and coauthoring papers.

## Network

A network is a group of individuals who communicate through formal and informal channels and willingly promote one another for mutual benefit. The network members trade services, ideas, recommendations, and "tips" to further their own development and success. The various state and national professional associations are examples of networks.

## Peer Pals

Peer pals boost one another's careers by sharing information and strategies. They share one another's strengths and weaknesses because they are on the same developmental level.

## ▶ Clinical Affiliation/ Clinical Practice Program and Contract

Healthcare organizations typically include education and research in their mission. In developing their client base, managers include healthcare practitioners who are in training. These clients are identified in the clientele network as secondary clients whose needs are important and deserving of attention. Practitioners-in-training also become a source of potential employees, thus helping the managers in their recruitment outreach. Supervising practitioners-in-training is part of managers' leadership role as well; they are effective role models through their support of the educational efforts of colleges, universities, and specialty training programs. Managers recognize the importance of clinical rotation because of their own experience as students. They appreciate and understand the professional association/credentialing requirements that include clinical practice.

## Organizational Responsibility and Coordination

There is on-going interaction among peer professionals about shared interests and concerns. The need for clinical rotation is one recurring topic. The initial discussion of, and request for, developing a clinical rotation sequence often starts at this informal level. Formal responsibility and coordination are the next steps, usually involving the chief academic officer of the healthcare facility. This executive-level manager develops policies and procedures, including legal guidelines, for accepting student practitioners in the clinical setting. The department manager determines the availability of the department for specific kinds of rotations, their length, and their scope. When an agreement has been reached between the academic institution and the healthcare site, department managers prepare their employees for the presence of a student observer/participant. This manager assumes responsibility for on-site supervision of the student. The academic institution maintains responsibility for students as well. For example, the outline and description of the content and sequence of the clinical rotation is developed by the academic department, and the assignment of a grade for the coursework is the responsibility of the faculty.

## Elements of the Clinical Affiliation Agreement

There are a number of considerations about placement of a student in the clinical site. Although these formalities may seem bureaucratic, their purpose is the mutual protection of the healthcare organization, its patients and workers, and the academic institution and its students. The affiliation agreement is developed to address aspects of the training and typically includes the following elements:

1. Organizational name of the parties to the agreement.
2. Length of agreement. A certain number of students (*n*) are accepted for a specific time period (e.g., September 1–November 30) for the particular activities associated with the clinical rotation. The names of the students are listed.
3. Stipulations of trainee status. Students are not employees or independent contractors, even if they are receiving a stipend. They are not eligible for any fringe benefits, unionization eligibility, or workers' compensation. A student should sign a statement indicating this so that there is no misunderstanding.
4. Stipends or support (e.g., room and board, meal plan). If either is provided, either by the academic institution or the healthcare organization, the tax consequences to the recipient are the responsibility of the recipient.
5. Liabilities. The healthcare organization restricts its arrangements with academic institutions, accepting students only if the academic institution carries proper insurance to cover field placement of its students. Furthermore, a student receives orientation about the healthcare organization's policies, procedures, and rules about standards of conduct; use of social media; protection of patient privacy; and confidentiality provisions about patient care

interactions. The privacy of the employees is also emphasized. The use of organizational assets and information, prohibition about political activity, and similar limits on behavior are included in the initial briefing. A student must sign a confidentiality agreement, pledging to maintain confidentiality about the site, the patients, and the workers. They must also sign the sexual harassment policy, including a statement that they have reviewed the policy and received a copy of it.

6. Removal from clinical placement. The healthcare organization reserves the right to have students recalled by the educational institution if they do not carry out the agreed-on activities or behave in a nonprofessional manner.

7. Intellectual property and copyright considerations. Reports, computer software development, data, photographs, and images and similar material covered by the usual concept of intellectual property become the property of the healthcare organization. Students shall be permitted to use such material in their academic reports, without identifying patients, workers, or the organization. Subsequent use of the material shall be covered by the usual understandings of intellectual property and copyright considerations. The director of affiliations of the healthcare organization coordinates the requests for such approval.

8. Designated contacts. The academic institution shall provide the name and title of the faculty coordinator for clinical placement. The healthcare organization provides the name and title of the department manager who is accepting the supervision of the student while on-site.

9. Contract. This is dated and signed by the officials from each party to the agreement.

# Appendix 9-A

## Frequently Asked Questions About Sexual Harassment

*Note: Nothing in this discussion is intended to be legal advice.*

As a department manager, you are responsible for the ongoing training of your staff. The discussion presented here illustrates a training method—frequently asked questions (FAQ). This training module might be used to update assistants and supervisors. The topic is a sensitive one, with many details and nuances. Using the FAQ method allows the presenter to break up the information into specific topics. The questions, with the answers, range from highly specific to more generalized responses as the topic is having ongoing interpretation and applicability.

1. What is the origin of the policy regarding sexual harassment?

    It stems from the overall issues covered by the Civil Rights Act, Title VI. This federal law prohibits discrimination, including gender discrimination. Gender discrimination includes sexual harassment. There are companion laws at state level. Counties and municipalities have similar prohibitions, as do accrediting agencies. The organization develops policies as part of its corporate compliance program.

2. Who is responsible for developing and monitoring the sexual harassment policy?

    The chief executive office, acting on behalf of the governing board, has primary responsibility. The CEO will, in turn, designate specific operational responsibility to one of several units who work together to formulate, implement, and monitor relevant policies, such as the chief compliance officer and the human relations department, along with legal counsel.

3. What are the duties and responsibilities of a department manager?

    The first duty is to know the policies, understand them, and obtain clarification as needed.

Remain up to date about changes in the policy and its interpretation.

    The second duty is active and continual monitoring of the departmental environment. This includes employee compliance with such aspects as dress code, behavior, and general rules about office accessories (e.g., posters, calendars, photos, mugs, decorations, computer screen displays).

    Third, follow reporting requirements by promptly responding to oral or written reports given to you by an employee.

    Fourth, actively intervene to stop harassment behavior. In case of a potentially violent situation, call security.

4. What is Sexual Harassment?

    In general, sexual harassment refers to sexual advances, requests for sexual favors, and verbal or physical conduct of a sexual nature. More specifically, the definition includes such aspects as sexual jokes; written or verbal references to sexual conduct or activity (either about one's own activity or another's); comments about another person's body or attire; posting, sending, forwarding, or displaying materials, documents, or images (as on a mug or T-shirt, poster, banner, magazine, bumper sticker, computer screens); leering, staring, whistling, or cat calls; making lewd or derogatory comments; gestures with sexual overtones; and physical touching (hugging, massaging, pinching).

    Furthermore, sexual harassment may include inappropriate behavior that violates the general standards of behavior in the workplace. It may include the situation wherein the attention was originally welcomed (e.g., request for a date; general social interaction) and is now unwelcomed.

    No list of examples is complete. Simply because an action or behavior is not listed, that

210

does not mean that it is acceptable. Follow the basic principle: unwelcomed behavior.

5. To Whom Does the Policy Apply?

The concept and policy about sexual harassment is gender-neutral. It applies to female–male, female–female, and male–male interaction. There are several groups included in policy application, for example, clients, visitors, and employees. In this discussion about sexual harassment in the workplace, the focus is employee behavior, and a manager's duties. It is useful to follow a framework to determine the employment status of an individual and the location at which the event occurred. Here are three major elements to consider: Is this person an employee of this organization? Is this person at the job site in another capacity, such as a contractual agent or vendor? Did the behavior occur at the job site or other designated work site (e.g., home care work or traveling together to and from the client's home) during working hours? Also note the arrival/departure times and places (e.g., parking lot, bus stop).

An employee's status is well defined in terms of hiring date, job title and assignment, location, and hours of work. There are other individuals who come to the workplace by specific arrangement made by the manager. These individuals are not employees of the organization. Examples include contractual workers, temporary agency workers, independent contractors or consultants, embedded nurses, operating room technicians from equipment companies, outsourced contractual services, vendors, students in affiliation rotation, and volunteers. These individuals have a primary organization to which they belong (e.g., a temporary agency service, individual corporation, equipment company for vendors, educational institution for students). Volunteers are under the coordination of the organization's volunteer services. These primary organizations or units are responsible for briefing their employees about sexual harassment. As an additional safeguard, a compliance officer, or, by delegation, a middle manager, might give a specific briefing (documented) about the relevant policies.

6. What Are Some Examples of Situations Involving Employee–Employee Interaction?

Note the primary characteristics of the interactions among employees. Some situations are clear-cut and the policy definitely applies:

a. Day-to-day interaction by employees, on the job, at the designated workplace.

b. Attending a conference or training workshop (offsite location) regarding job-related topics, fees and related expenses (e.g., travel) paid for by organization.

c. Participating in a department-sponsored social event during the work day, on the premises, in the department. Worker is not required to attend, but if he or she chooses not to participate, worker continues with regular work. Examples of such events include retirement farewells, celebration of successful work projects, celebration of national profession's annual spotlight event.

These next examples reflect more ambiguity; a manager would review such instances with a designated official (HR, compliance officer) to obtain a definitive answer:

d. Senior management officials arrange an organization-sponsored fund raiser, with an officially sponsored social event: the event is held off premises; is not part of scheduled work hours; employees are *expected*, but not officially required, to attend. Management expects employees to be supportive of such endeavors.

e. Manager's holiday party at his or her home or other off-job-site venue selected by the manager: all department employees invited; after-hours event; not work time; not work-related activities. Attendance is *voluntary*, but *expected*. (A manager would be well advised not to have such an event; he or she should definitely review the situation with a designated official; some organizations permit and even encourage such events as part of team building; other organizations prohibit these.)

f. Employee-sponsored activities and events: several employees regularly get together for lunch once a week; group is limited to employees of the department only; lunch time is the regularly scheduled time; group goes off-premises. In assessing this situation, determine whether workers are free to come and go during their regularly scheduled lunch time; even if they are free to use lunch time as they wish, they are still expected to follow organization's policies.

g. Employees who are neighbors: as neighbors, they carpool, share many activities in common in their neighbor-to-neighbor relationship. They are not engaged in work activity, nor are they at the work site. A situation could, however, develop: if they bring into the workplace conversational references, photos, and so forth or when referring to personal, private behavior, teasing, innuendo, and so on, the policy is applicable.

7. What Is the Process Relating to Sexual Harassment Complaints?

A complaint may be filed verbally or in writing. The written complaint may be in the worker's own writing, or an official report form may be used. An organization must make report forms and instructions available by placing them in readily accessible locations (e.g., at designated employee-information bulletin boards, employee break-rooms). The materials are to be displayed prominently. A manager would give the form and instructions to the employee, should he or she request it. There must also be a clearly designated contact (e.g., HR, compliance officer) listed, showing location, and job title of contact, phone number, and e-mail address so that the process is unencumbered and nonthreatening.

8. Is the Complaint Report Confidential?

In general, yes, but when a formal investigation is conducted, the information necessarily is shared (e.g., the accused and his or her representatives need to have information in order to prepare response/defense).

9. What Is Involved in the Official Investigation?

The designated official (e.g., HR, compliance officer) conducts an investigation, including an interview with the alleged offender. When a complaint is received, it is assessed to determine whether a violation has occurred. If the situation does not rise to the level of a potential violation of policy, the complainant is so informed. If the situation does rise to the level of a potential violation, it is further investigated. Some organizations specify a timeline for completion of each step, and a required response time.

10. What Are the Rights of the Accused?

These are to be safeguarded. The same right of appeal as used with any disciplinary action apply.

11. What Is the "No Retaliation" Provision?

It is, quite simply, that no retaliatory action may be made against an employee who, in good faith, files a complaint or cooperates with the investigation of a complaint.

# Appendix 9–B

# Training Design: Release of Information

## ▶ Background Information and Needs Assessment

The department manager completed a thorough review of the release of information function as part of a quality improvement study. The study included the following areas of focus:

1. Risk management study: HIPAA breach prevention with more than satisfactory compliance.
2. Review of licensure and accrediting standards: no problem area identified; no plan of correction required.
3. Turnover rate in the unit: 30% higher than the department as a whole.
4. Management inventory review: potential problem identified. No one is cross-trained for the release of information (ROI) positions; no one has been promoted internally to ROI positions for the past 4 years.
5. Productivity standards: adequate to above average for most functions except those associated with in-person and telephone requests, with only an 80% level achieved by workers.
6. Patient/client satisfaction survey results: reflected significant dissatisfaction with ROI responses to in-person and telephone requests. Typical comments included the following: "it was confusing—all those details; how are we supposed to know the rules?" "I felt like I got the run-around; it was overwhelming … all those details," and "worker was very impersonal; kept referring to the policy. It all seemed like a huge mess of red tape to me."
7. Worker satisfaction survey results: reflected satisfaction with most working conditions. Workers felt well-trained in the technical functions of their work but expressed concerns at being "put on the spot," "feeling bullied by aggressive or upset clients who did not understand the consent and fee requirements," and "feeling badly that they could not help the patient/client who clearly had a pressing need for the requested information." They felt poorly trained to deal with difficult situations and expressed the desire to transfer out of this area of work because of this stressful aspect.
8. Focused study: determined which kind of request and what steps in the process were generating the most difficulty. Findings showed that, with the success of the regional health information exchange, information for continuing care was not problematic. The gradual implementation of the electronic health record and the related portal-access processes were satisfactory. The three areas of concern, reflected in both patient and worker surveys were these:
   a. The fee structure and its application
   b. Release of information for records of deceased patients
   c. Dealing with one-to-one interactions with upset or angry clients

## ▶ The Redesign of the Training Program

In light of the background findings and needs assessment, the manager added an initial phase of training to emphasize the value and importance of the ROI function. With the assistance of the social service department and the human relations department, the manager developed a training module for communicating with distressed patients/clients. This initial phase was then followed by the technical training module (see below).

## Phase One: Valuing Our Mission—Valuing Your Role

The objectives are to assist the trainee in understanding and valuing the overall mission: service to the patients/clients and their role in this process. To emphasize the interpersonal nature of the work, this presentation is made in a small group setting; the manager presents the key points in a discussion format rather than as a formal lecture. Role playing is used to provide the trainees with interactive experience reflecting the challenging aspects of dealing with difficult situations. Key points include the following:

- Identifying examples of difficult situations, such as a client who needs information immediately because:
  - He or she is late in filing a benefits claim and will miss the final deadline.
  - He or she is receiving bill collection notices from the hospital for failure to pay.
  - He or she needs immediate assistance relating to disability claim or workers' compensation claim and has no other means of support.
  - He or she is eligible for special program assistance (e.g., learning disability) but the deadline for providing support information is next week.
  - He or she is a family member of a recently deceased patient but is not the executor of the estate and does not understand why he or she cannot have information.
- Acknowledging the conflict experienced by worker who wants to help but must follow the designated procedures. Small-group discussion of this topic: when you are the perceived source of the "red tape" and your role in offsetting the impersonal aspects of formal organizations.
- Valuing the worker's role as facilitator in assisting patients/clients in navigating the system.

## ▶ Communication in Stressful Situations

A social service or human relations specialist presents information about communication in such situations. This is applied to the common situations (identified above) through role playing. After the completion of Phase One, the trainee continues with learning the technical aspects of the work (Phase Two). An excerpt of a training design for processing written requests follows.

## Phase Two—Release of Information Functions

- Purpose
- Overall training objective
- Assumptions
- Resources
- Training sequence and performance level
- Methods

### Purpose

This training module is designed to enable the trainee to perform the release of information duties as delineated in the job description and prescribed in detail in the applicable policies and procedures.

### Overall Training Objective

The objective is to gain the ability to process written requests for release of information from the patient health record maintained by this facility.

- In accordance with the healthcare organization's policies and procedures as well as applicable federal and state laws and accrediting standards
- With 100% accuracy
- Within the established time frames and priority indications
- Within the work standards parameters

### Assumptions

1. The trainee meets the job qualifications except for knowledge and skill in release of information.
2. The trainee has successfully completed the training modules for:
   - Computer competency in job-related heath information systems software utilization
   - Privacy and confidentiality, including applicable laws and regulations
   - Overview of release of information function
   - Patient health record content and sequence
3. There is a comprehensive policy and procedure manual for release of information.
4. There are validated work standards.

### Resources

During this training process, the trainee will use

1. The release of information policy and procedure manual, including the reference grids for the following items:
   - Authorization requirements and examples

- Content and format of acceptable authorizations
- Fee schedule and transmittal forms
- Cover letters and sample responses
2. Software for tracking and completing each request
3. Fictitious requests and health records

## Training Sequence and Performance Level

The training sequence is based on the steps described in the procedure manual. The trainee learns to process standard requests, followed by nonstandard requests.

1. The trainee processes a standard request by performing each step with 100% accuracy, then proceeds to the next step.
2. After having demonstrated the ability to complete each separate step, the trainee processes a standard request through the complete cycle with 100% accuracy.
3. The trainee processes a nonstandard request by performing each step with 100% accuracy, then proceeds to the next step.
4. After having demonstrated the ability to complete each separate step, the trainee processes a nonstandard request through the complete cycle with 100% accuracy.
5. After having demonstrated the preceding abilities, the trainee is given a mix of standard and nonstandard requests to process with 100% accuracy within the work standards parameters.

## Methods

An in-basket exercise is used to introduce the material. Lecture and demonstration are used to explain each step.

## CHAPTER 10

# Adaptation, Motivation, and Conflict Management

## CHAPTER OBJECTIVES

- Address the necessity for properly and thoroughly integrating each individual employee into the organization and describe the common techniques of integration.
- Introduce the theories that address present-day employee motivational concerns and provide the manager with insight into the conditions and circumstances that inspire employees to perform.
- Specifically address the motivational concerns arising in conjunction with reengineering, reorganizing, and other practices resulting in downsizing of the workforce.
- Develop an understanding of the origins of conflict, especially in the organizational setting, and describe how to address conflict constructively.
- Describe the essential need for discipline within the organization and introduce the concept of progressive disciplinary action, differentiating between problems of performance and problems of conduct relative to rules and policies.
- Briefly examine the role of the collective bargaining agreement (union contract) in the avoidance of and as necessary the control of conflict.

## ▶ Adaptation and Motivation

To get work done efficiently and effectively, managers must motivate workers and assist them in their adaptation to organizational demands. Individuals must fit into the organizational framework. There is a close relationship between the manager's concern for employee motivation and the adaptation activities and controlling function of the manager. The worker who fits into the organization and who values an assigned role is likely to be motivated more readily than one who does not experience such feelings of belonging. In turn, when workers fit into the organization, the need to control or modify activity or behavior through disciplinary action is reduced.

## Adaptation to Organizational Life

Two specific conditions that exist as a result of organizational structure illustrate the need for an explicit management process to help integrate the individual into the organization:

1. The need to offset the effects of decentralization
2. The need to coordinate the many individual functions that result from departmentation and specialization

Overall goals and policies are established at the highest levels of the organizational hierarchy, but the actual work is carried out at every level. Occasionally, conflicting directives, or what seem to be conflicting directives, are issued from the central authority.

Additionally, the number of individuals who enter the organization and the different manner in which these individuals react to the complexities of organizational life must be taken into consideration. These individuals not only have different values, different personalities, and different life experiences, but they also belong to other organizations, some of which may have values that compete and even conflict with the values embodied in the workplace. Some of the patterns of accommodation to organizational life may be functional for the organization but dysfunctional for the individual. Potential conflict must be offset, and the personality mixes of workers and clients must be melded into smoothly functioning interpersonal relationships.

## Techniques for Fostering Integration

Events and conditions should be anticipated as fully as possible, and the courses of action to be taken for designated categories of events and conditions should be described. Authorization of the course of action applicable to any category may be permissive; it may spell out several series of steps from which the employee can choose. To prevent undesirable actions from arising, sanctions or penalties should be established for those who commit these offenses. The policy manual, the procedure manual, the employee handbook, the medical staff bylaws, and the licensure laws for the various health professionals are all routine management tools for guiding behavior and fostering integration.

### Work Rules

Rule formulation has generally been accepted as a management prerogative embodied in the control function. Work rules are related to motivational processes because they contribute to a stable organizational environment. They serve several functions in an organization:

- They create order and discipline so that the behavior of workers is goal oriented.
- They help unify the organization by channeling and limiting behavior.
- They give members confidence that the behavior of other members will be predictable and uniform.
- They make behavior routine so that managers are free to give their attention to nonroutine problems.
- They prevent harm, discomfort, and annoyance to clients.

- They help ensure compliance with legislation that affects the institution as a whole.

The organization has a positive duty to protect both clients and workers with regard to health, sanitation, and safety. In addition, it must seek to prevent behavior that has the potential of alienating or offending clients. Because they deal with patients and their families in stressful situations, healthcare organizations have specific obligations in this area.

### Incentives and Sanctions

Both incentives and sanctions can be used to induce compliance. Incentives include bonus pay, merit increases, special time off, and student loan assistance. Sanctions include demotion, suspension, and written reprimands. An essential element in any system of sanctions is the development of adequate feedback mechanisms and correction where needed. Employee evaluation and training processes can provide feedback and correction on a routine basis.

### Selection

Managers may increase the likelihood of worker satisfaction with the organization by developing recruitment and selection strategies to enhance this possibility. By recruiting from groups with a positive predisposition toward the organization, such as students in training rotations at the organization, managers will be able to attract employees who already value the organization's mission. When an organization has a long-standing relationship with its surrounding community and is recognized as "the best place to work," managers are able to recruit and select individuals who are accustomed to the presence and practices of the organization. The more selective an organization is, the more effective the involvement of its members tends to be. Their commitment to organizational values is deeper, and they need fewer external controls.

In recruiting members, the highly selective organization seeks to appeal to an audience composed of individuals who are favorably disposed toward the values of the organization, even at the preselection stage. Recruitment information may indicate, either implicitly or explicitly, the need to conform.

### Training

Workers who are unsettled because of rapid changes in work processes, or potential employees who have been out of the workforce, will benefit from an active, well-publicized training program geared toward these needs. For example, their technical skills can be modified so that they will perform the work according to the specific procedures unique to the organization. Orientation programs have been developed in hospitals to familiarize professionally trained individuals (e.g., technologists) with particular routines. Businesses often use rotating management internships to foster integration of newly graduated management majors. Training that enhances internal transfer and promotional opportunity is yet another motivational tool.

### *Identification with the Organization*

Managers tap into the human need to belong by using tangible expressions of organizational identity to help foster identification with the organization. Recall the early stages in the life cycle of an organization: a well-developed expression of mission is reflected in a motto, a logo, or some other readily identifiable symbol. A manager seeks to use these icons as sort of internal advertising telling employees, "You are a part of this excellent organization." The manager uses these simple but effective means of building up identification with the organization—yes, the coffee mug, the cap, and the T-shirt are all small but effective means of keeping the organization and its mission at the forefront. They are used because they work. The development of a sense of identification is good for the organization, and it can also be good for each individual.

### *The Work Group*

An employee's particular mindset is continually reinforced by his or her work group. Through the work group, the individual becomes assimilated into the organization—or is perhaps prevented from being properly assimilated. In addition to the formal prescriptions regarding work activities, informal patterns of behavior arise among members of the group. The individual learns the unwritten rules as well as interpretations of the written rules. The informal organization of the work group also satisfies an essential human need—the need to belong. Nonconformity with group norms could lead to expulsion from the group, which would eliminate a vital source of information and communication as well as an arena in which to air conflicts that stem from the formal organizational role demands.

## ▶ Theories of Motivation

On the one hand, the manager seeks to develop a workforce that fits the organization; on the other

hand, the manager must remain aware of the basic needs of the workers. The art of motivating is built on this recognition of human needs. Motivation is the degree of readiness or the desire within an individual to pursue some goal. The function of motivating or actuating is essentially a matter of leading the workers to understand and accept the organizational goals and to contribute effectively to meeting these goals. In motivating or actuating, the manager seeks to increase the zone of acceptance within the individual and to create an organizational environment that enhances the individual's will to work. As self-motivation increases, the need for coercive controls and punishment decreases.

## Bases of Motivation

Needs are the internal, felt wants of an individual (they are also referred to as drives and desires). Incentives are external factors that an individual perceives as possible satisfiers of felt needs.

A manager may gain insight into aspects of motivation in several ways:

- Observation of existing work situations
- Review of cultural expressions concerning work
- Studying the work of management theorists who have addressed the concept

## Observation of Existing Work Situations

Consider the response in your work setting to these two basic questions: Why do the employees (including you) work? Why do they work in this specific setting? The answers surface quite readily. One employee might say, "I work because I need the money. I need money to procure basic goods and services for daily life and for those additional items that constitute 'the good life.'" Another might give as the reason, "I don't really have to work but I want to keep involved; this work is meaningful to the community and it gives me a reason to get out of the house and be around people." Attractive and necessary fringe benefits might be the magnet for still other workers—the college tuition benefit and/or educational loan forgiveness programs for a worker or a member of the family, health insurance coverage, special discounts on pharmacy products, or day care for dependent children or aged parents.

In answering the question "Why work at this specific organization?", workers might offer a variety of responses. "Everyone in our family started out here; it is our tradition," says one worker. Another might indicate he or she is feeling stuck, even trapped: "It's the only place that is hiring right now and we can't relocate, so here we are for now; we will move on when there is opportunity." "It is a résumé enhancer," states a new entrant into the workforce. "It is the place to be if you want to be on the cutting edge of practice," says another. Yet another person might belong to the sponsoring religious or fraternal organization and enter the workforce of its organizations because of this affiliation. As noted earlier, generous fringe benefits, including flexible work schedules, may be the main source of attraction.

When managers sort through these reasons, they can readily see a mix of internal and external motivators they can then use to enhance worker satisfaction. The satisfied, motivated worker more readily contributes to the organizational mission than the dissatisfied or indifferent employee.

## Cultural Expectations about Work

Another avenue for considering work and motivation is the study of cultural expectations about work. These cultural attitudes are readily expressed in classic literature, art, and drama. They are evidenced in music—everything from coal miners' roots music lyrics, to seafaring chanteys, to 9-to-5 contemporary offerings. Television and movies represent the full range of the work setting, presenting both the comical and the dramatic aspects. One can identify repeated themes: the worker as hero, the manager as remote, the team as valuable, or the work setting as uplifting or repressive. Such cultural influences seep into everyone. The management team remains aware of this potential and develops positive motivational practices to offset what is negative and enhance what is good.

## Motivational Theories

In reviewing published works concerning theories of motivation, a manager will see that studies of motivation tend to deal with several broad questions: What satisfies human needs? And, therefore, what satisfies workers' needs? When one or several basic needs are met, what is the next level of motivators to be activated? Is motivation internal to the worker, part of our basic human makeup, dependent on external practices, or a combination of all these factors? Undertaking individual research into the various available theories of motivation can provide the manager with insight into a number of aspects of employee behavior.

## ▶ Practical Strategies for Employee Motivation

Motivation may be described as the drive, impetus, or initiative that causes an individual to direct his or her behavior toward satisfaction of some personal need, using "need" in the broader sense of the word to describe something one pursues because its attainment represents fulfillment of a sort. Considering motivation in this light, we might question whether it is possible for anyone to "motivate" another human being to do anything or pursue anything.

It is, in fact, not strictly possible to motivate another person. The best that can be done is to create the circumstances under which an individual can become self-motivated. It is much like the old saying, "You can lead a horse to water but you can't make it drink." One can create what would seem to be ideal conditions and structure seemingly perfect circumstances, but these alone provide no guarantee of successful employee motivation because there is no way of making someone respond appropriately if the person does not care to respond. Most people in work organizations are subject to the same overall collection of needs, but the mix of needs—that is, the differing emphasis on the various needs that drive an individual—may vary greatly from person to person. In brief, what "motivates" one person may have little or no effect on another individual. This necessitates generalizing to some extent and recognizing that any particular motivational strategy may work with some people and fail to work with others who are similarly situated.

## Motivators

The true motivating forces, or at least the strongest of the genuine motivating forces, are to be found in the work itself and are all describable as opportunities. The genuine sources of motivation are the opportunity to:

- Accomplish or achieve and be recognized for doing so
- Acquire new knowledge
- Do work that is both challenging and interesting
- Do work that is meaningful or that makes a societal contribution
- Assume responsibility
- Be involved in determining how the work is done

The foregoing opportunities are likely to include the primary motivators for a great many employees, provided that these employees are at least nominally satisfied with the environmental factors surrounding their employment—that is, the potential dissatisfiers.

## Dissatisfiers

The potential dissatisfiers are the environmental factors that exist in all aspects of an employee's relationship with the organization. They generally do not motivate workers, but they can easily lead to employee dissatisfaction if they are not maintained at a level acceptable to the employee. These potential dissatisfiers can be grouped in five categories:

1. *Salary administration*, primarily the perceived overall fairness of salaries and benefits
2. *Potential for promotion and growth* and the extent to which this is or is not present
3. *Personnel policies,* or how each employee is treated both as an individual and relative to other employees
4. *Working conditions* and the extent to which they promote well-being relative to what is expected
5. *Communication* in all of its forms, including knowledge of the organization's plans and prospects, regular feedback on performance, individual confidentiality, and higher management's responsiveness to employee questions and concerns

## Motivational Strategies

The first four of the five dissatisfiers listed previously have much to do with the overall organization and are perhaps mostly beyond the control or direct influence of the department manager. The final one on the list, communication, depends in part on the organization's policies and practices but also depends to a considerable extent on the individual manager's behavior. Any specific motivational strategy must take into account the relative strength of potential dissatisfiers, so it might be said that an initial—and continuing—motivational strategy is the maintenance of the environmental factors so as to minimize their potential effects as dissatisfiers. Other active motivational strategies that might be used include the following:

*Performance appraisal.* Making full use of the organization's performance appraisal process, preferably including self-appraisal participation and faithfully including appraisal interviews, serves a number of communication needs and can also provide recognition for work well done (only very rarely is it not possible to convey something positive in an appraisal). However, the formal appraisal done annually or perhaps semiannually is not enough; the manager should

dispense praise when earned and in general maintain an ongoing communicating relationship with each employee.

- *Job rotation, job enrichment, and job enlargement.* These strategies generally involve expanding or enlarging jobs or rotating duties. Such actions provide employees with the opportunity to gain new knowledge and can serve to inject increased interest and challenge into the work.
- *Delegation.* Related to the foregoing strategy concerning job expansion, proper delegation well administered can provide employees with added interest and challenge, the chance to acquire new knowledge, and the opportunity to take on increased responsibility.
- *Awards and honors.* Employee awards and honors programs provide visible recognition that can go a long way toward satisfying some employees' needs for recognition and appreciation. Such programs often include "Employee of the Month" and "Employee of the Year" selections.
- *Career ladders and parallel-path progression systems.* Such systems provide the opportunity for capable individuals to advance themselves professionally without necessarily seeking entry into management, thereby satisfying a continuing need for learning, growth, status, and recognition.
- *Incentives and bonuses.* Although it may be argued that in and of itself money is not a particularly strong motivator, it nevertheless looms large as a driving force for some workers. Often the monetary value of an incentive or bonus does not count nearly as strongly as the act of achievement. For some employees, it can truthfully be said that the money becomes primarily the "score" in the quest for accomplishment.
- *Employee participation.* Allowing employees to participate in establishing or revising methods, procedures, and processes is potentially one of the strongest individual motivators. In addition to involving the employee in determining how the work is done, doing so provides increased responsibility, adds interest and challenge, and promotes the acquisition of new knowledge.

## Motivation in Critical Incidents

From time to time, an organization experiences difficult situations in which workers, along with management, may experience a sense of defeat. By way of example, consider the long-term care facility with a history of excellence. Year after year, it passes the licensure review with flying colors. Then there is one unfortunate incident: a caregiver fails to report a patient-to-patient altercation until 2 days after the incident. This omission is noted by the on-site surveyors, who flag the organization for the incidence of patient abuse. The staff is devastated because they have taken such matters seriously and have had no prior instances.

A second example of a difficult situation stems from ever-increasing external regulations: the organization works diligently to comply with these requirements, only to find more regulations to follow. Consider the emphasis on disaster rehearsal to the point of failure; this is well meaning, but down in the trenches, it is hard to be enthusiastic when one is set up to fail.

A third example may be found in the difficult situation of budget freezes or cuts. There may be a season of dry promotions, no raises, and cutbacks in fringe benefits. Yet despite these measures, the worker is expected to give full effort.

A fourth example occurs when one or a few caregivers commit extensive fraud in billing. This serious infraction attracts extremely bad publicity for the facility. Other workers may bear the brunt of this criticism in their community and social settings: "Oh, you work at that place—was your department involved in the fraud?"

In each of these situations, particular attention must be given to motivational practices, starting with fostering a climate of trust. Trust is enhanced by transparency: "Yes, this happened. Yes, this is what management did about it. Yes, here is information you may share with others." Timely and accurate information, the presence of feedback, and the encouragement of all workers that things are going well—these are all motivational strategies that are appropriate for critical incident situations.

## ▶ Appreciative Inquiry

Appreciative inquiry (AI) represents yet another tool that can be used in critical situations, because it helps shift the focus back to the good done by the employees. AI is an approach to organizational change and development that begins with examination of what is working well and appreciation, through active recognition and expression, of the best of the individual and the group or organization's experience. Developed in the mid-1980s by Dr. David Cooperrider, Suresh Srivastva, and their colleagues at Case Western Reserve University, AI has been applied in a variety of organizational settings, including large federal agencies, business ventures, and professional associations.[1]

## The Appreciative Inquiry Process

When a manager uses the AI approach, the focus is on the values and mission of the organization and the positive experiences of the individual members of the organization. In the healthcare setting, this can be broadened to include client or patient groups as well as the professional, technical, and support staffs. The operative assumption is the understanding that something—perhaps even many things—are working well. These positive experiences are explicitly recalled and actively noted as successes. The starting point is to reframe the situation in terms of what is going well? What is working? The manager avoids using phrases such as "what went wrong?" "Why was the goal not met?" "Who is responsible for these errors?" Using these positive accomplishments, the group then builds on them to envision improvements. A set of goal statements is developed, or updated, based on the newly energized vision of the organization's efforts.

By way of example, consider the difference in two methods of dealing with patient safety, risk management, and incident reporting and review. In a more traditional approach, the emphasis is on the number, causes, and characteristics of the problems relating to patient safety—for example, number of falls, medication errors, or misdiagnoses. In an AI approach, the emphasis is on the goal of making this organization the safest possible environment for patients, staff, and visitors. The review process would still include specific data such as those noted earlier. However, the data would be cast in the context of all the care that is given without mishap. Specific problem areas will usually decrease simply as a result of positive efforts at improvement of safety practices.

## Motivational Aspects of Appreciative Inquiry

Appreciative Inquiry is a planning and assessment process which, by its very nature, includes motivation through positive reinforcement of that which is good. The process diffuses potential conflict because the best results of both individuals and departments or divisions are emphasized. Cooperation and enthusiasm for participation are enhanced.

Managers have many opportunities in their ongoing work to apply AI. Consider, for example, the usual concerns associated with preparation for outside surveys and reviews, such as accreditation or licensure inspections. The preparation of the survey report necessarily involves fact gathering. Instead of using the mindset that many vague problems will come to light, the management team could start by reaffirming the organization's best practices, noting them, and then isolating those areas needing improvement. Consider a report prepared by a consultant. The areas of compliance, which represent the majority of the day-to-day practices, are clearly listed, following which the areas needing improvement are identified.

Another situation of potential concern and conflict is associated with periodic labor contract negations. Typically, each party brings to the table its list of concerns and demands. Using an AI approach, however, the starting point would be a reflection of those areas of management–labor relations and those provisions of the contract that have enhanced the accomplishment of the organization's mission.

When an organization as a whole, or a group within an organization, has experienced much change and yet another major change must be absorbed, AI can be used to coalesce the positive energy needed to carry on. For example, the implementation of the Health Insurance Portability and Accountability Act regulations involved major changes affecting budgeting, vendor selection, collection, processing, and release of patient care information. In taking on this challenge, the health information manager and the professional association as a whole recalled its long-standing commitment to privacy and confidentiality with the concomitant successes in these areas. These managers were easily motivated to take leadership roles in implementing these requirements regarding confidentiality and security of patient care information.

Another example of the use of an AI approach is reflected in the employee evaluation process.

Using an AI approach, a manager carries out an employee performance review using as a starting point the employee's assessment of the work and his or her contribution to the department's mission. The manager would invite the employee to identify all the areas where he or she is performing well and then discuss those areas where performance could be improved.

Using the framework of AI, a manager continually seeks to take advantage of opportunities to express public appreciation for all that is going well. The customary declaration of a week highlighting one or another department is an example of this practice. The nomination of employees as "Employee of the Month" or similar recognition events reflect an AI attitude.

The celebration of milestones in a professional organization's life cycle is yet another opportunity to reflect on past accomplishments, leading to emphasis on future endeavors.

# ▶ Motivation and Downsizing[2]

Reducing labor cost is usually the most common goal of reengineering or reorganizing or other organizational restructuring efforts that result in "downsizing" (i.e., the reduction of the workforce). A considerable amount of thought and effort are required in structuring and implementing a staff reduction in a manner that will be as fair as possible to all concerned while supporting the organization's primary responsibility for delivering quality health care. However, the effort associated with downsizing cannot end simply when the employees who have been identified for separation have been released. For those at all levels who remain with the organization—and in essentially all workforce cutbacks, the people who remain are far more numerous than those who leave—the implementation of a reduction-in-force (RIF; sounds like "riff" in the language of human resources management) is the beginning of a completely new work situation in what will, and what in fact must, become an altered organization culture. Although many will tend to seek a "business as usual" state of affairs following a staff reduction, they will find that this is not possible.

## What Follows Downsizing?

A significant downsizing will forever alter many employees' beliefs and attitudes concerning their employment. Consider the following:

- For many years, healthcare workers saw reductions occurring in other industries in their communities while feeling relatively safe against the likelihood of ever being laid off. For a long time, many felt certain that health care, as an absolutely essential service, would remain untouched by the economic concerns that plagued other industries.
- Many healthcare workers long enjoyed a sense of employment security that has now been severely damaged.
- Healthcare workers have been awakened to the fact that health care is now subject to many of the external forces that plague other industries. That is, there are forces beyond their control that are causing permanent changes to health care.

The immediate responses to a healthcare organization's downsizing can include the following:

- Many employees may initially—and permanently, if positive steps are not taken—feel more like they are a "cost of doing business" rather than valued members of a work organization. They come to view themselves as simply another commodity that the organization will probably purchase less of in the future.
- Employee commitment to the organization will tend to erode as perceived employment security is diminished.
- Employee morale will be automatically reduced.
- Some key staff the organization desires to retain may resign to seek employment in environments they may perceive as more stable, further negatively affecting the morale and outlook of those who remain.
- Managers, with their thinking still governed by former ways of doing things, may try to compensate for lost staff by increasing the use of overtime and temporary help. They will experience additional frustration as controls are placed on hiring and on the use of overtime and temporaries.

In the time immediately following downsizing, there is a severe risk of cost reduction's becoming universally perceived as a higher priority than people. It is true that cost control is an essential element of survival; the healthcare organization that cannot adapt to financial reality will not survive to employ anyone. People, however, still remain the driving force. It is people working together who must bring the organization into line with financial reality, yet the same organization's continued existence then and forever will depend on serving people.

What must follow downsizing is a revitalization of the remaining workforce. An organization cannot and should never attempt to simply lay off a number of employees and call on those who remain to close ranks and continue as before. All who remain have a more difficult and more responsible task looming before them, and the organization's top management should endeavor to give all of the support and assistance that can reasonably be provided in making the transition to a leaner, more purposefully directed organization.

## The Necessity of Reducing the Workforce

Although the scenarios have differed to some extent from state to state, healthcare provider organizations across the nation have been experiencing reductions in revenue from most payment sources or revenue increases that fall short of covering increasing operating costs. Further significant revenue shortfalls will likely be occurring because of additional limitations placed on reimbursement levels by most payers. The simple fact of the matter is that the healthcare system is being forced by external circumstances to continually deliver the best of care while holding down increases in costs. Because the demand for service remains as high as ever and, in many respects continues to grow, the system is called on to accomplish more results with limited resources.

One may hope that realistic cost-containment activities, pursued as a normal course of business, would help an organization avoid or at least lessen a major financial crunch. However, the problem remains the same regardless of its immediate magnitude, and it must be dealt with. The communication issues are difficult enough when faced squarely with realistic data on a year-to-year basis; they become all the more difficult when the workforce has long been conditioned to believe that nothing serious is amiss.

In brief, when downsizing is planned and before the cuts occur, the workforce must be given every opportunity to understand why this is going to happen. The more openly the employees have been treated all along and the more frankly they have been advised of the organization's real circumstances on a continuing basis, the easier it will be to communicate why.

Any downsizing, while preferably designed and recommended by senior management and the medical staff leadership and approved by the board of directors, should proceed after all other reasonable efforts to reduce costs have been explored as follows:

- All realistic short-term savings opportunities should be identified and implemented.
- Before the actual reduction occurs, maximum effort should be expended to reduce staff through attrition by freezing hiring in most positions and, as much as possible, transferring current employees into areas of greatest need.
- Overtime should be severely curtailed, essentially reserved for true emergencies only and approvable by only a select few. Also, the use of temporary help should be curtailed (along with overtime, agency temporary help can tend to increase under staff reduction pressure if not closely monitored).
- Supply inventories should be reduced to levels conforming to the true needs indicated by reduced levels of activity.

It must be stressed that no matter how much cost-control effort precedes downsizing, the reduction itself is never the end of the process. For the organization's continued financial viability and effectiveness, it becomes the job of all employees to pursue continuous cost control in concert with continuous quality improvement if the organization is to prevail as a quality provider of health care.

## The Employees Who Remain

A RIF instantly establishes two different groups of employees: those who leave and those who remain. Except in rare instances, those who remain far outnumber those who leave. Judging from many of the healthcare staff reductions that have occurred in recent years, it is not unusual for the "survivors" to outnumber those leaving by eight, nine, or ten to one.

Management must recognize that the manner in which it deals with the reduction's survivors has a considerably greater bearing on the organization's future than how the terminations related to the RIF have been addressed. Those who have departed are gone, probably forever, but the survivors are there and are critical to the organization's future.

Stress and stress-related fear among those who remain following a layoff is natural, predictable, and essentially universal throughout the organization. A fully understandable feeling among survivors is the fear that they may be the next to go. To counter this fear, some top managers have essentially promised that "this is it—no more layoffs" or allowed employees to believe that the condition is only temporary and that employees will most likely be called back. Any belief in either of these scenarios must not be encouraged; more than a few managers who have promised "no more layoffs" have been severely contradicted by worsening reality.

It becomes necessary to unite the remaining workers into a forward-moving team and to motivate them to work harder in a leaner, more efficient, and yet initially a completely alien situation. Through a concentrated and continuing communication program, the survivors of the reduction need to learn:

- Why they remain and what will be expected of them, why the old organization is gone forever, and how they can help shape the new organizational culture that will be emerging
- That as the survivors of the reduction they are among the best in their occupations and that is essentially why they are still in place
- That a future in which continually doing more with less will remain critical to organizational survival and continued employment

## Immediate and Natural Reactions to Downsizing

The issues emerging in the wake of downsizing are all essentially "people" issues. The major issues that surface usually include the following:

- The short-term loss of talent in the form of productive employees the organization would wish to retain. At special risk are valuable "free-agent" employees, those professional and technical workers whose primary loyalty is to an occupation and whose movement between and among organizations may be governed more by labor market circumstances than by ties to a specific organization.
- An immediate drop in productivity, precisely at a time when productivity increases are needed for the sake of long-term survival. This occurs because morale has dropped and employees are preoccupied with issues of security and concern for their future.
- Increases in the use of sick time, healthcare benefits, on-the-job accidents, medication errors, and other lapses in quality. These are often experienced during and after downsizing, again because of employees' concern for their employment.

## Employee Motivation Following Downsizing

Under normal circumstances—without the direct prospect of a reduction in the workforce and with each employee's reasonable expectation of continued employment—job security and wages are not particularly active motivating forces. Rather, as noted earlier, they are potential dissatisfiers; as long as wages and job security are perceived as "reasonable," the concern for them is largely secondary. However, when these are disturbed—when raises are eliminated, for instance, or when security is perceived as threatened—these become factors in heightening employee dissatisfaction, which in turn negatively impacts motivation.

It becomes necessary to help the surviving employees reestablish a sense of equilibrium with their altered surroundings and achieve a relative sense of security. An employee who may come to work each day wondering "Will I be next?" will be neither effective nor productive. As long as an employee is preoccupied with personal survival, individual productivity will decline at the time its improvement is needed more than ever.

It is necessary to communicate with employees fully, completely, and repeatedly until they understand that:

- Nobody—neither the organization nor a labor union—can absolutely guarantee continued employment.
- A certain amount of stress is inevitable regardless of what management does following downsizing, but stress can be energizing as well as debilitating and can serve as a spur to improvement.
- A future emphasis on improved productivity is essential to survival as an organization.
- Employees' aggregate job performance is the organization's best survival guarantee, and as far as individual employees are concerned, their performance is their own best job security.

The most potent motivating forces—perhaps the only true long-run motivating forces—are inherent in people's work. These forces are, of course, the opportunity to learn and grow, to do interesting work, to contribute, and to feel a sense of accomplishment and worth. However, these motivators can work only when employees are able to feel relatively secure and reasonably compensated. Management needs to provide conditions under which all employees can become self-motivated and then act on that belief.

Attendant to employees' motivational needs, the organization might also consider the creation of incentive programs and other flexible rewards to encourage and acknowledge innovation, commitment, and enhanced productivity. Overall, top management should at all times let employees know what is expected of them and tell them exactly how this desired behavior will be rewarded.

## Changes in Managers' Roles

Any significant downsizing is bound to include the elimination of some management positions or the combination of selected management positions. In the presence of a generally flatter management structure, managers and their superiors are both likely to find their roles enhanced. They will essentially assume new roles, roles that are more challenging and that require more direct decision making.

The individual who directly supervises others will be the organization's primary conduit for communication with staff. At each management level, the manager is always a critical link in the movement of information up and down the chain of command. The first-line manager is the primary communicating link between each direct reporting employee and the rest of the organization. As the one member of management who the employee knows best and the one whose role it is to be the employee's communicating link, the manager influences the attitudes and outlooks of a significant portion of the organization. Thus, as the individual employee views the manager, so too is he or she likely to view the organization. In other words, if a manager of 15 people is seen as distant, uncommunicative, and uncaring, then 15 people are likely to see the total organization as distant, uncommunicative, and uncaring. Because the size of direct reporting work groups generally increases following downsizing and flattening of the organization, the influence of the individual manager becomes even more significant.

Some of the manager's key concerns after downsizing are:

- The need to be conscious of the employee's motivational needs and to work to control turnover both immediately and over the long term.
- The need to function as a strong advocate for the staff—to achieve the best for those who must leave as well as for those who remain.
- The need to begin preparing to work with the survivors, helping them to internalize the dramatic change well before the reduction is fully implemented.
- The need to actively encourage employee participation more than ever before, stressing involvement and drawing all possible employees into the decision-making processes. More than ever, the supervisor's focus needs to be "we," never "I" or "you."
- The need to develop and use employee teams to the maximum possible extent.
- The need to communicate, communicate, communicate at all times, remaining in touch with employees' fears and concerns even when some of the answers have to be "We simply don't know yet, but we'll keep you informed."

## ▶ Conflict

Conflict is an inevitable component of cooperative action, and the effects of conflict are felt by all participants in organizational life. Indeed, in a sense organizational life largely consists of carefully orchestrated conflict, so much so that one of the classic functions of a manager is to ensure coordination, which includes promoting cooperation and minimizing conflict.

Dictionary definitions of *conflict* use terms such as "variance," "incompatibility," "disagreement," "inner divergence," and "disturbance." Conflict is basically a state of external and internal tension that results when two or more demands are made on an individual, group, or organization. Even as managers remain aware of the pervasive, almost unnoticed presence of cooperation, they are attentive to the dynamics of conflict.

## The Study of Conflict

The manager and healthcare practitioner seek to understand the phenomenon of conflict within organizations so that they can make it acceptable, predictable, and therefore manageable. Conflict must be accepted as an inevitable part of all group effort. The causes of conflict are found primarily in the organizational structure, with its system of authority, roles, and specialization. The clash of personal styles of interaction can be analyzed so as to deal more effectively with such clashes.

Conflict can be accepted as an element of change, a positive catalyst for continual challenge to the organization. Aggression may be accepted and channeled to foster survival. If conflict is not channeled and controlled, it may have negative effects that impede the growth of both the individual and the organization.

In certain situations, conflict may clarify relationships, effect change, and define organizational territories or jurisdictions. When there has been an integrative solution, resulting from open review of all points of view, agreement is strengthened and morale heightened. Conflict tends to energize an organization, forcing it to keep alert, to plan and anticipate change, and to serve clients in more effective ways.

## ▶ Organizational Conflict

Managers can assess organizational conflicts by using a theoretical model, which frees them from the bias created by their own immediate involvement in the conflict. By analyzing conflict in a relatively objective manner, a manager can deal with it more positively and more easily. The following is a basic model for such an analysis:

1. The basic conflict
   a. Overt level
   b. The hidden agenda
   c. The source of conflict
2. The participants
   a. Immediate and primary participants
   b. Secondary participants
   c. The audience
3. The provision of an arena
4. The development of rules
5. Strategies for dealing with organizational conflict

**Exhibit 10–1** is an example of the use of this model.

## The Basic Conflict
### Overt Level

As a starting point, the manager analyzing a conflict describes the obvious problem. This process of naming the conflict elements provides focus and clarifies

---

**Exhibit 10–1 Conflict Model with Example**

| *The Basic Conflict* | |
|---|---|
| Overt issue | Habitual lateness and/or absenteeism of employee |
| Hidden agenda | Growing employee resistance to managerial authority |
| Sources | Human need versus organizational needOrganizational structure |
| *Participants* | |
| Immediate | Unit supervisor and employee |
| Secondary | Chief of service, personnel director |
| Audience | Other employees with similar problems with work schedule, other managers with similar employee disciplinary problems, and higher levels of management who monitor organizational climate |
| *Arena* | Grievance procedure |
| *Rules* | Work rules related to attendance, procedures for filing grievances |
| *Strategy* | Limitation of conflict to unit members |

the issues that are at stake. Examples include the following problems: clients, rank and file employees, and managers all experience the effects of conflict such as these; several of these examples reflect a rather low level, chronic conflict that saps energy from the workplace and could lead to greater conflict.

- Habitual lateness by an employee
- Coworker who is ineffective and uncooperative
- Delays in transport of patients from inpatient services to physical therapy or occupational therapy services
- Lack of clarity about job responsibilities
- Delays in treating patients, causing patients to wait unduly for their appointments
- Confusing and/or delayed billing for care received months before
- Mandatory job rotation to alternate care sites due to the acquisition of new sites
- Effect of seniority provisions on vacation and holiday time off. Newer employees are almost never able to take prime-time vacations or holiday time off.

### The Hidden Agenda

Although the overt issue may be the true and only substance of the conflict, there is sometimes another area of conflict that constitutes a hidden agenda. This hidden agenda may be the true conflict, or it may be an adjunct issue. The process of naming the conflict and describing its elements helps bring to light any hidden agenda that may exist.

Conflict issues are buried for several reasons. For instance, they may be too explosive to deal with openly, or subconscious protective mechanisms may prevent a threatening subject from surfacing until the individual in question has a safe structure and the necessary support to deal with it. Within an institution, the climate may not be appropriate for accepting conflict, or organizational resources may be insufficient to deal with it.

The subtleties of intraorganizational power struggles cause certain aspects of conflict to remain hidden. Individuals may choose to obscure the real issue as a means of testing their strength, of determining points of opposition before plunging ahead with an issue, or of checking the intensity of opposition. Periodic sparring over issues that never seem to be resolved is a clue to the existence of a hidden agenda. For example, the hospital budget issue of billing a medical group practice for certain administrative services may surface each year and be subjected to temporary

resolution. The root of the problem is not the allocation of money, but rather the creation of a new institutional structure. As a consequence, organizational control of outpatient services is at stake.

## The Sources of Conflict

The analysis of a conflict begins with identifying its primary sources, including competition for resources, authority relationships, and extraorganizational pressures. As discussed earlier, organizational conflicts are ultimately due to the individuals who participate in organizational activities.

### The Nature of the Organization

Organizations with multiple goals face competing and sometimes mutually exclusive demands for available resources. A hospital, for example, must safeguard against malpractice claims through active risk control management, yet it must also contain costs. The medical staff must give priority to the best-care practices, yet avoid potentially unnecessary tests. The rules, regulations, and requirements imposed by the many controllers of the organization identified in the clientele network may be a source of conflict. Shifting client demand and changes in the degree of client participation in the organization may lead to conflict when an increase in the allocation of resources for one group is a loss for another. The authority structure is another clue to potential conflict; members of coercive organizations are more frequently in conflict with the organization than are members of normative institutions.

### The Organizational Climate

An emphasis on competition as a means of enhancing productivity, as in the use of the "deadly parallel" organizational structure or the use of a reward system that emphasizes competition among individuals or departments, may cause conflict. The intentional overlap and blurred jurisdiction of units can produce continual jockeying for organizational territory. Competition for scarce resources may be sharp, with resulting conflicts, coalitions, and compromises. The subtleties of an institution's power struggles, the shifting balance of power (e.g., a growing union movement), and the need to demonstrate power constitute another facet of organizational climate. Denial of conflict is a potential source of trouble, because it removes a safe outlet for the resolution of conflict before it becomes a serious problem.

## The Organizational Structure

The complex authority structure of healthcare organizations (i.e., a dual track of authority coupled with an increasing professionalism among the many specialized workers) creates situations of potential conflict. Professional practitioners, such as nurses, physical therapists, clinical psychologists, and social workers, are trained to assess patient needs and to take actions within the scope of their licensure or certification; however, their ability to make decisions is limited by the hierarchical organizational structure. This problem is compounded when the individual practitioner has a legal duty to act or refrain from acting that is in direct opposition to the hierarchical system, such as when a nurse refrains from giving a medication that would be harmful to the patient even when the physician has (inadvertently) ordered such a dosage.

Physicians, in holding staff appointments, find themselves required to shift regularly from their roles as independent practitioners when functioning outside the healthcare facility to more limited roles as members of the organizational hierarchy. This regular role shift may also be required of the physical therapist, nurse practitioner, or occupational therapist who functions as an independent agent in private practice and at the same time participates in the patient care process as a staff member of a healthcare institution.

Conflict may also arise from specialization within the organizational structure when individuals attempt to carry out their assigned activities. For example, the social worker might seek to place a patient in a long-term care facility, but the utilization review coordinator must impose strict guidelines in terms of days of care allotted under certain payment contracts. The health information manager must develop a system of record control, although many users of records find it more practical to retain records in restricted areas of their own. The purchasing agent must comply with certain regulations on deadlines, budget restrictions, and auditing procedures in spite of individual needs. Specialization within the complexities of bureaucratization leads to frustration, misunderstanding, and conflict.

Superior–subordinate relationships constitute another area of potential conflict. The organizational chart is, in fact, a suppression chart that specifies which positions have authority over and literally suppress other individual jobs or units. The legitimacy of a leader's claim to office is continually assessed. The power, prestige, and rewards built into the hierarchical system all represent gain for some and related loss for others. The erosion of traditional territory associated with line management results from activities clearly intended to remove some authority from line managers. These activities include client or worker involvement in decision making.

The process of management by objectives, in which workers are directly involved in setting and assessing objectives, commands much attention for its motivational value. Also, streamlined processes, such as central number assignments or patient bed assignments, have much merit as systems improvements, and a central pool of patient aides, assistants, and transporters is an alternative to assignment by department. Yet each of these processes erodes the distinct territory of one or several managers, whose ability to make decisions is affected by such changes. Increased specialization in some technical areas leads to a more frequent use of functional specialists. Although the line manager retains authority, the specialist must be included in the planning and decision-making process; the line manager is no longer the sole agent in charge.

Unions may move into management territory in several areas relating to personnel management and direct work assignment. In the collective bargaining process, the nature of the work, who will do it, and how much will be done may be issues. Union gains may be management losses.

## Individual Versus Organizational Needs

Human needs and values must be welded into the organizational framework. A large number of clients and workers enters the organization, and they have different values, experience, motives, and expectations. The degree to which each individual internalizes the values of the organization and accepts a primary identity derived from the institution varies greatly. Individuals who do not participate directly in the accomplishment of organizational goals or in the institutional authority structure tend to identify less with the organization and view its demands less favorably than those who participate more fully in direct, goal-oriented activities.

## Solutions to Previous Conflicts

New problems may arise from solutions to previous conflicts. The use of compromise as a strategy in dealing with conflict tends to leave all participants somewhat dissatisfied. At the next opportunity, one or more participants may seek to reopen the issue in an attempt to regain what was lost, particularly if the loss was acute. The loser may build up resources and enter into an active state of aggression when such resources have been accumulated, such as a nation defeated after a war (e.g., Germany after World War I). When there is a consistent denial pattern, the conflict may "go underground" for a time, then emerge again with greater force. Again, managers should realistically examine the negative consequences of conflict resolutions so as to minimize their recurrence.

# The Participants

The immediate participants in the conflict can be identified readily as the individuals or groups caught in the open exchange.

The secondary participants are the individuals called in to take an active role, such as persons at the next level of the hierarchy. A manager may consult with a senior official to whom the individual involved in the conflict reports or with a staff adviser, such as a labor relations specialist. A unit manager may be required in some instances to refer conflict to the next level for resolution, as in some grievance procedures. In the case of a unionized employee, a representative of the union, such as a shop steward, may be involved. A "neutral" party may be called in by both sides in a labor dispute (e.g., a mediator or an arbitrator). Occasionally, a manager may consult informally with certain "marginal" individuals, such as those in the department or organization who have an overlapping role set, a supervisor whose domain spans several activities, a client who is also on an advisory committee, or another department head who has faced similar situations. Because they link groups, these individuals are sought out to test a potential solution or to obtain information and even advice.

A third category of participants may be classified as the audience. This category may include the following:

- *The clients.* If the conflict is overt and severe, the clients may turn to other organizations for the necessary services so as to avoid the conflict. Uncertainty may cause tension within this group, however, and clients may become active participants (e.g., protests, unofficial boycotts, class-action lawsuits). A client group alienated from the institution may develop its own system to meet its needs.
- *The public at large.* This group may seek action through recourse to some government agency, and an agency's intervention into the conflict may take the form of additional regulation of the organization. The conflict may be brought into the public arena; for example, a labor dispute may be taken to court. The net effect of intervention by some agent on behalf of the public at large is the opening or broadening of the conflict, which removes it from the immediate control of the original parties to the dispute.
- *A potential rival or enemy.* While one group and its opponents are absorbed in conflict, a third group whose energies are not drained by conflict may seek to expand its services and attract the clients of the groups locked in the dispute.
- *Individuals or groups with similar complaints.* Some observers may seek to press a similar claim if "the right side" wins. In the case of employee unrest, a labor organizer may consider more active unionization attempts. Independent practitioners who seek greater autonomy in the practice of health care may monitor changes in organizational bylaws or state licensure regulations and find gains made by one individual or group of practitioners to be the catalyst needed to obtain similar gains. In malpractice cases, jury awards are monitored and publicized. As the basis for a certain kind of claim is expanded through a trend in court decisions, more individuals may advance their cases. Without extensive publicity of the benchmark cases, this basis of claim might not have arisen. A worker who sees another worker win a concession from the manager about some work rule will more readily press a similar claim.
- *The opportunist.* Some individual or group may seek to enter the conflict as champion or savior. Such action may be undertaken by individuals seeking to raise themselves to leadership positions.

In many cases, members of the audience not only cheer and jeer, but they also become active participants, thereby expanding the conflict in terms of the number of individuals or groups who must be satisfied in any solution.

Conflict should be resolved at as low an organizational level as possible. The facts are better known by the immediate participants, who are able to communicate directly. Also, because the number of participants is limited, agreement on a solution may be more easily obtained. Top levels of management should be involved only rarely in conflicts within the organization, because their involvement might give undue weight to the problem, establish precedent, and force the setting of policy that escalates resolutions to a higher level. The resources of top management should generally be reserved for critical issues.

# The Provision of an Arena

The development of a safe, predictable, and accessible arena tends to create a sense of security and to keep the problems from becoming diffuse. The aggrieved know where to turn and what to do to seek redress. The provision of an acceptable arena is also efficient. The individuals involved give their attention to it in a highly structured manner, and it establishes clear boundaries to the conflict: It is legitimate to bring issues of conflict to *this* place, through *this* structure, at *these* designated times. The court system and legislative debate are such arenas in the larger society. In organizations, arenas include the structured grievance process for employees (**Exhibit 10-2**), the appeals process for the professional staff member seeking staff appointment, or the complaint department for customers. Committees in which multiple input is invited are also common arenas for the resolution of conflict.

# The Development of Rules

Rules serve to limit the energy expended on the conflict process. The provision of rules has a face-saving and legitimizing effect; it is permissible to disagree,

---

## Exhibit 10–2 Excerpts from Grievance Procedure

Any grievance that may arise between the parties concerning the application, meaning, or interpretation of this Agreement shall be resolved in the following manner:

Step 1: An employee having a grievance and his Union delegate shall discuss it with his immediate supervisor within five (5) working days after it arose or should have been made known to the employee. The Hospital shall give its response through the supervisor to the employee and to this Union delegate within five (5) working days after the presentation of the grievance. In the event no appeal is taken to the next step (Step 2), the decision rendered in this step shall be final.

Step 2: If the grievance is not settled in Step 1, the grievance may, within five (5) working days after the answer in Step 1, be presented in Step 2. When grievances are presented in Step 2, they shall be reduced to writing on grievance forms provided by the Hospital (which shall then be assigned a number by the Department of Human Resources at the Union's request), signed by the grievant and his or her Union representative, and presented to the Department Head and the Department of Human Resources. A grievance so presented in Step 2 shall be answered in writing within five (5) working days after its presentation.

---

equal time is guaranteed, and each point of view is aired. The rules also provide a basis for the intervention of a referee or neutral party. The rules may be developed to allow a cooling-off period so that the issues can be put in perspective. The time frame given by the rules reduces uneasiness, because participants are assured of a legitimate opportunity to present the issues. Conflict remains under control.

# Strategies for Dealing with Organizational Conflict

Two strategies for dealing with conflict are opposite in nature: limitation and purposeful expansion. A manager assesses a conflict situation and makes a judgment. Is the wiser course of action one in which the conflict is allowed to become greater? With this approach, there is the risk that the organization could lose control as conflict is widened, and it is unlikely that both sides will be reinforced equally. Conflict is best kept private, limited, and therefore controllable. Yet there might be an advantage to conscious expansion. The underlying purpose of the intentional expansion of conflict is to demonstrate its immediate effect on the clients or the public, who in turn will bring pressure on the opposing party to end the dispute. The immediate involvement of the client group is sought in the hope that it will act as a catalytic factor, forcing quick resolution. For example, a teachers' union may go on strike at the beginning of a school year, a coal miners' union may strike during the winter, and traffic officers may conduct a slowdown or job action during the height of the Fourth of July traffic to the shore.

The routinization of conflict is an additional strategy wherein conflict is accepted as a normal part of organizational life. Thus, the conflicts are anticipated. Certain conflicts are identified and contingency plans are developed. For example, a strike plan is developed in anticipation of possible conflict arising at the conclusion of a contract cycle. Such an event may be short-lived, with more of a symbolic value as a kind of catharsis as a biennial event. The energy associated with such conflict is brought to the surface and played out in a scripted fashion; it is predictable and therefore manageable. Other strategies for the routinization of conflict include, for example, co-optation, strategic leniency, preformed decisions through policy and procedure development, and the selection of individuals who fit the organization.

In addition to such conscious strategies, a manager should make use of the general principles of sound organization. When used properly, these principles bring about stability and reduce conflict. Known policies and rules, sufficient orientation and training of members, proper authority–responsibility designations, and clear chains of command and communication—all of these practices foster cooperation and mutual expectation, with the attendant reduction of undue conflict.

Finally, awareness of "burnout" and programs to prevent it can contribute to the reduction of conflict and enhance motivation. Such programs are discussed in another section on this topic.

## ▶ Conflict Model Applied to Whistleblower Action

A manager uses the model presented in this chapter to recognize and deal with conflict. As a final example of the application of the conflict model to contemporary work settings, consider the laws, policies, and procedures relating to whistleblower activity.

1. *The basic conflict*: a whistleblower might have concerns about reimbursement fraud, supply chain mismanagement, accrediting standards violations, or harassment issues. In general, these represent activities that are illegal, dishonest, or unethical.
2. *The participants*: the whistleblower bringing the complaint is the primary participant. Other participants include members of the internal chain of command, and human resources official as designated in organizational policy. There is the potential for an external audience when the situation becomes public.
3. *Provision of Arena*: the policy and procedures indicate the appropriate reporting process for both internal and external arenas. Tip lines, dedicated phone numbers, and names of contact officials are provided. Some aspects of the processes allow for anonymity of the whistleblower. Unless required by law, it is customary to provide anonymity in order to encourage a whistleblower to come forward. However, some organizations require that a written report be made to the chief executive officer before initiating a report to an external body. This report triggers the necessary internal review process.
4. *The Rules*: there are two major rules protecting the whistleblower: maintenance of confidentiality of the proceedings and prohibition of retaliation.

    The whistleblower, in turn, must not make false or unfounded accusations. Severe penalties apply to individuals who fail to follow "good faith" understanding.

5. *Strategies for dealing with conflict*: clearly delineated policies and procedures generally contain conflict within the organization, but permit the expansion of conflict when internal resolution is lacking.

## ▶ Discipline

The attitudes, emotions, and motivations of each employee within an organization affect not only the degree to which goals and objectives are attained but also influence the behavior of other employees. The manager of any unit or department must be concerned with the conduct or behavior of all employees within that unit or department. A manager's guidance of a work group is best supported and facilitated by: (1) establishing reasonable standards of conduct, or work rules, and informing employees of these standards, and (2) enforcing all rules consistently and humanely.

The word *discipline* has acquired different and sometimes less-than-favorable connotations over the years. In the military context, the word is usually associated with order, consistency, and unquestioning obedience. In the context of the work organization, however, the word is strongly associated with the use of authority, and it carries the disagreeable connotation of punishment. However, a brief foray into the origins of the word reveals that *discipline* comes from the same root as *disciple* and as such actually means "to teach so as to mold." Thus, at one time, teaching was the primary intent of discipline, the process of shaping or molding the disciple. Nevertheless, for the most part, in the context of the work organization, people have come to associate discipline—and therefore disciplinary *action*—with punishment.

Although much disciplinary action necessarily includes elements of punishment, its primary objective must never be punishment itself. Rather, the principal purpose of disciplinary action should be *correction of behavior*. Therefore it is a requirement of disciplinary action that for all but the most serious infractions, the transgressing party be afforded the opportunity to correct the offending behavior. The obvious exceptions are those instances of behavior that are sufficiently serious to prompt "correction" by removing (that is, terminating) the offenders without a second chance. These exceptions arise in a relative minority of disciplinary situations; for the greatest part, disciplinary action is properly directed toward correcting errant behavior.

In addition to using disciplinary action to improve employee behavior, at times it can help motivate employees so they become self-disciplined and thus more effective in the performance of their jobs.

However, no matter how skillfully it is applied, disciplinary action will always carry something of a negative connotation for many employees, so in the long run calling attention to correct behavior is more effective in promoting self-discipline and cooperation than calling attention to incorrect behavior. In other words, disciplinary action is necessary and has its place, but praise ultimately proves more powerful in inspiring acceptable performance and behavior. Even in an organization where employees exhibit a high degree of independence and self-discipline, a manager must occasionally apply disciplinary action of some kind because rules have been broken.

At this stage of the discussion, it is necessary to make a distinction between two kinds of employee problems with which the manager may be confronted: problems of performance and problems of conduct or behavior. When a manager speaks of taking disciplinary action, he or she is talking of addressing problems of conduct or behavior—that is, problems that involve the breaking of rules or the violation of policies. In addressing these kinds of problems, although it is usually his or her purpose to correct the errant behavior, the process frequently involves "warnings" of various kinds. Thus, the process can acquire a negative connotation and be perceived as including "punishment." Most, if not all, problems of conduct or behavior involve violations that are willful or that at least result from carelessness or indifference. Such violations are considered the fault of the perpetrators.

Problems of performance are an entirely different matter. The warnings, suspensions, and other measures described within a progressive disciplinary process are inappropriate for problems of performance. Such problems, which usually encompass an employee's failure to meet the minimum expectations of the job, are not considered willful violations of rules. Therefore, problems of performance must be addressed through counseling and retraining as necessary, using a process that is entirely corrective in nature and not punitive in any respect. The progressive disciplinary process, then, is applicable only to problems of conduct or behavior and not to problems of performance.

Distasteful as the application of disciplinary action may be, it is the manager's responsibility to act promptly, firmly, and consistently when action is called for. Disciplinary action should follow the misconduct as closely in time as possible. The only significant reasons for ever delaying disciplinary action even briefly are to allow tempers to cool, perhaps to investigate a situation and decide how to proceed, or to take the time and opportunity to secure a private one-on-one meeting with the offending individual.

Every instance of disciplinary action must be treated as a confidential matter, handled in private; it is, quite bluntly, nobody's business but that of the offending employee and the manager.

# Progressive Disciplinary Action

Several steps constitute the progressive disciplinary process. Not all of these steps will be applicable in all instances; at which step the process is entered and how many steps are applied will depend on the nature of the specific infraction. The steps comprising a complete progressive disciplinary process are described next.

## Counseling

The initial step taken to address a number of kinds of noncritical errant behavior should be counseling. In a one-to-one meeting with the manager, the employee should be told the nature of the perceived problem, why it is a problem (or how it can become a problem), what the rules are concerning this behavior (with specific reference to handbooks and policy manuals), what the possible consequences of this kind of behavior are, and within what period of time correction is expected. This should be accomplished without reference to any kind of "warning"; it is simply an important, job-related discussion between manager and employee.

The manager should document each counseling session. Some organizations use a specific form for documenting counseling sessions, but a simple handwritten note retained in departmental files should be sufficient.

## Oral Warning

Repeated problem behavior following counseling should be addressed using the more formal early stages of the progressive disciplinary process, specifically the oral warning. The oral warning stage, often regarded as involving a "counseling" session itself, should be used only after the employee has failed to respond to informal counseling.

The oral warning should be documented by the manager, preferably on a form created for that purpose. **Exhibit 10–3** presents an example of a simple oral warning form.

Often someone will argue that if the "oral" warning is documented, it is actually a written warning. It may seem so, but the difference between a written warning and an oral warning lies in what goes into the employee's personnel file. The record of an oral warning should be retained in department files; it should

**Exhibit 10–3** Record of Oral Warning

Employee Name _____ ID No. _____

Department _____ Hire Date _____

Job Title and Grade _____ Job Date _____

Infraction or incident; policy reviewed and discussed:


Dates of counseling sessions or discussions concerning the same policy:


The employee must take the following action:


Employee Signature _____ Date _____

Manager Signature _____ Date _____

This record will be maintained in departmental files. If further action is required for the same offense, it will be forwarded to Human Resources for inclusion in the personnel file.

go into the official personnel files only as part of a subsequent warning for the same kind of behavior.

One might logically ask that if it is truly to be an "oral" warning, why document it at all? This is done because the oral warning is a step in the published progressive disciplinary process. When an employment relationship breaks down and legal problems result, it can become necessary to provide evidence that every step in the process was followed.

## Written Warning

The written warning follows the oral warning as necessary, with this documentation automatically included in the employee's personnel file. **Exhibit 10–4** is an example of a written warning form.

An employee whose improper behavior has not been corrected following counseling, oral warning, and written warning is in a position in which failure to change is likely to lead to loss of income via suspension and perhaps eventual loss of employment. By this stage, the manager and the employee have been together on the subject of the employee's behavior problem at least three or more times. It is time for the manager to bring other resources into the process.

## Before Suspension

Before proceeding to the suspension step, the manager should consider referring the employee to one of two available sources of assistance: the employee health service or the human resources department. If in any of their numerous contacts, the employee has

given the manager reason to believe that he or she may be experiencing health problems of any kind, a referral to the employee health service is in order. If the problem appears to possibly lie in the employee's attitude or in other difficulties unrelated to health, the referral should be to human resources. In the ideal system, the human resources department will include an employee relations specialist or employee ombudsperson, but in the absence of such specialists, most human resources generalists can fill the employee relations role.

This referral puts the employee in contact with someone who may be able to point the way toward resolution of some underlying problem. Also, a knowledgeable person other than the manager is brought into the process, and this new participant may be able to get through to the employee where the manager could not. This step provides the employee with a more distinct opportunity to correct the problem behavior. Also, the involvement of human resources can be helpful in instances in which tension or strain exists between the department manager and the employee.

## Suspension and Discharge

If the referral step described previously proves unsuccessful, suspension without pay, which in many systems ranges from 1 to 5 days, may follow. Eventually, discharge will likely be necessary if nothing up to and including suspension without pay is successful in changing behavior. **Exhibits 10–5** and **10–6** are

## Exhibit 10–4 Written Warning

Employee Name _____ ID No. _____

Department _____ Hire Date _____

Job Title and Grade _____ Job Date _____

Infraction or incident; policy reviewed and discussed:


Dates of previous actions related to the foregoing:


The employee must take the following action:


Employee Signature _____ Date _____

Manager Signature _____ Date _____

This record puts the employee on notice that additional violations will result in more serious disciplinary action such as suspension without pay or discharge.

## Exhibit 10–5 Suspension Without Pay

Employee Name _____ ID No. _____

Department Hire _____ Date _____

Job Title and Grade _____ Job Date _____

Infraction or incident, and rule or policy reviewed and discussed:


Previous Disciplinary Actions:

  Date:          Action Taken:


Suspended for ____ days from the above date. Report back on regular shift on ____.

Or

____ Time off waived by manager for the following reason (waiver does not lessen the severity of the action):


Employee Signature _____ Date _____

Manager Signature _____ Date _____

This is a final warning. Failure to respond appropriately may result in discharge.

examples of forms used to document suspension and discharge, respectively. However, a well-functioning referral program for employee behavior problems will significantly reduce the use of the clearly punitive steps of suspension and discharge.

There is an important point to address concerning suspension without pay. Note that in Exhibit 10–5, the manager has the option to waive the time-off requirement of a suspension. The manager is permitted to use this option on occasions when the enforced

**Exhibit 10–6** Notice of Discharge or Dismissal

Employee Name _____ ID No. _____

Department Hire _____ Date _____

Job Title and Grade _____ Job Date _____

Your employment is being terminated for the following reasons:




Previous Disciplinary Actions:

    Date:              Action Taken:




_____ Check here to indicate whether the employee desires an exit interview to discuss benefits status. If this opportunity is declined, continuation-of-benefits information will be mailed to the employee's home address.



Employee Signature _____ Date _____

Manager Signature _____ Date _____

time off for a suspension would leave an important job untended or an area critically understaffed. However, the employee must be strongly advised that waiver of time off does not lessen the severity of the disciplinary action as far as the official record and future actions are concerned.

The manager who believes there is cause to discharge an employee should take the case to the human resources department for thorough review before initiating action. Given the legal environment of the times, most organizations today require human resources or administrative review and concurrence for most discharges. This review is conducted to determine whether all bases have been covered from a legal perspective and whether the record clearly demonstrates that the employee was given the opportunity to correct the inappropriate behavior. Because of the time required to accomplish it, this review serves another extremely important function in ensuring that no employee is ever fired on the spot or otherwise terminated in the anger of the moment.

Some severe infractions must, of course, be dealt with as they occur. However, immediate firing is never the answer. The offending employee should instead be sent home on indefinite suspension pending investigation and resolution.

Not all kinds of infractions will require the application of all the foregoing steps. A mild infraction, such as tardiness (within a few minutes of starting time) may, if it becomes chronic, eventually require all of the steps described previously. A more serious infraction, such as sleeping on duty, may call for a written warning or suspension on the first violation and discharge on the second violation.

The organization's human resources department ordinarily provides guidance for determining the severity of disciplinary action for specific infractions. Differences exist among organizations as to which kind of action applies to which sort of infraction, but guidelines might include the following:

- For typical minor infractions such as chronic tardiness, absenteeism, or perhaps discourtesy, the progression might consist of first, oral warning; second, written warning; then 1-day suspension without pay; then 3-day suspension without pay; and finally discharge.
- For more serious infractions, such as conducting personal business on work time, unexcused absence, or failure to report for work when scheduled, the progression might consist of written warning for the first offense, then 3-day suspension, and finally discharge.
- For still more serious infractions such as insubordination, falsification of records, or violation of confidentiality, the complete progression

might consist of a written warning for an initial offense and discharge for a second offense.

- For the most serious infractions, there is no progression; these incidents call for discharge on the first and only offense. Typical serious infractions include theft, fighting on the job, possessing or using alcohol or illegal substances on the job, bringing weapons onto the premises, deliberate destruction of property, and absence without notice for three consecutive scheduled days (considered job abandonment).

## Heading Off Infractions Before They Occur

The manager who observes an employee apparently headed toward a point where disciplinary action will be necessary is advised to introduce counseling before true progressive discipline is necessary. For example, if the manager sees that a particular employee is developing a poor attendance record and is closing in on the point at which disciplinary action is called for, the manager should address this problem via counseling with the employee before such action is necessary. It is the unfeeling manager who, observing that an employee is approaching the point where disciplinary action is necessary, will allow the circumstances to continue until action is unavoidable. It is better by far for both manager and employee to use counseling in an effort to head off the problem before it fully develops.

## Appeal Procedure

Numerous organizations use appeal procedures to address employee complaints about work-related matters. Such matters can include, for example, disciplinary actions, performance evaluations, and decisions based on specific interpretations of policy. A typical appeal procedure might include the following steps or some variation of them. The time frames given are simply what one organization might specify.

- An employee with a complaint should first address the issue with the immediate supervisor.
- If the employee is not satisfied with the supervisor's response, within a week of the meeting he or she may complete a simple appeal form (obtained from human resources) and schedule a meeting with the appropriate department head (the manager to whom the supervisor reports). If the department head is the immediate supervisor, this step and the following step are omitted.

- Within 2 weeks the department head will review all facts and circumstances, investigating as necessary, and render a decision in writing on the appeal form.
- If not satisfied with the department head's response, the employee may take the appeal to the member of administration to whom the department head reports. As in the previous step, within 2 weeks the administrative representative will render a decision in writing.
- If the employee remains unsatisfied with the response, the appeal is then taken to the director of human resources, who will convene a three-party ad hoc appeal committee consisting of one staff employee, one management employee, and one human resources representative. Within 2 weeks this committee will submit a confidential recommendation to the director of human resources.
- As necessary, the director of human resources will review the complaint and recommendation with administration or legal counsel for legal or other significant implications. Once cleared at this level, the recommendation becomes final and binding.
- The employee does, of course, have external options for appeal, such as the Equal Employment Opportunity Commission and the State Division of Human Rights. However, if the organization's representatives have applied the appeal procedure honestly and impartially, the chances of a successful external challenge are severely limited.

## Grievance Procedure

The word *appeal* was used throughout the foregoing procedure to differentiate the process from that which might be embodied in a collective bargaining agreement (union contract). Collective bargaining agreements invariably use the term *grievance* in the same sense that *appeal* might be used in a nonunion context. As in the nonunion appeal process, a union grievance procedure uses several steps that take the complaint up through succeeding levels of consideration. The essential differences arise from the involvement of union officials and perhaps outside arbitrators or mediators.

One form of grievance procedure is presented in **Appendix 10–A**, Sample Collective Bargaining Agreement. In that document, Article Fifteen covers the grievance procedure.

# ▶ The Labor Union and the Collective Bargaining Agreement

Since the National Labor Relations Act was amended in 1975 to remove the exemption of not-for-profit hospitals, workers in healthcare organizations have been permitted by federal law to organize into labor unions. The specific exemption of not-for-profit hospitals had been in place since 1947, so between 1947 and 1975 the only active union organizing that occurred in not-for-profit institutions was that made possible by the labor relations laws of a few states.

The typical collective bargaining agreement reflects management's and the union's efforts to contain and control conflict and provide a framework for the resolution of disagreement. Appendix 10–A contains a typical collective bargaining agreement. This sample agreement is included to provide the complete context of the formal relationship between employer and union. This sample agreement is a "bare bones" example. A union contract typically includes additional items covered under memoranda of understanding (MOAs). These MOAs are developed to clarify issues as they arise and to settle low-level conflict situations. They are also used to deal with issues that arise during the life of the contract. If the issues are of continuing concern, they are incorporated into the next contract, and/or next set of official work rules and/or employee handbook. For example, some workers are expected to be "always on," checking and responding to cellphone calls, texts, or e-mails even when they are off duty and are not in supervisory or management jobs. Another example reflects clarifications about fringe benefits. For example, does the childcare benefit cover only the parent of the child, or may a grandparent take this benefit for a grandchild for whom they are caring, although no formal guardianship designation has been made. Yet another example, is there a mileage reimbursement provision for workers who are detailed to alternate sites?

With specific reference to conflict both actual and potential, attention is called to the following articles:

- Articles Six and Seven, in which the contracting parties agree to the limitation of conflict during the life of the agreement
- Articles Fourteen and Fifteen, which provide for the orderly resolution of disciplinary actions and complaints by employees against management
- Articles Eight through Twenty, which address the specifics of working conditions, hours of work,

benefits of employment, and other employment-related matters in a manner intended to provide clear guidelines for practice and, therefore, to avoid conflict or minimize the chances of conflict occurring

Note also the provisions about union security. Traditional contract provisions fostered strong union membership by means of mandatory membership, or the payment of an agency fee by nonmembers. Over the years, individual state laws have been passed, prohibiting mandatory membership and agency fees (right-to-work laws). The 2018 Supreme Court decision, the Janus decision, limits a union's ability to charge agency fees for some categories of workers. Because unions face some weakening as a result of these factors, they continue to expand their own member benefits, including workforce retraining, and educational support (beyond what management provides.)

Although some members of the healthcare organization, especially managers and professionals, may find a collective bargaining agreement restrictive because of the apparent limitations it places on actions of various kinds, the overall clarity of the provisions in a well-written contract, plus the fact that the contract has been negotiated by management and workers together, so that both sides "own" the agreement, can sometimes foster positive organizational relationships. When the occasional conflict does occur, the provisions of the contract can guide its resolution.

# ▶ Labor Unions in Health Care: Trends and Indicators

Since the initial development of labor unions in health care in the 1970s, unions have become a permanent feature in the healthcare setting. Efforts to increase membership are an ongoing focus for any labor union. In healthcare settings, current outreach initiatives focus on home care workers, namely home health aides, noncredentialled caregivers, and housekeeping aides. With the growth of this type of care, there is a natural pool of potential new union members.

Why is unionization continuing to increase in health care, and why do some of the unions seem to be concentrating on healthcare employees? Consider the following factors:

- Healthcare employment is large and growing. Health care has long since passed manufacturing and is presently second only to government in number of employees. Large groups of non-unionized employees attract union attention.

- Health care has for several years been in an especially unsettled state. Mergers, acquisitions, closures, systems formation, and various downsizing activities have resulted in layoffs or displacements of employees as healthcare delivery patterns have changed. This unsettled state renders many employees susceptible to union overtures.

- Health care was once considered by many to be essentially recession-proof, but that is no longer the case. With all of the changes occurring in health care, employees have seen many of their fellow workers laid off as a result of the effects of the aforementioned circumstances plus the ever-tightening web of financial constraints placed on the healthcare system. There are now fears concerning job security where no such fears existed in the past.

- In numerous hospitals, cutbacks in staffing have raised nurses' concerns over both the safety of patients and the well-being of nurses themselves. Complaints about the effects of long shifts, extra shifts, and mandatory overtime have driven some nurses closer to unions, and the nurses' unions have taken up these staffing issues on their behalf.

Many of the foregoing circumstances, plus healthcare employees' concerns for other employment-related matters, are reflected in the issues emerging prominently in union contract negotiations. The industry is seeing—and for a while should continue seeing—discussions, disputes, and demands addressing the following issues:

- Job security, as new patterns of care delivery continue to evolve and uncertainty concerning continued employment prevails. The introduction of new technologies and the increased use of robots and AI along with increased use of outsourcing contribute to concerns about job security.

- The employer's share of the cost of employee health insurance. As health insurance rates continue climbing, employers are endeavoring to shift a greater portion of these costs to

employees—a move strongly resisted by employees and unions. In addition, there may be limits placed on the selection of providers, restricting choice to in-network, pre-approved providers.

- Pension plans and associated employer contributions to them, as organizations continue to abandon defined-benefit plans and increase their reliance on defined contribution plans, such as 401(k) plans.

- Staffing levels, especially from nurses but possibly from other professional groups as well.

- Pay rates, which are always a source of contention, although in many instances these concerns may be secondary to some of the other issues. As minimum wage requirements increase, workers with several years of employment may seek wage adjustments to offset the impact of newer workers' higher wage.

- Mandatory (or expected) overtime presents an issue for some employees who cannot easily accept additional hours because of family obligations.

- For long-term employees, vacation day accrual often has a set limit (e.g., 240 days). Rather than lose additional days, workers want to "cash out" some or all of these days for their dollar value.

- Disciplinary concerns such as those concomitant with the increased focus on sexual harassment, where workers want clarity about acceptable and unacceptable behavior, mandatory orientation and training, along with periodic updates about these issues. They want uniformity of application rather than variable interpretation from one unit or department to another.

Unions of all stripes—in health care and elsewhere—continue to work together to push a national legislative agenda. As noted above, there is continuing debate over the right of individuals to join or not join a union. The union's position is that, with strength in numbers, it is in a stronger negotiating position. Furthermore, benefits won by the union are enjoyed by all the workers in the designated work categories. Unions continue to seek limits on right-to-work laws and limits on agency fees.

A complete sample bargaining agreement is provided in Appendix 10–A.

# Appendix 10-A

## Sample Collective Bargaining Agreement

(Fictitious in all respects—for training use only to illustrate various aspects of contract agreement; assumption: sample hospital is located in a state that does not have a right-to-work law)

| Article | Content |
|---|---|
| One | Intent and Purpose |
| Two | Recognition |
| Three | Union Security |
| Four | No Discrimination |
| Five | Management Rights |
| Six | Union Activity |
| Seven | No Strike; No Lockout |
| Eight | Hours of Work and Overtime |
| Nine | Rate of Pay; Shift Differential |
| Ten | Probationary Employees |
| Eleven | Seniority; Layoffs and Promotion |
| Twelve | Safety and Health |
| Thirteen | Resignation |
| Fourteen | Discipline and Discharge |
| Fifteen | Grievance Procedure |
| Sixteen | Arbitration |
| Seventeen | Holidays |
| Eighteen | Vacation |
| Nineteen | Sick Leave |
| Twenty | Leave of Absence |
| Twenty-One | Insurance and Pensions |
| Twenty-Two | Terms of Agreement |

COLLECTIVE BARGAINING AGREEMENT BETWEEN JGL MEMORIAL HOSPITAL AND THE CLERICAL AND TECHNICAL HOSPITAL EMPLOYEES' GUILD OF GREATER NEW CITY METROPOLIS, AFL-CIO AND ITS AFFILIATE LOCAL 123B

This agreement dated January 4, 20N1, to be effective as of February 1, 20N1, is entered into between JGL Memorial Hospital (herein called the "Hospital") and Clerical and Technical Hospital Employees' Guild of Greater New City Metropolis AFL-CIO and its affiliate, Local 123B (herein called the "Union").

(Note: this fictitious hospital is a non-profit, privately sponsored institution.)

## ▶ Article One: Intent and Purpose

1.1 Whereas, the Hospital is engaged in furnishing an essential public service vital to the health, welfare, and safety of the community and more particularly of the patients seeking and receiving service at the hospital; and

Whereas, both the Hospital and its employees have a high degree of responsibility to provide such services without interruption of this essential service; and

Whereas, both parties recognize this mutual obligation, they have entered into this Agreement to promote and improve the mutual interests of the Hospital and its employees and to establish and maintain cooperation and harmony between the Hospital and its employees;

Therefore, in consideration of the mutual promises and obligations herein assumed, the parties agree as follows:

# ▶ Article Two: Recognition

2.1 The Hospital recognizes the Union as the sole collective bargaining Agency for all technical and clerical workers including messengers, mailroom workers, unit clerks, clerks and clerk typists, data entry staff, secretaries, and other technical workers as certified in the State labor relations board certification of December 11, 20N1.

2.2 The Unit specifically excludes supervisors, temporary workers, casual workers, and students.

2.3 Part-time work employees who work 20 or more hours per week shall be covered by the terms of this agreement on completion of the probationary period.

2.4 The number of part-time employees shall not exceed 5% of the total number of bargaining unit employees in each department as of February 1, 20N1. Temporary employees and students and independent contractual employees may not be hired for a period longer than 4 months per job per year.

# ▶ Article Three: Union Security

3.1 It shall be a condition of employment that all employees of the Hospital covered by this agreement who are members of the Union in good standing on the effective date of this agreement shall remain members in good standing and those who are not members on the effective date of this agreement shall, after the 60th day actually worked, following the date of signing this agreement, or its effective date, whichever is later, become and remain members in good standing in the Union. It shall also be a condition of employment that all employees covered by this agreement and hired on or after the date of signing or its effective date, whichever is later, shall, after the 60th day actually worked following such date, become and remain members in good standing in the Union.

3.2 The failure of any employee to become a member of the Union at the required time shall obligate the Hospital, on written notice from the Union to such effect and to the further effect that Union membership was available to such employee on the same terms and conditions generally available to other members, to forthwith discharge such employee. Furthermore, the failure of any employee to maintain his Union membership in good standing as required herein shall, on written notice to the Hospital by the Union to such effect, obligate the Hospital to discharge such employee. Following such notification to the Hospital, the employee shall be given a period of not more than 30 days during which he shall be given an opportunity to reestablish his membership in good standing with the Union. Management and union officials recognize the religious/conscience exemption from required membership and this provision does not apply to workers who claim this exemption.

3.3 The Union agrees that the payment of regular monthly membership dues and initiation fees shall constitute membership in good standing.

3.4 The Hospital shall for the term of this Agreement deduct union dues and initiation fees from such employees who are members of the Union and who individually and voluntarily notify the Hospital through written authorization to the Hospital for deductions from any wage paid to such employee. The Hospital agrees to make such deductions on the first payday of each month or at such other time as both the Hospital and the Union shall mutually agree and shall remit such monies promptly to the designated officer of the National Union. The Hospital shall supply the Union with a list of those employees for whom deductions were made and the amount of deductions per current month.

3.5 The Hospital will furnish the Union each month with the names; addresses; Social Security numbers; classification of work; dates of hires; names of terminated employees, together with their dates of termination; and the names of employees on leave of absence and specific kind of leave of absence. Employees shall promptly notify the Hospital of changes in their names and addresses.

3.6 The Union shall indemnify and save the Hospital harmless against any claims, demands, suits, and other forms of liability that may arise out of action taken or not taken by the Hospital for purposes of compliance with these provisions.

# ▶ Article Four: No Discrimination

4.1 There shall be no discrimination against or for an employee because of race, color, creed, national origin, political belief, sex, age, Union membership, or nonmembership by the Hospital or by the Union.

# ▶ Article Five: Management Rights

5.1 Unless expressly included in this Agreement, nothing herein contained shall be construed to limit the Hospital's right to exercise the functions of management under which it shall have, among others, the right to employ, supervise, and direct the working force; to discipline, suspend, and discharge employees for just cause; to transfer and lay off employees because of lack of work; to require employees to observe reasonable work rules and regulations not inconsistent with this Agreement; to determine the extent to which its properties, equipment, and facilities shall be maintained and/or operated or shut down; to introduce new or improved methods and/or procedures; to determine the services to be rendered to patients and the schedules of maintaining such services; and otherwise to manage or conduct the facility, provided that these provisions shall not be used for the sole purpose of depriving any Hospital employee of work. The above rights are not all inclusive, but indicate the type of matters or rights that belong to and are inherent to Management. Any of the rights, power, and authority the Hospital had prior to entering this collective bargaining agreement are retained by the Hospital except as expressly and specifically abridged, delegated, granted, or modified by this Agreement.

# ▶ Article Six: Union Activity

6.1 Except for Union activity expressly provided for in this agreement, no employee shall engage in any Union activity, including the distribution of literature, and mass e-mail or instant messaging alerts which could interfere with the performance of work during working time or in working areas at any time.

6.2 Union representatives (or designees) shall have reasonable access to the Hospital for the purpose of administering the provision of this agreement, provided they obtain clearance from the designated Hospital official, who shall not unduly restrict such access.

6.3 The Hospital will provide bulletin boards and internet access for Union use for the purpose of posting Union notices. Such bulletin boards shall be located at places readily accessible to the employees' place of work. The Union will be permitted to post on these boards and/or on the internet site such notices of a noncontroversial nature, copies to be submitted to the Labor Relations manager prior to posting.

6.4 The work schedules of employees elected as Union Delegates shall be adjusted so far as practicable as to permit attendance at regularly scheduled meetings after normal working hours, provided the Hospital's operations shall not be impaired. The Union shall give reasonable notice to the Labor Relations manager of such regularly scheduled meetings and the names of such delegates.

# ▶ Article Seven: No Strike; No Lockout

7.1 During the terms of this agreement, neither the Union nor the employees shall engage in any strike, sit-down, sit-in, slow-down, cessation, stoppage, interruption of work, boycott, or other interference with the operations of the Hospital.

7.2 The union, its officers, agents, representatives, and members shall not in any way, directly or indirectly, authorize, assist, encourage, participate in, or sanction any strike, sit-down, sit-in, slow-down, cessation or stoppage or interruption of work, or other interference of the operations of the Hospital, or ratify, condone, or lend support to any such conduct or action.

7.3 Should any strike, slow-down, picketing, or other curtailment, restriction, or interference with Hospital functions or operations occur that the Union has not caused or sanctioned either directly or indirectly, the Union shall immediately:

a. Publicly disavow such actions by the employees or persons involved.
b. Advise the Hospital in writing that such action has not been caused or sanctioned by the Union.
c. Post notices on the Union bulletin boards stating that it disapproves of such actions and instruct the members to return to work immediately.
d. Take such other steps as would reasonably ensure renewed observance of provisions of this Article.

7.4 The Hospital shall have the right to discharge or otherwise discipline all employees or the Union on their behalf without having recourse to the grievance procedure and arbitration, except for the sole purpose of determining whether an employee participated in the prohibited action.

7.5 During the terms of this Agreement, the Hospital shall not engage in any lockout of any employee.

## ▶ Article Eight: Hours of Work and Overtime

8.1 A period of 8 hours shall constitute a regular day's work, and 40 hours shall constitute a regular week's work in any one day or in any one week. A work day is defined as the continuous 24-hour period beginning at the employee's regular starting time.

8.2 All work performed by an employee in excess of 40 hours in any 1 week shall be paid for at the rate of time and one-half.

8.3 The Hospital shall distribute and allot overtime work to best suit the efficient operation of a department and will make every reasonable effort to distribute in a reasonable way the overtime work equitably among the employees of the department in which the overtime occurs, provided the employee is qualified to perform the work.

8.4 All employees shall receive a 1-hour paid lunch period, which shall be counted as time worked. The Hospital will schedule this lunch period.

8.5 There shall be no pyramiding or duplicating of overtime rates. Hours compensated for at overtime rates under one provision of this Agreement shall be excluded as hours worked in computing overtime under any other provision. When two or more provisions requiring the payment of overtime rates are applicable, the one most favorable to the employee shall apply.

8.6 Employees shall be required to work overtime when assigned for the proper administration of the Hospital's operations.

## ▶ Article Nine: Rates of Pay; Shift Differentials

9.1 Job classifications and rates of pay and progression in existence on the day of this agreement are set forth in the Job Classification and Wage Scale which is made part of this agreement.

9.2 If during the term of this Agreement new job classifications are established or substantial changes are made in existing job classifications covered by the bargaining unit, the Hospital will put the new or changed job classification into effect and establish a rate of pay therefor. Such rate will be discussed with the Union in advance, with the objective of obtaining its agreement. The Hospital may then install the rate

with or without agreement; when installed after agreement, no grievance may be filed with respect to the rate. If installed without agreement, the employee(s) affected or the Union may within 30 days present a grievance protesting the rate if that rate does not bear a proper relationship to existing rates. If no grievance is filed within the 30 days or if the grievance is settled, the new rate will become part of the Job Classification and Wage Scale and shall not be subject to challenge under the grievance procedure.

9.3 Full-time employees working on a shift that begins on or after 3:00 P.M., and before 4:00 A.M., shall be paid a shift differential of ($n$ amount) per hour. An employee who is entitled to a shift differential for work on his regular shift shall receive the shift differential for overtime hours that are an extension of the regular shift. A shift differential shall not be paid when employees are authorized to exchange shifts temporarily for personal reasons.

9.4 A shift differential shall not be gained or lost as a result of an extension of a shift caused by overtime.

9.5 If an employee is regularly assigned to a shift receiving a shift differential, the differential shall be included in calculating the employee's vacation, holiday, and sick leave pay.

## ▶ Article Ten: Probationary Employees

10.1 New employees and those hired after a break in continuity of service of more than 6 months will be regarded as probationary employees until they have actually worked 60 days and will receive no continuous service credit during such period. During this period of probationary employment, probationary employees may be disciplined, laid off, or discharged as exclusively determined by the Hospital, and the Hospital shall not be subject to the grievance and arbitration provision of this Agreement.

Continuing employees who apply for and are accepted into another job/position are considered probationary employees for 25 working days. See Article 11.9 for related stipulations.

10.2 The rate of pay for new employees and those hired after a break in continuity of service of more than 6 months shall be the hiring rate for the job. The rate of pay for continuing employees shall be the grade level rate of pay.

# ▶ Article Eleven: Seniority; Layoffs and Promotions

11.1 Seniority is defined as an employee's length of continuous regular full-time Hospital service last date of hire. Employees who were hired the same day shall have their seniority established by lot and carried subsequently on the seniority list.

11.2 Seniority is computed from the day of last hire, on completion of the probationary period delineated in Article Ten.

11.3 Seniority shall accrue
a. During any authorized leave of absence with pay
b. During an authorized leave of absence without pay because of personal illness or accident for a period of 6 months or less, or maternity leave for a period of 1 year
During military service, as provided by federal law, an employee will not accrue, but will not lose, seniority during an authorized leave of absence without pay.

11.4 An employee will lose seniority when he/she
a. Voluntarily terminates his or her full-time employment
b. Is discharged for cause
c. Willfully exceeds the length, or violates the purpose, of an authorized leave of absence
d. Is laid off for a period of 6 months or the length of the employee's service with the Hospital, whichever is less
e. Fails to report in accordance with a notice for recall from layoff within 48 hours of the time specified in the notice sent by certified mail to the last address furnished to the Hospital by the employee. The Hospital shall send a copy of the notification to the Union.
f. Fails to report for recall to the assigned job
An absence from work for three consecutive work days without notice or permission shall be deemed a voluntary resignation.

11.5 An employee who is or has been promoted or transferred out of the bargaining unit and who is later transferred back into the bargaining unit by the Hospital shall be credited on returning to the bargaining unit with the seniority he /she would have had if he/she had remained continuously in the bargaining unit.

11.6 In the event of a layoff in a department, temporary employees shall be laid off first, then probationary employees, then regular part-time employees, and then regular full-time employees on the basis of their Hospital-wide seniority. In the event a full-time permanent nonprobationary employee is scheduled to be laid off from a department, he or she may either bid for a posted vacant position in accordance with the provisions of Section 7 or displace another employee within the department of equal or lesser grade on the basis of Hospital-wide seniority, provided he has the ability to perform said job within 25 working days. The immediate department manager shall determine the employee's acceptability.

11.7 Employees on layoff shall be recalled as follows:
a. To a position, if open, previously held successfully in department by the employee regardless of place on the recall list
b. In reverse order of layoff on a Hospital-wide basis to other open positions with the following provisions:
   1. Employees may not upgrade from the recall list.
   2. The employee must be acceptable to the hiring supervisor.
   3. The employee must have the ability to perform the open position. The hiring supervisor shall determine the employee's acceptability for that position during the applicable probationary period for a newly hired employee in that grade level.
   4. When probationary or part-time employees are laid off, they shall have no recall rights.

11.8 Promotional opportunities
a. Openings for bargaining unit positions shall be posted for five (5) work days.
b. Employees within a department will be given preference for promotion to a higher-paying job in the department.
c. All bids must be submitted in person and in writing to the Office of Human Resources within the five (5) work days.
d. An open position shall be defined as a position that has been posted and for which no acceptable bidders have been found.
e. An employee who has been promoted in pay grades six (6) to ten (10) shall not be eligible for further promotion for six (6) months.
f. An employee who has accepted a promotional opportunity shall have twenty-five (25) working days to prove that he or she can perform in the new position.
g. An employee who has accepted a promotional opportunity and fails the probationary period shall return to his or her previous position. If this position has been filled, the employee may be offered an open equivalent position. If none is

available, the disqualified employee shall be laid off, subject to recall according to the provisions of Section 11.7.

11.9 The rate of pay during the probationary period is that of the grade level of the job.

# ▸ Article Twelve: Safety and Health

12.1 The Hospital agrees to provide reasonable safeguards on the premises for the health and safety of its employees. Two employees from the bargaining unit mutually agreed on by the Hospital and the Union shall serve on the Hospital Safety Committee.

# ▸ Article Thirteen: Resignation

13.1 An employee who resigns shall give the Hospital 2 weeks advance written notice.

13.2 An employee who fails to give such notice or whose employment is terminated shall forfeit unused vacation time, provided it was physically possible for the employee to give such notice.

# ▸ Article Fourteen: Discipline and Discharge

14.1 No employee who has completed his or her probationary period shall be discharged or disciplined without just cause. If disciplinary action becomes necessary in the interest of proper operation of the Hospital, care of the patients, and general employee welfare, such actions of the Hospital shall be subject to the grievance procedure. The Hospital agrees to furnish copies to the Union of disciplinary notices resulting in suspension or discharge of an employee.

14.2 Any grievance resulting from action taken as outlined in the preceding section must be filed in writing according to the grievance procedure outlined in Article Fifteen.

# ▸ Article Fifteen: Grievance Procedure

15.1 Any grievance that may arise between the parties concerning the application, meaning, or interpretation of this Agreement shall be resolved in the following manner:

Step 1. An employee having a grievance and his Union delegate shall discuss it with his /her immediate department head within five (5) working days after it arose or should have been made known to the employee. The Hospital shall give its response through the department head to the employee and to his or her Union delegate within five (5) working days after the presentation of the grievance. In the event no appeal is taken to the next step (Step 2), the decision rendered in this step shall be final.

Step 2. If the grievance is not settled in Step 1, the grievance may, within five (5) working days after the answer in Step 1, be presented in Step 2. When grievances are presented in Step 2, they shall be reduced to writing on grievance forms provided by the Hospital (which shall then be assigned a number by the Office of Human Resources at the Union's request) signed by the grievant and his or her Union representative, and presented to the Department Head and the Department of Human Resources. A grievance so presented in Step 2 shall be answered in writing within five (5) working days after its presentation.

Step 3. If the grievance is not settled in Step 2, the grievance may within five (5) working days after the answer in Step 2, be presented in Step 3. A grievance shall be presented in this step to the Office of Human Resources. The Office of Human Resources shall hold a hearing within five (5) days and shall thereafter render a decision in writing within 5 days.

15.2 Failure on the part of the Hospital to answer a grievance at any step shall not be deemed acquiescence thereto, and the Union may proceed to the next step.

15.3 An employee who has been suspended or discharged, or the Union on his behalf, may file within five (5) business days of the suspension or discharge a grievance in writing in respect thereof with the Office of Human Resources at Step 3 of the foregoing Grievance Procedure. Any prior written warnings applicable to the employee shall be mailed to the Union by the Hospital within five (5) working days after the employee is notified of his or her discharge.

15.4 All time limits herein specified shall be deemed to be exclusive of Saturdays, Sundays, and holidays.

15.5 Any disposition of a grievance from which no appeal is taken within the time limits specified herein shall be deemed resolved and shall not thereafter be considered subject to the grievance and arbitration provisions of this Agreement.

15.6 A grievance that affects a substantial number of a class of employees may initially be presented at Step 2 or Step 3 by the Union. The grievance shall then be processed in accordance with the Grievance Procedure.

# ▶ Article Sixteen: Arbitration

16.1 A grievance that has not been resolved may, within ten (10) working days after completion of Step 3 of the Grievance Procedure, be referred for arbitration by the Hospital or the Union to the designated official arbitration association for resolution under the rules of arbitration currently in effect.

16.2 The fees and expenses of the arbitration association and the arbitrator shall be borne equally by the parties.

16.3 The award of an arbitrator hereunder shall be final, conclusive, and binding on the Hospital, the Union, and the employees.

16.4 The arbitrator shall have jurisdiction only over grievances after completion of the Grievance Procedure, and he or she shall have no power to add to, subtract from, or modify in any way any of the terms of this Agreement.

# ▶ Article Seventeen: Holidays

17.1 The following days are recognized as paid holidays for full-time and part-time employees who have completed their first 25 working days of employment:

| | |
|---|---|
| New Year's Day | Martin Luther King, Jr. Day |
| Memorial Day | Labor Day |
| Independence Day | Thanksgiving Day |
| Christmas Day | Presidents' Day |

Two additional days that may be scheduled in accordance with the employee's preference.

17.2 The additional days shall be taken at a mutually agreeable time and shall be requested in writing at least five (5) working days in advance. Once scheduled, these days shall not be canceled by an employee without the consent of the Hospital. These additional days must be taken within the calendar year and are not cumulative.

17.3 Employees shall receive their regular rate of pay for each holiday observed, provided they are on active pay status.

17.4 To be eligible for holiday benefits, an employee must have worked the last scheduled work day before and the first scheduled work day after the holiday (or the day scheduled in place of the holiday) except in the case of accident or illness preventing employee from working. The Hospital may require a written certificate from a physician or other proof.

17.5 If a holiday falls during an employee's regularly scheduled day off, the employee shall receive an additional day off or an additional day's pay, as the Hospital may decide.

17.6 If an employee is required to work on a holiday, he shall be compensated at $2\frac{1}{2}$ times his or her regular rate of pay for time worked or shall be given a compensatory day off at regular rate of pay, as determined by the Hospital. An employee shall not be considered as working on a holiday if the shift he/she is working started prior to the holiday.

17.7 If the holiday falls during an employee's vacation, he shall receive an extra day's pay or an extra day off with pay, as the Hospital shall decide.

# ▶ Article Eighteen: Vacation

18.1 Employees shall be granted vacation with pay according to the following schedule; vacation pay rate will be at the current straight hourly rate, including shift differential, for the number of hours indicated.

| Period of Uninterrupted Service | Vacation Pay | |
|---|---|---|
| One (1) year | 10 working days | 80 hours |
| Five (5) years | 12 working days | 96 hours |
| Six (6) years | 13 working days | 104 hours |
| Seven (7) years | 14 working days | 112 hours |
| Eight (8) years | 15 working days | 120 hours |
| Nine (9) years | 16 working days | 128 hours |
| Twenty (20) years | 20 working days | 160 hours |

18.2 Employees whose vacations occur during a period in which a holiday occurs shall receive an extra day's pay for the holiday, or an extra day off with pay, as the Hospital shall decide.

18.3 Employees must take their vacations during the 12-month period following their vacation eligibility year. No vacations may be carried over and employees will not be compensated for vacation time not taken.

No part of an employee's scheduled vacation may be charged to sick leave.

18.4 Vacations shall be scheduled by the Hospital, in order to meet the staffing needs of the Hospital. Insofar as practicable, vacations will be granted to meet the requests of employees. Employees in each department with the greatest seniority shall have first choice of vacation period. The Hospital maintains the right to limit the number of employees permitted to be on vacation at any one time. The Hospital reserves the right to change the vacation schedule as needed.

18.5 Employees shall submit their vacation request to their Department Head in writing at least 2 weeks before date of desired period of vacation.

18.6 On written request 2 weeks in advance, an employee will be paid his or her vacation pay before starting vacation.

18.7 Employees who give 2 weeks' notice of voluntary termination and employees terminated involuntarily shall be entitled to accrued vacation pay.

## ▶ Article Nineteen: Sick Leave

19.1 "Sick leave" is defined as the absence of an employee from work by reason of illness or accident that is not work connected or is not compensable under the workers' compensation laws of the state. Full-time workers are paid for an 8-hour day; part-time workers are paid for a 4-hour day.

19.2 Eligibility and Benefits. An employee who has completed his or her probationary period is eligible for one (1) day of sick leave earned at the rate of the said day for each full month of continuous service retroactive to his or her date of hire but not to exceed a total of 10 days for any 1 year. As of July 1 of each year, employees with at least 1 year of service shall be credited with 10 days of sick leave.

19.3 Unused sick leave may be accumulated up to a maximum of 150 days. Unused sick leave will not be compensated on termination.

19.4 Pay for any day of approved sick leave shall be paid at the employee's regular rate of pay.

19.5 Employees with accumulated paid sick leave will continue to earn vacation while out on paid sick leave. Holidays falling within an employee's paid sick leave will be treated as a holiday, and a sick leave day will not be charged to that day. An employee cannot receive both holiday pay and sick leave pay for the same day.

19.6 To be eligible for the benefits of this Article, an employee must notify his or her supervisor at least 1 hour before the start of his or her regularly scheduled work day unless proper excuse is presented for the employee's inability to call. The Hospital may require written certification by a physician or other proof of illness or accident. Employees who wish to return to work after sick leave may be required to be examined by a physician designated by the Hospital before returning to work.

## ▶ Article Twenty: Leave of Absence

20.1 Maternity leave, military leave, funeral leave, and jury duty shall be the same as described in the Employee Handbook (November 20N1 revision) and shall remain in effect and may not be reduced during the life of this contract.

## ▶ Article Twenty-One: Insurance and Pension

21.1 The provisions for life insurance, health and accident insurance, pension plan, and related benefits outlined in the Employee Handbook (November 20N1 revision) shall remain in effect and may not be reduced during the life of this agreement.

## ▶ Article Twenty-Two: Terms of Agreement

22.1 This Agreement constitutes the entire agreement between parties until and including January 20, 20N3, and shall continue in full force and effort from year to year thereafter unless and until either of the parties hereto shall give to the other party notice in accordance with applicable law, but in no case less than 60 days prior to expiration of the contract. Such notice shall be given in writing.

IN WITNESS THEREOF, the parties hereto have hereunto set their hands and seals.

# Notes

1. David L. Cooperrider, Peter F. Sorensen Jr., Diana Whitney, and Therese F. Yaeger, eds. *Appreciative Inquiry: Rethinking Human Organization Toward a Positive Theory of Change* (Champaign, IL: Stipes Publishing, 2000).

2. Portions of this section are adapted from C. R. McConnell, *The Effective Health Care Supervisor*, 8th ed. (Burlington, MA: Jones & Bartlett Learning, 2015), Chapter 25, "Reengineering and Reduction in Force," 466–472.

## CHAPTER 11

# Communication: The Glue That Binds Us Together

## CHAPTER OBJECTIVES

- Provide a working definition of communication.
- Address the manager's critical role in employee communication.
- Review the common means of communication used in the work setting.
- Provide guidelines for the proper use of electronic mail (e-mail) and social media.
- Examine the components of individual and small-group communication, including verbal (oral) and nonverbal communication.
- Enumerate the essential components of successful interpersonal communication.
- Review means of fostering, enhancing, and improving interpersonal communication and overcoming barriers to individual communication.
- Provide guidelines for personal improvement in using written communication in its various forms.
- Present the fundamentals of organization communication, including both formal and informal communication.
- Differentiate between formal and informal communication in the organizational setting.
- Review the commonly encountered barriers to effective communication in the organizational setting.

## ▶ A Complex Process

It is necessary to begin this discussion with an important disclaimer: what follows is no more than a once-over-easy treatment, an effort to hit the high spots of a topic of extreme importance to every manager—professional or otherwise. Each heading and subheading in this section could be the subject of an entire text in its own right and yet leave much unaddressed. This section provides an introduction to the basics of communication within the healthcare organization as experienced from the perspective of the individual manager.

In a relatively large healthcare organization—for example, the average hospital—decisions are frequently presented as orders or instructions, and members whose activities are affected are expected to comply with those directives. Organizational roles may be specialized, and much communication occurs through relatively formal channels such as memos, policies, procedures, or regulations.

In a relatively small organization such as a group medical practice of fewer than 20 employees, the communications environment may be considerably different. In the small organization, work roles overlap and are likely to be far less specialized. In this setting, communication is less formal and the opportunity for the direct sharing of information is greater than in a large organization. Formal communication in the small organization may be minimal. The single factor of size can influence the quality and kinds of communication employed within an organization.

There are, however, many factors other than organization size to consider. Communication is a complex process, requiring particular skills on both individual and group levels. Also, as an individual interacts with more and more people, the overall complexity of the interactions increases. Whether considered in an individual or organizational context, communication is a far more complex process than many at first imagine. Therefore, to be optimally successful, communication requires conscious effort by managers.

Communication may be described as the exchange of ideas, thoughts, or emotions between or among two or more people. It may be literally described as the transfer of meaning or, in a somewhat broader sense, the development of mutual understanding. Concerning the transfer of meaning, the intent is to take information that exists in a specific form in one person's mind and ensure that it is duplicated in another's mind. In the broader sense, the development of mutual understanding, the intent is for two or more people to share whatever information they have about a specific subject and arrive at an agreed-on meaning, whether that meaning is an opinion, a decision, or a course of action.

From the perspective of the individual manager, communication in the organizational setting ranges from the highly informal to the strictly formal, from on-the-run spoken remarks to structured presentations, from quick e-mail, text message, or voice mail messages to formal reports, and from one-on-one contacts to the necessity to address large groups. In other words, as experienced by the individual manager, communication in the organizational setting can occur in nearly any form or format.

## ▶ Communication and the Individual Manager

Many of the problems encountered in communicating with others arise because the majority of human beings take their communications capacity for granted. After all, communication is basic to all human activity. Except when asleep, most people are usually in one of four fundamental communicating modes: talking or writing (i.e., sending information out) or reading or hearing (i.e., receiving information). Note that the fourth mode is identified as hearing rather than listening, suggesting the source of a great many problems and misunderstandings—one can hear without truly listening. In any case, one who is awake is in one of the four fundamental communicating modes, with hearing being the "default" mode.

Whether in the workplace or any place, people cannot function adequately without communicating. For the individual manager, communication in any of several forms is essentially constant. Consider communication in the context of the essential management functions of planning, decision making, organizing, staffing, directing, coordinating, and controlling. Once formulated, plans and related decisions must be communicated in a form appropriate to the situation. To be complete, organizing, staffing, coordinating, and controlling all require communication. Also, the basic function of directing is itself largely communication. Truly, communication holds everything together.

In their day-to-day activities, managers must be involved in communication in one form or another for the following reasons, among others:

- Receiving orders, instructions, and direction from above
- Delivering orders, instructions, and direction to employees
- Coaching, counseling, and disciplining employees as necessary
- Interviewing and selecting candidates for employment
- Relating to managers and employees of other departments
- Relating to patients, visitors, clients, customers, vendors, and others from outside as necessary
- Reporting to higher management on departmental activities
- Responding to questions and requests coming from any of a number of sources

Depending on the situation, the manager's communication under the foregoing various circumstances might be spoken or written, or formal or informal. In addition, it might make use of any of several common communications practices or media, which are described (along with the significant advantages and disadvantages of each) in the following subsections.

### Face-to-Face

Face-to-face interaction is potentially the strongest means of communication available to the manager. The word "potentially" is appropriate here, however, because far too many face-to-face contacts are neither efficient nor effective. Properly used, the face-to-face contact has some important characteristics going for it. A message is transmitted not only in words but also with vocal tone and facial expression and other body language. Because it occurs in the here and now, the opportunity for feedback is immediate; questions and answers can flow back and forth until understanding is achieved. Properly used, the face-to-face contact is the most effective means of fulfilling most of the communication needs that arise during the workday: it appeals to multiple senses, offers immediacy of feedback and response, and ensures the maximum likelihood of establishing mutual understanding.

The disadvantages of this method are few. Face-to-face contact is frequently more time-consuming than other means because it involves bringing the parties together physically. Because it is immediate, there is always some risk of instant disagreement. Also—and this may be a minor consideration in most instances but once in a while can become extremely important—there is no physical record resulting from the conversation unless positive steps are taken to create one.

## The Telephone

As an aid to business communication, the telephone offers several advantages. A telephone call provides for immediate feedback and response; views can be exchanged, and mutual understanding can be achieved without delays between messages. A message comes through not only as words themselves but also as vocal tone and general manner of speaking. And for many purposes, the telephone is faster than most other means.

Consider, though, what is lost in using a telephone call instead of meeting face-to-face. What can often be a significant part of one's "message"—facial expressions and other body language—are completely lacking. Because one's body language is not always communicating the same message as the words one uses, the telephone call is generally less reliable than the face-to-face conversation. Technological advances that provide visual elements to telecommunication partly overcome this disadvantage. One additional consideration relates to making a record of the transaction. Unless a record is deliberately created or a call is recorded, there is no official record of the transaction. Reminder: permission to record or a notice that the conversation is being recorded is customary, and, in some states, required.

## Voice Mail

Voice mail represents the telephone call with one critical omission: immediacy of feedback and response, extremely important in interpersonal communication, is absent. A clear advantage of voice mail, when it is frequently accessed, is speed of transmission; a message is quickly left in a voice mail box, and the originator moves on to other matters. (Undoubtedly some also see it as an "advantage" to speak to a voice mail system rather than a live person; when delivering bad news, criticism, or something controversial, many a caller is happy to simply "drop it and run.") One clear advantage of voice mail is that many issues can be successfully addressed via messages and responses without the parties having to connect directly.

One disadvantage, of course, lies in having to wait for someone to respond to a message. Also, as noted, there is no immediacy of feedback and response, so voice mail is a still weaker means of communication than the telephone. Again, there is no record unless positive steps are taken to create one.

## Letters and Memos

When a communication takes the form of a letter or memo, everything has been removed except the words themselves. There is no vocal tone, facial expression, or body movement; there is no immediacy of feedback and response. The words are made to carry the entire message, so to do so with reasonable accuracy the words must be well thought out. The primary advantage of a letter or memo is the creation of a record that can be read again, shared with others, and retained in a file. Also, the permanent record is often important because of legal implications.

The principal disadvantage, as already noted, is the absence of all the dimensions of an effective communication except the words themselves. Another disadvantage lies in time; it invariably takes longer to write an effective letter or memo than to use most other means. Other disadvantages include the dislike of writing shared by many in the workforce and the carelessness with which some apply the written word.

Written communication is addressed further in a later section of this chapter.

## E-mail and Instant Messaging

E-mail and instant messaging have probably become the most actively used means of message transmission, for messages both from person to person and from individuals or groups to other individuals or groups. In some respects, however, it is one of the weaker means of communication available. Response to an e-mail is generally faster than response to a letter or memo, but as with letters and memos, e-mail is dependent on words only. And often—although certainly not always—e-mail messages are prepared with considerably less care than their paper counterparts and are thus more susceptible to misinterpretation.

E-mail and text messaging are rapid as far as message transmission is concerned, and feedback can—but does not reliably—occur quickly. The availability of instant messaging offers very nearly the same advantages as the telephone call.

Other aspects of e-mail and social media are addressed later in this discussion of communication.

Consideration of the characteristics of these several communication methods provides some guidance for structuring one's communications according to need. That is, the means chosen for a particular communication may be governed by the following considerations:

- The time available—that is, how quickly resolution is needed
- The importance of the issue
- The complexity of the issue
- The sensitivity of the issue
- The need for negotiation or problem solving
- The need for documentation (a paper trail)

# ▶ Verbal (Oral) Communication

Spoken communication, which may be correctly referred to as either "oral" or "verbal" communication, is of critical importance in all aspects of health care. The practitioner and the client need to understand each other's thoughts and ideas. An oral exchange includes the voice (its tone, such as friendly and supportive or crisp and blunt, accents, speed or pace of speaking). Content, such as the choice of words, degree of formality, level of technical detail, and specificity of instructions, is another factor. Pauses, the use of silence and nonverbal cues (nodding, hand gestures), are additional elements to note. Some of these factors (such as voice quality) are genetic, and certain others (such as speed of speech) are cultural. Health practitioners must also understand that their professional education has trained them to express ideas in a selective fashion.

The unconscious aspects of verbal communication are frequently overlooked.

## Nonverbal Communication

Nonverbal communication is included in the discussion of verbal communication because the two are inseparable parts of many interpersonal exchanges. Nonverbal communication, both intentional (conscious) and spontaneous (unconscious), augments the verbal exchange. Body language includes nodding, hand gestures, facial expression, the "knowing look or glance," physical distance between the individuals, and posture.

## Components of Communication

Communication includes four principal components: initiation, transmission, reception, and feedback. For communication to occur, there must be a sender, someone who begins the interaction. Initiation, which includes the preparation for the interaction, might begin on a nonverbal level and move to a verbal exchange. Transmission is the movement of the communication from one party to another; it depends on verbal and nonverbal sharing methods. Reception is the manner in which the message is received. The receiver's perception shapes the way in which a message is decoded and acted on. To ensure that the sender and the receiver are truly sharing ideas, the receiver offers feedback, which is a verbal or nonverbal signal that acknowledges the message. Acknowledgments include modification, suppression, or nonacceptance of the information.

Interpersonal communication depends on assumptions, perceptions, feelings, past experiences, and present surroundings. Although people frequently talk, communication may prove taxing and difficult. People must transcend personal and cultural barriers that obstruct their understanding of an exchange.

## Methods of Improving Communication

Communication is improved by observing, attending, responding to requests, and checking information. Each of these strategies depends on an objective analysis of an exchange.

Observation is the activity of perceiving events, objects, and people. Skilled observers are objective. Accurate observation is dependent on self-knowledge, because inner reality can make someone "see" an event that did not occur. An event can be "real" in the mind of the person who really wants to "see" it.

Attending helps people hear or see events as they are. During a conversation, instead of planning their next remark, those who are attending direct their energy toward listening or empathizing with the other person. Attending is also referred to as active listening.

Responding is the behavior an individual selects to address the needs or requests of the other person. The behavior may be verbal or nonverbal, and the quality of the response shapes the remainder of the communication. If a person asks for the time and receives a pleasant answer, that person may decide to continue the exchange. In contrast, unpleasant replies may inhibit further communication.

Communication is also improved by checking information through repeating with exactitude, paraphrasing, and/or asking for feedback.

## Communication Barriers

Communication can be blocked by internal or external forces. Internal forces, including both conscious and unconscious thoughts, may preclude listening, sharing, and caring so that the meaning of the exchange is confused and misinterpreted. Conscious behaviors that limit communication include facial expressions that are perceived as negative or inappropriate (e.g., smiling when reprimanding a subordinate), body postures that are perceived as rejecting or critical of the person (e.g., folding one's arms over one's chest although expressing a desire to share ideas), verbalizations that interrupt the flow of the exchange (e.g., saying "Terrific!" or "Great!" every time a speaker pauses), and interruption or disruption of the speaker's thoughts (e.g., changing topics abruptly, such as interrupting a request for assistance with a comment about football scores; going off on a tangent).

External forces may also impede communication. Distractions, such as noise, motion, and confusion, may compromise the quality of an exchange. The context for a communication may either add to or subtract from the interaction. For example, a crowded room with flashing lights and loud music is designed for sensory stimulation, not verbal communication. In this environment, intimate conversations are taxed and labored; communication is limited to nonverbal cueing.

## Speaking to Groups

Much of a department manager's verbal communication—surely an overwhelming majority for most first-line managers—involves one-on-one, face-to-face interchanges with individuals or with collectives of perhaps two or three people at most. There are, however, regularly occurring needs for the manager to address larger groups, such as an entire department or perhaps the organization's management group. Speaking before groups is unavoidable, yet some managers who do very well in face-to-face situations experience considerable problems with addressing groups. This is unfortunate because public-speaking ability is extremely important to the career-minded manager who wishes to advance in an organization.

The following story suggests the value of a manager's capacity for public speaking. To afford all managers with some development opportunity, the administrator of a small community hospital established the practice of rotating the chairmanship of the

monthly meeting of the facility's 24 or 25 managers. Given a broad outline, each manager would develop a specific agenda and chair the meeting, making the month's announcements and calling on other participants as needed. It was believed that experience with speaking and with leading meetings could be acquired as painlessly as possible in this friendly, familiar setting in which everyone knew one another.

On the day when the supervisor of the hospital's small business office was to chair the meeting, she called in sick. Having missed her turn, she was assigned the next month's meeting; that time she scheduled a day off for personal business. When spoken with privately by the administrator, she admitted her intense fear of public speaking. When asked how she conducted department meetings, she pointed out that with just three employees other than herself a department meeting was more like four friends getting together. She declared she could not possibly address a group as large as the management team. Over the following few weeks she resisted all of the administrator's efforts to get her some assistance in overcoming her fear. She claimed that the mere thought of speaking to a group made her physically ill.

Shortly thereafter, the hospital's board of directors voted in favor of a merger with another, slightly larger, community hospital. Most department managers from the two facilities were put in the position of having to compete for the resulting single position for each combined department. The process involved having each pair of managers prepare proposals describing how they would administer the combined department; each proposal was to be presented orally before the administrators and senior managers of both facilities, a group of five or six in total.

As one might expect at this point in the story, the supervisor who feared speaking was not chosen to head the combined department. She did everything possible to duck the appearance, and, when essentially trapped into it, delivered a brief, stammering start before excusing herself, pleading illness.

The person who was chosen as the department head was actually her equal in education and qualifications and had less experience. Yet the fearful speaker accepted a staff position in the combined department in the knowledge that she would probably never return to management.

At the very least, every group supervisor and department manager will have to conduct meetings of his or her own staff. In most organizations, it is also likely that from time to time one will also have to present a proposal or deliver an oral report to a management team or perhaps even to an administrative group or board of directors. Any person who dodges assignments that involve speaking had best appreciate that doing so is decidedly a career-limiting practice.

It should not be news for many readers to learn that fear of public speaking is both common and widespread; it is one of the most frequently encountered fears in the population at large. However, it may be news to most to learn that the majority of individuals who regularly, capably, and comfortably speak before groups of people once struggled with this same fear. To be sure, some natural speakers may be encountered now and then—fortunate individuals who never had reservations about addressing many people at one time. But these natural speakers are a minority. Most people who regularly speak in public had to overcome a certain amount of apprehension about doing so.

The keys to success in public speaking are preparation, practice, and repetition. Preparation should always go without saying; there are not a great many speakers who can go in cold and simply "wing it," especially on an important topic. Preparation—knowing what one will say and how it will be said—helps moderate the uneasiness felt by the new speaker. Practice simply makes sense, at least for the inexperienced speaker; it also helps quell the new speaker's apprehensions. The most significant key, however, is repetition. For most people, the more public speaking you do, the better you become at it; also, the more speaking you do, the less fearful you become about speaking. Getting started requires preparation and practice, and getting better and becoming less fearful and more confident require preparation and repetition.

## The Meeting

Meetings, particularly those of smaller groups, are where most managers acquire their early experience in both speaking to groups and leading discussions. For convenience, we can consider the department manager's meetings as being of two kinds: staff meetings and general meetings (all others). Staff meetings are those the manager convenes with his or her own employees. General meetings include problem-solving meetings or meetings held for various other purposes with people from a variety of departments or activities.

### The Staff Meeting

The manager has considerable flexibility in determining how and when staff meetings are scheduled, how they are conducted, and what is covered at them. Some managers find it advisable to bring the staff together on a weekly basis; some do so monthly and occasionally even less frequently. Staff meetings may

take different forms: Sometimes it is necessary for the manager to carry most of the meeting for providing information and updates, sometimes it is appropriate to have each staff member report on his or her recent activities, and sometimes one or two staff members will provide most of the meeting's substance. Regardless of frequency or form, however, some fundamentals should be observed:

- Employees should expect staff meetings to occur on some regular, planned frequency (except for the occasional emergency meeting).
- Staff meetings should occur; there should be only a few special circumstances under which a meeting is skipped or canceled. (For activities in certain professional areas, regular meetings—and minutes thereof—are a requirement of regulatory and accreditation bodies.)
- Staff should be advised that meetings will start on time, that starting will not be delayed for the sake of latecomers, and that information will not be repeated for latecomers.
- Meeting length should be limited, holding to specific starting and quitting times. Ending early is fine if all pertinent business has been transacted, but ending late should occur only under exceptional circumstances and then as seldom as possible.
- The meeting leader—assuming that this person is the department manager—should not dominate the meeting but rather make every effort to secure employee participation.
- If decisions are made or specific subsequent actions are required, they should be committed to writing.

### The General Meeting

Every manager should expect to become involved in specially scheduled meetings held for a variety of purposes—information sharing, exploratory discussion, problem solving, and so on—as both meeting convener and participant. Specific guidelines for calling and holding such meetings are as follows:

- Define the issue or problem and determine whether a meeting is truly required. Depending on the number of people who must be involved, the required timing, and other means of communication available, it might be possible to avoid a meeting. The most efficient meeting is the meeting that never takes place.
- Determine a goal for the meeting, deciding what must be accomplished. It is necessary to be able to identify what one desires from the

meeting—the solution to a problem, a group decision, the group's acceptance of an idea, or whatever.

- Select the participants, taking care to include the people who have the necessary knowledge of the topic and those who have the authority to commit to a solution, if this is necessary.
- Give participants sufficient advance notice—no last-minute surprises that create conflicts—and distribute needed materials, if any, along with the initial notice (it is highly inefficient to wait until meeting time to provide handout material pertinent to the meeting).
- Make certain a proper meeting area is secured well in advance of the meeting; it can be highly frustrating to have a group ready to meet with no place to gather.
- Prepare an agenda. It need not be elaborate; a brief list of points to cover will usually suffice.
- Start the meeting on time and reiterate its purpose. Describe up front what you wish to accomplish and by what time you expect to end the meeting.
- As meeting leader, do not lecture or otherwise dominate the meeting. Encourage participation by all; stimulate discussion.
- Do not let any particular participants monopolize or dominate the meeting; likewise, if possible do not allow anyone to remain silent the entire time.
- End with a decision, a plan, a schedule of subsequent activity, or whatever concrete results come of the meeting.
- Arrange for the production of meeting minutes, if necessary, or otherwise ensure that significant results are documented.
- If a follow-up meeting is necessary, if at all possible, get it scheduled before the participants leave. If it cannot be scheduled then, schedule it as soon as practical.
- Recall also the guidelines relating to enhancing committee, team, and group deliberations presented in the earlier sections on these topics.

# ▸ Written Communication

## The Importance of Written Communication

Written communication is essential to the conduct of business in any organization. Some ways of doing business require that letters and memoranda pass between individuals and organizations, and in spite of advances in electronic record storage there remain many needs for filed hard copy. Also, written copy of various kinds must be produced and maintained for purposes of satisfying legal, regulatory, and accreditation requirements.

Many people who work in the delivery of health care can attest to the volume of writing required of them. Complaints about "paperwork" are common and widespread, and there is undoubtedly much more paper generated than is truly needed. Nevertheless, much of the written material that is produced is inescapable; hard copy documents of various kinds will remain in existence for the foreseeable future.

Just as many professionals and managers resist speaking in public, so do many frequently resist writing. Thus, many professionals and managers who resist writing chores do not write especially well. It could perhaps be argued forever whether some dislike writing because they are not especially good at it or whether they are not especially adept at writing because they dislike it. This problem is often compounded by widespread dislike of writing because it seems to consume more time than many wish to devote to it. The resulting resistance to writing is such that any number of professionals and managers will write a letter or memo only when absolutely necessary and even then will react to the pressures of time and write something once through and send it on its way.

The biggest problem concerning writing in business is not that it takes too much time but rather that it is allowed to consume too little time. Writing well requires more time and effort than simply dashing something off to get it sent and out of the way. Writing well requires editing and rewriting—admittedly time-consuming activities but activities that will usually pay for themselves in improved understanding and fewer problems of misinterpretation.

## E-mail: Helpful, but the Source of Many Problems

E-mail carries a high volume of nonbusiness material, and it tends to carry business information in a generally informal fashion. Appropriate use of e-mail requires attention to the handling of both that which is received and that which is sent.

In addressing incoming e-mail, heed these guidelines:

- First be attentive to deleting rather than reading. In most instances, a quick look at the subject line along with one's knowledge of the sender will indicate whether a message should be read in full or discarded at once.

- Become familiar with frequent senders and know what they are likely to be sending. There has never been, and there will never be, a beneficial technology that does not have a downside: the downside of the personal computer is its appeal to some users as more of a toy than a tool. Learn where many of the important messages come from and who is likely to be sending junk.
- Similar to the age-old advice about handling each incoming piece of paper only once, try dealing with each e-mail message once and only once. On reading a message, reply to it, forward it, delete it, or store it in an electronic folder. Messages should not be allowed to accumulate; they fill up the inbox and increase the chances of importance messages getting lost in the clutter.

In sending an e-mail message, follow these guidelines:

- Use a clear, understandable subject line that tells the addressee in a few words what to expect of the communication.
- Write, edit, and rewrite each message as though it were an important letter or memo (more on this to follow).
- As a safeguard, prepare the content of the message before filling in the address, as this allows for a more careful response and reduces the chance for a misdirected missive.
- Inform employees of the proper business use of e-mail and train them in proper handling of incoming mail. Consider reminding employees that e-mail is not as private as they might believe; messages are regularly misdirected accidentally, and it is easy for some computer users to tap into others' e-mail. It helps to imagine that any particular message could conceivably become as public as a bulletin-board notice. Your e-mail messages are never truly private; most organizations must archive all e-mails transmitted on company equipment or servers.

Concerning the seemingly prevalent "casual" (or, less euphemistically, "sloppy") use of e-mail, it often seems that e-mail brings out the worst in many writers of business communications. E-mail is such a readily available and easily usable means of interpersonal communication that it is easy to overlook its relatively severe shortcomings. When speaking with someone in a face-to-face interchange, in addition to words, one has the benefit of facial expression, vocal tone, and immediacy of feedback. Even in a telephone conversation, there is vocal tone and immediacy of feedback.

However, an e-mail message is like a letter or memo in that all that is available to carry the message are words someone must read.

Misunderstandings abound because so many users simply "dash off" messages without using the care they might apply to letters or memos. Some who would never allow a letter to go out containing obvious errors think nothing of e-mailing unedited ramblings devoid of capitalization and normal punctuation and overflowing with misspellings and incorrect terms.

Editing a letter takes time. Although this task is often ignored, it is not ignored nearly as often as editing an e-mail message. What's different about an e-mail message that causes its writer to forget the need to edit and clarify? Perhaps it is the seeming immediacy of e-mail, the feeling it provides of talking directly to someone via the computer screen. But it is easy to forget that the key element present in dealing with someone face-to-face, with the immediacy of feedback, is missing in e-mail. Feedback is delayed, and all too often it becomes necessary to trade messages back and forth to achieve the appropriate transfer of meaning. It is far better to edit and rewrite—and certainly spell-check—before sending each message. Clarity of content is most likely to accompany clarity of presentation.

E-mail is perhaps best thought of as one of a subset of tools in that versatile toolkit known as the personal computer. Like any good tool, to retain its usefulness it must be kept in good order and used for its intended purposes only. The observations made about e-mail also apply to text messages, instant messaging, and similar communications.

## Some Guidelines About Social Media Policies and Practices

The topic of social media policies and practices is an evolving one. A related issues into the topics provides the manager with insight into these issues. As a starting point, one might simply assert that, as with other issues relating to employee conduct, the worker is hired to be productive. Activities that reduce or interfere with productivity are usually limited, or even prohibited. Another obvious premise is that the equipment, physical space, support technologies, and services belong to the employer who may stipulate the conditions under which they are used.

For example, a cellphone or laptop computer may be provided as part of job-related equipment (e.g., a social worker assigned to home-visit duties). As with other equipment (e.g., fax machines, copiers, telephones) the organization owns the equipment and directs the use of these. Top-level management will put in place an organization-wide policy about the use of social media. Other members of the management team who share the development and implementation of these policies include the chief compliance officer and public relations manager. Within the public relations unit there may be a designated social media manager who oversees the official web presence of the organization, thus promoting outreach, marketing initiatives, and information for the public. Legal counsel is part of the team, as is a representative of human relations division, with particular attention given to union liaison designate.

Many of the issues relating to social media use are already in place. Existing law, regulation, and standards, plus codes of ethics and rules of conduct apply to social media. These include HIPAA, civil rights, sexual harassment, bullying and intimidation, safety, conflict of interest, copyright and intellectual property protections, NLRB rulings, and the general obligation that management maintain a nonhostile work environment. Workers, as well as clients, are entitled to a psychologically and physically safe environment.

Even in permitted personal use of social media, an employee would be prohibited from claiming to be a spokesperson for the organization, or an official endorser of a product or practice. A disclaimer might be required as a condition of employment. Through orientation and training as well as employment agreement, an employee will be briefed about the confidentiality of internal reports, documents, surveys, research, marketing plans, and other information about the organization.

Middle managers have input into the organization' social media policies and should look into what is working and what needs clarification. They may also need to develop department-level policies and training materials. These must be cleared with the higher levels of management to ensure consistency and compliance with the constraints noted. The middle manager may encourage the use of cellphones and other personal communication devices as a matter of safety for certain workers, for example, those performing tasks in remote settings of the facility, or evening and night-shift duties. A home health aide's safety is enhanced by ready contact with supervisors. In addition to direct work-related use, a manager might want to provide a humane and pleasant, worry-free work environment. Many workers have family responsibilities; permitting a short phone or text message from children arriving home from school or an elderly family member returning safely from an adult day care program gives workers peace of mind. This, in turn, enables them to focus on their work.

"Your presence is requested." In some organizations, a middle manager is expected to be part of the social media outreach. One might be asked, even required, to provide a short summary of their work, training, and experience for the organization's home page.

## Some Additional Considerations

General provisions of social media policies and guidelines often include these elements:

- Workers have personal cellphones and social media accounts; during work hours and when on premises (arriving, leaving, on break) certain limits might be placed. (Again, a reminder to clear any practice with the designated officials in your organization; nothing in this discussion constitutes legal advice. The discussion is intended to simply alert the manager to the kind of issues that arise.) In general, a manager might implement a policy that broadly states: no use of these devices during work time; no interference with productivity of the worker or other workers; no intrusion into the privacy and safety of the clients.

- Prohibition of use of these items in any location where clients/patients and their families might see or hear these activities. This includes such areas as lobbies, coffee shops, dining rooms, and outside seating areas. Clients might feel uncomfortable in their vulnerable state (ill, limited mobility, accessing behavioral care) if they see workers with cameras, cellphones, and similar devices.

- Union contracts, employee handbooks, and work rules often include specific provisions about social media use. These provisions often include specifications, or at least, examples of personal time provided to workers during their scheduled shifts (e.g., break time, lunch time). Personal social media access may be permitted during such personal time (e.g., internet shopping). However, the usual prohibitions that apply to all communication remain in place (e.g., bullying, teasing, harassment).

- NLRB decisions prohibit management from discouraging or interfering with union activity through social media. For example, a worker is free to give out information about his or her wages and benefits. This is distinctly different from a worker taking organizational information about a unit's wages and salaries, including workers' names, and sharing these details.

An employee is not permitted to do this. However, the union officials are usually provided with such information and (usually omitting personal identification details) may share it with members and potential members as part of union outreach or negotiating strategies.

These and similar issues continue to be subject to clarification. The manager therefore gives ongoing attention to these developing matters.

## Memos and Letters[1]

Letters and memoranda are essential—and unavoidable—in the operation of any business or other organization. To many people who work in various healthcare settings, it often seems that more than enough paperwork is already required without adding more by creating documents in addition to necessary charting, covering the organization legally, and responding to external requirements. However, even though the paper volume seems almost overwhelming at times, much of this paper is nevertheless necessary. Many organizations function quite well in spite of hefty amounts of paperwork, but just try to run an organization completely without paper.

Any written communication serves one or more of several important functions. Specifically, a given written communication may be used to advise (or inform), explain, request, convince, or provide a permanent record. Letters and memos may be used for any one or a combination of these purposes.

No matter how well it is written, any letter or memo possesses a serious drawback: it is essentially a one-way communication, providing no opportunity for immediate feedback. The individual who writes a letter or memo is unable to amend, correct, clarify, or defend what is being written based on the reactions of the audience.

Because of the one-way nature of a letter or memo, the need for clarity in writing becomes critical. However, clarity is an attribute frequently lacking in written communications in the organizational setting.

This section offers some guidelines for communicating more clearly via letter or memorandum. However, although these guidelines will help improve the clarity of one's writing, following a few pages of advice in a work such as this book is unlikely to make a person become a "good" writer. To become a writer of effective business communications, two things are needed: (1) the desire to write better letters and memos and (2) the help provided by practically oriented teachers of business writing and good references on writing.

Numerous books on writing techniques are available, but the writer who wishes to use one single straightforward reference should turn to The Elements of Style by William Strunk, Jr., and E. B. White. This classic volume contains solid, usable advice.

For better letters and memos, conscientious use of the following guidelines will improve your writing in a minimum amount of time.

### Write for a Specific Audience

A particular letter or memo may be going to one person, or it may be intended for several people. Before writing, the writer must decide to whom, specifically, the missive is to be directed. The person for whom the message is primarily intended is the primary audience. However, there may also be a sizable secondary audience—others who will receive, read, and perhaps make use of the communication.

Many managers write as though they believe that anyone picking up a particular document will completely understand its contents. Targeting a specific audience is a difficult task at best, however, and it becomes nearly impossible in the presence of a sizable secondary audience, including people of widely varying backgrounds and different degrees of familiarity with the subject.

Write specifically for the primary audience. No person can successfully write for everyone. If there is difficulty identifying the primary audience, it is necessary to sift through the likely recipients of the message with one question in mind: who of all these people needs this information for decision-making purposes? Often the primary audience will be a single person, but it could just as well be two, three, or more people. For example, a nursing supervisor writing about the need for a specific change in departmental policy would likely be making all of nursing management aware of the issue, but it would be the supervisor's immediate superior—the director of nursing service—who would be the primary audience because this is the person who wields the decision-making authority concerning departmental policy. In contrast, if the director of nursing service is releasing a new policy with which all supervisors are expected to comply,

---

1  Portions of this section were adapted from Charles R. McConnell, *The Effective Health Care Supervisor*, 8th ed. (Chapter 19, "Communication: Not by Spoken Words Alone") (Burlington, MA: Jones & Bartlett Learning, 2015), 347–360.

then the memo announcing the policy will have all supervisors as its primary audience.

Use what is known about the primary audience in deciding how to structure a message. Can it be on a friendly, first-name basis? Must it be a formal letter, or will a brief, casual note suffice? Does this person prefer detail, or would a concise overview be enough? Let knowledge of the primary audience suggest how to communicate.

## Avoid Unneeded Words

Understanding and exercising one simple concept—that of the "zero word"—will go a long way in removing excess words from one's writing. Every word in a given piece of writing can be placed in one of three categories: necessary, optional, or zero. A necessary word is essential to getting the basic message across. An optional word, as the name suggests, can be used at one's option to qualify or modify a necessary word or phrase. A zero word contributes nothing and should be removed.

Consider the following sentence:

Mary is certainly an exceptionally intelligent woman.

This sentence contains only three necessary words: Mary is intelligent. Note, however, that even with all zero words and optional words removed, what remains is still a sentence.

The word "exceptionally" is the only optional word in the sentence. It may well make a difference in what you are trying to communicate to say that "Mary is exceptionally intelligent" rather than simply "Mary is intelligent." Although this is perfectly acceptable, it is necessary to watch out for the excess use of such modifiers and qualifiers; after a while, they not only become tiresome but also lose much of their impact.

The example sentence includes three zero words: certainly, an, and woman. At least they are zero under normal circumstances, assuming that Mary is a woman. The word "an" is there for structural reasons, and "certainly" is certainly unnecessary, because in terms of what the writer is trying to convey, Mary either is or is not intelligent, and certainly does not make that judgment any more binding. Zero words abound in most business writing, but they are relatively easy to get rid of with conscientious editing.

Almost any sample of business writing will yield at least a few zero words. If in doubt about a word, try the sentence without it. If the sentence remains a sentence and continues to convey the intended message, the word is probably a zero word. One can usually find a surprising number of zero words, among which are often many uses of the, that, of, and other simple words.

Unnecessary words are often used in phrases of several words, where they do the work that could be done by one or two words. This is especially common in business correspondence in which some phrases have reached cliché proportions. Consider these examples:

- The use of "due to the fact that" when one can simply say "because"
- Saying "be in a position to" when all that is needed is "can"
- Saying "in the state of California" when "in California" says the same
- Using the stuffy "with reference to" when the job can be done by "about"

Such phrases are to be avoided; they simply add bulk without adding clarity. In fact, such words not only fail to add clarity, but they also can actually harm the message by surrounding and obscuring the real meaning.

## Use Simple Words

Almost every technical and professional field has its own jargon, with jargon defined as "the technical terminology or characteristic idiom of a special activity or group." However, this is the second definition of jargon appearing in several dictionaries—the first is "confused unintelligible language."

It is one thing for a laboratory technologist to write to an audience of other laboratory technologists; in this instance one can get away with the free use of the language of the field. It is another thing to write to all employees of the healthcare organization simultaneously; this audience usually includes highly educated, specialized professionals; unskilled and semiskilled workers; and numerous levels in between these two extremes. Also, an organization's staff includes people in many different but medically related fields, all of which have their own "languages."

Medical and technical professionals are among the worst offenders when it comes to sprinkling correspondence with jargon. The excuse that the writing is "in the language" of a field should not allow one to cut across departmental lines to any considerable extent. As already suggested, technologist-to-technologist communication may be a safe channel for the use of jargon. In contrast, technologist-to-finance director is a channel calling for a completely different approach. Again, consider the primary audience in preparing to write.

## Edit and Rewrite

During editing and rewriting, zero words, roundabout phrases, and other verbal stuffing should come out of the intended correspondence. Few pieces of writing cannot be improved by careful editing or rewriting. Most people—and this statement includes professional writers—cannot go from thought to a completely effective finished message in a single pass. In fact, professional writers do much more editing and rewriting than do most writers of day-to-day business correspondence. This reveals the problem: much of what is wrong with our writing is wrong simply because not enough time and effort are put into it. It often takes more time to write a shorter letter than it does to write a longer one.

Anyone who might think that better writing is too time consuming should think also of the cost of misunderstanding. Many a manager has had to spend valuable time and effort smoothing out some problem that developed because a written message was misunderstood. Many memos can be edited in the time it takes to solve a couple of knotty problems arising from missed communication.

## Change Old Habits

In their day-to-day writing, many people are unconsciously still trying to please English teachers of years gone by. Throughout several decades of the 20th century, students were taught to write letters using a highly formal style. Depending on one's organization, a less formal style and tone may be the norm. Many practices that are acceptable (and even improve) business writing today would not have been approved in the recent past.

**Be Friendly and Personal.** Feel free to use personal pronouns in letters and memos. People use "I," "you," and "we" when they are speaking to each other, so why not use them when writing? Many people were taught to avoid personal pronouns, and this warning sticks with them. Students were once taught never to use "I" in academic writing. But for clarity and directness, "I" is far preferable to archaic affectations such as "the undersigned" or "the author."

Most letters and memos should strive for a conversational tone. Once this is achieved, correspondence will be direct, friendly, and personal.

**Use Direct, Active Language.** Ask direct questions when the situation warrants it. Some writers may have been taught to go out of their way to avoid questions and thus say things like, "Let me

know whether you will attend." It is much more direct to ask, "Will you attend?"

Statements should be kept in the active voice, avoiding the likes of "The contract was signed by your representative." How much cleaner it is to say, "Your representative signed the contract."

**Use Contractions.** It is preferable to use contractions such as "don't," "wouldn't," "can't," "shouldn't," and so on, even though this usage in business was long discouraged. Contractions contribute to the natural, conversational tone one should be working to achieve. Even so, many writers of business correspondence squeeze the contractions out of their writing without realizing what they are doing. The result is a formalistic style, stilted and stuffy, that merely serves to create more distance between writer and reader.

**Write Short Sentences.** Although it is difficult to set firm guidelines for sentence length, consider that any sentence much longer than 20 words is edging into questionable territory. Some teachers of business writing have suggested 20 words as maximum sentence length, and others suggest that 14 or 15 words as the maximum. Regardless, it is safe to say that the longer the sentence, the more opportunities there are for misunderstanding.

**Forget Old Taboos About Prepositions and Conjunctions.** It is likely that most people were repeatedly and sternly warned against committing three terrible transgressions: ending a sentence with a preposition, starting a sentence with a conjunction, and the practice of beginning a sentence with "and" or "but." The freedom to open a sentence in this manner can help avoid long sentences and needless repetition.

**Say It and Stop.** Avoid starting a letter by repeating what was said in the letter being answered. Also, avoid opening with standard stuffing such as "In response to your letter of the…"

Simply state the message. If the point of the letter is to tell a potential supplier that the bid was rejected, do not spend two paragraphs describing the evaluation process and building the rationale for the "no" to be delivered in paragraph three. Deliver the answer in the opening paragraph, preferably in the first sentence. Then go on to explain why, if necessary.

Having delivered the message and explained it as necessary, do not spend another paragraph or two winding down by repeating what has already said. Simply say it—and stop. Also, watch out for standard closing lines that mean little or nothing. It may be quite all right to say, "Call me if you need more information"; this statement is thoughtful and shows interest. But avoid phrases such as "We trust this arrangement meets with your complete satisfaction." If the reader is not completely satisfied, the writer is likely to hear about it.

Consider also the use of the collective "we" in the foregoing example. Few words are more likely to make a letter more impersonal to a reader than one who is made to feel that the communication is coming from a crowd. The "we" has its place—for instance, when writing to someone outside the organization and speaking on behalf of the organization. However, rather than being organization-to-person or organization-to-organization communications, most of one's writing will consist of person-to-person messages. As long as the thoughts are your own and yours is the only hand pushing the pen or tapping the keys, say "I."

## Sample Letter: Wrong and Right

Following is the text of a letter sent to a number of hospital chief executives by the director of a regional office of a state health department:

Dear Administrator:

I would like to call your attention to Section 702.4 (c) of the State Hospital Code, which requires nosocomial infections in hospitals be reported immediately to the Regional Health Director.

We have recently experienced several hospital outbreaks in this region, which have not been reported to this office by the hospital. It is recommended that you review Section 702.4, Infection Control and Reporting, of the State Hospital Code so that you understand what your responsibilities are regarding increased incidence of hospital infections or disease due to chemical or radioactive agents or their toxic products in patients or persons working in the hospital.

In counties where there is an organized county or city health department or a Commissioner of Health, it is also required that a report of communicable be made immediately to the County or City Health Commissioner. In the unorganized counties or districts, a report must be made to the District Health Officer immediately. This is no way eliminates or excuses the hospital from reporting immediately to the Regional Health Director.

Please note that failure to report nosocomial infections is a violation of Section 702.4(c) of the State Hospital Code. Violations of the Code are subject to penalty. In the future, such violations will leave us no alternative but to recommend that appropriate sanctions be taken against a hospital for violation of this section of the State Hospital Code.

Very truly yours,
Regional Health Director

It is certainly possible to correctly extract the true message from this letter, although a telephone call or two might be necessary before a recipient would feel comfortable about its meaning. Also, there is no denying the scolding tone and the threat contained in the letter (with threats of sanctions or punishment of some kind seemingly incorporated in a great many communications from government agencies).

Now consider how the text of the letter could read if more thoughtfully written:

The State Hospital Code calls for the reporting of nosocomial infections to the Regional Health Director as soon as they are discovered. However, several recent outbreaks in this region have not been reported.

Please review Section 702.4 of the Code (Infection Control and Reporting) concerning your role in helping to control infection or disease resulting from the exposure of patients, staff, or others to chemical or radioactive agents or their toxic products.

If your community has a Department of Health, your timely report should go to the local Commissioner. If you have no local health department, your report should go directly to the District Health Office.

Please assist us in ensuring that Section 702.4 of the Code is observed as intended. Your cooperation will be appreciated.

Why should the author have bothered to edit and rewrite the original letter? One good reason for doing so is for clarity. In its rewritten form, the letter is far less likely to be misunderstood. Also, the scolding and threatening have been removed; there is always the opportunity to communicate more sternly later with recipients who might remain noncompliant. And consider this as well: the text of the original letter contains 230 words, and the rewritten version contains 126 words. This amounts to a reduction in length of 45%. Not only is the rewritten letter clearer, but there is also less to read. Is this at all important? It has been estimated that most business documentation contains anywhere from 25% to 100% more words than are actually needed. This suggests that the 2-inch-thick stack of documentation in the manager's inbox need be only 1–1.6 inches thick if properly written.

Time spent editing and rewriting is time well spent in making a message more readily understood while greatly reducing the chances of misunderstanding.

## Formal Writing and Reporting

Letters and memos constitute a significant percentage of most managers' writing chores. However, it may occasionally be necessary or desirable to tackle larger writing tasks such as informational or analytical reports, educational presentations, speeches, or perhaps even journal articles.

Many elements of the personal, direct style preferred for correspondence are applicable to other writing. For instance, some speeches or educational presentations can, and should, be handled with the same personal touch. However, some additional rules apply in writing more structured material such as formal reports, and still more rules apply when writing for publication in trade magazines or professional journals.

Sample reports such as annual reports, consultant findings, and due diligence reviews are included in the section on comprehensive planning and accountability documents in Chapter 12.

If you need to author a formal report, obtain a manual or handbook on the subject and do some studying, paying particular attention to outlining schemes if the report in question is likely to be lengthy. Also, be aware of the advisability of using one of the commonly recommended report formats, one that calls for a tight summary of objectives, conclusions, and recommendations early in the report. Within an organization, there are generally accepted style and format guidelines for report writing.

Whether you are writing a letter, memorandum, or formal report, never lose sight of the fact that the initial step in preparing to write anything is to get a clear image of the intended audience, both primary and secondary.

## ▶ Communication in Organizations

Considering that communication between two people may be difficult at times, and small-group communication may frequently be taxing, the task of communicating with a large group may at first seem overwhelming. As bureaucracies began to emerge at the dawn of the 20th century, when industrialization promoted the growth of large organizations, the need to develop complex communication patterns became more pressing as organizations added more and more members. Put simply, communication had to keep pace with production. The resulting strategies to increase organizational communication can be divided into two categories: formal and informal.

## Formal Communication
### Verbal

An organization is a stratified social system with a hierarchy of roles. The roles are arranged according to the degree of power and status assigned to each, and the assignment is based on the goal-oriented needs of the organization. Formal communication is sanctioned by the organization and is shared along communication channels established by the hierarchy of roles. The arrangement of roles determines the direction of the communication.

Formal communication is directional. The four traditional channels of communication are upward, downward, diagonal, and lateral. Examples of each direction are these:

| ■ Upward | Staff person communicating with supervisor |
|---|---|
| ■ Downward | Staff therapist giving directions to an aide |
| ■ Diagonal | Head of social work conferring with patient registrar in admissions |
| ■ Lateral | Nurse sharing night orders with another nurse |

Formal verbal communication in organizations takes place through orderly channels. The exchanges are directional and promote organizational goals, such as a verbal exchange of orders or instructions. Department meetings can also be formal. An aide who wants to register a complaint must go through a series of formal channels; the aide cannot walk into the president's office and discuss the grievance.

Because the size of organizations precludes face-to-face interaction among the majority of group members, they must rely on less personal means of communication (e.g., written and transmitted communication). Common examples include goal statements, policy and procedure manuals, directives, direct mailings to employees, mass e-mail communications, organizational bulletins, newsletters, magazines, bulletin boards, posters, and handbooks.

## Nonverbal

The use of space is a form of nonverbal communication. The goals of the organization determine the location and quality of space assigned to group members (who may resist adjustments and reassignments). The way that furniture is arranged, the selection of ornaments, and the care given to the space all reflect the values of the group. If an organization has an elaborate waiting room but sloppy offices and treatment units, it can be inferred that the company is more interested in its public face.

The arrangement of furniture can stimulate or stifle communication. Managers rely on spatial relationships to strengthen their communication. For example, asking for a raise while the manager looks over a desk is more difficult than asking while both parties are seated next to each other.

# Informal Communication

Because informal communication is not sanctioned by the social system, it may or may not promote the goals of the organization. Informal communication is not directional; it may—and frequently does—circumvent formal channels. Informal communication is frequently anonymous, and more often than not sources cannot be verified.

Informal communication, such as small talk and gossip, may not be accurate. Even so, the use of informal communication should not be neglected. Managers can use this type of communication to determine the success of formal communication patterns. Rumor and gossip, although inaccurate, may gauge the feelings of group members. Perceptions about events can also be examined. Informal communication is a barometer of the organization, because information can travel at a fast rate. Future events may be foreshadowed by listening to information communicated informally.

Informal communication within the organization may be accurately described by a single familiar term: the grapevine. This may perhaps be more accurately described as the communications network of the informal organization. Every organization has a formal structure of relationships governing relationships within the workplace. In addition, every person in the organization has a number of informal channels of communication, relationships with friends, acquaintances, and others with whom one might speak. Furthermore, many of the relationships partially define the informal organization, with the implied structure being based on numerous interactions between and among people.

The informal organization is at work, for example, when two or three employees happen to stand out from the group, perhaps even speaking for others, although they have no official standing. This effect is also evident when a single manager is regarded as senior by the work group over a number of others at the same level because of longevity or perhaps because of strength of personality or some particular trait or combination of traits. In brief, interpersonal relationships and people's regard for one another describe the informal organization, which is at best a phantom structure that is always shifting and realigning.

People will talk. The grapevine spontaneously develops; it is not controlled by management. It moves back and forth across departmental lines and rapidly changes its course. The grapevine is dynamic but unreliable. It carries a great deal of misinformation, but it is in the organization to stay.

It is best to remain acutely aware of the grapevine. Tune in, listen to what it is carrying, and learn from it. A manager is likely to be isolated from some of the bits and pieces the grapevine carries, or at least miss a few things until they have been around awhile. How much one hears is frequently dependent on how well one relates with employees, peers, and others.

When tuned in to the grapevine, a manager will inevitably hear some things that he or she knows are simply not correct. A manager who hears something that is disturbing or inappropriate should check it out if possible. Each manager is responsible for setting the facts of the story right whenever the opportunity to do so presents itself. One must be sure, however, to have the story straight—do not heap more speculation onto a growing rumor.

The grapevine sometimes possesses the distinct advantages of speed and depth of penetration. Some bits of news can travel through the organization at an astonishingly rapid rate and often reach people who would never think to read a bulletin board or look at an employee newsletter. The grapevine can carry the good as well as the bad, and because it will always be around, it is best to feed it some real facts whenever possible so it will have something useful to carry.

# Tools for Improving Communication

A number of formal and informal tools can be used to promote communication within the organization. Assessment instruments require analysis of the conscious and unconscious goals of group members. Some can be used to assess individual interaction styles, members' perceptions of one another, perceptions of leadership, roles that members play relative to one another in the work group, and members' feelings about the organization. Group members complete questionnaires, and the results are compared and discussed. The goals of the members are compared with the goals of the leaders. The results are discussed in nonthreatening ways. Strategies for promoting change can be generated in the group.

Sometimes group communication becomes so difficult that outside experts are brought in as facilitators to resolve the issues. Professional facilitators are trained in a number of disciplines, including business, psychology, education, and sociology.

## Barriers to Communication in Organizations

A number of obstacles can block communication or distort the goals of organizational exchanges:

1. Language. There may be a lack of common understanding of certain important terms. The use of slang, jargon, or technical language can create problems.
2. Unconscious motives. Personal thoughts, ideas, and emotions not readily available for examination may cloud a group's ability to perceive or interpret events. A group may share a collective mentality that may not be based on real events. Such collective thought has been shaped by emotions.
3. Psychological factors. Past experience and ideas impinge on the communication process. Feelings such as mistrust, fear, anger, hostility, or indifference may shape group perceptions.
4. Status. Real or perceived differences in rank, socioeconomic status, or prestige may detract from the communication process. People develop preconceived notions about others and act on their preconceptions instead of reality.
5. Organizational size. The larger the social system, the greater the number of communication layers. Each layer provides an opportunity for additional distortion.
6. Logistical factors. Groups may lack the time, place, or space to communicate clearly. Feedback may be neglected because it is difficult to collect.
7. Overstimulation. Members may be bombarded with so many events that they are unable to process any more information. People who are stressed must be managed carefully so they are not additionally burdened.
8. Cultural clashes. One group may misinterpret another's ideas because of a difference in cultural factors, such as age, socioeconomic status, the region of birth, and education level.

9. Organizational structure. Communication may be blocked by the structure of the communication channels. One person's role may serve as a bottleneck for open communication. In another instance, roles may overlap, and some groups may not receive the information that they need.
10. Phase in the life cycle of the organization. Communication may be taxed during the organization's developmental stage. In later stages in the life cycle, the old channels may not have been adapted to new situations. Sometimes organizations rely on one type of communication and ignore other methods.
11. A manager has a number of means to offset these barriers and enhance communication. These include attending to one's availability so that there is an ease to communication exchanges. For example, if a manager arrives exactly on time for a meeting, uses the break time to answer messages, and leaves immediately, he or she is signaling a lack of availability. Much of the informal, but important, communication flows within these settings because of the face-to-face nature of the interactions. A modicum of social–business interaction yields dividends; colleagues easily share information that would not be conveyed in formal memos. These opportunities for easy colleague interaction lead to enhanced cooperative ventures.
12. Attention to clarity is another means to enhance communication. Simple, direct, brief missives help offset information overload and prevent misunderstanding. A meeting announcement, for example, might be shortened to read: Utilization Committee meeting—Wednesday, April 10, 20n2 at 10:00 A.M. The meeting will last approximately two hours. Notice that the specific ending time is not listed, and there is minimal possibility of someone misreading the ending time for the start time.
13. Timing and timeliness are important factors. When crucial information is time-bound, it must be conveyed quickly. For example, weather-related closure notice should be disseminated well before workers leave home. In situations in which there is preliminary information available, notice of anticipated time of posting for additional details and updates is given. Another aspect of timing relates to a well-intentioned, but possibly problematic, practice of clearing the desk and e-mail inbox with a late Friday afternoon dumping of material into other workers' inboxes. They face a Monday morning deluge of missives. Thoughtful

managers provide a regular flow of communication throughout the work week to avoid these situations.

14. Concise communications are usually a welcomed feature in a busy work setting. While one seeks to be cordial and thoughtful, one should avoid over-communicating. An e-mail message is received, the prompt at the bottom of the page gives the option of reply, and sometimes we end up replying to the reply, as in, thank you for your message. If there is no new information to exchange, it recommended to not reply.

15. In direct patient care (and in support services to some extent) a simplified, concise hard-copy form is often used when handing off the patient from one service to another (e.g., from ambulance to intake, from care unit to medical imaging). The SBAR method is one such form: S for situation—the basics such as patient identification; B for background—working diagnosis, code status, allergies, time of last medication and food intake; A for assessment—checklist of key factors including fall risk, disorientation, isolation precautions; R for recommendations—care needed while in transit (e.g., IV drip; oxygen) and off the primary care unit.

16. Finally, one should remain aware of the need to be prudent about casual comments. A few examples illustrate this. During an open microphone event, a group of staff members meet for grievance review and casual remarks are made such as, "I am glad that one's gone," "she is not the nicest person you will ever meet," "she surely will never be employee of the month." At another meeting, one might casually say, "No, we can't get started yet, we have to wait until his highness arrives with his big red book of rules and regulations (referring to the senior level manager representing the CEO)." And one more example: Before the official meeting begins with a client and his or her attorney, a staff member (in a closed-door setting) says to the other staff members, "They do not need to know about our settlement in the other case relating to medication errors." These conversations are easily overheard. Open microphones often broadcast into corridors and waiting areas. Without being paranoid, a prudent worker remains aware of the growing use of virtual personal assistant devices with a capacity to record conversations. In a similar vein, one remains aware that other individuals may be inadvertently or purposefully using smart phones to record conversations and proceedings. In home care settings and some offices, personal assistance technologies record continuously.

## Special Consideration: Directional Flow Barriers

Communication within a work organization moves downward with far greater ease than it moves upward. The downward channels of communication are largely controlled by management and tend to be exercised at management's option. Letters and memoranda to employees, general e-mailings to employees, employee meetings and staff meetings, informational stuffers in paycheck envelopes, bulletin boards (except for occasional boards placed solely for employee use), policy and procedure manuals, most newsletters and employee newspapers, and public address systems all represent downward channels of communication controlled by management. Perhaps the most potent downward channels reside in the vested authority that each level of management has over its subordinates; in any vertical relationship in the chain of command, the person higher in authority is seen as exerting the greater measure of control in the communication that occurs within the relationship.

When a bit of information is set in motion in any of the downward channels, barring occasional breakdowns in flow, it moves as does anything moving from higher to lower—as though readily assisted by gravity. Moving a message up the chain of command, however, is often like attempting to make a physical object rise in spite of gravity. One can, of course, make an object rise in spite of gravity, but doing so requires the effort of lifting it plus whatever extra effort is required to overcome gravity. The same is true of communication: it usually requires a bit of extra effort to make a message travel upward against the normal downward-flowing tendency of organizational communication.

To obtain communication from employees, the manager can, and indeed should, through techniques such as proper delegation, build in requirements for all reasonable forms of employee feedback. If an employee clearly understands that he or she is to report to the manager on a given matter at a given time, then reporting usually takes place. It is likely that a large part of the effective group manager's time is consumed in the basic management function of controlling—ensuring, through regular follow-up and correction, that work is getting done as intended. This function requires employee feedback.

Despite such efforts, the manager can never secure all of the most valuable information by mandating feedback. Information that frequently remains hidden from the manager can include both personal and work-related employee problems. It can also include difficulties employees experience with management and coworkers, problems understanding or adhering to certain policies and practices, ideas for improvement that employees may not know how to structure or transmit, complaints about treatment from the organization, and numerous other indications of unmet needs. These kinds of information may be essential, or at least helpful, to the manager in running the department. Yet the manager may obtain such information not through mandate but rather by being visible and available to the employees and by earning the trust and confidence of the employees to the extent that they will volunteer such information.

Thus, the manager may ordinarily communicate downward at will because of position in the hierarchy. In contrast, employees can communicate upward effectively only if the manager makes it possible for them to do so.

## ▶ Orders and Directives

The manager's role is to direct the employees toward achieving the goals and objectives of the department and the institution. Regardless of the leadership style used, the manager must issue orders and directives to convey what must be done. The terms "orders" and "directives" may be used interchangeably, although "orders" has a more autocratic tone.

Giving orders is a major function of the manager's day-to-day operation of the department. Too often it is taken for granted that every manager knows how to give orders. Unfortunately, this is not true. The manager must remember to convey to the employees what is to be done, who is to do it, and when, where, how, and why it is to be done. At times, some of the components are implied or omitted. As an example, consider this announcement: "Effective July 1, John Doe will be the Senior Physical Therapist of the Amputee Service." This statement answers the what, who, when, and where but omits the how and why.

### Verbal Orders Versus Written Orders

The form of an order depends on the situation. The verbal (actually, oral) order is the most frequently used.

Because it is given on a one-to-one basis with immediate feedback possible, the manager can observe the employee's reaction, ask questions, and appraise the degree of understanding. Disagreements can be handled immediately. Observation of the employee's body language provides additional feedback.

When permanence is important, written orders are more appropriate. This form is most effective when information is to be disseminated to employees as a group. Written orders are more carefully thought through, because there is less opportunity for explanation. The use of long sentences, excessive adjectives, and involved word patterns should be avoided. The written order also carries a degree of formality not present in the verbal order. It is difficult, however, to keep written material up-to-date and impossible to clear up obscure meanings.

### Making Orders Acceptable and Effective

The issuing of effective orders requires attention to timing as well as to language. Planning to issue an order involves content, format (oral or written), and the manner in which the order is actually issued. When there is rapport between manager and employee, a simple request may be suitable; an implied order is sometimes given with the same informality. When certain action must be taken, precision is involved, and misunderstanding must be avoided; the written, direct order is the best method. The sense of command may be foreign to many managers, yet commands may be needed on some occasions, such as emergencies. Although policies, work rules, and procedures may not be considered orders, they do set required courses of action as determined by management.

Because a critical aspect of the manager's function is communicating, effort must be applied to making orders acceptable and effective. Acceptability is enhanced by the general processes of leadership that the manager has developed over time. In effect, the manager prepares the employees in many ways so that when orders are actually given, they are normally both acceptable and effective in terms of essential communication.

## CHAPTER 12

# Comprehensive Planning and Accountability Documentation

## CHAPTER OBJECTIVES

- Identify the responsibilities of middle managers in developing comprehensive management documents, including the strategic plan, annual report, executive summary of the annual report, project proposal, due diligence report, and plan of correction.
- Examine the essential elements of each plan and its importance to the organization.
- Identify the special considerations related to the development of a business plan.
- Identify the special considerations relating to due diligence review reports.
- Describe the typical content of each of the foregoing documents.
- Provide examples of suggested wording for these essential planning and accountability documents.

Managers formulate comprehensive plans to reflect trends and respond to change. These plans and reports reflect the corporate culture of transparency, of the celebration of success, and a commitment to accountability. They constitute an historical record of the organization's development. Some plans are mandated by law or regulation, for example, a plan of correction resulting from licensure survey. Some are required by the organization's charter of bylaws (e.g., an annual report). In formulating these plans, managers apply the principles of planning, decision making, organizing, continuous performance improvement, budgeting, and resource allocation. This chapter focuses on the application of these concepts to comprehensive plans and related reports: the strategic or long-range plan, the annual report with executive summary, and the major project proposal. The narrative explanations of these documents include reminders of concepts from the foundational chapters. Examples of these plans or reports are included in the chapter appendices. In addition, the general concepts of a business plan, due diligence review, and plan of correction are described. The first several chapters of this text lay the foundation for these concepts. The earlier discussions on planning include a 500-day plan with a major project, and the earlier discussion on consulting includes an example of report development and summarization.

Within an organization, the top management provides specific guidelines about content and format for internal documents and reports. When developing a project proposal or a business plan for which external funding is being requested, the manager follows the specifications given by the funding agency.

The fictitious examples presented are intended to assist the middle manager by providing ideas, sample wording, and expression of level of detail.

# ▶ The Strategic Plan

Managers develop a proactive response to change by developing long-range plans, including strategic steps to advance the mission of the organization. This plan ties together the mission with the means of fostering it. A strategic plan combines idealism, expressed in the mission and values, with realism, expressed in statements of goals and objectives. Such a long-range plan lays out the desired outcomes to be accomplished over several years. Strategic planning is the process of determining long-term objectives along with the strategies for accomplishing them. The activities and objectives lead to action today in light of desired outcomes.

Part of the realism of strategic planning involves a frank assessment of both the internal and external environments. Risk factors, strengths and weaknesses, threats and challenges, and opportunities are all identified during this process.

Top managers initiate the strategic planning process and provide guidelines for its development. Middle managers develop details to reflect the particulars of their departments. In an integrative step, the master plan is augmented by the various department plans.

When is a strategic plan developed? Usually this long-range plan is prepared early in the organization's life cycle, when the organization moves from the gestational to the youth stage. During this process, the organization hones its mission and commits to an action plan; a forecast of objectives to be pursued over the coming 5 or 10 years is typically created. After this initial phase in the life cycle, the master plan is updated periodically. As the organization evolves, the dynamics of goal succession, expansion, and multiplication come into play. Which goals will be kept or modified, and which will be set aside temporarily or permanently? Throughout the long phase of middle age, the plan is reviewed and routinely adjusted. When major changes (e.g., a merger, a change of ownership) occur, when a new opportunity becomes available, or when the organization's leaders express a desire for revitalization, a new plan is developed.

## Content of Strategic/Master Plans

There are a variety of ways to formulate a master plan. **Appendix 12–A** presents one version of a strategic plan for a healthcare agency. In general, the typical content includes all or most of the following elements:

- A vision and mission statement
- Core values and principles
- A strategic overview of current status
- Major strategic goals
- An action plan or detailed objectives
- The resources needed and their probable source
- An evaluation process

### Vision and Mission Statement and Core Values

The organization's charter and statement of underlying philosophy include foundational principles, usually stated as vision, mission, and core values. Subsequent plans reflect these elements. The corporate culture, expressed in these statements, provides the impetus for the plan. The details of the plan should clearly reflect these values.

### Strategic Overview of Current Status

This element is a brief, factual statement of the organization's legal configuration (e.g., nonprofit corporation), its full legal title and its familiar or shortened name, its tax-exempt status if applicable, the year it was founded, and its sponsorship. Sources of financial support are identified in a general way. A brief summary of strengths, weaknesses, threats or challenges, and opportunities is provided.

### Major Strategic Goals and Action Plan or Detailed Objectives

Major goals are stated; these are usually limited to the most critical goals. For example, a hospital might have three major goals: provision of patient care, teaching, and research. For each of these major goals, managers develop specific objectives and action plans. The master plan is supplemented by departmental or division plans, usually laid out as a series of annual plans with measurable outcomes with specific timetables.

### Resources Needed and Their Probable Source

The statement of resources needed includes the usual categories of personnel, financial, equipment, and space requirements. Potential sources of trained workers, local job market characteristics, and availability of specialty education programs are noted.

In addition, calculations relating to fee structure, number of potential clients, and public and private reimbursement schedules are delineated. Middle managers provide detailed support data relating to their unit. If there is a plan to participate in major grants, projects, or fund-raising programs, managers state this expectation.

### Evaluation Process

To effectively control the implementation of the strategic plan, it is necessary to monitor the implementation process closely. The key point is to determine how well the action plan is progressing toward meeting the objectives. The assessment may lead to reconsideration and possible refinement of objectives, modification of activities, and alteration of resource allocation. For additional commentary on the evaluation process, see the evaluation section later in this chapter, in the discussion of major projects and proposals. The evaluation and monitoring system can involve several approaches. Refer to the material covered in Chapter 5 about decision making, the cycle of evaluation, and evaluation of major projects. Also, see the discussion in Chapter 13 on total quality management that includes examples relating to this process.

## The Strategic Planning Process

The strategic planning process consists of several steps. It begins with a preliminary phase, often described as the period devoted to "planning to plan." In this initial step, the strategic planning team is identified and brought together. Top management, department heads, and support staff establish the framework of teams, tasks and responsibilities, and timelines for provision of status reports. Interdepartmental coordination is built into the team structure. At the department level, the manager usually involves associate and assistant directors and unit supervisors in the planning effort. Given its comprehensive nature, the strategic planning process may take 3 or 4 months or even longer, depending on the complexity of the organization.

Step two is the in-depth assessment of the organization's current circumstances and conditions that may have changed. A useful tool for describing these aspects of the organization is a review of the organization's life cycle: how its mission developed and changed, what the past and current relationships to stakeholders are, and how client characteristics have changed. An update of the clientele network will reveal valuable information related to these elements. Factors and constraints are again noted, but are now challenged: is this limiting factor a continuing one or is the way open to undertake some new initiative?

During the assessment phase, managers carry out a SWOT analysis—a brainstorming technique that focuses on the organization's strengths, weaknesses, opportunities, and threats. The working notes of this analysis reflect raw, blunt, unfiltered responses by team members. Team leaders take care to allow issues and ideas to surface without censoring and without concern for level of formality. From this initial set of responses, themes are clustered and gradually filtered into a formal summary. For example, in the working notes under the topic of weaknesses, participants might list the following items, in no particular order: lack of competitive wage structure, poor working conditions (e.g., lack of parking space), absence of security escort for night shift, minimal opportunity for advancement, and competitor's attractive location and working conditions. In the follow-up session, all issues relating to personnel and working conditions might be grouped together. Under the topic of strengths, the organization's positive track record of licensure and accreditation compliance might be noted, its specialty outreach programs highlighted, and its staff development and training programs emphasized.

Threats to organizational survival and success are also identified through the SWOT analysis. This is another topic for which the clientele network (competitors and adversaries) and the concept of bureaucratic imperialism—which organizations are competing and in what manner—provide easy access to the pertinent issues.

Financial stability and reimbursement patterns present another aspect of concern. Changing licensure requirements or changes in government initiatives (e.g., phasing out specialty hospitals or assisted living facilities) represent other threats needing a response from healthcare organizations. Some managers may prefer to use the term *challenges* instead of threats. Opportunities arise, often from these same external agency requirements (e.g., increased emphasis on home care or domiciliary care, new funding for specific clinical conditions such as memory care or autism). Trend analysis and response to change figure prominently in this part of the discussion. Data gathering and analysis are major aspects of step two of the strategic planning process.

Step three features the development, or the reaffirmation, of the organization's mission and core values. In light of the factual analysis from step two, these foundational statements are put in place.

Step four focuses on the development of the specific objectives, and identification and plans for obtaining the necessary resources. Chapter 5 includes discussions of mission, values, goals, and objectives.

Step five is the implementation of the plan, usually through a year-by-year delineation of objectives, stated in measurable terms and with evaluation processes noted. The annual report, which will be discussed in the next section of this chapter, is the usual adjunct document in which progress toward achieving this plan is described in detail. Communication of the plan is an obvious part of implementation. The master plan, often in abridged form, may be shared by top management with key stakeholders as part of its marketing and public relations outreach. When special funding requests are made (e.g., major projects, grant proposals, fund-raising initiatives), the abridged version is included with the request. Department plans are shared internally among related departments but are not made available to the general public.

## ▶ The Annual Report

The annual report is a detailed summary of the organization's efforts during the designated fiscal year. It reflects the annual plan, which was derived from the long-range master plan. Middle managers prepare the portions of the report dealing with their respective departments. Top management then compiles these departmental reports into one overall report to present to the governing board. Sometimes this master summary is distributed to key stakeholders outside the organization. In addition, licensure and accrediting agencies may request access to these reports as part of their review process. Internally, department managers share their reports with closely related departments.

The annual report is part of the evaluation process and, therefore, includes specific information about goal achievement, whether full, partial, or nonachievement. In this regard, it is an accountability review. The reasons for partial or nonachievement of planned goals are provided without excuse or blame. These reasons give the management team insight into the various factors and constraints that either impede or foster success. And yes, these results reflect on a manager's performance. Analysis of the annual report, coupled with evaluation of reports from prior years, can help the management team identify trends. Data from these reports may be used effectively in budget justification. For example, if unexpected equipment failures of significant proportion occur, or if unforeseen major problems with physical space arise, the existence of a series of annual reports means that

the management team has ready access to data with which to support a request for special funding to address these recurring problems. Wheel book entries from the current and past year are useful references to develop the back story concerning such issues.

The annual report incorporates some aspects of public relations, including a comprehensive report reflecting the overall organizational performance, highlighting accomplishments, and celebrating success. An easy-to-read, attention-getting device is *By the Numbers* displays. This upbeat approach emphasizes data-driven reporting as well as capturing the dynamic atmosphere of the organization. A middle manager, in preparing departmental reports, would include capsule information (e.g., number of new patients, number of emergency responses, reduction in days lost due to accidents, number of volunteer hours, number of community outreach programs) to correspond to this style of report presentation.

In writing an annual report, some managers might feel they are stating the obvious: the department carried out its designated functions. However, not everyone in the organization has the same grasp of detail about a particular department. As part of their leadership role, department managers use the opportunity afforded by the annual report to present the successes and challenges of their departments in a strong light.

The content of the annual report for a healthcare organization is arranged under several major categories: licensure and accrediting review results, performance improvement and quality control efforts, budget issues, staff development and training, interdepartmental coordination, patient or client education, and special projects. A useful practice is to set up a file for each of these major topics and add to it on a regular basis so that compilation of the annual report is an easy task. Attachments are used to keep the report short and to the point, yet comprehensive.

As with all reports, the name and title of the manager responsible for producing the report is included. The date of report preparation is also listed. **Appendix 12–B** provides an excerpt from a health information department's annual report.

## ▶ The Executive Summary

The executive summary is a condensed version of the detailed annual report. In this abridged version, major topics are highlighted for rapid perusal. The department manager prepares this one- or two-page summary as the cover document for the annual report.

Wise managers make this summary the "headliner" to emphasize those activities most critical to the accomplishment of the organization's mission. The time and effort devoted to writing a succinct document, presented in the format prescribed by the top management, often pay handsome dividends: a short, to-the-point report is much more likely to be read. **Appendix 12–C** provides an example of an executive summary based on the annual report presented in **Appendix 12–B**.

# ▶ Major Project Proposal

Project proposals are the logical result of strategic planning that incorporates the statement of opportunities. The middle manager becomes involved in the development of project proposals, for either internal or external consideration, in two ways: (1) by assisting other members and departments of the organization through the provision of support data or as part of the project team and (2) by initiating projects related to the manager's area of interest. Project proposals are developed in response to a request for proposal from a public or private agency. Eligibility guidelines, along with specific requirements and deadlines, are published in the sponsoring agency's notice of funding availability. Sometimes project funding comes from within an organization. In such instances, managers follow the designated internal process for requesting this funding, usually through a process kept separate from general operating budget requests.

## The Development Officer

Within the organization, a development officer is designated to coordinate project proposals. This individual, who may perhaps head a staff department if the organization is large and complex, monitors funding availability and makes initial contacts with potential donors to garner support. In addition to helping other managers prepare their proposals, the development officer makes sure that requests are coordinated; individuals and groups within the organization should not compete with one another, and certain potential funding groups will be subject to restrictions on the frequency of requests and may prohibit requests for funding of more than one proposal in a funding cycle. In addition, managers may need to heed unwritten rules such as avoiding competition with closely associated agencies.

The development officer provides assistance with questions such as those dealing with the following areas: institutional review board or ethics committee review requirements, ownership of research or project results, ownership of equipment acquired under grant provisions, and eligibility review for the funding being requested. Boiler-plate information (e.g., short history of the organization, statistical profiles, and the like) may also be obtained from this department. The final approval of the proposal request is given by the development officer before it is submitted to the chief executive officer.

## Background Preparation

Success in receiving funding correlates with thorough background preparation. Project proposals require exacting detail; concise wording is the norm. Background preparation includes identification of need and development of supporting data. The usual management materials are reviewed for adequacy to meet funding proposal requirements—for example, job descriptions, assessment of physical space and equipment availability, and projections of staffing needs.

Matching the proposal with the appropriate funding source is another aspect of background preparation. Some funding agencies will limit their support to direct care projects only and do not fund projects falling within the categories of training or equipment. In contrast, some other agencies provide equipment or supplies as their way of providing support. Eligibility factors need assessment as well; some grants are limited to projects in a geographic area, and some require accreditation by a specific agency.

The timeline should receive careful attention. Prudent optimism is needed so that, if the project is funded, it is reasonably possible to meet prescribed deadlines. In preparing support data, it is necessary to look for unusual changes in data. For example, if a major increase or decrease occurs in the number of clients served or in budget expenditures, an explanation for these variations should be prepared. If a pilot program or demonstration project was carried out, a description of how it relates to the new request should be included. This reflects the accountability aspect of reporting: How were requested resources used? How successful were these efforts?

## Content of Project Proposals

Many of the required elements in the project proposal are the same as those included in the strategic plan—for example, title, mission, values, and goals. Thus, they may be carried forward, largely intact, into project proposals. The history might be slightly amplified to show that the organization is capable of providing the proposed model of care. The eligibility for the funding is clearly specified. If the funding source is based on a federal or state law, the specific law is named. The statement of need reflects client or community need, based on support data.

The core of the proposal is the statement of objectives, the methods or plans to achieve those objectives, and the timeline. Budget calculations are presented in summary form; an appendix would include (if requested) the detailed calculations. The basis of calculations are noted, such as the assumption that wage and benefit estimates are based on area-wide patterns. The donation-in-kind category might include volunteer hours (with an equivalent dollar value assigned to this resource), space, equipment, information technology support, and support personnel. If support personnel are loaned to the project, the percentage of time contributed by these personnel is noted, along with its dollar value.

Fund-raising activities and estimated results are specified if they are part of the financial plan for the project. Plans for becoming self-sustaining are included. For example, staffing costs might be absorbed because of planned retirement of higher-paid employees; the break-even and then profit level of income from the reimbursement structure is projected. One-time, start-up costs are identified as part of first-year expenses, with funding needs then decreasing in subsequent years.

The evaluation process is tied to the objectives. The manager should prepare a comprehensive evaluation process consisting of early assessment followed by periodic review so that corrective action may be taken, should the plan need it. Final review is accomplished at the conclusion of the program. Both internal and external review processes should be identified within the project plan, including systematic feedback from clients. Use, where possible, externally established standards, measures, and benchmarks. Agency publications and websites offer examples of evaluation methodologies.

**Appendix 12–D** provides an example of a project proposal for a healthcare agency. See also the 500-day plan/project plan in Chapter 5 in the section on the project plan for a neighborhood health center.

## ▶ Business Planning for Independent Practice

Although most healthcare professionals work as employees in nonprofit healthcare organizations, some venture out of this traditional setting into the world of entrepreneurship. An entrepreneur is, quite simply, a person who owns, organizes, manages, and assumes the risk for a business enterprise.

What might cause a practitioner to make such a career change? Some respond to an opportunity: a federal or state law includes a mandate for a particular program; a region's demographics change, with more families with young children or more elderly residents; a colleague offers to bring in another practitioner as a partner or offers to sell the practice; or a practitioner is asked to help with a one-time consultation that develops into an ongoing contract. Other practitioners develop heightened awareness of a need. Perhaps they have a passion for helping a special client group, such as developmentally challenged youth, home-bound elderly, or hospice patients. As a consequence, they may decide to offer customized services to the specific client group. Yet other practitioners may be motivated by simple necessity because of downsizing or a change in family obligations such as young children or aged relatives needing care. Full- or part-time private practice often provides the necessary flexibility to meet these personal responsibilities.

Potential independent practitioners need to consider various aspects of forming a business. Doing so is a complex process for which formal legal and financial guidance is required. This short introduction is simply intended to help practitioners prepare for interaction with their legal and financial advisors. "One size does *not* fit all" is surely the case with business undertakings. The following key points are offered with the attitude, "ask a better question; get a better answer." When practitioners are ready to consider entrepreneurship, the following factors should be kept in mind.

## The Need for a Business Plan

Business owners need to plan for success; they need to comply with legal and taxation requirements, and they need to raise start-up funds. The business plan is the foundational document detailing the purpose of the business, its product or service, its clients, and its revenue. If owners apply for bank loans, public funding (e.g., Small Business Administration funding), or private venture capital, they will need to present formal business plans to the potential lender. Sources of information for, and examples of, business plans include the federal Bureau of Census, Department of Labor, and the Small Business Administration. State government bureaus make available similar information for business owners in their respective jurisdictions. In addition, county or regional development or commerce agencies carry out studies, develop regional plans, and sometimes have seed money available for start-up operations. National and regional chambers of commerce are yet another source of information and ideas. Moreover, professional associations sometimes offer workshops on the topic of independent practice. Local colleges typically offer courses and workshops on these issues.

## Three Reminders

If practitioners are full- or part-time employees of an organization, they need to obtain the necessary clearance to engage in outside activity. Some organizations encourage this kind of "moonlighting" because it builds up good interagency cooperation; other organizations have limits on the amount of time that may be devoted to self-employment. If practitioners decide to follow this course of action, they should remember to follow the conflict of interest provisions and remember to clarify their own role as independent contractors, not as agents of their primary employer. (See Chapters 6 and 9 for further information.)

## Self-Employment Considerations: Income and Taxes and Other Issues

When you discuss your plans with your legal and accounting advisors, be sure you ask about the following topics:

- *Taxes* (i.e., local business tax, income tax, wage tax, sales tax on services, state and federal tax income taxes). How these are calculated and when (e.g., quarterly, yearly) are they due?
- *Business expenditures and income.* What is the definition of each? What is needed to justify home office or personal automobile use, how is equipment amortized, which travel and continuing education expenses are allowable, and what documentation is needed for each of these items?
- *Operating at a loss.* It is not uncommon during the early phases of a business to operate at a loss or just below the break-even point. What is the allowable time limit for this and what documentation is needed to explain this circumstance?
- *Social Security, workers' compensation, health insurance mandates.* Which of these is required and what is the payment schedule relating to them? If the business employs others, what are the applicable rules?
- *Zoning codes and business permits.* What are the requirements for these?
- *Liability insurance. This is to cover practitioners, coverage of accidents on the physical property, and motor vehicle coverage if the worker uses a vehicle as part of assigned work (e.g., travel to and from home care site).*

## Articles of Incorporation and Bylaws

Articles of incorporation and bylaws are formal documents that provide the framework within which owners implement their business plans. These documents are augmented by the usual organization chart, job descriptions, and policies. Key points to consider when drafting these documents are summarized here. Official wording can be provided by a practitioner's legal counsel.

### Name of Organization

As an entrepreneur, you should select a name that immediately tells the public what service or product you are offering. Marketing and advertising firms recognize this need, which explains why millions of dollars are spent in developing product or brand names. Consider the easy-to-remember names you encounter every day. They are, generally speaking, short and informative. They fit easily on a logo, a promotional item, or a business card. When an employee answers the phone, the name is easy to say. If the name is shortened, or if abbreviations are used, the product or service is still properly represented. Look in the telephone book or enter a key word in a search engine. Which names have prominence? Which have informative, easy-to-remember names?

Give some thought about using your personal name as part of your business name; if you later decide to sell your business, you may lose control over your name. Consider the implications of including a regional name (e.g., Northeast Kansas Physical Therapy Associates); what happens if you later want to expand to another region? Avoid the use of a name that implies that your business is part of, or affiliated with, some other entity—for example, avoid using a name such as Madison County Occupational Therapy Services. You may have intended to convey the idea that your general outreach area is this county, but to many people, the name will imply that that the organization is a county agency. Take care also to avoid names that imply a relationship with a well-known university, professional sports team, or some other incorporated name.

### Legal Status or Configuration

Decide whether your business is a sole proprietorship, a partnership, or a corporation. Specify the ownership, the date of incorporation, and any changes to configuration associated with the business' development. For example, a sole proprietorship company might later become a partnership.

## Service or Product

Clearly identify the type of service or product you are offering. If your scope of practice is a specialty (e.g., sports rehabilitation; home care for elderly), state this fact.

## Board of Directors and Officers

Identify who is eligible to hold positions as directors and corporate officers. Provide a list of duties, and specify the term of office and whether consecutive terms may be served. Make provision for both appointment and removal, along with replacement. Include a detailed succession plan and the circumstances in which it would be activated.

## Executive Officer

If this position is filled by someone other than the owner, specify that the incumbent is hired and terminated (following proper processes), by management. Identify to whom he or she reports. Clarify that the officer is an ex officio but nonvoting member of the board.

## Meetings

Specify that there is at least an annual meeting. Delineate the requirements for notice of meetings, who may call a meeting, quorum requirements, documentation of the proceedings, and, usually, the adoption of *Robert's Rules of Order* (current revision) for the conduct of meetings.

## Finances

Adopt a business year and provide for a timely annual audit. Indicate who may authorize routine and exceptional expenditures.

## Formal Bylaws

Specify how bylaws are adopted and later, amended; define the process of notification of proposed changes; and describe how voting is to be carried out (written ballot or electronic voting), as well as the provision for absentee voting. Add the date of adoption, and then list the dates of subsequent revision as they occur.

## Dissolution of the Business

What is the process of notifying the public of dissolution? If there are health records, how can the clients obtain their own records? If there is public or private funding, what is required by those agents? What is the plan of distribution of assets among owners?

Once the foregoing organizational issues are addressed and articles of incorporation and related bylaws are developed, the business plan is ready for submission to appropriate parties (e.g., a bank for obtaining a loan, a government agency for obtaining special funding).

## Content of the Business Plan

The business plan is a straightforward document but one developed from detailed fact gathering and projections. As noted earlier, sample plans are available from both public and private sources. The major headings within a business plan are as follows:

- The legal name of the business, its ownership, and its legal structure.
- The product or service being offered.
- The proposed market, along with a marketing plan. This often includes assessment of both competition and support; details of number and types of clients, reimbursement agents, and calculations (e.g., Medicare, Medicaid, private insurance); and related schedules of charges and payment details.
- A financial plan. This includes sources of funding; break-even analysis; budget from past years if applicable; and current budget, with a projection for, usually, 3 or 5 years.

The appendices of a business plan usually include the organization chart, succession plan, job descriptions for the officers, résumés of owners, and support data with detailed calculation.

## ▶ The Due Diligence Review

When the owners or board of directors consider plans to merge with or acquire another organization, they need correct, complete background information about the target organization's assets and liabilities. They must seek to meet the *reasonable person* standard of due diligence by obtaining and assessing this information before entering into formal agreement. Due diligence review (DDR) is the usual descriptor for this intense review of legal and financial matters. It represents an aspect of accountability about these practices. The purpose of the DDR is to prevent undue harm to either party. It reflects the need for transparency and is part of good *faith* negotiations. This practice is patterned after that of the banking and securities industries, for which it is a requirement. Businesses have adopted modified versions of this practice for their own purposes. Although DDR is not usually mandated for these organizations, it is certainly a wise step; thus, both profit and nonprofit healthcare organizations follow similar practices when mergers or acquisitions are being considered. Although the term *due diligence review* might not be used, the purpose and process are similar to the traditional DDR.

A mid-level manager participates in the DDR at the direction of top management. Although this process is a rare occurrence, middle managers are required to contribute input into the report; they have detailed knowledge of actual and potential problem areas as well as corrective steps that have already been implemented. Middle managers will recognize several points of emphasis, realizing that they already engage in sound managerial practices and carry out many of these studies on a routine basis. They want everything to be found in good order during the DDR—that is, routine practices and studies, done in the normal course of business, with accuracy and completeness.

## Focus and Content of the Due Diligence Review

The external auditing agent, in concert with the board of directors or owners, provides specific guidelines. The major categories include some or all of the following:

- *Licensure and accrediting reviews:* past and current reviews and plans of correction and status of compliance
- *Financial status and obligations:* assets and liabilities, budget reviews and audits, the reimbursement cycle, recovery audit results, denials management and prevention practices, revenue cycle and cash flow, pension funding, and union contract obligations
- *Grants and special endowments:* any restrictions on the use of endowments or the transferability of grants and the current status of these financial instruments
- *Pending and recent lawsuits:* suits by clients, by current and recent employees, or by government agencies (with emphasis on fraud and abuse); risk management studies with emphasis on hospital-acquired conditions and accidents; data breach analysis; and medical identity theft. Sometimes a review of a sample of patients is carried out to ensure that there are, in fact, real patients; such a review identifies proper registration of patients, date(s) seen, by whom seen, proper documentation, and accuracy of coding and billing.

- *Patents, royalties, and intellectual property:* institutional policies, proper registration of customized software, and ownership of results of medical research
- *Equipment inventory:* all items properly logged and accounted for, date of lease or purchase, and status of lease or contract. For proprietary software, it is essential to ensure that there are appropriate license agreements, no pirated software, and no non-work-related software installed
- *Human resources considerations:* payroll obligations; health insurance funding; union contract provisions; and outsourcing arrangements, with particular attention paid to compliance with relevant laws and regulations.
- *Closure of facility:* close out all employee files and inform employees how they may request information from these files; finalize continuing health insurance coverage plans; close out pension plans; retire the license, charter, and related accounts; end service contracts and leases; arrange for closure of the physical plant along with final inventory and disposition of equipment; arrange storage and retrieval of business records and client records; inform clients where their records will be located and how to request information from them; ensure that no business or client data remain on retired or recycled computer equipment; make arrangements for continuity of educational programs for professional staff-in-training (e.g., medical residencies or nursing rotations); arrange financial audit of present assets, and a final audit when all the obligations have been met.

To uncover or prevent inadvertent omissions or purposeful fraud associated with employment, the DDR team reviews a sample of employees from their initial applications for employment through their current status (i.e., still employed, on leave, voluntary or involuntary separation). Payroll and time sheets are matched; paychecks are traced from issuance to final clearance.

The due diligence report is to be considered highly confidential; it is not made public. Middle managers may not necessarily receive copies of such reports.

## ▶ The Plan of Correction

The plan of correction (POC) is a formal document developed and submitted to federal or state licensure and/or provider reimbursement programs (e.g.,

Medicare) in response to citations made during official onsite surveys. Accrediting bodies may also require such documentation. It is a mandatory response, becomes part of the public record, and is displayed within the organization.

As a starting point, a middle manager will become thoroughly acquainted with the site survey process, from preparation of annual survey report through the development and implementation of the POC. The relevant standards (e.g., licensure requirements, billing and reimbursement provisions) and their interpretive guidelines are reviewed. These agencies provide sample reports and frequently asked questions with clarifications and further examples.

The next step taken by the manager is the review of previous POCs, with particular attention to those deficiencies that recur year after year.

During the site visit, managers take notes about the site reviewer's questions and observations (e.g., what resident records were pulled for audit, what aspects of activities therapy were questioned.) Should there be a citation noted that involves patient safety, corrective action is usually made immediately. For example, if the surveyor noted a broken bed railing, a call to maintenance would be made by the manager for immediate action.

After the surveyors have left, an after-action/hot wash review is made immediately to note the following:

- Positive and negative impressions
- Factual information (e.g., what resident records were audited)
- Deficiencies noted by surveyor(s)
- Time and date of in-depth after-action review to be scheduled immediately after receipt of surveyor's formal report
- Assignment of responsibilities for report development
- Immediate plans to fix any major deficiency (e.g., anything relating to patient safety)

After the formal report is received from the surveyor, the management team reviews it to determine the validity of the citation. If there is an appeal process, the time frames and stipulations are noted.

The surveyor report is highly stylized, as are the POC responses. The citations are keyed to the precise section of the law or regulation. The basis of their citation of deficiency is provided (e.g., that menus and meal plans were compared to resident records that showed food allergies or special nutritional considerations).

The surveyor report includes required response time frames and information about the appeal process.

Writing the POC report is a joint effort, with each manager developing appropriate responses regarding citations relating to their departments. The CEO compiles the final, official report and submits it. Major points for writing a response include:

- Key the response exactly to the deficiency cited.
- No defensive or accusatory language.
- Precise wording; what corrective action has been and/or continues to be implemented, along with time frames.
- No expansion of the issues (e.g., if the citation refers to residents receiving pain-control medications, this category of residents is reviewed, not the plan of care reviewed for "all" patients).
- Supportive evidence (e.g., dates of training session, its content, the attendees, and measurement of outcome of training. Topics might include proper positioning of bedridden patient to prevent pressure ulcers; methods to prevent falls; follow-up studies to determine success of the training).
- Plans for ongoing monitoring to prevent reoccurrence of deficiency (e.g., POC review at end of first week of admission, monthly reviews, and *prn* reviews when a major change occurs such as a hospitalization).
- Assignment of individual, team, and committee responsibilities.
- Provision of sample wording of response such as the following:
  - Incomplete minimum data set: carried out audit of (*n*) sample to determine nature of incomplete entries; training session on (dates) for intake/admission staff and unit clerks using the state agency's webinar self-study module; quality assurance committee's focused study at end of each month for that month's admissions, with recommendations for follow-up.

    At time of preadmission and admission processing, obtain full demographic details from the patient and their family; update this during the POC/patient–family conference. If family members are not available for in-person participation, use teleconference. Responsibility: admissions/intake, social service, nursing representative, health information.
  - Pressure ulcers: review of assessment and POC process: director of nursing; training of

staff regarding proper positioning of patient and wound care (dates of training, attendees; content).

- Medication and therapeutic diet coordination: director food service, dietician, and director of nursing; review of each resident's medical record regarding medications and contraindications concerning food; timing of food intake and relationship to instructions about medication use (e.g., do/do not take with food). Schedule ongoing review with any change in medications.

- Activity therapy: citation noted that 20% of residents do not actively participate in AT.

Review AT offerings: timing; content; review medical records of ($n$) sample to determine reasons for attending or declining to attend, or attending but not actively participating; discuss reasons with individual residents (social service and AT). For bedridden patients offer bedside AT appropriate to their ability to function—($n$) times per week. Review POC (routine monthly review) for all residents to include AT services (review done by physician, nursing, and AT team).

# Appendix 12–A

# Newman Eldercare Services, Inc.: Strategic Plan

July 1, 20n1–June 30, 20n5

Revised and adopted by the Board of Directors, April 25, 20n1

The Board of Directors of Newman Eldercare Services, Inc. (NES), has adopted this strategic plan for implementation over the next 5 years. In keeping with its mission of promoting excellence in elder care, NES has reaffirmed its core values, reviewed its strengths and weaknesses, and assessed related threats and opportunities. This plan outlines the major goals and objectives resulting from this in-depth assessment. The departments and divisions within the organization have developed supplemental plans appropriate to their functions. These include specific objectives and activities for each of the 5 years.

## ▶ Mission

Newman Eldercare Services, Inc. is committed to providing high-quality, affordable, comprehensive care to the elderly population through a network of coordinated programs. These services encompass both residential and nonresidential programs, including the integration of e/health and virtual health programs.

## ▶ Core Values

Our mission flows from the following core values:

- A person-centered approach to care
- Respect for the elderly
- A family-centered emphasis
- Enhancement of the quality of life and independence
- Coordination of care within programs and with other care providers including the integration of e/health and virtual health programs
- Commitment to sound management and fiscal practices
- Commitment to continuous quality improvement
- Innovative approaches to care to foster client decision making about the rhythm of their day and level of participation in activities

## ▶ Strategic Overview

A tax-exempt, nonprofit corporation, NES was established 6 years ago as a specialty division of Lakeview Continuing Care Community Inc. (LCCC). LCCC sponsors and owns the elder care facilities and programs. NES is licensed under applicable state laws to provide home care and older adult day care services. It is accredited by the national accreditation commission for continuing care and retirement communities.

NES receives its financial support from fees paid by clients, charitable endowments, and donations. It has operated at a break-even level for the past 3 years, having operated at a loss during the first year due to start-up costs and having received special offset funding in the second year.

NES concentrated on the home care services during the first 4 years and has gradually increased the older adult day care program. The home care program is stable and operates at a break-even level. The older adult day care program is the focus of expansion over the next 5 years. One area of emphasis will focus on respite care programs for both week days and weekends/holidays and family caregiver vacation or illness relief. Both full and half day options will be offered.

To further enhance coordination of health care, programs will be offered about developing and maintaining one's personal health record.

# SWOT Analysis

Assessment of strengths, weaknesses, threats, and opportunities reveals the following:

- *Strengths:* licensure and accrediting requirements are routinely met; NES is financially stable; location is ideal (within a 10-mile radius of 15 major employers); there is a potential client population of 2000; NES is part of a continuing care community that is the only one in the county; a major medical center is nearby, as are a community hospital and two universities with healthcare educational programs; there is ample physical space for renovation to meet day care specifications; and NES possesses creative management and direct-care staff who are willing to innovate
- *Weaknesses:* NES offers traditional pattern of adult day care, with 9-to-5 care (no early morning or early evening care); wage and benefits are locally noncompetitive; there are limited transportation services in the area; and there is a lack of client and family understanding of adult day care services (versus general senior center programs)
- *Threats and challenges:* proposed expansion of adult day care services by the regional medical center will occur within 3 years; changes are proposed in federal and state reimbursement allocations for home care and adult day care, but details will not be available for at least 2 years
- *Opportunities:* state government promotion of home care and adult day care services; state government offer of program innovation opportunities through a special funding option; collaborative efforts with faculty and students from area colleges and universities to develop innovative programs; collaborative efforts with regional vocational–technical programs to develop training programs; partnership with area businesses, industries, schools, and healthcare employers to meet the needs of workers who depend on reliable adult day care for their elderly family members

# Goals and Objectives

1. Provide a comprehensive range of programs that meet licensure and accrediting requirements for home care and older adult day care for the elderly:
   - Develop and maintain a network of nonresidential programs.
   - Coordinate these programs with the residential services of LCCC (independent living units, personal care, rehabilitation care, skilled care).
   - Coordinate these programs with non-LCCC providers.
2. Provide innovative programs to meet the needs of clients and their families:
   - Expand the hours of day care service from 6:30 A.M. to 7:00 P.M. 7 days per week.
   - Expand days of care to include weekends.
   - Expand respite care module for holidays, caregiver vacation or illness relief.
   - Offer modules of care to correspond to the client care plan and their decision making about the rhythm of their day.
   - Assist clients with telehealth appointments and personal health monitoring programs.
   - Offer programs to assist clients in developing conceptual and motor skills to easily use computer technology, including the various monitoring devices relating to their care, and telemedicine interactions; also, programs to facilitate their use of social media to enhance their interaction with family, friends, and social groups.
   - Offer programs on developing personal health record (assist clients and caregivers in this effort).
   - Educate families about the flexible program options for respite care to enhance the care of the client and the well-being of the caregiver.
3. Ensure sound management and fiscal practices to maintain quality and affordability:
   - Select, develop, and retain qualified and competent professional, support, and administrative staff.
   - Develop and implement long-range plans for fiscal stability through maximum participation in third-party payer programs; dedicated fund-raising endeavors; grant requests; and marketing, including a strong web presence.
   - Implement continuous quality improvement programs both in client care and in management activities using, as much as possible, externally benchmarked standards.

# Resources Needed and Their Provision

- *Staffing:* Recruit from regional vocational–technical program, colleges, and universities;

collaborate with them in training programs; and develop flexible work hours and part-time options for potential employees.

- *Financial support:* Meet requirements for Medicare and Medicaid reimbursement, participate in private health insurance reimbursement systems, educate families about their insurance options, develop one major fund raiser to raise $50,000 per year, seek state agency demonstration program funding, apply for foundation grants for targeted projects (e.g., physical renovation, subsidy of meal program), and seek donations of money for equipment from two area business whose charitable giving includes this focus.

- *Physical space:* Renovate first floor of existing personal care building (former assisted living facility), renovate second-floor dining area and east wing rooms, and reconfigure driveways to create a safe traffic patterns resulting from increased traffic flow.

- *Equipment:* five computer stations/modules designed for use with telemedicine, e/health and social media interactions; must meet privacy requirements and handicap accommodation.

# ▶ Action Plan

See the attached detailed plans from departments and divisions. (These documents would be attached as appendices.)

# ▶ Evaluation

Participate in, and meet requirements of, licensure and accrediting and reimbursement agencies for home care and adult day care.

Develop and implement continuous quality improvement efforts, including the following:

1. Patient care review: monthly
2. Risk management review: monthly
3. Budget monitors and reconciliation: monthly
4. Financial audit by external agent: annually

Develop and implement a plan to assess client satisfaction with all aspects of care:

1. Monthly client and family satisfaction questionnaire
2. Annual survey of healthcare providers, business and industry about level of service offered

# Appendix 12-B

# Annual Report of the Health Information Services

Fiscal Year July 1, 20n1–June 30, 20n2

Prepared by Teresa Bissette, Director, Health Information Services, August 15, 20n2

(Note to user: this is an excerpt only.)

Health Information Services completed another successful year in support of the hospital's mission. The following major activities represent the department's efforts in the areas of its jurisdiction and responsibility. These activities flow from the organization's current strategic plan.

## ▶ Licensure and Accreditation

Health Information Systems met or exceeded the required standards for both state licensure and Joint Commission accreditation for all department systems. No citations were associated with the health information systems.

## ▶ Health Information Systems Review

A comprehensive audit of the Master Patient Index was completed as scheduled. The process was based on the protocols developed by the national professional association for health information practice.

Release of information practices were improved through patient and client education. Approximately 30% of all requests lacked proper authorization, which in turn delayed final responses. An educational presentation was prepared using the closed-loop system in patient care areas and waiting rooms. A companion brochure was prepared and distributed. Funding for this project was provided through a grant from the regional Patients First Foundation as part of its community outreach. The presentations included explanation of, and assistance in, enrollment in the regional data base for health information coordination.

Storage and retrieval processes continued as routinely planned with one exception. There was an incident of inadvertent record destruction in February due to the major ice storm. Approximately 3000 records from 18 years ago were destroyed because of flooding in the remote storage area. With the cooperation of Risk Management, the record of inadvertent destruction was filed internally. The statute of limitations was met for these records. However, the hospital's policy of a 30-year retention was not met.

The goal of implementing a complete system audit and productivity review for the entire department was postponed until summer 20n2. We had planned to partner with a faculty member from a health information program. This individual's study leave program was postponed until July, 20n2. This project is currently under way.

## ▶ Client/Patient Outreach

In addition to the release of information project noted earlier, we carried out an educational program on the personal health record. The closed-loop system in patient care areas and waiting rooms was utilized. The local cable television network donated time on its channel, resulting in 10 presentations to the general public. In addition to the presentations on release of information, topics included the use of, and access to, the electronic health record system. These efforts supported national initiatives associated with electronic health records.

# Budget and Resource Allocation

The department did not utilize all of the planned allocation. The purchase of the word processing system and related space renovations were postponed until next year. A superior system will be available in January of next year. The unused funds were allocated to another department, with the understanding that the necessary funds will be reallocated at that time. All other line items were held at the planned level.

One special note about the cost of clean-up from the inadvertent record destruction: costs for this project were covered by administration from special funding and not charged to the regular operating budget of the department.

# Staff Development and Training

One hundred percent of those employees eligible for national certification programs in the areas of coding and cancer registry met these requirements. Certified positions include Coding and Billing Compliance Auditor, Clinical Documentation Improvement Practitioner, and Certified Health Data Analyst (AHIMA certifications). Regular in-service training programs for each systems area were carried out on a monthly basis. In addition to raising the level of competence for the department workers, motivation has been enhanced: there has been no turnover in the department staff due to lack of opportunity to develop new skills and to advance within the department. This represents a major reversal from a chronic high turnover.

An additional positive outcome has resulted from the department's training: workers have also advanced to positions in other units of the healthcare enterprise, including both inpatient and outpatient units, physicians' group practice, and finance/billing department. While this has required time and resources from the health information department, there has been an increase in timeliness, accuracy and completeness of documentation and systems integration with these units.

# Professional Leadership

Each member of the management team was involved in at least one external activity in a leadership position. One member is president of the regional association; one coauthored an article on the personal health record initiative. One member presented a paper at the national association meeting, and two gave poster presentations. One member is chair of the national association's committee for the development of the next version of international coding systems. All of the team participated in an area peer group for the study of health information implications of the current federal laws and companion regulations.

The department continues to mentor students from the area college and university programs in health information. Six students completed their clinical affiliation rotations (14 weeks each) in the department, one management-level health information management student completed a 1-month rotation, and one healthcare administration student completed a 2-month rotation.

# Appendix 12–C

# Executive Summary: Annual Report of the Health Information Services

Fiscal Year July 1, 20n1–June 30, 20n2

Prepared by Teresa Bissette, Director, Health Information Services, August 15, 20n2

The Health Information Services completed another successful year in support of the hospital's mission. Eight of ten major goals for year two of the strategic plan were met. These include compliance with licensure and accrediting standards, staff development and training, budget and resource allocation at or under budget, and improvement of revenue cycle support resulting in a 15% increase in revenue recovery. The department continues to implement the electronic health record according to the facility-wide plan.

Two goals were not met. First, the comprehensive systems and productivity review was postponed to this fiscal year due to the unavailability of a key participant. The study leave program of a faculty member from the area health information management program was delayed until July. The study is underway at this time. A second unmet goal relates to 100% percent compliance with our internal record retention schedule. The February ice storm resulted in unprecedented flooding in the remote storage area, with the inadvertent destruction of approximately 3000 records from 18 years ago. The statute of limitations was met, but our internal 30-year retention policy was disrupted. With the cooperation of Risk Management, the record of inadvertent destruction was filed internally. No external filing was required.

Three areas of success stand out. First, 100% of those employees eligible for AHIMA certification programs in the areas of coding and billing auditing, cancer registry, clinical documentation improvement, and health data analyst met the requirements. This directly contributes to an improved revenue cycle.

Second, patient or client education outreach on the topics of the personal health record was presented, as was education on requesting information from the health record. These efforts used both internal and external media. External funding was obtained for these projects.

Third, the management team continues to provide leadership through both regional and national activities, including presentations at national conferences and publication in national journals. The department provides mentoring and training to students in health information and health administration from the regional colleges and universities. The management team and the support staff of the department participate in hospital-sponsored public relations events throughout the year. Our goal of 100% participation was reached.

We recognize that our success is tied to that of the other departments. We acknowledge their ongoing cooperation with us as we all strive to carry out our overall mission.

The complete Health Information Services annual report is attached to this summary.

# Appendix 12–D

# Sample Project Proposal for Funding

Request for Funding: Older Adult Day Care Center Program

Prepared by Edna Ray, Administrator, Lakeview Continuing Care Community

Submitted: September 30, 20n1 for January 20n2 funding cycle

Lakeview Continuing Care Community (LCCC) has as its mission the provision of high-quality, affordable, comprehensive care to the elderly population through a network of coordinated programs. These services encompass both residential and nonresidential programs. The home care and older adult day care services are part of the program offerings and make up Newman Eldercare Services, Inc. (NES), a corporate division of LCCC. LCCC was founded as a nonprofit, tax-exempt corporation 6 years ago. The residential services of independent living housing, personal care, and skilled care opened 5 years ago and continue to operate. NES opened with financial endowment from the Newman Trust, which specified that the funds were to be used for the home care and older adult day care programs. These programs became operational 5 years ago, with primary emphasis on the home care services. The home care program is stable; the older adult day care service is the focus of expansion over the next 5 years.

## ▶ Need for Program Expansion

We seek to meet the needs of an expanding client population. There are approximately 2000 older adults in our catchment area (according to the state government's latest statistical report) who potentially need day care on a full- or part-time basis. There is one comprehensive center in the region, serving approximately 80 clients per day. Although it offers excellent care, clients must travel an hour or more to reach it, and its hours are 8:30 A.M. to 4:30 P.M., WEEK DAYS ONLY; NO HOLIDAY OR WEEKEND SERVICES. Moreover, to receive services at this center, a client must be a member of the sponsoring healthcare center's insurance plan.

NES currently serves approximately 20 clients per day. We conducted marketing research in December of last year, using focus groups and questionnaires. We included potential clients and their families, business, industry and service organizations, and healthcare providers within a 10-mile radius of our facility. These groups included a major medical center, a community hospital, three skilled care facilities, one state hospital for behavioral care, two regional high schools, four middle schools, four grade schools, and three industrial plants.

All of these groups need workers for a 7:00 A.M. starting time. One-third of their workers have direct responsibility for the daily care one or more elderly relatives. Lateness, absenteeism, and overtime for other employees result from the lack of availability of early-morning day care options. In spite of economic downturns, significant numbers of skilled workers (usually women) have left the workforce to meet this important family responsibility.

The clients themselves expressed reluctance about attending day care programs; their own words convey the core of this resistance: "We can't get up and get going, take our diuretics and insulin, eat that balanced meal, get our oxygen levels up to speed, and stay cheerful through it all! And besides all that, we don't want to leave our spouses alone all day; they don't need the kind of care we need." In the focus groups, the clients and families, along with representatives from the professional caregiver team, explored ideas for meeting these needs.

Summaries of the focus group proceedings and questionnaires are attached.

## ▶ Meeting the Need

We have renovated physical space to accommodate an increase of 25 clients per day, bringing the projected daily census to 45 clients per day Monday through Friday (approximately 11,000 clients per year).

We have developed an innovative program for older adult day care with the following features:

- *Early morning opening:* open at 6:30 A.M. Monday through Friday.
- *Extended hours:* open until 7:00 P.M. Monday through Friday.
- *Weekend and holiday hours:* same as above; will be offered, starting next fiscal year.
- *Customized schedule for early morning care:* medication supervision and nutrition plan with particular attention to diabetic needs, bathing, and grooming assistance. Instead of centralized dining and recreational areas, smaller, more private units have been established to increase the privacy aspect of early morning care. Clients are able to ease into the day's activities at their own pace.
- *A support program for spouses and older adult relatives who reside with the client:* provision of breakfast at our center and transportation to and from the senior adult center located 5 miles away. For those who are able and who express an interest, there are volunteer opportunities at our center.
- *Telemedicine, e/health, and Personal Health Record initiatives:* clients and families will receive support training in the use of interactive telehealth; when a client has a scheduled appointment using telehealth interaction, he or she will be assisted with this process. Family caregivers will not need to take time off from work to bring family member to an appointment, or remain home to accept the telehealth call. Training relating to developing and maintaining one's personal health record will be offered on a regular basis as part of care plan.

This plan reflects our values of a person-centered approach and family involvement to foster client decision making about the rhythm of the day. These values reflect the underlying philosophy of your foundation as well as the state and accrediting agencies' emphasis on fostering quality of life and independence for older adults. A certified registered nurse practitioner, with certification in gerontology, will be recruited as program director.

## ▶ Timeline

### January 20n1

- Implement marketing plan (attached)
- Recruit professional and support staff
- Orient and train support staff
- Complete renovations

### February 20n1

- Begin new hours: 6:30 A.M. to 7:00 P.M.
- Begin customized early morning care program
- Begin spouse/relative support program

## ▶ Budget Considerations

The detailed budget for the program is attached; it reflects the customary categories of personnel, space, equipment and supplies, and technological support. Income from fees, in-kind donation of services and space, and third-party reimbursement calculations are provided. These calculations are based on a projected participation rate of 45 clients per day, 5 days per week. There are four line items for which we ask your support; these are one-time costs associated with the first year of program operation. The total request is for $40,000. The breakdown of these costs is:

Marketing costs (TV ads; web site development; brochures): $10,000

- In-kind donation of advertisement content from LCCC

Training of additional aides: $8000

- Two-week course sponsored by local university (January 20n1)
- Needed to bring staffing ratio up to state requirements
- 10 attendees at $800 each

Subsidy of salary for Certified Registered Nurse Practitioner—annual salary with benefits: $52,000 based on area rate

Systems and equipment upgrades: $11,000

Using our current fee structure and estimates of continuing charitable donation level, we have a shortfall of $40,000.

## ▶ Plan to Become Self-Sustaining

In October 20n1, we will launch our major fundraising event for NES older adult day care. Based on past success, we plan to raise $45,000 each year for this purpose. An additional grant was received from a private donor to cover the cost of computer modules and stations to support the telehealth initiative; the funds from this one-time donation cover these costs plus upgrade and maintenance for the next 5 years. An annual replacement cycle will be initiated so that there will be no outlay of this magnitude in subsequent years.

# ▶ Program Evaluation

Components of program evaluation are as follows:

1. Participate in, and meet or exceed standards of, external licensing and accreditation.
2. Implement a comprehensive care plan to achieve 100% client compliance with emphasis on four areas:
   - Prescribed medication
   - Nutritional plan
   - Personal health record maintenance
   - Ease of use of technologies relating to telehealth
3. Monitor care plan outcomes through weekly review of pattern of compliance by client.
4. Provide client education about the necessity for compliance through weekly one-on-one sessions with the registered nurse practitioner.
5. Obtain feedback about program effectiveness through semiannual focus groups and questionnaires to be filled out by clients, families, healthcare providers, and area employers.

(*Note*: The attachments would be included with the proposal.)

## CHAPTER 13

# Quality Improvement and Control Processes

## CHAPTER OBJECTIVES

- Define the management functions of quality improvement and controlling.
- Introduce the concept of the search for excellence and examine its relationship to the function of controlling.
- Describe the characteristics of a thriving organization.
- Relate controlling to directing in an essential cycle that affords ongoing attention to follow-up and correction.
- Describe the concept of benchmarking and its place in the management process.
- Describe selected techniques for improving quality.
- Enumerate the essential characteristics of adequate controls, and introduce some commonly used tools of control.

## ▶ Quality, Excellence, and Continuous Performance Improvement

Headlines and key phrases that reflect a strong organizational commitment to quality include the following:

- *Committed to Excellence*
- *Your Safety Comes First*
- *The 30-Minutes-or-Less ER Service Pledge*
- *Memorial Nursing Care Facility Granted 5-Star Rating*

These are signs of the continuing search for excellence and a climate of continuous improvement. These phrases and similar ones reflect the overall theme of performance improvement initiatives associated with the management functions of quality improvement and controlling. The search for excellence flows from

the healthcare organization's fundamental vision and purpose: the timely and thorough care of the patient. Its values of stewardship and integrity further infuse the organization with energy directed toward continuous quality improvement (CQI). Effective managers engage in this pervasive process of continuous performance improvement that, in turn, fosters a thriving organization.

## ▶ The Characteristics of a Thriving Organization

When individuals or groups interact with an organization over time, they become aware that it is healthy, thriving, and effective. Conversely, when an organization seems to lack quality, vigor, and effectiveness, certain characteristics are missing. Some of the indicators of a thriving organization are the following:

- Client care or service is readily available, including options about choice of location and/or provider.
- Loyal and supportive clients return with regularity and refer others to the organization.
- There is stability along with innovation.
- Financial aspects are sound (routine finances reflect break-even or profit levels).
- The organization is linked to its surrounding community; it partners with local groups, sponsors events, and provides educational opportunities.
- The physical facilities are clean, well-maintained, and safe.
- Less tangible indicators include a welcoming and accommodating atmosphere; workers reflect competency and are loyal to the organization.
- The tempo is busy, but not chaotic.

Four additional characteristics are noteworthy:

1. There is a common understanding of the end state, that is, the overall purpose and mission of the organization.
2. Every employee is responsive to tasking, that is, they receive the tasks/duties/work/role sets and carry out the assigned work easily and routinely.
3. Members of the organization are receptive to feedback, that is, flow of communication through all levels is effective.
4. There is the assumption of noble intent, that is, there is abundant good will, cooperation, and trust; conflict is rare; mutual respect is the norm.

What other factors occasion the emphasis on quality? There are several—some positive, some challenging. The fundamental commitment to excellence includes full compliance with the applicable laws, regulations, and standards. Thus, any area with less-than-full compliance receives review and corrective action to achieve that basic goal. The response to major legislation or regulation (e.g., Health Insurance Portability and Accountability Act [HIPAA], Affordable Care Act, electronic health record [EHR] mandates, recovery audit programs) brings renewed attention to the systems and functions affected by these mandates. When management chooses to make a major systems change (e.g., complete automation of information system, adoption of advanced technology), new concerns arise; in these examples, the related issues of identity theft, date security, and antihacking measures become the focus of quality review. During any major changeover in a system (e.g., migration from hard copy to EHRs; a shift from one coding system to a newly required one), the manager must attend to the issues associated with phasing out legacy systems.

Topics relating to patient care studies reflect new concerns and therefore special studies about these topics. By way of example, note the increased attention paid to sports-related injuries (e.g., concussions, hand or knee injuries) in professional and high school athletes. Another aspect of quality improvement studies relating to patient care is reflected in the emphasis on outcomes and predictive analysis. Or an external event (e.g., a superstorm, a pandemic) might result in a review of the disaster response findings: what went well; what needs upgrading? Finally, negative publicity about a particular issue (e.g., rising infection rate, a scandal arising from employee behavior, an accident resulting in improper disposal of medical records) may require the management team to prepare a proactive response, including a renewed commitment to quality.

Just as there is negative publicity from time to time, there is also the opportunity for sharing positive accomplishments with the internal and external communities. For example, public relations releases feature the achievement of a five-star rating, the ($n$) number of days without accidents, excellence awards by specialty groups for certain diagnostic categories (e.g., cancer, stroke, neonatal care), peer-reviewed score for hospital safety, and ranking in top 25 hospitals nationally in supply-chain management. All of these issues reflect managers' concerns about maintaining quality in every aspect of organizational life.

This continuing search for excellence has a long and varied history. A review of this history provides managers with a framework within which to consider effective approaches to CQI.

# ▶ The Search for Excellence: A Long and Varied History

Emerging with a vengeance in the late 1980s, *quality* became the most fashionable business term of the 1990s, just as the term *excellence* had dominated much of the 1980s. The total quality management (TQM) movement and the earlier excellence movement had somewhat different origins, but so far the results of the quality movement have been much the same as the visible results of the excellence movement, although more widespread. In each instance, a basically sound, well-intentioned philosophy has been adopted, promoted, and implemented with extremely mixed results.

Many of the organizations that attempted to adopt dedication to excellence as a guiding philosophy ran into the same problem that has stymied many otherwise effective organizations: how to instill a *philosophy* in people so that it will cause them to behave in the desired manner.

Between the philosophy, which may initially be accepted by a few members of top management, and the actual practice, which involves many employees living out the philosophy, lies a matter of *process*. There has to be some process available to successfully transfer the philosophy from the few to the many.

Many people never see past the process and are thus unable to truly adopt the philosophy. They simply go through the motions, appearing to do what they perceive top management wants them to do. Invariably, when a philosophy is proceduralized—that is, when a process is superimposed on something as ethereal as a concept, idea, or belief—something essential is lost. Those who simply adopt the process as part of the job without buying into the philosophy will not truly reflect the philosophy in their behavior.

When a philosophy of management is overproceduralized, overpromoted, overpublicized, and overpraised, it could become a fad and fashionable for its own sake. Sustained commitment to quality improvement is, therefore, essential so that these practices remain relevant.

## Quality Control, Quality Assurance, and Quality Management

For years, many of the manufacturing and service industries used *quality control*. Quality control ordinarily concentrated on finding defects, rejecting defective products, and providing information with which to alter processes so they would produce fewer defects.

Healthcare organizations used the term *quality assurance*. It consisted largely of record scrutiny during which errors consisting of departures from some dictated standard were counted, providing information that subsequently directed which steps would be taken to reduce the frequency of recurrence of the same kinds of errors.

In addition to correcting the processes that produced the errors, both quality control and quality assurance were often responsible for instituting more frequent quality checkpoints so that errors might be caught earlier. The most important similarity between quality control and quality assurance, however, was that both focused primarily on finding errors after the fact. Both were retrospective processes.

During the 1980s, using philosophical grounding and methods exported from the United States to Japan decades earlier and later brought back as "new, revolutionary management techniques," the emphasis on quality began to shift from catching errors before they went out the door to avoiding errors in the first place. Thus we have the basis of the quality movement embodied today in labels such as TQM, CQI, and *performance improvement initiatives*.

Many of the tools and techniques included under the performance improvement umbrella are familiar to those who have been in the workforce for a few years. Many of the "current" tools and techniques have been around for a considerable amount of time—some for decades. They have been resurrected, revitalized (especially through computer technology), and in some instances renamed. Team-oriented problem solving (TOPS) or *self-directed work teams* and *team-oriented process improvements* are some of the renamed initiatives. Quality circles, methods improvement, productivity, and quality programs are other designations associated with quality improvement.

Even many of the specific tools used by today's performance improvement problem solvers go back 50, 60, or as far as 70 years. Industrial engineering techniques already existing for decades scored a number of modest, if not long-lasting, successes when implemented in hospitals from the second half of the 1960s to the mid-1970s. Renamed *management engineering re-engineering*—probably because of a general aversion in health care to anything perceived as "industrial"— these practices (process flow, control charts, and cause-and-effect diagrams, for instance) are part of today's performance improvement programs.

## The Common Driving Force

Regardless of how many previously popular techniques are returned to the spotlight or how many genuinely new features are added, there are two essential ingredients for successful performance improvement. The first crucial ingredient is top management commitment. The second is participative leadership/management style. The importance of top management should come as no surprise. Top management commitment to new ideas and approaches has been a prerequisite to complete success for as long as organized enterprise has existed. Without sufficient top management commitment, most organized endeavors are destined to, at best, generate results that fall short of intentions, or, at worst, fail altogether and cause harmful results or leave residual damage.

None of today's total quality programs will work as intended unless top management is actually involved and actively promoting the concept. Superficial commitment at the top results in similarly weak commitment at lower organizational levels.

Participative leadership/management style and approach includes a commitment to training supervisors and line workers regarding the quality assurance/improvement processes. A total quality program also will not work if managers, especially first-line supervisors, will not let go and truly delegate to employees. This means not simply giving employees the responsibility for doing different tasks or determining more efficient methods; it means also giving them the authority to make the decisions to implement their own findings once these changes have been vetted by the manager. Letting go as just described is difficult for the majority of managers. A manager might inadvertently possess a streak of authoritarianism; the reasons for a fairly strong presence of residual authoritarianism are understandable. Modern management—true, open participative management—is a phenomenon of the past few decades. Although the spread of participative management has been steady, it has also been gradual; there remain many areas of organized activity in which employees have yet to experience any management style other than straightforward "bossism." However, the ultimate responsibility still falls on the manager.

Managers learn about management mostly from other managers, and especially from those organizational superiors who, for good or ill, were by virtue of their positions role models for those persons newer to management. At one time, virtually all management everywhere was authoritarian; even now, management that is at least partly authoritarian predominates. Most management role models thus convey at least a modicum of authoritarianism. Subtle proof of the existence of the authoritarian streak can be experienced by the manager who might ponder his or her reaction to being pushed abruptly into a fully participative management situation. The manager may feel that participative management exhibits weakness and that delegating decision-making authority to subordinates is somehow abrogating his or her responsibility.

Managers may also have trouble letting go and adjusting to a truly participative environment because this runs contrary to classical organizational theory and old notions about how a work group is to be managed. Classical theory stresses structure, lines of authority, and the chain of command, and it suggests that as far as each level is concerned, someone just above it is in charge. In classical organizational theory, one works *for* the manager; in contrast, in a truly participative environment, one works *with* the manager.

It remains clear, however, that changes in management style and approach may have to occur for a quality management program to be successful. In most instances the manager will need to shift from being the boss—from planning, telling, and instructing—to being the leader of a team—to counseling, teaching, coaching, and facilitating.

Management's commitment, then, can be seen as a total commitment not only to participative management and employee empowerment but also to intradepartmental and interdepartmental teamwork and improved communication throughout the organization.

Will quality assurance and performance improvement continue? The answer to this question is yes: the focus on quality is a mandate flowing from the very purpose of the healthcare organization. However, its forms and approaches will vary from time to time.

In the healthcare setting, quality improvement has become the norm. It flows from the organization's overall vision: quality patient care, with emphasis on timely, effective care given in a climate of safety. The Joint Commission as well as state and federal regulatory bodies mandate performance monitoring and improvement. Examples include the Centers for Medicare and Medicaid Services (CMS) quality of care initiatives for hospitals and other healthcare facilities; the American Recovery and Reinvestment Act (ARRA)/Health Information Technology for Economic and Clinical Health Act (HITECH), which gives additional mandates concerning the protection of patients' privacy; and the Federal Trade Commission and its regulations concerning medical identity theft prevention. In addition, Congress passed the Patient Safety and Quality Improvement Act of 2005 ("Patient Safety Act"). The Joint Commission reflects this mandate in its standards for patient safety. Quality, excellence, and continuous improvement have become the permanent underlying themes in the healthcare setting.

## Performance Improvement Focus

Studies relating to performance improvement generally fall into one of seven categories:

1. Mandates resulting from laws, regulations, and standards. Within these laws and regulations there are specific target areas requiring attention—for example, the payment-error review requirements of the CMS, which includes a user's guide indicating the type of quality study needed to satisfy the review of payments. Topics for study include same-day surgery discharges, readmission within

30 days for same diagnosis, septicemia, simple pneumonia, and chronic obstructive pulmonary disease. Also, any topic reflected in the Plan of Correction for licensure or accreditation would receive particular focus. Many of the mandates have been noted in earlier discussions (see Chapters 1, 2, and 5) and in the opening discussions in this chapter. Recall the guidelines provided in Chapter 6 under the consultant report that uses a priority system of action.

2. CQI, focusing on *maintaining* the quality of standard operations—for example, the quality of medical transcription, detection of fraudulent line counting, completeness of documentation, and spoliation of medical evidence in documentation. These studies become routine and frequent (e.g., monthly).

3. Periodic studies, stemming from external requirements as well as internal commitment to excellence—for example, an accrediting agency's quarterly reports or the state agency's annual licensure survey.

4. Adoption of a new process or approach, focusing on the "debugging" of such undertakings and eventually moving it into routine practice. Examples include "dry runs" using the tracer methodology advocated by The Joint Commission, following the course of care and services the patient received during the course of hospitalization, with real-time review involving several departments. Quality review protocols would be used in a major project such as the overhaul of the master patient index, culling out duplicate numbers, and consolidating the related medical record documents. Once the solution has been found to this problem, the topic becomes one of routine focus.

5. Critical areas of interest stemming from internal or external concerns. From time to time, an issue demands intense review. Examples include:

   a. *Patient safety.* Although this has been an area of focus of risk management for many years, fresh impetus has been given to this topic, as noted earlier. The Patient Safety Act, The Joint Commission standards, internal malpractice-related reviews, infection control concerns—all of these have led to renewed interest in studies such as those focusing on wrong-site surgery, medication errors, "read back" requirements, and any of the events emphasized by The Joint Commission in its adverse patient occurrences topics. The ECRI Institute continues to develop patient safety–quality improvement programs to support risk management activities.

   b. *The revenue cycle.* Efforts in improving both the timeliness and the accuracy of billing, along with the prevention of fraud, is a multidepartment effort including the physicians, the admitting department, the emergency service, the finance office, and health information management. Studies typically include such topics as:
      - Tracking the time elapsed from the time of clinical events through the final payment of a bill.
      - Analysis of billing rejections along with comprehensive error rate testing as it relates to accuracy in payment.
      - Selection of high-priority coding and billing (e.g., a $200,000 inpatient bill versus a $500 clinic visit). All are important, but priority effort devoted to rapid, high-revenue return is sometimes indicated.
      - Comparison of present organizational practices to the planned reviews announced by the Office of Inspector General and its efforts at fraud control, with emphasis on the IG's regularly published schedule of focus.

   c. *Disaster and emergency preparedness.* A major catastrophe (e.g., hurricane, tornado, blizzard, fire) brings renewed attention to this aspect of organizational plans. The after-action reports, with lessons learned noted, provide the management team with valuable focus points. In addition to overall preparedness as reflected in the disaster/emergency plan, topics of study could include:
      - Aspects of the business continuity plan for patient care and financial records
      - Compliance with the HIPAA/Department of Health and Human Services (DHHS) guidelines for release of information about the aged and persons with disabilities during a disaster event
      - The proper use of the condition modifiers in coding and billing relating to catastrophic or disaster-related events

   d. *Patient privacy and medical identity theft.* HIPAA, ARRA, and HITECH legislation mandate a variety of security compliance assessments, prevention of breach analysis studies, and development of practices to prevent and mitigate compromises of patient privacy. The increased use of smart phones, laptop computers, and other devices that are often used off site (such as by home care personnel) is an area needing particular attention when these devices are lost or stolen. When equipment is leased, or recycled, these items must be securely "scrubbed" of confidential data. The Federal Trade Commission has promulgated regulations (the "red flag" rules) focusing on the detection, prevention, and mitigation of the effects of medical identity theft. Regular auditing of workers' access activity and their history of access/attempted access to health record information is another area of monitoring.

    e. *Patterns of care.* Various federal and state government initiatives include provisions concerning the reduction of rates for preventable readmission. The frequency and causes of readmission are aspects of this mandate. Related topics include transition from acute to post-acute care and observation unit utilization. Such initiatives also include requirements to monitor and report elder abuse, making this a topic ripe for fresh scrutiny.

6. Patient satisfaction studies. Questionnaires (using a mix of anonymous and identifiable responses) provide feedback about the effectiveness of quality initiatives as well as processes in need of improvement. The incidents may describe seemingly small concerns, but from the client's perspective, these are the tangible effects of practices. The care per se may have been excellent, but the related processes might cause discomfort, anger, or confusion. Examples include being unable to easily access health record information because of HIPAA rules but being asked over and over to state one's date of birth within earshot of other patients, giving an overseas 14-digit telephone number of the next-of-kin/power-of-attorney (POA) holder to registration personnel only to be told that phone number field is limited to 10 digits, difficult-to-read/use computers for self–check in, and no weekend or holiday campus transportation to remote parking sites.

7. Employee satisfaction studies. As with patient satisfaction studies, these questionnaires and interviews provide information to assist managers in maintaining a culture of excellence. Topics include general working conditions (noise levels, temperature, proper equipment in good working order) and related concerns such as safety, parking, lack of flexibility in working hours, lack of adequate training and therefore promotion opportunities, and lack of easy-to-contact "help

desk" for computer support. An analysis of grievance issues provides another source of information about topics of concern.

There are many resources available to the manager for carrying out performance improvement studies. Examples include American Health Information Management Association (AHIMA)'s Information Governance Principles for Healthcare, National Hospice and Palliative Care performance outcomes and measures, Medicare's allowable/nonallowable cost compliance checklist, and performance measures and quality improvement core set for cultural and linguistic services. See also the interpretive guidelines of federal and state regulations.

Managers of each department develop and carry out such studies within their immediate organizational jurisdiction; they also partner with other units in the organization through committees, teams, and special projects to achieve the goals relating to organizational excellence. The management function of *controlling* is the traditional term associated with these detailed processes.

# ▶ The Management Function of Controlling

Controlling is the management function by which performance is measured and corrective action is taken to ensure the accomplishment of organizational goals. Performance improvement, continuous quality efforts, TQM—all of these initiatives make up the controlling function. It is an oversight operation in management, although the manager seeks to create a positive climate so that the process of control is accepted as part of routine activity. Controlling is also a forward-looking process in that the manager seeks to anticipate deviation and prevent it. It is an overarching activity, involving all the functions of management.

The manager initiates the control function during the planning phase, when possible deviation is anticipated and policies are developed to help ensure uniformity of practice. Goals and objectives include quality measures. During the organizing phase, a manager may consciously introduce the "deadly parallel" arrangement as a control factor. Job descriptions include reference to maintaining excellence through performance of duties. Training and retraining programs are provided in order to prevent poor performance. Motivation, reduction of conflict, and the promotion of team effort support quality initiatives. Two styles of leadership are necessarily blended in this function:

- Close supervision and a tight leadership style reflect an aspect of control. Through rewards and positive sanctions, the manager seeks to motivate workers to conform, thereby limiting the amount of control that must be imposed. Finally, the manager develops specific control tools, such as inspections, visible control charts, work counts, special reports, and audits.
- Participative management/leadership style, with wide participation in the quality cycle, is the generally accepted principle in performance improvement initiatives.

Does this comprehensive focus on quality consume all or most of the manager's time? No, not necessarily—studies and oversight processes can be combined, efficiently scheduled, and carried out by designated individuals, teams, and committees. For example, when budget preparation is undertaken, a review of just-in-time inventory practices could be an adjunct activity. When a project to clean up and consolidate the master patient index is implemented (including timely and accurate updates of identifying information), a related study might focus on registration processes regarding unconscious patients or trauma and emergency admissions. A comprehensive study of clinic appointments might include the reasons for "no shows," cancellations, late arrivals, and those who "leave without being seen." A review of related support systems such as on-campus and other transportation issues would contribute to the comprehensiveness of the study. Elderly patients who depend on community-based driver services might silently resist certain follow-up appointments because of timing. A simple entry into their care plan to indicate preferred appointment time (and clinic location on multisite campuses) easily eliminates this concern.

A manager might focus on one system at a time through a comprehensive review, including the positive and negative results of work productivity, error types and rates, HIPAA compliance, standards of conduct annual briefing, safety of equipment, worker safety, employee satisfaction survey, turnover rates, and overall process and methods improvement.

A study relating to payment denials logically includes a review of coding accuracy, completeness, and timeliness; this, in turn, relates to the quality of data entries, studied routinely in clinical data reviews. Some additional data mining relating to patterns of denial would usually lead to the identification of problem areas.

# When Improvements Fail

Using the results of the feedback step in controlling, the manager assesses the results of the planned improvement, noting immediate results along with the long-term effects. If the effects are starkly negative, spontaneous feedback may occur, requiring the manager to reassess the change. Two caveats are in order:

1. The manager must respond to the feedback, making the necessary adjustments or providing clients with assistance in adjusting to the changes.
2. The manager must be willing to abandon a change when the data indicate clearly that the new, hoped-for improvement has not come to pass.

Consider these examples:

*Situation 1:* A university decreases resources for part-time and evening students in favor of full-time students. The new goal is to eliminate the longer cycle of degree completion (average of 6 years) in favor of the traditional 4-year cycle.

*Outcome:* The university had as its founding mission the education of part-time and evening students. Full-time, day students are the secondary clients. The primary endowment funds are restricted for use with the part-time and evening programs and cannot be distributed without a return to original mission of emphasizing part-time and evening students.

*Situation 2:* An acute care hospital has undergone renovations of three inpatient care units. One of the goals was making the environment "softer" and less clinical. The color scheme was changed to reflect this goal. The typical red crash cart was given a new look, including changing its color, and equipment, including the crash cart, was placed inside closeted areas or behind screens.

*Outcome:* The crash carts were difficult to find in an emergency when personnel from other units were deployed. The standard routine—color and location of crash carts—was disrupted, leading to delays in their use at critical times.

*Situation 3:* A continuing care facility streamlined various services, including maintenance, transportation, and reception. All maintenance personnel were reassigned to one central location, and all requests were processed through an online/telephone commercial clearinghouse service. Also, transportation was centralized, with bus-stop style pickup and drop off replacing the door-to-door service on campus. Transportation to the local hospital and clinics was changed to a 2-hour shuttle service.

*Outcome:* Response time for maintenance requests increased from 2 hours to 2 days. Certainly not an improvement. Transportation shuttle to hospital and clinics resulted in early arrival of patients (usually about 1 hour ahead of schedule), thus crowding the clinic waiting areas; return pickup was delayed on average by approximately 2 hours, again causing crowding in clinic waiting areas. Patients/residents evidenced higher rates of anxiety because of the waiting time. The population of frail elderly had an increase of falls on wet- or snow-covered sidewalks at the pickup points.

The unintended consequences of hoped-for improvements in efficiency and cost savings outweighed any positive benefits. Managers reworked their plans, thus removing the negative outcomes. See Chapter 5 for additional examples of unintended consequences.

## Participants in the Planning—Controlling Process

The governing board's commitment to excellence, stated in the vision or mission statement and overall organizational goals, is the starting point for such initiatives. Relying on both external benchmarks and internal assessments, the board takes the lead in CQI. The chief compliance officer, at the executive level, often takes the lead in these matters.

Process improvements and routine quality control initiatives are the purview of the line managers who are involved in day-to-day operations. These managers do not work in isolation but rather partner with other stakeholders and superusers. Physician satisfaction surveys as part of the annual strategic plan review are one major source of input. The findings can be used to set priorities and outline strategic initiatives to improve the working environment (e.g., space allocation, renovations) and systems improvements (e.g., upgrading technologies).

Quality improvement teams and committees are yet another common approach: patient care providers and support department managers cooperate in a variety of reviews such as patient safety and risk management, infection control, and medication error prevention. Employee involvement through

quality circles is a long-standing feature of performance improvement. These workers, close to the daily routines, provide important insight and feedback to operational managers.

Clients are included in quality improvement initiatives. Patient satisfaction questionnaires are used routinely to capture information about wait times and adequacy of information provided about such delays. Privacy considerations, intake processing procedures, and related aspects of admission are commonly included in such questionnaires.

## The Basic Control Process

The control process involves three cyclic phases: establishing standards, measuring performance, and correcting deviations. In the first step, the specific units of measure that delineate acceptable work are determined. Basic standards may be stated as staff hours allowed per activity, speed and time limits, quantity that must be produced, and number of errors or rejects permitted. The second step in the control process, measuring performance, involves comparing the work (i.e., the goods produced or the service provided) against the standard. Employee evaluation is one aspect of this measurement. In manufacturing, inspection of goods is a routine part of this process; studies of client satisfaction are key elements when services are involved. Finally, if necessary, remedial action is taken, including retraining employees, repairing equipment, or changing the quality of the raw materials used in a manufacturing process.

## Characteristics of Adequate Controls

Several features are necessary to ensure the adequacy of control processes and tools:

- *Timeliness.* The control device should reflect deviations from the standard promptly, at an early stage, so there is only a small time lag between detection and the beginning of corrective action. *Example:* Patients with chronic conditions have repeat visits; a coding-billing error, with resulting denial of payment, should be addressed immediately so that the same denials do not recur in the repeat-visit billing. *Example:* Frail, elderly residents of a skilled care center need regular update of POA and next-of-kin notifications when these individuals are, themselves, frail and elderly. *Example:* A required change in billing systems, with a related change in the coding system, has a deadline for claims submissions under the old coding system. Failure to meet the deadline will mean no claims payment. Any problems in denials and related appeals needs to be monitored throughout the changeover, with rapid feedback and correction processes in place.

- *Economy*. If possible, control devices should involve routine, normal processes rather than special inspection routines at additional expense. The control devices must be worth their cost.
- *Comprehensiveness*. The controls should be directed at the basic phases of the work in addition to later levels or steps in the process; for example, a defective part is best inspected and eliminated before it has been assembled with other parts. Furthermore, the controls need to include focus on workers, equipment, and processes.
- *Specificity and appropriateness*. The control process should reflect the nature of the activity. Proper laboratory inspection methods, for example, differ from the financial audit and machine inspection processes.

   The setting itself should be taken into account when developing controls. For example, a rural critical access hospital needs to monitor its billing and payment systems to reflect services provided via telehealth and distant-site practitioners. Studies relating to unnecessary medication, along with positive outcome measures for behavioral interventions are topics for continuing review.

- *Objectivity*. The processes should be grounded in fact, and standards should be known and verifiable. External reviewers and auditors should augment line managers' observations.
- *Responsibility*. Controls should reflect the authority–responsibility pattern. As far as possible, the worker and the immediate supervisor should be involved in the monitoring and correction process.
- *Understandability*. Control devices, charts, graphs, and reports that are complicated or cumbersome will not be readily used.

## Types of Standards

Standards may be of a physical nature, in terms of both quantity and quality (e.g., the number of charts processed according to the required regulations). Such standards make it easier to develop inspection processes because such information can be recorded relatively simply on visible control charts, work logs, and similar tools. Standards may also be set in terms of cost; a monetary value is attached to an operation or to the delivery of a service (e.g., the cost per square

foot per employee, the cost per patient per visit, or the cost per object in a factory). Occasionally, the standard is expressed somewhat intangibly, such as the success of a volunteer drive, competence or loyalty in an employee, or ability in a trainee. Whenever possible, however, a quantifiable factor should be introduced. For example, behavioral objectives could be developed for each level of trainee functioning.

## The Intangible Nature of Service

Healthcare organizations face a special difficulty in that their primary activities are services, which do not always lend themselves to quantifiable measurement. Furthermore, it is difficult to monitor the delivery of a service because of its dynamic nature. Patient privacy is a major consideration. Another dilemma stems from attempts to delineate services in terms of cost; many services must remain available even if the patient census has dropped during a given period. For example, an emergency service must have adequate coverage no matter how many patients come for service at a particular time.

## Selected Strategies

Traditional approaches to developing control processes may be further refined through the use of additional strategies and methods. Examples include:

- The Six Sigma approach to TQM and continuous performance improvement, which is based on statistical analysis of variations in performance measures. Sigma, the Greek symbol, is used in statistics to measure variation (standard deviation) from the mean. In the Six Sigma approach, process improvement teams seek to minimize variation from the desired norm. The target is six sigma (99.999%) or less of variation from this desired level of performance. The emphasis is on prevention of error, reduction of variation, zero defects, and continuously increasing customer satisfaction. This management strategy, applying proven management principles, was widely used in the 1990s and continues to be implemented. Managers acquire certification in the principles and practices of lean enterprises, streamlining processes, reengineering total systems, and focusing on cost reductions, while at the same time increasing productivity and quality: these are characteristics of Six Sigma. Measurement and statistical analysis are central. The ongoing analysis focuses on process variation and then rapid response to correct undesirable variations.

- Root cause analysis. The emphasis in this approach is the search for fundamental cause of problems rather than only treating the symptoms. Developing the in-depth review of a situation requires thoroughness. It often involves working with other departments because of the interconnectedness of both problem and cause.
- Waterfall or cascading impact review. The emphasis is early detection and correction so that one error is not repeated and compounded throughout the system. For example, an error made during the intake/registration process, if not detected and corrected, may remain dormant, surfacing later as a compound problem (e.g., duplicate numbers; misidentification of patients, with resulting errors in care).
- Rapid improvement cycle. The emphasis is short implementation time (e.g., a few months), with continual improvements made during the same time period. Federal and state agencies have guidelines and examples of such processes for the healthcare setting. A plan of correction associated with a licensure site visit might indicate a specific time frame within which corrective action must be made. A rapid improvement cycle provides such methods.
- Dashboard reporting. The emphasis is timely, concise data capture, along with real-time updates. Such reporting is especially useful in emergency situations (e.g., an unexpected weather-related emergency). Consider the situation of a large, acute care hospital, with multiple clinics; a once-in-a-century hailstorm developed in the early afternoon, around the time of shift change and at the height of outpatient clinic traffic. The storm damage occurred in a short outburst but with great intensity. Traffic came to a standstill; storm damage was extensive (cars, windshields, windows, signs). Management of the related disaster response was facilitated by the immediacy and accuracy of data. Other examples of dashboard reporting include monitoring flu or pandemic cases or virus outbreaks (numbers, locations, patient population affected).

Healthcare organizations have a long history of monitoring performance and seeking continuous improvement. Risk management reviews, infection control monitoring, clinical audit studies, patient safety analysis, coding error rates, reducing accounts receivable delays, filing accuracy studies—all are examples of ongoing quality reviews that are suitable for these types of application. Projects relating to compliance measures mandated by licensure and accrediting agencies are yet another set of examples of continuous control and improvement. For example, the quality-of-life indicators associated with long-term care of the frail elderly or the core compliance areas of The Joint Commission provide ideas for topics of study. Coding–billing–documentation correlation in the revenue cycle is another suitable focus for studies. Studies reflecting key indicators related to rationing or focused review as mandated by state law or regulation need development (e.g., number of C-sections, or number of medical imaging above a set limit). Dashboard reporting, with a focus on timely, concise summaries, is a useful method to combine financial and clinical information to foster rapid response to a problem area.

The various control charts presented here provide working tools for tracking data for such studies. By coupling the Six Sigma approach with the motivational aspect of appreciative inquiry, a manager helps foster a climate of success. This culture of celebrating success, giving it tangible expression in results-oriented projects, sets up a chain reaction in the organization, with each part of the system becoming fine-tuned and continuously improved. These approaches to quality reflect the fundamental values of the organization, spelled out in its vision and core values statement. CQI helps reduce cost, prevents errors, enhances the climate of patient safety and satisfaction, and fosters positive communication among the caregivers and support staff. The motivational aspect of appreciative inquiry is discussed in Chapter 10.

# ▶ Benchmarking and Best Practices

Benchmarking is simply comparison of one's own activity or results with the level of activity or results of another department or organization. This involves as a "benchmark" the experience of some other entity, the operating results of which appear to be reasonable or perhaps to represent a desirable target. Benchmarking frequently involves adopting various organizations' best practices and comparing with their results in an effort to improve results in the benchmarking organization. Benchmarks may be derived internally from data obtained from peak performance analysis.

The present-day emphasis on benchmarking activities provides the manager with the impetus to develop standards of practice, deriving them from and comparing them with organizations having characteristics similar to one's own.

## Sources of Benchmarking Measures

Managers use benchmarking measures developed by external groups, develop measures unique to their organizations, or combine external and internal sources for comparison. Examples of external sources include those taken from federal agencies, national associations, and specialty groups—for example, the core performance measures or the patient safety practices of The Joint Commission, the ECRI Institute's guidelines for emergency care, and the American Society for Testing and Materials and its standards for medical transcription quality programs. National associations of the various credentialed practitioners offer benchmarking studies appropriate to given fields of practice, such as AHIMA's best practices model. Regional associations (such as a regional hospital group) have benchmarks custom-tailored to the particular characteristics of patient care in the geographic area.

## Sample Benchmarking Studies: Health Information Management

The four studies profiled here reflect various aspects of benchmarking as found in typical health information management activities. **Table 13–1** uses internal benchmarks and reflects issues of interest to medical staff review groups. **Table 13–2** relates to personnel management, specifically turnover rate comparisons. **Tables 13–3** and **13–4** focus on specific systems within the department. For the purposes of these studies, the data should be considered fictitious. The examples include both internal benchmark sources as well as external sources.

## ▶ Tools of Control

Certain tools of control may be used in combination with the planning process. Management by objectives, the budget, and the Gantt chart are examples of tools used for both planning and controlling. Other techniques may also be used in planning workflow or assessing a proposed change in a plan or procedure. They may also be adapted for specific control use, such as when a flowchart is used to audit the way in which a task is actually being done as compared with the original plan. Some controls are directed at employee performance, such as the principle of requalification, whereby the employee is tested periodically to ensure quality standards are met. Specific, quantifiable output measures may be recorded and monitored through a variety of control charts. In addition to these specific tools, the manager exercises control through the assessment and limitation of conflict, through the communication process, and through active monitoring of employees. Specific tools of planning and control are dealt with here.

**Table 13–1** Adequacy of Discharge Summary Content

**Department of Health Information Management, Memorial Hospital**

**Source of Benchmark**: Hospital policy manual and medical staff bylaws concerning documentation standards
**Participants**: Active Medical Staff—Internal Medicine Service
**Study Prepared by**: Quality Assurance Coordinator, Department of Health Information Management
**Time Frame Covered**: January, February, March 20N1 discharges
**Date of Study**: April 15, 20N1

| Elements Noted | January (%) | February (%) | March (%) |
|---|---|---|---|
| Diagnosis and procedures stated in acceptable terminology | 92 | 90 | 96 |
| Brief summary: reason for admission; chief complaint | 94 | 94 | 91 |
| Summation of pertinent laboratory and diagnostic studies | 80 | 82 | 87 |
| Statement of negative findings and special conditions | 50 | 57 | 51 |
| Summation of treatment rendered and brief justification | 94 | 95 | 95 |
| Condition at discharge | 91 | 91 | 90 |
| Instructions to patient or family | 82 | 84 | 82 |
| Final disposition | 82 | 83 | 83 |

**Table 13–2** Turnover Rate: Clerical Workers in Job Grades 3–6 in Health Information Department

**Department of Health Information Management, Memorial Hospital**

**Source of Benchmark**: Area-wide turnover rates for hospitals in greater metropolitan area; data developed by hospital council and labor union representing hospital workers in geographic area

**Participants**: Management Team: Department of Health Information Management assisted by Director of Human Resources

**Study Prepared by**: Director, Department of Health Information Management

**Time Frame Covered**: October–December 20n1; January–March 20n2

**Date of Study**: April 20, 20n2

| | | | | Department Rate | | |
|---|---|---|---|---|---|---|
| **Turnover Rate** | **October** | **November** | **December** | **January** | **February** | **March** |
| **Area Rate (%)** | **20n1** | **20n1** | **20n1** | **20n2** | **20n2** | **20n2** |
| 5% | 3% | 8% | 4% | 0 | 6% | 2% |

**Table 13–3** Medical Transcription Productivity

**Department of Health Information Management, Memorial Hospital**

**Source of Benchmark:** consortium of five medical school hospitals in urban area, using productivity standards developed by systems engineers through special contract

**Participants:** Medical Transcription divisions in each of the five hospitals

**Study Prepared by:** Medical Transcription Coordinator, Memorial Hospital

**Time Frame Covered:** March 20n1

| Work Standard Met | Memorial Hospital (%) | Hospital One (%) | Hospital Two (%) | Hospital Three (%) | Hospital Four (%) |
|---|---|---|---|---|---|
| | 87 | 94 | 89 | 95 | 94 |

# Gantt Chart

A visual control device, the Gantt chart was developed by Henry L. Gantt (1861–1919), one of the pioneers in scientific management. Sometimes referred to as a scheduling and progress chart, it emphasizes the work–time relationships necessary to meet some defined goal. The time needed for each activity is estimated, and a time value is assigned. This information is plotted on the chart. As the work progresses, entries are made to reflect the work completed. The chart focuses on the interrelationships among the phases of work within a given task. The Gantt chart may be used to reflect different aspects of the work:

- Machine or equipment scheduling (in this application it is also called a load chart)
- Overall production control
- Individual worker production
- Project management

## Basic Components of Gantt Charts

Each Gantt chart contains the same basic components regardless of the application. The estimated time allotted for the work is plotted against a time scale that shows the appropriate time frame in days, weeks, or months, as well as calendar dates. The calendar legend may be placed at the top or bottom of the chart. As work progresses, items completed are entered and compared to those planned. In using the chart as a visual control tool, the manager uses shading or color coding to enter lines proportional in length to the percentage of work accomplished.

## Standard Symbols

Standard symbols are used for plotting the Gantt chart:

1. The "opening angle" is entered under the date an operation is planned to start.

**Table 13-4** Release of Information: Adequacy of Consent

**Department of Health Information Management, Memorial Hospital**

**Source of Benchmark**: State Legislation—requirements for ROI consent; federal regulation—requirements for drug and alcohol ROI consent; hospital policy manual—requirements for adequate consent
**Participants**: Release of Information Team: Supervisor and day-shift ROI specialists
**Study Prepared by**: Supervisor of ROI unit
**Time Frame Covered**: May 20n1
**Date of Study**: June 6, 20n1

| Elements Noted | Week of | | | |
|---|---|---|---|---|
| | May 8 (%) | May 15 (%) | May 22 (%) | May 29 (%) |
| Name of patient | 100 | 100 | 100 | 100 |
| Addressed to this facility with full title and address | 96 | 92 | 94 | 94 |
| Purpose of release stated | 92 | 92 | 90 | 90 |
| Kind of information to be released specified | 78 | 78 | 81 | 76 |
| Name and title of person to whom information to be released | 40 | 42 | 45 | 45 |
| Signature of patient or parent or guardian, as applicable | 94 | 95 | 95 | 95 |
| Date signed: current within 6 months | 93 | 92 | 89 | 92 |
| HIV restrictions applicable? If yes, additional authorization provided to cover HIV/AIDS–related information | 96 | 96 | 97 | 97 |
| Drug/alcohol requirements applicable? If yes, additional authorization provided to cover drug and/or alcohol information | 98 | 98 | 98 | 97 |

2. The "closing angle" is entered under the date the operation is planned to be completed.
3. A straight line joining the opening and closing angle shows the time span within which the operation is to be done.
4. A heavy line shows work completed. This progress line is usually proportional to the amount of work completed.
5. A check mark is placed at the date when the progress was posted and is entered on the time scale.

An additional entry may show cumulative work done as time progresses. Codes may be entered to show the reason for being off schedule, such as the following:

- W: worker unavailable due to illness or personal day
- M: lack of materials
- E: equipment breakdown

In constructing and reading any charts, codes should be used and interpreted consistently. **Figure 13-1** portrays the Gantt chart for planning and controlling

the filing backlog for laboratory reports in the remaining legacy hard-copy records.

# The Flowchart

The manager may use a flowchart to depict the chronological flow of work. A flowchart is a graphic representation of an ordered sequence of events, steps, or procedures that take place in a system. The following are various types of flowcharts:

- *Procedure flowchart:* a graphic depiction of the distribution and subsequent steps in processing work.
- *Program block diagram:* a detailed description of the steps that take place in computer routines. Specific operations and decisions, as well as their sequence in the program, are indicated.
- *Logic diagram:* a graphic representation of the data-processing logic.
- *Two-dimensional flowchart:* a depiction of complex workflow. This type of flowchart allows the procedures analyst to show a number of flows at the same time, such as a procedure that begins

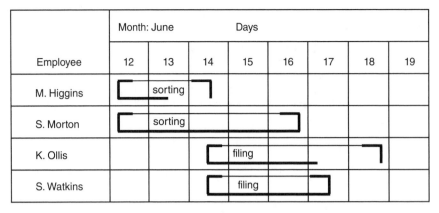

**Figure 13–1** Gantt Progress Chart—Filing Reports in Legacy Hard-Copy Files.

with a single action and branches out into several workflows.

- *Systems flowchart:* a display of the information flow throughout all parts of the system. These flowcharts may be task-oriented (i.e., emphasize work performed) or forms-oriented (i.e., depict the flow of documents through the functional structure).

## Uses of the Flowchart

Flowcharting is associated with computerized data processing because of its emphasis on logical flow, but it is not restricted to program documentation. The flowchart may be used to advantage by any manager who must analyze, plan, and control workflow.

The flowchart may be used for both planning and controlling activities. As a planning tool, it may be used for the following purposes:

1. *To develop a procedure.* The chart forces the manager to think logically, because it reveals how one aspect of the task is linked to others, which areas of workflow must be made consistent, and where coordination mechanisms are needed.
2. *To illustrate and emphasize key points in the written procedure.* The flowchart may be used as companion documentation to the written procedure, because it provides an overall picture of the workflow in concise form. Key points in the workflow may be emphasized by color-coding critical decisions or actions.
3. *To compare present and proposed procedures.* A comparison of a flowchart for a proposed procedure with a flowchart for the existing procedure may show that there are as many, or more, delays in the proposed procedure.

It is less costly to assess the probable outcome of a procedure before it is implemented than to find

that the procedure is not workable after it has been implemented.

As a control device, the flowchart may be used for these purposes:

1. *To compare the actual workflow with that originally planned.* For the charts to remain effective guides to actions, procedures must be updated and the workflow must be monitored for changes that occur imperceptibly. By developing a flowchart of a procedure as it is currently performed and comparing it with the original plan, the manager can see changes that have occurred in the workflow and may then decide whether to change the procedure so that it reflects existing practice or to enforce compliance with the original plan.
2. *To audit the workflow.* Every loop in a flowchart is a potential delay; the manager can pinpoint areas of delay, investigate the legitimacy of the delays, and determine how to shorten or eliminate them.

## Flowchart Symbols

On a flowchart, each distinctive symbol stands for a certain kind of function, such as decision making, processing, or input–output. Symbols provide a shorthand method of describing the processes involved in the work. These symbols, which have become standardized in data processing, are used for flowcharts in connection with both computer programs and with noncomputerized systems analysis. Commonly accepted flowchart symbols are shown in **Figure 13–2**.

## Support Documentation

Sometimes the flowchart is a companion document to a fully written procedure. When the flowchart depicts the overall systems flow or when the procedure has not yet been developed, support documentation is needed to complement the information on

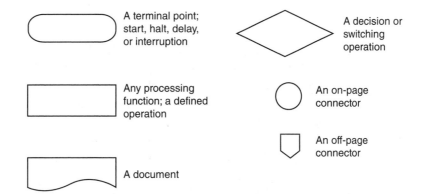

**Figure 13–2** Flowchart Symbols.

the chart. This documentation may be in the form of notes in the body of the flowchart or in the form of a narrative statement. Notes are brief, clarifying statements that supply information in conjunction with a process. They are keyed to their proper place in the chart by a number or a letter. Notes are placed in the side or bottom margins, where they will not interfere with the flowchart proper. A narrative statement covers assumptions, questions, and areas that need additional follow-up. A brief summary of the overall setting of the workflow may be included. Any special terms or abbreviations used are defined in this document.

## Total Quality Management Display Charts

A manager may use modifications of the TQM charts associated with the Deming approach to management and the TQM movement in general. These data display charts are those traditionally associated with TQM processes. The examples given here reflect application to health information systems.

### Run Chart

*Purpose*:   to identify trends over time (e.g., number of inpatient admissions from ER/observation unit).

*Display format*:   simple graph showing the element to be measured and the time period for the study.

### Histogram

*Purpose*:   to measure the rate and frequency of occurrences to determine the usual, most predictable pattern when averaging is not a reliable indicator (e.g., response time for release of information requests; reimbursement denials by inpatient clinical specialty).

*Display format*:   simple graph showing frequency distribution.

### Scattergram

*Purpose*:   to show the relationship between two variables or factors (e.g., number of "shadow charts" by clinical specialty).

*Display format*:   simple graph.

### Cause–Effect Chart ("Fishbone Diagram" or Ishikawa Diagram)

*Purpose*:   identify a major problem and its associated cause. Causes are usually clustered by category: people, procedure, equipment, and policy (e.g., times unavailable for appointments in day clinics).

*Display format*:   cluster diagram of causes, flowing toward the identified problem. Note: This chart is developed through team effort and it is displayed so that additions may be made as information becomes available.

### Pareto Chart

*Purpose*:   to determine priorities by comparing factors; to facilitate sorting the few critical elements from the less urgent (e.g., reasons for absenteeism).

*Display format*:   bar graph displaying factors from highest to lowest ranking.

The foregoing and similar graphic displays of data may be incorporated into dashboard reporting systems that provide at-a-glance summaries of findings. They are simple, flexible, and informative methods for supplying support to decision makers in the organization. Chapter 5 includes additional discussion of control processes in the section on evaluating project implementation.

## ▶ The Critical Cycle

In the opening portion of the chapter, three cyclic phases of the control process were noted: establishing standards, measuring performance, and correcting deviations. Standards were addressed in the information about benchmarking and the measurement of performance. The various means of measuring performance provide data about processes needing correction. The manager takes positive steps to implement corrective action. Controlling cannot be accomplished without active directing, which is ultimately a part of all management processes.

There are actually two cycles involved in controlling. One is the cycle already cited: establishing standards, measuring performance, and correcting deviations. In this cycle, the manager continually addresses the adequacy of the standards as well as the reliability of the measurements. Neither standards nor measurements are ever considered carved in stone; these must always be reevaluated as the environment changes.

The other pertinent cycle is the directing-and-controlling cycle, or, as it may be referred to, the cycle of directing, coordinating, and controlling.

Rarely are plans and decisions of any consequence implemented exactly as intended in every respect. Recall the examples of improvements that failed and/or had unintended consequences. Many changes, often from moment to moment, are required in pursuit of objectives. In this cycle, progress is evaluated against objectives, intentions, or needs and adjustments; new decisions are made as the work progresses. Perhaps the terms most descriptive of the complete controlling function are *follow-up* and *action*. The follow-up provides information; this is the observation or measurement of performance. Continually observing how things are going as compared with how they should be going and making new decisions provides new direction to effect corrective action.

Controlling is, quite appropriately, quarterbacking—observing the conditions of the moment and adjusting actions based on current information. It is sometimes simple and sometimes complex, but it is always cyclic.

# Human Resources Management: A Line Manager's Perspective

## CHAPTER OBJECTIVES

- Outline the functions of human resources and indicate how these relate to the role of the manager.
- Provide an overview of the individual manager's responsibilities in the management of human resources.
- Describe actions that the manager can take to ensure that he or she will obtain appropriate service from human resources when needed.
- Guide the manager toward the establishment of a working relationship with human resources that will lead to improved human resources service to the department.
- Review pertinent areas of legislation that the manager should know and that generally influence the manager's relationship with human resources.

## ▶ "Personnel" Equals People

As a professional managing the work of others, you are charged with the task of facilitating the work performance of a number of people. Quite literally, you are there primarily to make it possible for your employees to get their work done better than they could without your presence. In this role you are expected to ensure that the efforts of your group are applied toward the attainment of the organization's objectives. This must be done in such a way that the group functions more effectively with you than it would without you. And as a first-line manager, there are some days when you can use all the help you can get in fulfilling your basic charge. Help is where you find it in your organization—and one place where the manager can

find appropriate help in many instances of need is the human resources (HR) department.

HR is today's more comprehensive title for what most organizations once called "personnel." Whatever the label used, the true operative word is *people*. Management is frequently described as getting things done through people. People do the hands-on work and other people supervise them, and still other people oversee those who supervise and manage.

As surely as the most sophisticated piece of medical equipment requires periodic maintenance to ensure its continued functioning, so too, do the human beings who supply patient care and otherwise support the delivery of care require regular maintenance. Given that the human machine is generally unpredictable and varies considerably from person to person in numerous dimensions, the manager's maintenance encompasses many activities.

There are many places in the organization where the manager can go for help with various tasks and problems. For people problems, however, and for some straightforward people-related matters that cannot yet be described as problems, the manager's greatest source of assistance is the HR department. It remains only for the manager to take steps to access that assistance. It is to the individual manager's distinct advantage to know exactly what should be expected from HR and how to get it when needed.

## ▶ A Vital Staff Function

As a service department, human resources should be prepared to offer a variety of employee-related services in a number of ways. HR should anticipate numerous kinds of difficulties and needs and should communicate the availability of assistance throughout the organization. For example, a personnel policy manual dispenses advice and guidance in employee matters, and top management's instructions to managers to seek one-on-one guidance from HR in matters of disciplinary action are essentially "advertising" for human resources services.

Even though HR should be prepared to help in a variety of ways and should have so advised all levels of management, the HR department cannot anticipate every specific need of each individual manager. To truly put the HR department to work, the manager must be prepared to take his or her needs to that department and expect answers or assistance.

The terms *human resources* and *personnel* are still often used interchangeably and are currently used about equally as the designation for this particular service. This organizational function sometimes exists under other names—for example, employee services, employee affairs, and people systems. Fairly common, among a few other designations, are employee relations and labor relations. These latter two labels have also found use as descriptors of subfunctions of modern HR, with employee relations referring to dealing with employee problems and labor relations referring to dealing with unions. Regardless of label, however, the mission of this particular service department should remain the same—to engage in acquiring, maintaining, and retaining employees so that the objectives of the organization may be fulfilled. As a critical staff function, HR does none of the actual work of the healthcare organization; rather, it facilitates the work of the organization by concerning itself with the organization's most important resource.

## ▶ A Service of Increasing Value

The HR department has long been a source of increasing value to the organization at large and the individual manager in particular. Its value has increased because of rational responses to a number of forces, both external and internal to the organization, that have resulted in additional tasks for someone. Two major forces have been the expansion in the number and kinds of tasks that have fallen to HR and the proliferation of laws affecting aspects of employment. A third major force is the continuing trend toward organizational "flattening" evident among present-day healthcare organizations.

## ▶ Increase in Employee-Related Tasks

Like the majority of departments in a modern organization, there was a time when HR did not exist. Also, like other departments, HR arose to fill a need. The earliest HR departments, which were commonly known as *employment offices*, were created as businesses grew large enough to see the advantages of centralizing much of the process of acquiring employees. Employment and employment-related recordkeeping initially constituted all the work of the employment office.

When wage and hour laws came into being, the employment office absorbed much of the concern for establishing standard rates of pay and monitoring their application relative to hours worked. These tasks marked the beginnings of the compensation (payroll) function.

As organizations, in response to new laws and other pressures both internal and external, began to provide compensation in forms other than wages, the employment office took over the administration of what became known as fringe benefits. As organizations responded to labor legislation and to labor unions themselves, labor relations functions were added to the growing list of activities that shared a common theme: all had something to do with acquiring, maintaining, or retaining employees.

Other people-related activities were added as needed, and what had once been the employment office became personnel—the body of people employed by the organization. During the last quarter of the 20th century, the term *personnel* was increasingly replaced by the term *human resources*, but the essential meaning remains the same. All the while, the HR function grew in value as it took on an increasing number of employee-related functions.

## Proliferation of Laws Related to Employment

A number of laws were, of course, primary in causing much of the increase in employee-related tasks. For example, the establishment of Social Security, workers' compensation, and unemployment insurance all created tasks for HR, and much labor relations activity was brought about by laws affecting relationships with unions. In addition, various antidiscrimination laws, including the Civil Rights Act of 1964, the Age Discrimination in Employment Act, and the Equal Pay Act, brought with them much new work for HR.

The antidiscrimination laws have forever changed the way many organizations do business. They have created a strongly legalistic environment in which lawsuits and other formal discrimination complaints have become routine HR business. They have also turned employee recruitment in general, and specific processes such as employee evaluation and disciplinary action, into legal minefields filled with traps and pitfalls for the unwary. In the process, these laws have created more work for HR and have created myriad reasons for the individual manager to turn to HR on more occasions.

The passage of new major legislation affecting employment seems to have slowed, if only temporarily. Nevertheless, amendments to existing laws and "case law" arising from judicial decisions continue to expand the accumulation of potential legal obstacles that can influence how a manager runs a department and how HR serves the manager. For the most part, these continuing changes simply add to the regulations that affect employment; rarely do such changes remove or replace existing regulations.

## The Effects of Flattening

The tendency toward organizational flattening and its attendant elimination of entire layers of management has not appreciably added tasks to HR or increased the inherent importance of the HR function in and of itself. However, it has markedly increased the importance of HR to the individual manager.

Recent years have seen financially troubling times overtake many of the nation's healthcare provider organizations. As reimbursement is tightened and income grows at a lesser rate than costs, the resultant financial pinch is often felt in staffing, including numbers of management personnel. Usually the first managers to suffer, whether in health care or other settings, are middle managers.

Financial problems have caused significant reductions in middle management positions, but all such reductions have not occurred solely because of money problems. Increasing reliance on management approaches calling for increased employee participation and decision making also have resulted in the necessity for fewer middle managers.

Regardless of how it occurs, a reduction in the number of middle managers means that more decisions must be made closer to the bottom of the organization. As a consequence, certain decisions that might once have been made by a middle manager—such as sanctioning an employment offer that is higher than the normal entry rate or deciding how far to proceed in a situation that includes a high degree of legal risk—are forced down to the level of the individual first-line manager. The more employee-related decisions are forced to the first line of management, the more the first-line manager has to depend on the guidance and support of the HR department. Thus, the tendency toward flattening has increased the value of HR to the manager.

## Some Directions in Human Resources

Just as organizations have been flattened, management layers eliminated, and various activities combined or otherwise streamlined, so, too, has HR been affected in some organizations. HR has not been completely immune to the effects of mergers and affiliations and the general belt-tightening and other "downsizing" efforts undertaken in many healthcare organizations. Like other departments, HR may be called on to fulfill its responsibilities with fewer staff—to do as other departments are required to do in maintaining or improving service with fewer hands.

One effect of reduced HR staffing is a tendency toward decentralization of some activities, which effectively places more responsibility for certain HR-related activities with individual departments. For example, where once employment recruiters from HR would attend outside conferences and conventions in search of new employees, this task may now be done either jointly with or exclusively by professionals from the departments. Perhaps a major department such as nursing services or clinical laboratories now takes on the task of coordinating annual performance evaluations for its own employees—a job formerly handled centrally by HR. The upside of decentralization is that department managers become more intimately familiar with HR practices affecting their departments. The potential downside to decentralization is a significant one—it can lead to duplication of certain activities and especially duplication of records and files.

As HR department staffing becomes leaner in some organizations, it becomes increasingly important for the individual department manager to make it as convenient as possible for HR to provide its services. Any problem or issue taken to HR should be thought out in advance, with individual questions being refined and perhaps even possible solutions prepared. Advance preparation should also be seen as including appropriate familiarization with applicable personnel policies. For example, a manager facing the need for employee discipline should be able to determine from a brief review of policy whether the appropriate steps have been taken in support of the manager's proposed action.

In working with HR, as in working with one's own immediate superior, the age-old concept of completed staff work should apply. Do not simply submit a problem and ask in effect, "What should I do?" Rather, clearly define the problem, consider which possible actions might apply, indicate the option you believe may be best, and then request HR input.

## ▶ Learning About Your Human Resources Department

To be able to get the most out of your organization's HR department, it is first necessary to understand the nature of the HR function, know how HR relates organizationally, and be familiar with the functions performed by your particular HR department.

### The Nature of the Function: Staff Versus Line

Human resources has already been described in this chapter as a staff function. As opposed to a line activity, a function in which people actually perform the work of the organization (e.g., nursing or physical therapy), a staff function enhances and supports the performance of the organization's work. The presence of a staff function should make a difference to the extent that the organization's work is more effectively accomplished with the staff function than without it.

The distinction between line and staff is critical to appreciate because a staff function cannot legitimately make decisions that are the province of line management. Operating decisions belong to operating management; they must be made within the chains of command of the line departments. The primary

purpose of human resources in enhancing and supporting work performance is to recommend courses of action that are (1) consistent with legislation, regulation, and principles of fairness and (2) in the best interests of the organization as a whole.

It is not unusual for some managers to blame HR for decisions other than those they would have made themselves. Complaints such as "this is the HR department's decision" are not uncommon from managers whose preferred decisions are altered because of HR's recommendations. In general, however, HR does not—and should never—have authority to overrule line management in any matter, personnel or otherwise. If, as occasionally is the case, a personnel decision of line management must be overruled for the good of the organization, the overruling must be done by higher line management. HR may have to reach out and bring higher management into the process when a manager insists on pursuing a decision that HR has recommended against, but it must remain line management that actually makes the decision.

Whether line management really listens to its advisers in HR depends largely on the apparent professionalism of the HR function and HR's track record in making solid recommendations.

### The Human Resources Reporting Relationship

The modern HR department should report to one of the two top managers in the organization. Depending on the particular organizational scheme used, HR might report to the president or chief executive officer or perhaps to the executive vice president or chief operating officer. Generally, HR should report to a level no lower than the level that has authority over all of the organization's line or operating functions.

Human resources must be in a position to serve all of the organization's operating units equally and impartially. This cannot be done if HR reports to one particular operating division that stands as the organizational equal of other divisions. If, for example, HR reports to a vice president for general services who is the organizational equal of three other vice presidents, HR cannot equally serve all divisions because it is ultimately responsible to just one of those divisions and will likely be seen as "owned" by the division to which it reports.

Be wary if your HR department reports in the undesirable manner just described. Regardless of how well the HR function might be managed, at times of conflict, when inevitable differences arise concerning personnel decisions, you may conclude that the division that "owns" HR is usually the division that wins. Independence and impartiality are essential for HR to function effectively for the whole organization, and independence and impartiality are impossible in perception and unlikely in actuality if HR is assigned to one of several operating divisions.

Be wary also of the occasionally encountered practice of duplicating HR functions within the same facility. For example, one will encounter the occasional hospital in which the department of nursing has its own HR function while another HR office serves all other departments. Although there are sometimes advantages to be gained from basing some recruiting activity in the nursing department, splitting or subdividing other HR activities tends to create duplication of effort while increasing the organization's exposure to legal risks.

## The Human Resources Functions

There are almost as many possible combinations of HR functions as there are HR departments. A great many activities that may generally be described as administrative can find their way into the HR department. For purposes of this discussion however, the focus will be directed to the significant activities or groups of functions that are often identified as the tasks of HR. These basic HR functions are as follows:

- Employment, often referred to as recruiting. This is the overall process of acquiring employees— advertising and otherwise soliciting applicants, screening applicants, referring candidates to managers, checking references, extending offers of employment, and bringing employees into the organization.
- Compensation, or wage and salary administration. This is the process of creating and maintaining a wage structure and ensuring that this structure is administered fairly and consistently. Related to compensation, as well as to other HR task groupings, are job evaluation, the creation of job descriptions, and maintenance of a system of employee performance evaluation.
- Benefits administration. This activity is a natural offshoot of wage and salary administration, because benefits are actually a part of an employee's total compensation. Benefits administration consists of maintaining the organization's benefit structure and assisting employees in understanding and accessing their benefits.
- Employee relations. Generally, this activity may be described as dealing with employees and

their problems, needs, and concerns. It may range from handling employee complaints or appeals through processing disciplinary actions to arranging employee recognition and recreation activities.

These four general activities are at work in essentially every HR function, regardless of its size and overall scope. In a very large organization, these will be separate activities or groups within HR, each with its own head and its own staff and perhaps including multiple subdivisions. In a very small organization, these are likely to be the tasks of a single person who has other duties as well.

One additional basic function that might be encountered is labor relations. Although labor relations may be a functional title that identifies a whole department or simply an HR department activity, it is also a relatively generic label that applies to the maintenance of a continuing relationship with a bargaining unit—that is, a labor union. Again, depending on size, labor relations may be a subdivision of HR in its own right or simply one of several responsibilities assigned to one person.

Other activities that might be found within HR include the following:

- Employee health. Often part of HR, in healthcare organizations it sometimes will be a part of one of the medical divisions.
- Training for both managers and rank-and-file employees. With the exception of nursing in-service education, which is traditionally a part of the nursing department, if a formal training function exists it is most often part of HR.
- Payroll. In the past, payroll was often a part of personnel, but in recent years it has usually resided in the finance division; however, a working interrelationship of personnel and payroll has always been essential. Recent times have brought about integrated personnel-and-payroll systems, and have seen the beginnings of payroll's organizational shift back toward HR.
- Security and parking. With increasing frequency, these services, because of their strong employee relationships, are becoming attached to HR. At present, however, they are more likely to be found attached to an environmental or facilities division.
- Safety. As with security, safety is becoming increasingly attached to HR but is just as likely to be found in the facilities division.
- Child care. As an activity characterized largely as an employee service, an organization's child care function is most likely assigned to HR.

## Rounding Out Your Knowledge

Using the foregoing paragraphs as a guide, determine exactly which functions are performed by your organization's HR department. Furthermore, take steps to attach a person's name to each function. Strive to be in a position to understand how the HR department is organized—that is, who does what, who reports to whom, and who bears overall responsibility. Moreover, it is important to know the organizational relationships of the sometimes-HR functions (e.g., security) that belong elsewhere in your particular organization, to ensure that matters are taken to the correct department.

Next, take the time to make a list of the management activities or activities that can lead you to seek information or assistance from HR. The lists of most managers may have a great deal in common, such as:

- Employment—finding a sufficient number of qualified candidates from whom to fill an open position
- Benefits—providing information with which to answer employees' benefits questions
- Compensation—providing information with which to answer employees' questions related to pay
- Employee problems—determining where to send a particular employee who is having difficulty with a given problem
- Job descriptions and job evaluations—determining how to proceed in questioning the salary grade of any particular position
- Policy interpretations—determining the appropriate interpretation of personnel policy for any particular instance
- Disciplinary actions—determining how to proceed in dealing with what appear to be violations of work rules
- Performance problems—determining how to proceed in dealing with employees whose work performance is consistently below the department standard
- Performance appraisals—securing guidance in doing appropriate performance appraisals and finding out how much to depend on human resources to coordinate the overall appraisal process

The foregoing list can be expanded by each manager who may refer to it. One helpful method of expanding the list includes leafing through your organization's personnel policy manual and employee handbook; this activity will bring to mind additional areas of concern.

## ▶ Putting the Human Resources Department to Work

### A Universal Approach

The first, simplest, and most valuable advice to be offered for getting the most out of the HR department involves the age-old two-step process of initiation and follow-up. It is but a slight variation on a practice followed by most successful managers. The successful manager knows that any task worth assigning is worth assigning a specific deadline. Planning on doing things when you "have a little time to spare" or whenever you happen to think of something that needs doing breeds procrastination, delay, and inaction. An assignment—necessarily a well-thought-out, specific assignment—must be accompanied by a target for completion, a deadline that although perhaps generous or even loose leaves no doubt as to expected completion. When that deadline arrives and no results have been forthcoming, the manager then exercises the most important part of the total process—faithful follow-up. Faithful follow-up is the key; the manager who always waits a week beyond the deadline is behaving in a manner that tells the employees they always have at least an extra week.

Anything needed from the HR department should be addressed in a similar manner. Relative to the HR department, the process might be summarized as follows:

- Make certain the function of interest is part of HR's responsibilities, and determine, if possible, who in HR would be the best person to approach on the topic.
- Refine your question or need so that it is sufficiently specific to permit a specific response.
- If an answer is not immediately available, ask when one will be supplied.
- If the promised reply date occurs later than your legitimate need date, negotiate a deadline agreeable to both you and HR.
- If your agreed-on deadline arrives and you have not received your answer, follow up with the HR department. Follow up politely, follow up diplomatically, but follow up faithfully. Never let an unanswered deadline pass without following up.

This process should be applied not just to problems, issues, and concerns that you as a manager would consider taking to HR. It should also—and especially—apply to questions and concerns that employees bring to you. If an employee's question in any way involves HR concerns and you are unable to respond appropriately, then take the question to HR as if it were your own.

## Taking the Initiative

The HR department exists to assist individual managers and their employees—to assist, in fact, all employees from the chief executive officer to the newest entry-level hire. HR can be of considerable help to the department manager, but only if the manager is willing to reach out and request assistance when needed.

Expect the HR department to house the organization's resident experts on all organization-wide personnel practices. Respect HR's knowledge of personnel policy and procedure, and never hesitate to ask HR for clarification of any policy or practice that relates to employment and employee relations in any way. In those occasional instances when HR cannot immediately and completely respond to an inquiry— say, for example, the issue is one that requires input from legal counsel as well as HR—you should nevertheless expect HR to secure the answer.

When a personnel question has legal implications, as many such questions do, there is all the more reason to take it to HR to minimize management's exposure to the potential results of a faulty decision. It is far better to ask than to inadvertently put the organization at risk.

Often HR has exactly the information the department manager needs and is more than willing to share this information. Take the initiative to reach out and ask HR—and expect answers.

## ▶ Some Specific Action Steps

Any number of management needs present opportunities to put the HR department to work. The more frequently encountered of these are described here.

## Finding New Employees

There are any number of points in the employment process at which the manager and HR must work together. Fulfill your end of the working relationship, and expect HR staff to fulfill theirs. For example, if none of the candidates HR has supplied for a particular position is truly appropriate, ask for more; do not settle for only what is given if it is genuinely not enough. For your part of the arrangement, do not

continue to call for more applicants in a search for the "perfect" candidate if you have already seen two or three who meet the posted requirements for the job. Online recruiting and the use of social media platforms have become standard practice in recruiting and hiring efforts. Online recruiting sites offer a means of expanding the pool of applicants. For this potentially beneficial method to assist employers in their recruiting efforts, line managers need to hone the screening questions to attract more applicants as well as discourage unqualified applicants. Particular attention needs to be given to technical terms that have special meaning within a job set. For example, when recruiting for a coder, a manager in health information must specify that the position relates to clinical coding according to standard ICD-10 protocols, not merely "coding" as the term is used extensively in IT.

Another aspect on recruiting, and subsequent screening of applicants, relates to the access to, and use of, the applicant's social media presence. Should these sites be accessed without permission? Should applicants be required to allow access to their personal sites? Are applicants' comments from a few years ago, before or early in their work history, relevant at this stage in their career? These issues and questions are unfolding in the ever-increasing network of internet use.

Also, stay in touch with HR concerning the extending of offers, the checking of references, and the scheduling of pre-employment physical examinations and starting dates. Do not be unreasonable; recognize that these activities take time. By making your interest and attention known, however, you will encourage completion of the process.

## Bringing Job Descriptions Up-to-Date

The manager ordinarily has a significant responsibility in maintaining current job descriptions for the department. The HR department usually has the responsibility for associating a pay level with each job and for maintaining central files of up-to-date job descriptions. Job descriptions should be written in large part by those who do the work and those who supervise the doing of the work; however, it is important to involve HR deliberately in contributing consistency to every necessary job description and ensuring that each job is properly placed on a pay scale.

Once again, your visible interest in the process will encourage timely completion of HR's activities.

## Evaluating Employees

The HR department provides overall guidance about employee evaluation and performance appraisals so that there is uniformity across the organization. Guidelines typically include the time frames for evaluation (e.g., at the end of probationary term, annual review, final review). Generic content and standard forms are provided. Elements of the appeal process/disagreement with evaluation by the employee are delineated. The HR department monitors "evaluation inflation, or deflation," whereby a group of employees all receive above-average or excellent ratings, or, conversely, re-calibrating a point system whereby all the 4.0 ratings are reduced to 3.5 across the board. If a new rating scale is initiated, proper notation in employee files should be noted.

Line managers confer with HR specialists to customize generic content to reflect the aspects or elements unique to the department. Line managers benefit from periodically asking HR for rating profile information that reveals patterns in the manager's rating practices and shows whether those patterns are changing with time, and perhaps also show how this specific manager's rating practices compare with those of other managers.

Line managers provide the HR department with information about changing job requirements that may be affecting the application of criteria based on previous requirements.

The line manager has the responsibility of carrying out assessments of the department's employees. For supervisory and managerial positions, self-evaluation is a common practice. Training in the process of self-evaluation is provided. Highlights from the department's annual report are made available. Managers could use wheel book entries as a prompt to remind themselves, and the worker, of positive or problematic incidents. Key headers are listed on the evaluation form, for example, increasing acceptance of responsibilities, ability to work independently, ability to work as a team member, stability when working under stress, maintaining courtesy and tact in client and coworker interaction, acquisition of new skills, as well as training and development participation. Additional points of emphasis include special projects, critical incident response, and involvement in major initiatives associated with the organization's mission, goals, and strategic plans.

## Disciplining Employees

Regardless of the extent of HR involvement in the disciplinary process, it is not the HR department that decides on disciplinary action. The HR department disciplines no one except employees of the HR department, as necessary. Any employee deserving of disciplinary action must be disciplined through his or her immediate chain of command.

In most organizations, it is a requirement for the manager to take proposed disciplinary actions—at least those entailing actions more severe than oral warnings—through HR before implementation. Whether or not this is true for your organization, you are advised to always take your best assessment to HR and ask for advice. Expect sound advice, whether in the form of a single recommendation, complete with rationale for doing so, or as two or more alternatives, each with its own possible consequences fully explained. The decision is theoretically all yours, and if it is a poor decision you will bear much of the blame. Never let HR avoid responsibility by failing to provide specific direction; insist on complete HR participation in deciding on disciplinary action.

When separation from an organization is initiated by the employee, as in a voluntary resignation, or initiated by the manager, as in an involuntary separation, the line manager works closely with the HR department to ensure proper procedures and safeguards are followed. The employee handbook provides the employee with information about resignation, including time frame and manner of notification. Information about involuntary termination should also be included.

When an employee is physically present on their last day of employment, typical steps include cleaning out one's desk and locker; if the situation warrants it, a supervisor is present to monitor this activity; accounting for, and turning in, keys, pass cards, and official identification; computer access is frozen and passwords invalidated. The line manager completes a final evaluation and reviews it with the employee. The HR department carries out an exit interview with the employee, providing him or her with such information as continuing health insurance benefits, retirement benefits, and accrued leave time (sick leave, vacation, personal days) as well as the forms and deadlines associated with these issues. The HR department provides clarity about the official date of separation.

In the case of an employee who is unable to be present during these processes, a supervisor, with the assistance of another supervisor so that no question arises about impropriety of handling personal items, cleans out the work station and locker. The HR department makes an arrangement with the employee when or how to obtain these personal belongings.

In the event that a terminated worker presents a potential threat to the safety of employees and clients, the standard security alerts are activated through the joint action of HR and security.

## Dealing with Training Needs

If the HR department has responsibility for any employee training—and in most healthcare organizations there is a better-than-even chance that this is so—do not wait for needed training. If there are training needs in your work group, take them to HR. If, for example, several employees require training in basic telephone techniques, take your well-defined needs to HR, negotiate a timetable for providing the training, and offer to become personally involved in the training. (With appropriate HR involvement, every manager is a potentially valuable instructor in some topic.)

The foregoing are presented as a few specific suggestions but are offered primarily to convey a general idea to the manager. This idea is that the HR department exists as a service function for all employees and that it remains for the supervisor to take each legitimate personnel-related need to HR and to ask for—and expect—an honest response.

## ▸ Further Use of Human Resources

In addition to the previously mentioned activities, there are occasionally other times when the manager is well advised to turn to HR:

- When examining staff turnover patterns and attempting to determine what might be done to increase the chances of retaining key employees
- When planning for potential future staffing needs
- For periodically examining staff pay rates relative to the community, the region, and the occupations employed
- For using HR as a sounding board, a "safe harbor" for venting frustrations without involving employees, peers, or superiors
- When looking for confidential guidance in addressing difficult situations experienced with others
- For drawing on HR experience and resources in celebrating individual employees as appropriate (e.g., employee of the month) and in periodically recognizing various occupations (e.g., National Nurses Week, Physical Therapy Week)

## ▸ Wanted: Well-Considered Input

The most effective HR departments are not one-way dispensers of information and assistance. Effective HR departments are responsive to the needs of the organization's work force; however, the HR department can go only so far in anticipating needs and meeting them within the limits of available resources. To be fully effective, the HR department must learn of employees' needs from employees and managers and must in turn go to top management with solid proposals for meeting the most pressing needs.

Some employees, usually only a few, take their own questions, concerns, and suggestions to the HR department. But most employees will never do so for themselves; their needs, whether conveyed through words, actions, or attitudes, must find their way to HR and eventually to top management through their managers.

Among the kinds of information that the manager should pass along to HR are the following:

- Reactions to various personnel policies, especially when policies seem to have become less appropriate under changing conditions
- Employee attitudes concerning pay and benefits, especially perceptions of inequities and alleged instances of unfair treatment
- Complaints—and compliments as well—about employee services such as the cafeteria and parking
- Comments on the appropriateness of various employee benefits, and perceptions of benefits needed or desired as opposed to those currently given
- Potential changes in any or all means of acquiring, maintaining, or retaining employees who might afford the organization a competitive edge in its community

## ▸ Understanding Why As Well As What

It is relatively easy to determine what HR as a department does within the organization. However, it is necessary to go beyond what and develop an appreciation of why—that is, why HR does what it does and why it sometimes must espouse a position in opposition to a line department's position.

Consider the case of a manager who appeals to the HR department to help her resolve a seemingly unending series of difficulties by agreeing to the termination of a particular employee. The manager says,

> I simply can't do any more with this person. She's chronically late in spite of all my warnings. Her absenteeism disrupts staffing; she uses up her sick time as fast as she earns it. Her attitude is absolutely terrible; she's been rude to patients and families, and the way she talks to me borders on insubordination much of the time. Her clinical skills are just average at best, and she's a disruptive influence within the group. I've been patient longer than anyone has the right to expect me to be, but nothing has changed. I want to discharge her.

As often occurs in such circumstances, the HR practitioner hearing the manager's request briefly reviews the employee's background and immediately recommends against termination. This may understandably disappoint and upset the manager and leave her displeased with the HR department. She may complain, with some justification, that she ought to be supported in her efforts to get rid of an unsatisfactory employee. She may well view HR as obstructive and adopt an adversarial position, perhaps even attempting to solicit the assistance of her own higher management in opposing the HR position.

Why would HR be automatically protective of any employee whose relationship with work is as bad as described by this manager? The differences lie in, first, the manager's perspective versus the HR perspective, and second, the frequently cited employee personnel file—"the record."

The manager is legitimately focused on the good of the patients and the good of the unit, and the behavior of the employee in question threatens both. By contrast, HR must view the issues in two ways that conflict with the manager's perspective: (1) in micro terms, HR must be concerned with the rights of the individual and (2) in macro terms, HR must be concerned with the good of the total organization. The organization is, of course, no more than the sum total of a number of individuals. Nevertheless, in focusing on the one and the all, the HR perspective fails to match that of the manager, which is necessarily focused on more than one but much less than all.

Then there is "the record" to consider. In this example, it turns out that all of the manager's "warnings" concerning tardiness were informal oral warnings of which no record was made; the same was true for warnings for absenteeism, except for a single written warning that was far too old to give weight

to current disciplinary action. No other warnings appeared in the personnel file. In fact, although in the mind of the manager this employee had always been less than satisfactory, the personnel file included several performance evaluations that, while not glowing with praise, suggested at least nominally acceptable performance. In short, there was no basis for termination except perhaps in the manager's mind.

When it comes to problems such as that just described, the HR department is fulfilling two responsibilities:

- Defending the rights of the individual, not only because doing so arises from a sense of fairness but also because there are many laws requiring the organization to do so
- Protecting the organization from a multitude of legal risks

Whenever there is a risk that an employee problem or complaint will be taken outside of the organization, it is best to think of any criticism of employee conduct or performance in a single light: if it is not reflected in the record, it never happened. Except in instances of termination for major infractions calling for immediate discharge (and these days even many of these actions are successfully challenged), a discharge must be backed up with a paper trail describing all that occurred leading up to the termination. It is legally necessary to be able to demonstrate that the employee was given every reasonable opportunity to correct the offending behavior or improve the unsatisfactory performance.

## ▶ Legal Guides for Managerial Behavior

A number of areas of legislation—federal, state, and in some instances local—define how work organizations must deal with employees in certain respects. Any work organization is, of course, subject to many laws that bear on essentially all aspects of the conduct of business. A great many laws applicable to business are essentially invisible to the individual manager. For example, nothing done in the normal course of business by the manager of rehabilitative services has any bearing on corporate compliance with certain financial reporting laws. However, some laws directly shape the relationship between employer and employee. It is this collection of laws affecting employment that concerns the manager, and it is this general area of employment legislation for which HR is the source of most of the individual manager's guidance.

## Labor Relations

The National Labor Relations Act (NLRA) of 1935, known otherwise as the Wagner Act, originally provided the basis for most labor law in the United States. It was significantly amended in 1947 by the Labor Management Relations Act, otherwise known as the Taft-Hartley Act. Taft-Hartley is the primary reference applicable when discussing aspects of union organizing. Numerous references to the NLRA are actually references to the NLRA as amended by Taft-Hartley, which provides the framework for all modern labor law.

Before 1975, not-for-profit hospitals were exempt from all provisions of Taft-Hartley. However, in 1975 the act was amended to remove the not-for-profit hospital exemption. Before 1975, hospital employees were covered only in special sections of the labor relations laws of some states. The 1975 amendments provided hospitals, because of the nature of their business, with certain legal protections not available to other industries. For example, there is a requirement that 10 days' notice be provided prior to any picketing, strike, or other concerted refusal to work—a requirement not applicable in other industries. Overall, however, the effect of the removal of the exemption essentially made not-for-profit hospitals and certain other healthcare institutions equally subject to union organizing as organizations in other industries.

The individual manager needs to know the general impact of labor law as it applies to day-to-day operations within the department. If the organization's employees are not unionized and if there is no active threat of union organizing, labor law will be of little immediate concern, and common-sense management will prevail. If there is a union in place, much of the manager's behavior concerning employees will be governed by a collective bargaining agreement (contract). If there is no union, but active organizing is occurring, the manager's conduct in regard to employees will be governed by provisions of the NLRA. In either case, the manager's primary source of guidance will be the human resources department.

## Wages and Hours

Of primary interest is the Fair Labor Standards Act (FLSA), the federal wage and hour law, and as such the model for the wage and hour laws of many states. Occasional points that might not be addressed in federal law may be covered by pertinent state laws. Generally, if the same points are covered by both state and federal laws but differences exist between the two, the more stringent legislation will apply. For example,

the minimum wage required by some state laws may be higher than the one allowed by federal law in the amended FLSA, and employers in those states are required to pay the higher minimum wage.

In general, the wage and hour laws spell out who is to be paid for what and how. They specify who can be exempt and who must be considered nonexempt—where exempt literally means exempt from the overtime provisions of the law. Exempt employees—certain executive, administrative, and professional employees who meet special legal requirements—do not have to be paid overtime pay. Nonexempt employees as defined under the law must receive time-and-one-half the regular rate of pay for hours in excess of 40 in a week.

In 2004, a number of changes were made in the rules used for determining who is or is not eligible for overtime pay. Some significant issues surrounding these rules remain controversial. Many agree that the FLSA is antiquated and confusing, particularly the portions addressing overtime pay. The newer rules mandate overtime pay for more low-income workers but at the same time appear to render certain white-collar workers and professionals ineligible for overtime pay.

The entire overtime question can sometimes be confusing to the individual manager, but the status of overtime regulations at any given time is usually known in the HR department.

Human resources and the organization's payroll department are usually the manager's two primary sources of advice and assistance concerning the wage and hour laws. At the very least, the individual manager should be aware of the status (exempt or nonexempt) of each person in the work group and understand how time reporting and wage payment are handled for each. The wage and hour laws are actually extremely detailed and extensive, and fortunately only a relative handful of regulations will apply to any individual manager's situation.

## Equal Pay

A specific section of the FLSA, as augmented by the Equal Pay Act of 1963, requires covered employers to provide equal pay for men and women who are performing the same work. In 1972, coverage of this act was extended beyond employees covered by FLSA to an estimated 15 million additional executive, administrative, and professional employees, including academic and administrative personnel and teachers in elementary and secondary schools, and to outside salespeople.

# Civil Rights

Title VII of the Civil Rights Act of 1964, as amended by the Equal Employment Opportunity Act of 1972, prohibits discrimination because of race, color, religion, sex, or national origin in any term, condition, or privilege of employment. As enforced through the Equal Employment Opportunity Commission (EEOC), Title VII covers the following entities:

- All private employers of 15 or more persons
- All educational institutions, both public and private
- State and local governments
- Public and private employment agencies
- Labor unions with 15 or more members
- Joint labor–management committees for apprenticeship and training

The EEOC investigates job discrimination complaints. When it finds reasonable cause to believe that charges are justified, it attempts, through conciliation, to eliminate all aspects of discrimination revealed by the investigation. If conciliation fails, the EEOC has the power to take the employer to court to enforce the law. Discrimination charges may be filed by individuals (job applicants as well as active employees) and by organizations on behalf of aggrieved individuals.

Title VII was modified and strengthened by the Civil Rights Act of 1991 in an effort to reverse the effects of several U.S. Supreme Court decisions that had the effect of weakening the law. The 1991 legislation also made possible increased financial damages against organizations found guilty of discriminatory practices. It is civil rights legislation that causes the most potential difficulty for working managers. Therefore, it is in this area of concern that the HR department, usually backed up by the organization's legal counsel, is most prepared to advise and support department management.

# Americans with Disabilities Act

Passed in 1990 and largely made effective in 1992, the Americans with Disabilities Act (ADA) affirmed the right of persons with disabilities to equal access to employment; services; and facilities available to the public, including transportation and telecommunications. The ADA requires employers to provide "reasonable accommodation" for disabled individuals who are capable of performing the essential functions of the positions for which they apply. This may include altering physical facilities to make them usable by individuals with disabilities, restructuring jobs about

their essential functions, and altering or eliminating nonessential activities so that disabled persons can perform the work.

Amendments passed in 2008 placed new requirements on employers and the courts in deciding whether an individual can be considered sufficiently disabled to receive protection under the ADA. Also, a number of court decisions have had the effect of increasing the number of conditions that may be considered disabilities for ADA purposes.

The EEOC is responsible for dealing with complaints filed under the ADA.

# Family and Medical Leave Act

The Family and Medical Leave Act (FMLA) of 1993 makes it possible for an eligible employee (one who has been employed at least 1 year and has worked at least 1250 hours) to take up to 12 weeks of unpaid leave in a 12-month period for certain specified reasons without loss of employment. Qualifying reasons are as follows: for the birth of the employee's child or the care of that child up to 12 months of age; for placement of a child with the employee for adoption or foster care; for the employee to care for a spouse, child, or parent having a serious health condition; and for the employee's own serious health condition involving the employee's inability to perform the essential functions of the job. This law has expanded provisions to include military caregiver considerations and, in some states, an expanded definition of family and caregivers (e.g., grandparents). Some states provide greater flexibility in defining the caregiver–child relationship (e.g., de facto caregiver even when official foster care or next-of-kin considerations do not apply). An employee returning to work within the 12-week limit must be returned to his or her original position or to a fully equivalent position in terms of pay and benefits and overall working conditions.

The FMLA can be relatively complex in its interrelationships with other laws, conflicting in instances with the ADA, the FLSA, and various states' workers' compensation laws. Once again, HR, backed up with corporate legal counsel, stands ready to advise the manager.

# Sexual Harassment

Sexual harassment has been prominent in society for a number of years, and it continues to be an active concern in work organizations and elsewhere. The number of sexual harassment complaints filed with the EEOC and various state agencies continues to increase, as do the numbers of employers involved and the monetary penalties. In recent years, sexual harassment has been one of the two leading causes of legal complaints against employers (the other is age discrimination).

Sexual harassment is a form of sex discrimination under Title VII of the Civil Rights Act of 1964. It consists of unwelcome sexual advances, requests for sexual favors, or other conduct of a sexual nature in these conditions: if submission is either an actual or implied condition of employment, if submission or rejection is used as a basis for making employment-related decisions, or if the conduct interferes with work performance or creates an offensive work environment. A key concern in the foregoing resides in the word *unwelcome*; conduct is considered unwelcome if the employee neither solicits nor invites it and regards it as undesirable or offensive. Whether a particular occurrence is or is not sexual harassment sometimes depends largely on the perception of the victim.

Sexual harassment can take a number of forms. Sexually explicit pictures or calendars, offensive sexually related language, sexual humor, other sexual conduct that creates a hostile environment, sexually explicit behavior, indecent exposure, sexual propositions or intimidation, offensive touching, and participation in or observation of sexual activity are all examples of sexual harassment. Also considered sexual harassment is something as seemingly innocent (to some) as repeatedly asking a coworker or subordinate for a date after having been turned down. This adds the dimension of repetition to some harassing behavior; asking a time or two might be considered reasonable, but asking repeatedly after having been turned down may be considered harassing.

Sexual harassment is not limited strictly to the workplace; it is also sexual harassment if it occurs off-premises at employer-sponsored social events and at private sites if it involves people who have an employment relationship with each other. In addition to involving employees, sexual harassment can involve visitors, vendors, patients, and others as either potential perpetrators or victims.

To limit liability for sexual harassment, it is necessary for the employer to promptly and confidentially investigate all complaints, take appropriate corrective action, and create and retain complete and accurate records.

A sound prevention program is vital where sexual harassment is concerned. At a minimum such a program should include a published sexual harassment policy and a detailed procedure for investigating complaints. All employees, and especially all managers, should be educated in the recognition and prevention of sexual harassment. See also the section on training and orientation that includes frequently asked questions about sexual harassment.

# Violence in the Workplace

Violence in the workplace often results from stress. It frequently occurs when a person becomes stressed to what is for that individual an unbearable level. When stress becomes unbearable, some people become ill, some break down, some walk away from the sources of stress, and some become violent. Violence is similar to other forms of human behavior in that it is action in response to a condition, need, or demand.

Every change that alters employees' expectations becomes fertile ground for chronic anger, which can lead to reduced productivity and quality, increased fatigue, burnout, depression, and violence. One of every six violent crimes occurs in the workplace. Motor vehicle accidents are the leading cause of death for working men, but murder is the leading cause of death for working women.

The highest-risk areas for nonfatal assaults are the retail trades, such as grocery stores and eating and drinking establishments, and service organizations, such as hospitals, nursing homes, and social services agencies.

The department manager's best approach to workplace violence is awareness and prevention. There is no consistent profile to describe a person who commits violent acts in the workplace, but violence is often perpetrated by someone who has the following characteristics:

- Is experiencing family problems
- Has problems related to the abuse of alcohol or drugs
- Has a history of violence
- Is a known aggressive personality
- Is experiencing certain mental conditions (e.g., depression)
- Possesses a poor self-image or low self-esteem

People commit violent acts for a variety of reasons, which have been known at times to include these conditions:

- The inability to cope with what to the person is extreme stress
- Drug reactions
- Problems involving job, money, or family
- Reaction to the loss of employment
- Reaction to the loss of a relationship
- Frustration with long waits or rude or indifferent treatment

- Confusion or fear
- Perceived violation of privacy

One can never tell for certain who may resort to violence. However, there are steps to consider for preventing violence.

- Treat everyone with respect and consideration.
- Keep all potential weapons stored beyond the reach of patients and visitors.
- Take threats seriously and report them immediately.
- Know your security procedures, alarms, and warning codes.

Be extra alert to the possibility of violence if a person meets any of these criteria:

- Appears to be under the influence of alcohol or drugs
- Appears to have been in a fight
- Is brought into the facility by the police
- Is already being restrained

Visible indicators of potential violence include the following:

- Obvious possession of a weapon
- Nervousness or abrupt movements
- Extreme restlessness, such as pacing and obvious agitation

When observing an individual who appears to be on the edge of losing control, follow the safety and security protocols, including:

- Notify other staff and call security
- Stay alert but remain calm
- Maintain a safe distance, giving the person plenty of space; do not turn your back and do not touch the person
- Keep obstacles between you and the individual
- Be certain you have a way out; avoid dead end corridors or corners
- Listen; do not display anger or defensiveness and do not argue; speak slowly and quietly

Some departments, such as the emergency department, are more prone to violence than others, but violence is possible anywhere. Every department's staff should have some orientation in how to deal with violent behavior. If violence does occur:

- Protect yourself to the extent necessary
- Sound the alarm or call the appropriate code
- Help remove others from the vicinity, if necessary
- Do not try to disarm or restrain the person yourself
- Give the individual what he or she is demanding, if possible

## ▶ An Increasingly Legalistic Environment

Before 1964 there were not a great many legal concerns affecting the work of HR and department managers. As long as the organization was compliant with wage-and-hour law, labor law, and a few state regulations, there were not many legal requirements to be aware of. However, Title VII of the Civil Rights Act of 1964 was a major "game changer" in that it launched a legalistic phase of employee relations: a series of new employment-related laws came on line over three decades or so. Major new employment legislation slowed with passage of the FMLA of 1993, but there have been and most likely always will be periodic amendments to existing laws and changes wrought by case law as various legal challenges are dealt with in the courts. Present indications are that employers can expect to see increasing activity toward mandating paid sick leave in many organizations that do not offer this particular benefit. Overall, the effects of accrued employment legislation have been to legally make employers more socially responsible for their workers.

Although the issues described in this section are those of greatest concern to the manager (especially civil rights, wage and hour, and possibly labor relations), many other federal, state, and local laws can affect the employment relationship. It may seem at times as though this is excessive legislation and that all of these rules and regulations may not be truly necessary. Remember, however, that managers are employees as well and that the protections afforded employees under legislation such as equal pay and civil rights also extend to managers. All working managers should be willing to recognize that the laws affecting employment represent a well-defined part of management's boundaries, those limits within which it is necessary to learn to work in the fulfillment of management's responsibilities.

## The Work Environment: Hostile or Supportive?

In this increasing legalistic environment, a manger must remain alert to factors that directly or inadvertently create a hostile work environment. The manager seeks to create and maintain a positive environment, one in which workers feel psychologically and physically safe. A beginning point for a manager's assessment of dynamics of the workplace is this: what is the day-to day experience of the worker? Consider these factors:

- The adult worker spends a high percentage of available time at the workplace, e.g., the 40-hour work week; the "9 to 5" job.
- The workplace is a microcosm of interpersonal relationships; diversity in the work force is a day-to-day reality.
- Elements/aspects of organizational life mingle: the degree of bureaucracy, of central vs. decentralized structure
- Leadership styles are evident, and vary from department to department
- Aspects of motivation and demotivation surface; is this a "nice" place to work? Would I work want to work here? If I didn't have to work here and had other job opportunities, would I stay in this setting?
- The arena of conflict is localized in the department/unit.

The elements of a pronounced hostile work environment tend to be easily identified, overt, and well-defined. In general, such behavior is rare. Orientation, training, and re-training concerning standards of conduct help reduce such occurrences. However, there may be a low-level, chronic, unintentional fostering of a potentially hostile work environment. On the surface, the following examples might seem insignificant, even petty. Yet, workers pick up cues, both positive and negative, from these typical situations. When a manager is inattentive to seemingly small issues, there is a risk of escalation to the point of full-fledged, official complaints. Consider these examples through the lens of the legal framework (e.g., elements of gender, race, ethnicity, religion, disability, etc.).

1. Humor in the workplace: manager permits the posting of jokes, cartoon, posters, sarcastic quotes on mugs, calendars, plaques.
2. Unintentional, but jarring messaging: for example, a worker (or a visitor) might be facing a serious personal circumstance (e.g., terminally ill family member); he or she comes to the workplace and is bombarded with cheery signs and sayings and images on the elevator, on the doorways, at the work stations: SMILE! NO FROWNING ZONE; HAVE A NICE DAY; I'VE GOT MY OWN TROUBLES, THANK YOU.
3. Unintentional, but mild to moderate stressor such as constant pressure to participate in "causes", however worthy: wear red for heart health promotion; wear purple for memory impairment awareness; wear pink for cancer awareness; buy a flower for some special cause. Food or toy drives around seasonal holidays are yet another possible

point of pressure; not everyone observes certain holidays; some households have several family members, each of whom is also being asked to donate.

4. Pressure to donate to financial campaigns. Say, for example, an organization receives financial support from national or regional charitable fundraising organizations. During the annual fundraising campaign, managers are expected to achieve 100% participation from within their work group. What message does this send to an employee who does not wish to contribute because the fundraising organization also supports causes with which he or she does not agree and/or contradict one's religious tenets? "Team, we are only two people short of 100% participation; do your part; let's make our department part of the CEO's 100% list!"
5. Selective celebrations: birthdays (some religions do not observe this custom); engagements, weddings, baby showers…not every employee has these happy occasions.

## The Supportive Work Environment

Managers offset potentially unpleasant, even hostile, work environments through fostering one in which workers feel psychologically and physically safe. A group of managers and employee representatives brainstormed about improving ordinary work conditions. Their suggested practices include these topics; some of these topics may seem so basic, so obvious as to be overlooked. But when neglected, unpleasant, unsafe, and unhealthy situations may develop.

1. Confer with housekeeping/environmental services to ensure a clean, uncluttered work space. For example, an employee with visual impairment or using a wheel chair should be able to easily navigate the work space. Clean, properly supplied rest rooms: in more remote work areas, or during evening and night shifts, security is a paramount concern.
2. Offset negative work space elements such as windowless rooms or basement locations. Seek the assistance of environmental services to select proper lighting and painting to enhance the illusion of spaciousness; create more openness by use of partial partitions or interior windows.
3. Avoid sterile, institutionalized, bland wall expanses. Having put in place work rules about no posters, cartoons etc., the manager needs to provide a proper alternative. Use art work and

photographic images of the organization's building and grounds, such as historic images of its original buildings, thus providing an attractive visual display, and reinforcing identification with the organization.

4. Food: a most basic need: review the standard expectation that workers will take their breaks and lunch period at the scheduled time. Review the usual work rules: no food or drink in the work space (thus no garbage, no odors, no mice). Now consider the sheer logistics of getting to/from the centralized cafeteria. Where is it located? Are the lines so long during peak hours that workers do not have adequate time to eat? When there is inclement weather and cafeteria is in another building, workers might want to eat at their desks. Evening and night workers might not want to traverse long, empty corridors during off hours, a major safety and security circumstance. Workers who have certain health conditions (e.g. insulin dependent; specialty weight loss protocols) need to have reliable, convenient access to food. There is another overlay to these issues: managers often contradict their own work rules by taking coffee to meetings, having coffee and snacks in their own office, eating at desk. A double standard emerges: one set of rules for workers; one for managers. One solution to these issues is an in-department break room or alcove. Again, there are practical health and safety issues to consider, and employee cooperation is essential to successful implementation of such solutions.

5. The official social: instead of celebrations of birthdays, special events, and so forth for only some workers, a manager might consider a once-a-month, generic social event during a regular break or at lunch time. Sometimes a supplier or vendor wishes to contribute to a department by supplying food, but check with HR to be sure this is an acceptable practice. One final note: remember to have similar event for all shifts; do not overlook the evening and night work groups.

6. Casual Friday: yes or no? Does the dress code include this consideration? Are there clear-cut examples of acceptable casual attire? Consider the impact on clients and visitors. What impression does the casual appearance give? And again, no offensive or potentially offensive mottoes, cartoons, and others on clothing or accessories.

7. News of the day: managers need to offset rumors, provide accurate information, and build up a sense of team. A structured system of communication (e.g., the short daily meeting of supervisors and team leaders) provides for timely, accurate sharing. The big events such as results of the accreditation survey, the designation of the facility as a center of excellence, or a difficult circumstance (negative publicity) might occasion a more formal meeting in which to share details. Employees need to feel included in the life of the organization.

A periodic review of work rules, policies, and directives is an essential step in enhancing the work environment. Management cannot meet every personal need of employees, but there is much that can be done to make the organization a good place in which to work.

## ▶ Emphasis on Service

As a staff function, HR is organized as a service activity. Service activities render no patient care; they do not advance the primary work of the organization. Rather, they support the performance of the organization's work and in a practical sense become necessary. For example, if a pure service such as building maintenance did not exist, the facility's physical plant would gradually self-destruct. Similarly, without HR to see to the maintenance of the workforce, the overall suitability and capability of that workforce would steadily erode. Recognize HR for what it is: an essential service function required to help the organization run as efficiently as possible.

Learn what the HR department does, and especially learn why the department does what it does. Provide input and forge a continuing working relationship with the HR department, making it clear that you expect service from this essential service department. Challenge HR to do more, to do better, and to continually improve service—and put the HR department to work for you and your employees.

## The Manager's Wheel Book and The Management Reference Portfolio

As with each cluster of theoretical concepts and actual practice, a manager has two easy-to-use resources to plan and respond to the many issues of the day-to-day work: The Manager's Wheel Book (see excerpt in **Appendix 14–A**) and The Management Reference Portfolio (see excerpt in **Appendix 14–B**).

# Appendix 14-A

## The Manager's Wheel Book

These entries reflect many activities during the month of July, 20n2. Activities include major projects (QI studies; annual employee evaluation); systems and procedure issues; training and orientation; motivation. The usual, repetitive day-to-day operations were not included; assume these occurred in their usual way.

| Date | Activity |
|---|---|
| July 2 | Discussed concerns of supervisors about "always on" expectations, especially over holidays |
| July 5 | Completed HR department request for input into employee handbook revisions |
| July 6 | Agreed to accept an affiliation student: October through mid-November; agreement signed and returned to CEO's officer for external education programs |
| | State licensure (unannounced) visit |
| July 10 | Attended labor law workshop, sponsored by regional healthcare association; travel to workshop location at Paulsville |
| July 11 | Nominated lead coder for employee of the month award |
| | Presented "Privacy and Confidentiality" at regular monthly orientation for new employees of organization |
| July 16 | Work group meeting—department heads regarding finalizing social media policy |
| | Completed HR department request for input regarding sexual harassment policy |
| Week of July 23–27 | Evaluation of employees under new guidelines and timelines |
| | Carried out quality improvement studies: safety; infection control; accuracy of intake data; adequacy of transfer/hand off documentation, inter-departmental transfers; ER/observation unit admissions to inpatient. |
| | Forwarded studies to QI committee chair |
| July 27 | Reviewed strike plan regarding potential strike, midnight July 29 |
| July 31 | Completed plan of correction report regarding July 6 state licensure site visit |
| | Received whistleblower verbal report; forwarded to HR department designate |
| | Training needs assessment regarding new technology skills; reducing grievances; results of audit of legacy record storage |
| | Clarified "Casual Friday" dress code |
| | Received employees' concerns regarding seniority practices that limit prime time vacation choices |

# Appendix 14-B

# The Management Reference Portfolio

References and reminders reflect the topics of orientation and training, communication, conflict, comprehensive reports, and quality improvement. Each referenced document has its own complete file.

Orientation schedule and content
- General—by Human Relations; for all employees
- Departmental—by department head
- Some specific topics:
    - Modified Operations Schedule
    - Sexual Harassment
    - Internet use; social media

Training
- Long- and short-range plans and needs
- Cross training and succession plan aspects
- Training needs resulting from:
    - Vacation, holiday, leave of absence coverage
    - Quality improvement (QI) feedback
    - Grievance pattern review

Training Resources: internal; external

Clinical Affiliation
- Approval requirements—name and title of senior official
- Clinical affiliation contract specifications
- List of current affiliation agreements

Labor Union Contract and Memoranda of Understanding—list of contents

Employee Handbook—list of contents

Work Rules and Dress Code

Required process and forms:
- Grievances
- Disciplinary actions
- Whistleblower reports
- Sexual Harassment reports

Policy regarding internet use; social media

Standard content and time line—major reports

List of licensure and accrediting agencies
- Date of previous onsite survey
- Plan of correction
- Grants and special projects
- List of ongoing and planned grants/projects
- Name and title of review and approval officer (e.g., development office)

# CHAPTER 15

# Day-to-Day Management for the Health Professional-as-Manager

## CHAPTER OBJECTIVES

- Examine the dual role of the health professional working as a manager.
- Explore some potential problems and barriers often encountered by health professionals who enter management.
- Confirm the legitimacy of management, necessarily a second career for many health professionals, as a profession in its own right.
- Identify the nonmanagerial professional employee as a sometimes-scarce resource, suggesting a necessary focus on employee retention.
- Introduce the high-skill professional and review the special management problems of directing such personnel.
- Discuss several aspects of day-to-day management in which the manager must put more into the relationship with each employee because the employee is a professional.
- Establish the manager's critical role as the essential link between the employees' profession and the remainder of the organization.
- Address the need for the professional-as-manager to recognize the importance of self-development and active management of one's own career progression.

## ▶ A Second and Parallel Career

It bears repeating that the professional who assumes a management role is adopting a second and parallel career of equal importance to his or her profession. Most such managers are well trained in their specialties but enter management with little or no formal preparation for running a department or supervising others. Lack of preparation and inadequate understanding of the requirements of the management side of the combined role often lead to uneasiness and indecision in management matters. This condition subsequently causes some managers to seek refuge in the familiar by emphasizing the profession at the expense of attention to management duties. The professionals who become most successful managers are invariably those who develop the ability to appropriately balance the sides of the dual role.

## ▶ Two Hats: Specialist and Manager

The professional who is asked to assume a management position is being asked to take on a second occupation and perhaps even pursue a second career. Management positions turn over as other positions do, and vacant management positions are often filled from within the ranks of the work group. There are both advantages and disadvantages to having a particular member of a work group step up to the position of group manager. On occasion, however, the new manager of a group will come from outside of the organization.

Although familiarity with the specific organizational setting may be helpful to the new manager, such familiarity is certainly not a requirement of a group's new manager. There is one firm requirement of the individual who is to assume command of any work group: the individual must be intimately knowledgeable of the kinds of work the group performs. Because many work groups within the healthcare institution include professional employees and because the manager's technical qualifications must essentially be equivalent to the qualifications found in the department, the career ladder of a professional may logically be extended to include the management of that specialty.

The professional who enters management must exist ever after in a two-hat situation. This person must wear the hat of the professional—that is, the technical specialist—and render judgments on countless technical matters concerning the profession. At the same time, this person must also wear the hat of the manager and effect the application of generic techniques—processes that apply horizontally across the organization regardless of one's individual specialty. The professional in a management role must be both specialist and generalist. As a professional, the person is trained as a specialist in a particular field. As a manager, however, it remains largely up to the individual to recognize the need to become a generalist and to independently seek out sources of education and assistance.

The average employee who progresses from the ranks into management is usually well grounded in a working specialty. In this sense all employees—professionals and nonprofessionals alike—are functional specialists. For instance, the individual who works for several years in the housekeeping/environmental services department, performs a variety of tasks. This worker becomes a specialist in the work of that department and brings all this experience into the supervisory role when promoted. At the least, the nonprofessional is a specialist by virtue of experience.

Although the professional employee is usually also a specialist by virtue of experience, that is only a part of the professional's qualifications as a specialist; the remaining criteria defining the professional as a specialist are education and accreditation. The professional entering management brings both credentials and experience to the job. In this regard the person is usually eminently qualified to wear the manager's technical hat but may not be nearly as well qualified to wear the managerial hat.

The professional who enters management is usually extremely well trained in the specialty but trained minimally or not at all in matters of management. Healthcare professionals become professionals by seeking out appropriate programs, gaining entry to them, and working toward the necessary qualifications. In contrast, these same workers become managers by virtue of organizational edict; that is, they are simply appointed. Precisely at this stage some employees and organizations commit a classic error—assuming that because people have been promoted and given appropriate titles, they are suddenly managers in the true sense of the word. Unfortunately, organizational edict does not automatically make a manager out of someone who is not adequately trained or appropriately oriented to management, any more than the mere conferral of the title could turn an untrained person into a nurse, an accountant, a biomedical engineer, or any other professional.

The professional entering management, then, is usually well trained in wearing the hat of the specialist and trained little or not at all in wearing the hat of the manager. Although each aspect of the role is equally important, and even though one side or the other may dominate at times, many such persons exhibit a long-running tendency that is fully understandable under the circumstances. This is the tendency to favor the wearing of the hat that fits best, leaning toward the one of the two roles in which they find themselves more comfortable.

By listening carefully to some of the common complaints of certain managers, it is possible to identify the aspects of the management job that lie at the heart of these complaints. Such complaints will then identify the individuals on whom the management hat does not fit especially comfortably. Common areas of complaint that indicate the presence of ill-fitting management hats include the following:

- *Budgeting.* As one manager complained, "Budgeting is an annual chore that seems to come around every 2 or 3 months." If the management hat does not fit well, budgeting is likely to be a dreaded chore filled with frustration and only partly understood.
- *Performance appraisals.* Appraisals are also a common annual responsibility that seems to

come around sooner than it ought to. When the management hat does not fit well, appraisals are likewise dreaded, tend to run late or perhaps not get done at all and may make the manager feel uncomfortable and perhaps inadequate.

- *Employee problems.* The essence of the management role is getting things done through people, which requires maintenance of the manager's most valuable resource—the employees. When the management hat does not fit well, the manager may exhibit a tendency to shy away from people problems and resent them as intrusions that keep the manager away from the "real work."

- *Identification with the work group.* "Listen, gang, I know I'm the manager of this group but don't forget that my background is the same as yours and I'm a lot more like you than those people in top management." The tendency to identify with the group and join with them in condemnation of the infamous "they"—as in, "It's not my fault; they made me do it"—is another sure sign of the ill-fitting management hat.

- *Disciplinary issues.* Rarely is any manager completely comfortable with exercising the disciplinary process; indeed, he or she should never become completely comfortable with something of such importance. Often, however, out of discomfort the manager wearing the ill-fitting management hat will ignore disciplinary issues altogether or take action that is too little or too late.

- *Personnel policies.* The wearer of the ill-fitting management hat may have little familiarity with pertinent personnel policies and thus may simply tell employees to "call human resources" rather than help them answer policy questions.

- *Work priorities.* One sure sign of the ill-fitting management hat is the apparent inability to plan one's work and establish priorities. The manager so afflicted will often seem to be spending each day reacting to crises or continually responding to the demands of the moment regardless of their relative importance.

- *Delegation failure.* The manager who is constantly juggling an overload because of inability to delegate, or whose behavior seems to be saying, "If you want something done right, you'd better do it yourself," is wearing the ill-fitting management hat. This manager is failing to use staff to the full extent of their capabilities and is overlooking the important employee-development role of the manager.

This list could be longer, but the point is made. When such symptoms appear, the manager is feeling the pinch of the management hat, reacting out of frustration and insecurity, and taking refuge under the technical hat. Those processes that can be described as generic to management—because they apply across the organization regardless of the function managed, such as budgeting and performance appraisal—appear as mysterious, somewhat misunderstood activities. They come to be regarded as elements of interference rather than the vital elements of management. Disciplinary problems and other people problems are likewise seen as annoyances rather than as legitimate obstacles to overcome in the process of getting things done through people. What is seen as "real" work is the basic work of the technical specialty. Overlooked is the reality that the true task of the manager is largely to serve as a facilitator in the process of getting the real work done by the employees.

The signs of the ill-fitting management hat are numerous, and many managers continually take refuge under the hat of the technical specialist. This tendency is understandable considering the professional employee's degree of familiarity with the occupation and his or her unfamiliarity and discomfort with some of the processes of management. Yet simply being aware of the likely imbalance between the two halves of the role should be sufficient to inspire some managers to improve their capability and performance in the management sphere. Both sides of the manager's role are extremely important. A working knowledge of the technical specialty remains important at most levels in the healthcare hierarchy. Particularly in the lower levels of management, the generalist side of the role—that is, the management side—is neither more nor less important than the specialist side; it is simply different.

Although most managers in the healthcare organization's hierarchy have a need to be both technical specialist and management generalist, just as there is a place in the working ranks for the pure technical specialist, so there is also a place in the management hierarchy for the pure management generalist. However, the few management generalists in the organization are usually found in the upper reaches of the hierarchy in positions of multidepartmental responsibility.

In the healthcare organization, administration is the province of the pure management generalist. Administrators of health institutions come from a variety of backgrounds, with many of them arising out of the management of certain specialties and having perhaps broadened their scope through studies in administration. It matters little whether the institution's chief executive officer may have originally trained as an accountant, a registered nurse, an attorney, or a physician, as long as that person made the necessary transition from specialist to generalist while rising toward the top. Even so, it is rare to encounter, for example, a director of nursing service who is not a registered nurse, a health information manager who was not first a health information practitioner, a director of finance who was not an accountant, or a manager of physical therapy who was not a physical therapist.

## ▶ A Constant Balancing Act

Some professionals who take on the management of departments never completely adapt to the dual role of professional and manager and never develop an appropriate balance between the two sides of the role. Their behavior often sums up their attitude: once a specialist, always a specialist. Such persons tend to give the technical side of the role the majority of their interest and attention, their priority treatment, and certainly their favor. Never having become sufficiently comfortable with the management role to enjoy what they are doing, they take refuge in their strengths and minimize the importance of their weaknesses.

The dedicated professional often has far more difficulty than the nonprofessional in balancing the roles of professional and manager. The professional has devoted far more time, effort, and commitment to becoming a specialist and has probably done so at least partly because of an attraction to or an aptitude for that kind of work. Some may like their work so well that, although they do not necessarily refuse promotion to management, they show an inclination to subordinate the management side of the role so that it does not intrude too far into their favored territory.

Just as a liking for individual specialties is important to success in one's basic fields, so, too, is a liking for management essential for success in management. Usually a liking for a given activity is strongly influenced by one's degree of familiarity or level of comfort with the elements of that activity. Quite simply, the more a person knows about a given activity, the more the person is inclined to like that activity. Conversely, an individual may be more readily inclined to dislike an activity that seems bewildering, strange, or discomforting.

It has been suggested that the professional who enters management faces the challenges of becoming grounded in management and getting up to speed.

Once in management, the individual discovers that to remain effective both as a technical professional and as a manager, it is necessary to try to remain current in two career fields.

Staying current with the latest developments in a technical specialty is a sizable task in itself; getting fully up to speed and remaining current with the elements of one's management role is an unending task, considering the scope and breadth of management. Often, both sides of the role suffer to some extent. Nevertheless, the technical side is more likely to receive most of the conscientious attention. The professional employed as a manager has all the problems of any other manager as well as most of the problems that confront the working professional who is not a manager.

## ▶ The Ego Barrier

Probably few, if any, health professionals do not believe that their professions are of considerable importance to their organizations. This is to be expected; to find any significant measure of fulfillment in their work, healthcare professionals must regard their occupations as being of significant value to the organization and its patients. The potential for problems exists when an individual professional behaves as though his or her particular working specialty is more important than other occupations in the organization. If a professional who carries an inflated regard for the importance of a given profession happens to be the manager of a department, the potential for interdepartmental conflict is present.

Both generalist managers and technical-specialist managers can display self-serving tendencies at times. Managers, however, frequently differ in how they pursue their objectives of service according to whether they see themselves as generalists or technical specialists.

The generalist who is on a self-serving track often tends toward empire-building, working to acquire every function or responsibility that can in any way be connected under a common head. This manager is working toward elevation of self by achieving far-reaching control throughout the organization, much as some nations once extended their authority by acquiring colonies throughout the world.

The self-serving technical-specialist manager, by comparison, is often limited by the inability to absorb functions that are not technically related to the profession of the manager. Rather than building an empire, these managers act much like the feudal baron who remained in his castle but devoted most of his time and energies to making it the grandest and strongest castle in the country. That is, the manager strives to build an elegant structure whose glory will surely dwarf that of its neighbors. Thus the "most important" specialty eventually has the most well-appointed quarters, the most generous budget, the most favorable staffing relative to the amount of work to be done, and the strongest voice in influencing institution policy. These results convey the belief that the technical-specialist manager's own profession is somehow better than the other professions in the organization.

Another ego-related problem to which the technical-specialist manager may fall victim, and one of perhaps significantly more impact than the preceding effect, is found in the tendency to place management in an inferior role relative to the profession. This may also appear as a tendency to consider the profession itself as so necessary to management that one could not possibly be an accomplished manager of anything without knowledge of this particular profession. The behavioral message sent by some technical-specialist managers is this: knowledge of my technical specialty is critically important in healthcare management. Therefore, it is implied that you must originally be a social worker, psychologist, registered nurse, physical therapist, registered health information administrator, or other specialist to become fully effective as a manager in health care.

In fact, to become a well-rounded and effective healthcare manager, one need not be a social worker, speech pathologist, laboratory technologist, registered nurse, or any other healthcare specialist. It is automatically conceded that in all but the most general of support activities the manager must be some kind of specialist as well as a manager; in reality, no one specialty has a monopoly or even a modest edge regarding management expertise. The fundamental task of management—getting things done through people—is reflected in practices such as proper delegation, clear and open two-way communication, budgeting and cost control, scheduling, handling employee problems, and applying disciplinary action. All true management practices are transportable across departmental lines, and to believe otherwise is to fall into the ego trap of the technical specialist.

The professional employee who enters management is literally jumping into a second career. If a potential manager thinks of management as a profession—and to many people, management is, indeed, a profession of considerable breadth and depth—then he or she must recognize the necessity to enter management with as much preparation as possible. In their academic training, most professionals

receive a few credit hours in management courses. On this basis, some then claim expertise as management generalists. But consider the reverse situation: assume that a student of general business managed to take a couple of social work courses (perhaps as electives) and after graduation claimed to be a social worker as well as a management generalist. The individual's claim to social work expertise would be automatically rejected, of course. Yet time and again, the technical specialist who has had a management course or two lays claim to equivalent expertise in management.

To summarize, the ego barrier to managerial effectiveness can surface in two important dimensions:

1. An inflated view of the importance of one's profession relative to the importance of management
2. The failure to recognize management, devoid of all implications of any other particular occupation, as a specialty in its own right

The obstacles presented by ego are overcome with great difficulty. In fact, in many instances they are never overcome. This is unfortunate because the most significant effects of the ego barrier are the tendency to place organizational interests second to departmental interests, and the proliferation and perpetuation of middle-management mediocrity.

# ▶ The Professional Managing the Professional

## The Professional as a Scarce Resource

From time to time, some healthcare specialties experience conditions of oversupply. Conversely, on numerous occasions many parts of the country experience shortages of certain skills, and organizations are forced to compete for the services of available workers. Once a department's personnel needs have been met, however, the focus of the manager—and certainly much of the focus of the organization's human resources department—should turn from recruitment to the important matter of retention. In short, when certain human resources are scarce, it is necessary to concentrate on keeping the people who are already in the organization.

Consider, for example, professional nurses. The management of professional nurses, especially in the hospital setting, has become increasingly complex over the years. Financial restrictions, technological innovations, professional labor unions, and the changing attitudes of nurses have had a considerable impact on the practice of nursing. In some parts of the country, the recruitment of professional nurses has become highly competitive and is likely to remain that way for some time.

The retention of professional employees is emerging as one of the more challenging tasks faced by health administrators. Where once it was possible to accept relatively high turnover among some professionals—for example, many nurses were seen as entering or leaving the work force essentially at will—organizations have been finding supplies of help drying up and have therefore turned their attention to reducing turnover. Thus attention naturally shifts to factors and conditions that have a bearing on job satisfaction, such as better pay scales, more generous benefits, more attractive schedules, additional compensation for less desirable assignments, a more clearly defined role for the professional, and a stronger voice in matters of patient care.

Generally, the healthcare organization should be interested in retaining employees who are functioning satisfactorily, but the organization may not be inclined to do any more about retention than has already been done as long as replacement employees are available. When a particular specialty is in short supply, however, an organization should do what it can to retain those skilled employees—but always within limits, because to take steps that seem to favor one class or group of employees over others is to invite trouble; what is done for one group is often done for others as well.

There are costs associated with active retention efforts; after all, improved benefits and generous staffing patterns certainly cost money. For specialties in short supply, however, the cost of retaining employees is not nearly as high as the ongoing cost of continually recruiting, hiring, orienting, and training replacements. It is true that some professionals may be considered scarce resources because of their limited numbers; even so, it behooves the manager to consider all steadily and satisfactorily performing employees, professional and otherwise, as equally worthy of the best efforts at retention.

## The High-Skill Professional: Some Special Management Problems

The high-skill professional usually has extensive education, frequently possesses a master's degree or a doctorate (medical or otherwise), and is likely to work in a position that entails the exercise of a great deal of operating autonomy. High-skill professionals found in health care might include the following individuals:

- An employed physician or dentist
- A professional administrator engaged to operate a hospital or to run a major organizational unit
- A certified public accountant engaged to audit the organization or perhaps to oversee the organization's finance division
- A chemist, physicist, physician, or other scientist engaged in research or in day-to-day operations
- A management consultant engaged to solve a problem for the organization

Such persons have two obvious factors in common: they are extensively educated, and they are on their own much of the time in the performance of their work.

The high-skill professional often presents the manager with some special problems and unique challenges. Frequently these problems and challenges exist because of some of the same factors that contribute to the professional's ability to perform as desired.

The high-skill professional may generally be described by some or perhaps all of the following:

- Like many employees, the high-skill professional is accountable for results; however, this person is primarily responsible for getting things done and then later, if at all, reporting the results. There is only limited or occasional need for clearing actions or decisions in advance. In this regard the high-skill professional possesses a significant degree of operating autonomy.
- The high-skill professional may have a great deal of geographic mobility, ranging throughout an entire facility or, as in the case of a management consultant or an auditor, from organization to organization and even from city to city.
- Being a solitary operator much of the time, the high-skill professional must consistently exercise individual discretion and judgment.
- The successful high-skill professional generally exhibits a high degree of self-confidence and independence of thought and action.
- The successful high-skill professional is a self-starter who is also highly self-sufficient in work performance. He or she is able to function with minimal supervision or direction, sometimes for prolonged periods.

In general, the high-skill professional is a highly educated specialist who largely operates independently, determining what needs to be done and doing it without direct management. Yet many of the same characteristics that make for an effective high-skill professional also tend to make such an employee difficult to manage at times. This is especially true of the characteristics related to independence—that is, those factors that make an individual an effective lone operator. Although it is certainly important to cultivate independence in persons who work on their own much of the time, at times even the lone operator must be counted on to be a team player.

Some might say that a person should also have a healthy ego to be able to presume to operate in a mode that can often be described as that of the visiting expert. The high-skill professional is, indeed, often viewed as needing to be in control of the situation. The healthy ego, so helpful to the professional while on assignment, can sometimes be troublesome to the manager, however. For these reasons, the successful manager of the high-skill professional must adhere to a number of guidelines:

- Be thorough and cautious in recruiting and selection, ensuring that educational requirements have been met and that all necessary credentials are possessed. For an experienced candidate, the manager should look for a demonstrated record of success and for sound reasons for wishing to make a change. For a newly graduated professional, the manager should look for self-confidence and a strong desire to do that particular kind of work.
- Try to learn what most strongly motivates the individual. Often the effective high-skill professional has a strong liking for the work and a strong desire for achievement and accomplishment. The best independently functioning professionals like the work, are driven to do the work their own way, and have a great need to see the results of their efforts.
- Pay close attention to the orientation of every new employee. Even the well-experienced professional, when new to the organization, needs to be thoroughly oriented to the organization, its workers, clients, and policies before assuming the managerial role.
- In addition to knowing the rules and policies of the organization, make certain that the new hire knows the results expected on each assignment. The manager should take care to thoroughly define the boundaries for independent action, such that the individual is able to develop a sense for how much may be done independently and when it is necessary to call for management assistance.

- Once the boundaries for independent action are established, give the professional employee complete freedom to operate within those boundaries. Strive to develop trust in the individual and, by reflecting this trust, endeavor to instill in this person the belief that management has confidence in his or her ability. Do not violate the boundaries by trying to dictate from afar; besides generally not working, absentee management serves to frustrate the employee.
- Introduce changes—whether changes in policies, practices, operating guidelines, or whatever—with plenty of advance notice. If at all possible, allow and even encourage the employee to take part in determining the scope and direction of each change.

A number of characteristics that make a high-skill professional an effective employee may also make the same person difficult to manage at times. On the one hand, independence and self-confidence must be encouraged. On the other hand, the same characteristics must be controlled. The manager is most likely to succeed with the high-skill professional by applying an open, participative approach to management.

## Credibility of the Professional's Superior

When a work group includes professionals, there is always the potential for differences in professional opinion, and there is always the possibility that the professionals will demonstrate varying degrees of unwillingness to accept direction from the manager.

Whether such credibility problems exist in a given work group depends on the background and qualifications of the employees. Problems may arise from the presence of a certain amount of ego—from the belief that one's profession is at least a bit more important than other occupations. Some problems arise from a sense of territorialism exhibited by some professionals, the belief that no one should hold sway over any aspect of professional performance without being perceived as at least equal in professional status and capability to the perceiver.

Management credibility problems may exist when the manager is not of the same profession as the individual employee. For example, a professional trained as a chemist may have problems relating to an immediate superior whose background is that of a medical technologist. In all such cases there may be tendencies to differ on professional judgments—"He's only a medical technologist, so who is he to tell me what

I should be doing as a chemist?"—and there may be feelings of territorialism—"Chemistry is my area, and only a chemist can legitimately make judgments that involve chemistry."

Credibility problems are also likely to arise when the manager is thought to be on a lower professional level than the employee. Thus, the clinical psychologist with a doctoral degree may be less than completely willing to accept the leadership of a manager whose education stopped at the master's degree level, and the certified public accountant may balk at the direction of a managing accountant who is not similarly certified. It again becomes a matter of one person, the "higher" professional, being unwilling to accept the judgment of another person, who happens to be "lower" on the professional scale. In such situations, there are also more hints of territorialism: there appear to be more exclusive territories within broader territories that are mentally reserved for those of greater status.

Problems of management credibility are highly likely in situations in which employees see their managers as nonprofessionals. To fully understand such credibility problems, one must appreciate that many individual professionals do not regard management as a profession in its own right. Occasionally a nonmanagerial professional must report directly to a nonprofessional. In one organization, for example, a registered health information administrator and a utilization review coordinator who was a registered nurse reported to the director of health information services, who was a management generalist and held no professional credentials as a healthcare specialist. These two professionals were inevitably in some degree of conflict with their manager and frequently questioned the manager's direction. A direct reporting relationship between a nonmanagerial technical specialist and a generalist manager is often marked by many disputes concerning managerial judgments; in addition, it may be marked by strong territorialism on the part of the professional.

Automatic management credibility is likely to be greatest when the manager is a professional of obviously higher standing than the employee. At the other extreme, management credibility is most strained when the manager's standing is rejected by the professional as being nonprofessional.

# Leadership and the Professional

Leadership style may be simply described as that pattern of behavior projected by the leader in working with group members. Leadership styles run the gamut from completely closed to thoroughly open. At the closed end of the scale are the autocratic leaders, those who rule by order and edict. The harshest style is that of the exploitative autocrat, a leader who literally exploits the followers primarily in the service of self-interest. One major step along the scale takes one to the style of the benevolent autocrat. The benevolent autocrat also rules by order and edict, but it is a paternalistic rule imposed supposedly for the good of all.

Approaching the middle of the scale of leadership styles, one encounters the bureaucratic style. In many ways fully as onerous as the autocratic styles, the bureaucratic style ordinarily subordinates human considerations to the service of the "system" or the "book."

Toward the open end of the scale, one encounters the consultative style of leadership. Under this approach the employees are often given the opportunity to provide their thoughts, ideas, and suggestions, but the ground rules are such that the leader recognizes no obligation to use anything the employees provide. In this style, the guiding philosophy of management is "the buck stops here," and management reserves the right to make all decisions at all times regardless of employee input.

Consultative leadership often exists when management claims to practice true participative leadership, the most open style on the leadership scale. With participative leadership, all members are included in all decision-making processes so that all members own a piece of all decisions. The greatest flaw of participative leadership is the ease with which managers, most of whom grew into their positions under authoritarian role models, can unconsciously hinder participative processes such that they become consultative and perhaps even manipulative at times.

The higher the professional level of a work group, the more the manager will find it necessary to move toward the open end of the scale of leadership types to accomplish the work of the department. Given the nature of professional work and the advanced state of most professionals' education, the average professional does not willingly suffer authoritarian management. It falls to the manager to examine basic assumptions about human behavior, to get beyond mere verbal tribute to modern management, and to take some of the risks inherent in open leadership styles. For further discussion of aspects of leadership, see the earlier chapter on leadership.

Managers have assumptions and expectations about workers. In general, there are two opposing views. The first view flows from the assumption that workers must be actively managed through continual, close supervision. They need to be controlled, rewarded through incentives, and, if necessary, disciplined according to a set of corrective actions. This view also holds that workers, in general, do not want to take the initiative, preferring instead to be led.

The opposite view holds that workers are not passive participants in organizational efforts. Motivation, developmental potential, willingness to assume responsibility, and readiness to work toward organizational goals are present in most people. It is management's responsibility to enable people to recognize and develop these characteristics in themselves. The essential task of management is to arrange organizational conditions and methods of operation so that people can best achieve their own goals by directing their efforts toward the goals of the organization.

Professional or not, not every employee responds to the same leadership style; however, the average professional is generally more receptive to open styles. Thus, it is in the manager's best interest to begin a manager–employee relationship with reliance on an open style. Management style may depend largely on the individual circumstances, but in starting the relationship with an employee, the manager should initially extend every benefit of the doubt regarding the employee's motives.

The manager has a choice of leadership styles, ranging from extremely closed to extremely open. The trick is to know which style to apply and when to apply it. There may be a few who actually prefer to be led and have their thinking done for them. There may also be a number of people who are self-motivated and capable of significant self-direction. Their presence should be especially notable in departments employing large numbers of professionals. Although the same personnel policies apply uniformly to all employees, the manager deals differently with individuals in other ways. Some the manager consults with and invites their participation; others the manager simply directs.

Theories aside, a manager must avoid making assumptions about people. Rather, it is necessary to know the employees and to try to understand each one as both a person and a producer. By working with people over a period of time, and especially by working at the business of getting to know them, the manager can learn a great deal about individual likes, dislikes, and capabilities. Learn about the people as individuals and lead accordingly. If a certain employee genuinely prefers orders and instructions, and this attitude is not inconsistent with job

requirements, then use orders and instructions. Although many healthcare workers seem to prefer participative leadership, not everyone desires this same consideration. Sufficient flexibility must be maintained to accommodate the employee who wants or requires authoritarian supervision. It is fully as unfair to expect people to become what they do not want to be as it is to allow a rigid structure to stifle those other employees who feel they have something to contribute.

No single style of leadership is appropriate for all people and situations at all times. Today there are more reasons than ever to believe that the consultative and participative leadership approaches are most appropriate to modern healthcare organizations and today's educated workers.

Much can be said about what leadership is and what it is not, but in the end, only a single factor characterizes or defines a leader. That factor is acceptance of the followers. For this critical factor to be present in the manager—employee relationship, the professional employee must do the following:

- Respect the manager's technical knowledge
- Accept the manager's organizational authority and respect the manager's skill in utilizing that authority
- Respect the manager's ability to blend the technical and managerial sides of the management role fairly and justly

The manager accrues little, if any, acceptance by virtue of organizational authority. Most of what the manager acquires in the way of willing acceptance must be earned. It can thus be suggested that to lead the professional employee successfully, the manager must provide a broad framework for employee action. As a consequence, it is necessary to provide the employee with every opportunity to be self-led and to impose specific direction only after all else has failed and the employee has demonstrated the need to be taken by the hand.

## ▶ **The Professional and Change**

No single group or classification of employee has a monopoly on resistance to change. Indeed, rigidity and inflexibility are found at all levels of the organization. This being stated, the professional employee is expected to be on the average more amenable to change because of the professional's advanced education and broader perspective. Unfortunately, as many managers have discovered to their chagrin, the professional employee may be as fully resistant to change as any other employee. It depends entirely on how the employee is approached and how the particular change is presented.

## The Basis for Resistance

As far as the majority of people are concerned, change is threatening. Change threatens one's security by altering the environment; it disturbs one's equilibrium, the state of balance that most people automatically seek to maintain with their surroundings.

Most people tend to seek a state of equilibrium with their surroundings, and they continually make adjustments intended to preserve their equilibrium. Unwanted or unheralded change threatens to disturb this equilibrium, thereby posing a threat to a person's sense of security. People often react to change in completely human fashion by countering the threat with resistance. (See the section concerned with change.)

It is primarily the unknown that fosters resistance or intensifies what otherwise might be nominal resistance. In short, almost any change can generate resistance even if approached with full knowledge and plenty of warning, but if it comes by surprise, then intense resistance is almost certain. When a change is not a surprise, when it is approached in the full knowledge of everyone involved, much of the unknown becomes known and the chances of success are greatly increased.

## The Manager's Approach

In approaching the employees with a change, the manager can take either of three paths: tell them what to do, convince them of what must be done, or try to involve them in assessing the need for the change and in determining the form and substance of the change.

To enjoy the greatest chance of successfully functioning as a change agent, the manager should follow these guidelines:

- Inform employees, as early as possible, of what is likely to happen.
- Plan thoroughly.
- Communicate fully.
- Convince employees as necessary.
- Involve employees whenever circumstances permit.
- Monitor implementation and ensure that decisions are adjusted and plans are fine-tuned as necessary.

Employee knowledge and involvement are the keys to success in managing change. The employee who knows what is happening and is involved in making it happen is less likely to resist. For a comprehensive discussion of organizational change, see Chapter 2, The Challenge of Change.

## Organizational Change, the Manager, and the Professional

Recent years have seen significant organizational change in health care. Mergers and other affiliations, the formation of health systems, hospital closures, downsizing, and other reorganizing activities are altering what had been long-standing organizational arrangements. Many such changes have affected the ways in which managers run their departments and how they relate to individual employees.

Consider an example. Two small-town hospitals some 15 miles apart merged into a single corporate entity and combined activities such that each service became a single department with two locations. Where once there had been two physical therapy managers, a single manager became responsible for overseeing staff in two separate locations. The manager's span of control was significantly altered, so that this person was now responsible for more employees, approximately half of whom were 15 miles away at any given time. This arrangement, and a number of others like it, had the following effects on the relationships between manager and employees:

- The self-starting and independent-operating tendencies of the affected nonmanagerial professionals became far more important because direct supervision of their activities decreased significantly.
- Because employees now had to function more independently, the manager needed to pay more attention to effective delegation so that employees always knew what was expected of them, whether or not the manager was actually present at the site.
- The manager now had twice as many employees as previously under her span of control and thus had more employee-related activities to address (performance appraisals, for example).
- Running a two-location department necessitated—one might even say, "forced adoption of"—an open style of management; there was no possibility of providing close supervision to employees who were some distance away much of the time.

- With the manager permanently "spread thin," professional employees had to function as true professionals and the manager had to treat the employees as true professionals.

Such organizational changes will inevitably influence a manager's span of control and scope of responsibility and will necessitate the manager's increasing reliance on the self-governing, semi-autonomous professional employee.

## ▶ Methods Improvement

Every worker has a potentially valuable role in methods improvement. No one knows the inner workings of a job nearly as well as the people who do it every day. This detailed knowledge is essential in methods improvement activities. Precisely how a task is performed is the necessary starting point in working to improve the performance of that task. The professional, whether employee or manager, is especially important in methods improvement; the professional's depth of knowledge in the field, both theoretical and practical, is a critical source of work-improvement options. In addition, the creative nature of much professional work suggests that the professional knows not just what to do but also how to determine what to do.

The professional employee is often a key person in a methods improvement undertaking, such as in chairing a quality circle or leading a work simplification team. In all probability, the professional knows the work far better than the manager does. The manager, even though a professional as well, has necessarily been moving away from the technical work in some respects while growing as a manager. To succeed in improving the methods by which the work is accomplished, the manager must regard the department's professionals as the most potentially valuable source of improvement knowledge.

## ▶ Employee Problems

Occasionally, managers tend to treat their professional employees much like parents often treat the older children in the family: "you're more advanced, so we can expect more of you." The you-should-know-better attitude is fine as long as it is expressed properly and is not carried to extremes, at least in regard to the technical work of the profession. Conversely, this attitude is not generally appropriate regarding adherence to the policies and work rules of the organization.

Rules and policies must be applied consistently to all employees. The professional employee should not be held to more rigid standards of behavior simply because of being professional—but neither should the professional be allowed to get away with more simply because of his or her professional status. Rather, policies and work rules must apply equally to all employees regardless of their qualifications or classification, and the manager must take pains to ensure that all receive equal treatment.

The professional is as fully human and unpredictable as any other employee when it comes to the likelihood of personal problems, variations in personality, and behavior that might give rise to employee problems. The manager's long-run experience will likely demonstrate that professional employees are just as much of a source of discipline and behavior problems as nonprofessional employees. In fact, when the kinds of problems presented by employees are considered, one often finds that the problems presented by professionals are more complex and more difficult to deal with than the problems presented by others. Especially troublesome is the occasional professional who takes advantage of his or her professional status to demand professional treatment without extending the appropriate behavior in return.

## ▶ Communication and the Language of the Professional

For the professional who manages professionals, it would be pertinent to pass along all of the additional advice that can be offered about communication as it applies to the manager of any employees, professional or otherwise. This discussion, however, is limited to a few aspects of organizational communication in which professional status or professionalism may make a difference.

Each function within the modern healthcare organization includes a certain amount of what can be called "inside language." Those who work in rehabilitation services, for example, have special terms that they use regularly. A few of these terms may be unfamiliar to persons who work in other areas and completely foreign to persons not involved in health care. Likewise, health information practitioners, respiratory therapists, computer specialists, microbiologists, and numerous others have inside languages that have evolved within their respective disciplines.

Inside languages are an inevitable outgrowth of the development of any area of concentrated specialized activity. The more concentrated the specialty and, in the case of health professions, the higher on the professional scale an occupation resides, the more extensive this inside language is and the more incomprehensible it is to outsiders. Inside languages evolve for perfectly logical reasons: as advances are made in any aspect of life or any area of business activity, needs arise for describing concepts, conditions, problems, and even physical objects in a way that clearly identifies these within the context of the growing specialty as different from anything else in the world.

The needed words come from two sources: (1) existing words that are given new meanings for specific purposes and (2) new words that are coined to represent new concepts. Advancing technology has expanded the language, and every profession that has emerged and evolved has built its special language along the way.

Clearly, language must be dynamic; it must be able to shift and expand as knowledge increases. It is thus fully understandable that an inside language should develop within any activity. Such language serves a clear purpose in describing, in terms as specific as possible, what goes on within that activity. Some might also say, however, that the purpose of the inside language is to elevate the specialty and define it as a closed club of sorts. Although probably not a specific purpose of an inside language, this is undoubtedly an effect of such a language. An inside language heightens the mystique surrounding any given occupation and helps define the territory surrounding that occupation. Relative to territory, the presence of the inside language is a qualification—admittedly superficial but certainly highly visible—for entry into another's territory.

Nurses have a language of their own, and human resources practitioners have a language of their own. Laboratory employees, radiology employees, physical therapists, psychologists, social workers, occupational therapists, physicians, and many others have their own inside languages. Fortunately, many of these inside languages have some terms in common so they are not entirely different from one another. For example, some of the nurse's inside language is the same as part of the physician's inside language, and it is largely these areas of overlap that provide the interprofessional points of contact through which much communication flows. Occasionally, however, there emerges an inside language that has few, if any, points of overlap with other inside languages.

A glaring example of a highly restrictive inside language is found in computer science. This specialty area is filled with terms and abbreviations and acronyms that are used freely in normal interchange, often without explanation. Old, otherwise familiar words are used in new combinations and with entirely new meaning, such as terminal, disk, peripheral, online, and real time. Beyond the limited number of terms that many of us manage to absorb as computer users, "computerese" stands as very nearly a language in its own right.

One of the major problems commonly encountered in communication involving professionals is disregard for the need to structure any given communication to suit the needs and capabilities of the audience. In communicating, the professional:

- May freely use inside language when communicating with others in the same specialty
- Must use a lesser level of special terminology when relating to persons who are outside of the specific specialty but still within the realm of health care
- Must use a third and general level of language when relating to persons outside of both the specialty and the industry

The manager has a key role to fill in professional communication. It is all too easy for the manager to perpetuate foggy communication by simply joining in with other professionals in the group and relying on restrictive inside language in all contacts. This behavior is not unusual when the manager has risen from the ranks in the same profession. Ideally, however, it should fall to the manager to serve as a facilitator and a translator in communication between the professional group and others. This role should extend to instruction and guidance in how to structure reports, memoranda, and other documentation to best meet the needs of a specific audience and how to do likewise for the audiences for the professionals' oral presentations.

Some professionals tend to use language to make themselves appear knowledgeable and important, to elevate the mystique of the profession, and to isolate and protect their territory, but the primary purpose of language should be to communicate—that is, to transfer meaning. As a primary source of worker guidance and the department's major point of contact with the rest of the organization, the manager has a strong interest in ensuring that the department's contributions are presented so that they are completely understood by those who need to know.

# An Open-Ended Task

On any given day, the professional employee can present the manager with a problem or challenge that can be brought by the nonprofessional—and then some. Any advice that may apply to the management of anyone can apply to the management of the professional. Additional requirements on the manager call for the constant awareness of the sometimes subtle and sometimes glaring differences presented by the professional employee. In addition to the normal requirements of managing any employee, in the day-to-day management of the healthcare professional, the manager has several key objectives:

- Help the professional employee identify and pursue objectives that are consistent with the objectives of the department and the objectives of the organization
- Work to ensure consistency between the priorities of the employee's profession and the priorities of the department and the organization
- Strive to establish and maintain management credibility in a clear leadership role relative to the individual professional employee
- Establish and maintain a working communications link between the individual professional and all other employees

# The Next Step?

The growth-oriented manager cannot help possessing a split focus as far as employment is concerned. Although every manager should of course be largely attentive to the job at hand, the growth-oriented manager can be expected to have two important concerns: (1) performing the present job and (2) preparing for the next job.

Is it best to seek the next upward move within one's present organization or elsewhere? Some will extend their loyalty to a particular organization and seek to advance within that organization. Others, perhaps identifying more closely with a profession than an organization, will envision themselves readily going to another employer. Still others will remain open to either possibility.

It is not possible to say that either the inside focus or the outside focus is best. Although there can be distinct advantages to remaining with the same organization, this is not always possible. Also, staying with the same employer is not always advisable when one considers that more opportunity and more rapid advancement may exist elsewhere. When considering the next step, a manager would do well to take stock of his or her personal situation. The opening chapter of this text lays out the classic functions of a manager. It is helpful, in assessing career development, to review the classic functions of a manager and ask a rather stark set of questions: Am I a manager who carries out these traditional functions? Which functions are, for me, routine and relatively easy; which are neglected or outright avoided? Which aspects energize me? And yes, there is the most basic question: Do I want to be a manager? Reflecting on these questions, closing the loop between expected and actual management behavior, provides one with a factual basis to shore up day-to-day management activities and plan for further career development.

Managers have a variety of documents and guides to assist them in this assessment, such as the organization's master plan, annual strategic plans, past annual reports, annual performance review, and the individual's professional association's career guidelines, resources, and personal leadership plan. A review of the current and recent years' wheel book entries provides ready examples of management activity. **Appendix 15–A** Comprehensive Wheel Book with Analysis displays typical wheel book entries, with a comment section. When using the wheel book as a comprehensive review tool, as at the end of a fiscal year or during a personal assessment, a manager might code each activity to the predominant management function and identify areas of strength or weakness.

## A Private and Personal Assessment

There are a variety of highly personal factors in a person's life that contribute to developing a career plan. These factors are not "advertised" within the organization. They are simply an ethical, responsible, and practical assessment of the realities of one's circumstances that should be considered in a short- and long-range career plan. Here are some examples of prompts for a manager to consider; they are not in any particular order of importance nor are they interrelated examples. See also the examples noted in the section on leadership in Chapter 4.

- We are a military family; we will be rotated to new duty station at the end of 3 years. I want to consolidate my management experience before this move.
- I want to remain permanently in this geographic region, and at this expanding facility, so that I am close to extended family, and, as needed, help with the care of elderly relatives.

- I plan to request extended family/maternity leave next year. I hope to develop a skill set that enables me to then work at home for a year and return to management position at the end of a year.
- As a practical matter, I need to compare the salary benefit from increased pay at supervisory level with the loss of eligibility for overtime pay.
- This organization offers a wide variety of ever-increasing programs of service; the opportunities for advancement within the organization, and its excellent training programs, make it the best work setting for management advancement.

# Careers: Ladders and Tracks

Within certain areas of health care, the available career ladders or career paths may be perceived as both limited and limiting. There are a number of relatively short career ladders in health care. For example, in a mid-size hospital, the entire career ladder in the diagnostic imaging department may consist of only two or three levels, including the management level. The same may be true in the laboratory department. When a person reaches the top of a short career ladder, there are but a few steps remaining: moving to another hospital department that has a longer career ladder, working in general management or administration, or going to another organization that has a longer career ladder in one's specialty.

Moving to another department usually requires re-education in a completely new field. Entering administration also in most instances requires additional education and is a move not readily made. Moving to another, usually larger, organization that has a longer career ladder in one's specialty may work for some for a while. However, because the longer career ladder usually contains only an additional one or two steps, this eventually frustrates the growth-oriented individual, who again "tops out" and may again be faced with changing fields or striving for administration.

Career tracks are also affected by the essential pyramidal structure of most business organizations. As one goes up the pyramid, there are fewer positions available, so at each succeeding level, the competition is greater. This situation has been worsened in recent years by the tendency toward organizational flattening, which has resulted in the reduction in the numbers of available positions in first-line and middle management.

Whether you envision your next career step with your present employer or elsewhere, there is always the potential for a conflict in focus. If you think your next position will be in your present organization, the conflict of focus is upward versus downward. This is most pertinent to the positions of first-line and middle managers. If you think your next position will be in another organization, the conflict of focus is inside versus outside. The inside—outside conflict is most pertinent to department-head and top management positions.

## Upward Versus Downward

At any given time, the first-line or middle manager may tend to face upward, toward higher management and the rest of the hierarchy, or face downward, toward the work group. Certain factors may cause individuals to face in a particular direction at a given time, and certain tendencies in individuals favor one direction or the other. The pressures to face upward or downward are rarely equivalent, and there are no guarantees that one is facing in the appropriate direction.

*Facing Downward* The downward-facing pressures consist of the needs of one's direct-reporting employees; the needs of the department's clients, patients, or customers; and generally all of the responsibilities of one's present position. Downward is, in fact, the direction in which most managers of people should face most of the time. This is especially true of first-line managers, who may often be as much working professionals as managers. It is necessary to face toward the staff and be a functioning part of the staff to best fulfill the responsibilities of the position. Success in the management role depends on the manager's maximum visibility and availability to staff. However, facing downward runs counter to a number of frequently encountered tendencies resulting from pressure or forces that encourage many managers to face upward.

*Facing Upward* Facing upward is a natural inclination of many managers, but it occurs for a few largely personal reasons. In organizational hierarchy, it quickly becomes evident that one's reward and recognition and most positive strokes come from above. Therefore, to enhance one's chances of advancement, to assist in building a career, it is necessary to be known and appreciated at higher levels. Sometimes facing upward is appropriate and may even be essential. It is necessary in fulfilling responsibilities to one's immediate superior, and some is essential to the manager's growth and development through delegation and empowerment. However, facing upward must be accomplished in ways that do not detract from the manager's responsibilities to the employees.

## Which Way?

Which way the individual manager tends to face depends largely on that person's psychological needs. One's inclinations may be different whether the results tend to be upward or downward. For example, an individual who obtains the most personal satisfaction by doing hands-on work may well face completely downward and identify with the work group to the extent of being nearly invisible to the hierarchy. On the other hand, one who obtains maximum ego gratification through identification with higher management may face upward, even to the extent of ignoring the work group most of the time.

## A Matter of Human Motivation

It invariably becomes a matter of individual motivation when a person responds to what are essentially psychological needs. People are dramatically different from each other in terms of what they respond to most readily. In planning out a supposedly desired career path, it is not simply where a person—such as yourself—think he or she wants to go that is important. Rather, it is necessary with each move you make to reassess yet again where you are and where you want to go. This is so because your ultimate objective is only what you believe you want; you will never know for certain until you get there. Also, each intervening step on the way to your ultimate objective is something that you must be motivated to attain. However, each step has a different set of responsibilities and challenges that might represent a motivational turnoff (sending you in new career directions) or with insurmountable obstacles (suggesting you may have reached a career peak in spite of loftier desires). As far as career growth is concerned, that to which people think they aspire and that which they actually attain is most often not the same.

## Consolidate Before the Next Reach

It is unfortunately a fairly common circumstance for managers' aspirations to extend beyond their capabilities. Also, it is also fairly common to learn that what we managers think we want, we discover we do not really want when we get it. However, what some individuals believe they want can carry them too far too fast, setting them up for eventual failure. Some "fast-track" performers rise at a rate that outstrips the attainment of full control of their present positions. Beware of over-reaching and becoming incompetent in the new level of activity.

Perhaps managers become incompetent by being too focused on their next upward move to fully internalize and competently address their present roles. However, proper career advancement is somewhat like walking—it is not possible to step out with the left foot until the right foot is firmly planted from the previous step. It is always necessary to consolidate one's position and achieve working control of one's present job before addressing opportunities for climbing still higher.

## Dedication—and the Balancing Act

Total or near-total dedication to self over all else is of course an inappropriate strategy. Individuals who are fully focused on developing and advancing to the extent of subordinating all other considerations is making a number of crucial errors. However, because so many people ascribe, at least generally, to the perceived need to "look out for number one," there is a tendency exhibited by some to place themselves ahead of other considerations at all times. Individuals who behave in this manner are concentrating more on making the next upward move than on mastering their present roles.

However, total dedication to one's employer is not an appropriate strategy. Far too many managers allow themselves to become so completely controlled by the job that they are willfully managing very little. The job is managing them. Unfortunately, many work organizations readily accept, and some even demand, this total dedication, which can prevail to the extent of impairing or endangering people's health and family and personal relationships.

Some degree of dedication to both self and employer is of course necessary, but there must be a healthy balance between the two: loyalty of the employer to the employee and the loyalty of the employee to the organization. It might be suggested that loyalty of the organization to the employee is often more perception than reality, a product of a relatively stable period that some industries enjoyed over two, three, or four decades. It was only natural that as times changed and the perception of organizational loyalty diminished, individuals began to be less loyal to their employers. Loyalty in work life is very much a two-way street.

Many individuals, however, seem to need to be loyal to something or someone, even if only to themselves. This need frequently translates to a dedication to one's own career or to one's particular profession. It has become especially evident that a growing number of technical, professional, and specialized employees identify more with an occupation than with an organization. From the employing organization's point of view, this dedication to occupation translates into dedication to self.

Balancing one's own needs with the needs of the organization can be a difficult task. The majority of managerial and professional jobs are by nature somewhat open-ended; there is always something to be done, whether urgent, essential, marginally important, or just simply desirable. There is usually enough to be done in such jobs that one runs the risk of following an endless thread from task to task to task in a never-ending quest to get "caught up." In this direction lies the risk of being consumed by the job. A genuine balance of service to the job and to one's self is a necessity for personal health and survival.

## Goal Alignment

It has been suggested that the manager who wishes to advance throughout the course of a career must develop a workable mix of attention to one's present job and preparation for the next upward move. This mix is best achieved when one's goals are at least partly consistent with the goals of the organization.

You, the manager, should examine your goals and determine how consistent they are with your employer's goals. Will conscientious pursuit of your employer's goals also result in progress toward your own goals? If some of your goals seem to match up with some of the organization's goals, working toward these mutual goals will benefit both you and your employer. For example, consider the physical therapist and physical therapy manager who wishes to grow in that field and who is employed by a health system that has declared one of its goals to be the establishment and maintenance of the most comprehensive physical rehabilitation center in the region. Here, pursuing the goal of growth and advancement in physical therapy is consistent with pursuing the systems goal in physical rehabilitation.

However, if your goals do not align with those of your employer, you are faced with other necessary choices. Consider, for example, the environmental services manager who would like to work in accounting. Assume this manager is studying accounting part-time and is looking for ways to expand on job-related tasks that would support that particular goal. If this individual is significantly driven by this goal, the employer's goal for environmental services—keeping the facility sparkling clean—may well become secondary; pursuit of this organizational goal nets the

manager nothing toward the personal goal. This is, of course, an extreme example of goal inconsistency, suggesting that both individual and organization know it is likely this person will leave in the foreseeable future to pursue his or her personal goal. Fortunately, for most managers and professionals, the inconsistencies are not nearly this pronounced. So it is usually possible to uncover or perhaps even create a few areas in which some of your goals can be made consistent with some of the organization's goals.

## Some Unchanging Fundamentals
### Remember the Supporting Skills

Certain skills will always be important in helping managers perform their present job and making them more valuable for advancement. Certainly all of the basic management skills are applicable here, as are especially the communications skills. Any person who wishes to rise at all in management must of course master the basic management skills and must also develop a degree of mastery in writing, public speaking, and interpersonal communication.

Of course, interpersonal skills are important to managers and professionals at all levels. Writing and speaking are also important at all levels but seem to increase in importance as one ascends the organizational hierarchy. Public speaking, if only to the extent of running meetings, often presents a case in point. More than a few individuals have lost out on potential promotions by exhibiting unwillingness to speak in front of a group. This suggests immediately that the goals of one who would wish to rise in organizational life should include improvement in writing, making presentations, and dealing with other people.

Improvement in working with people is an aspect of job performance often overlooked or at least assumed out of existence. After all, managers do all tend, individually, to believe they are better communicators than they actually are. However, all managers constantly deal with people—employees, peers, superiors, clients, customers, whomever—and should ideally do so in ways that allow those they have contact with to feel respected and important. This is especially significant where employees are concerned. An age-old bit of anonymous wisdom suggests that a manager should be extremely careful how he or she deals with people at all times, because he or she might meet them again. For example, one manager who was twice demoted in successive reorganizing exercises said she never fully appreciated the truth of this until she wound up working side by side with people who had previously reported to her. She was very glad she had always treated people as she wished to be treated herself.

## Become Valuable

In pursuing goals of career advancement, it surely helps one's cause if he or she has a superior who delegates well, truly empowers, and generally believes in employee development. In fact, a good manager with strong feelings for employee development, who is confident and unafraid of having sharp, strong, fast-moving subordinates, is one of the greatest advantages individuals can have at work.

One way in which any individual can be valuable is to know enough about the manager's job to make him or herself useful, to make it easier for the manager to delegate. Much of what a person may be able to do of course depends on the kind of manager he or she answers to. One of the most valuable functions a person can perform, preventing the boss from making an obvious mistake or stepping unknowingly into a

dangerous situation, is appreciated by a strong, confident manager.

Pursuing one's desire to advance may be more or less difficult depending on the attitude of one's immediate superior's toward employee development and on one's relationship with that manager. Although advancement is the goal, first get one's present job responsibilities well under control. A deliberate downward focus may be necessary to obtain full control of one's basic responsibilities. When that control is achieved, however, it is possible to then carefully select those opportunities to focus or upward that seem to hold the most potential to do good. However, while balancing downward with upward, it helps to appreciate that in the long run the best and most lasting way to career advancement is through a track record of demonstrated success in fulfilling job responsibilities and meeting the expectations of employers. The Manager's Wheel Book provides managers with an on-going account of successful activities relating to their role and function as managers. See **Appendix 15–A**, a comprehensive Manager's Wheel Book. **Appendix 15–B** displays a fictitious calendar for use with case problems and wheel book entries.

# Appendix 15–A

## Comprehensive Wheel Book

This excerpt reflects a variety of management activities for September, 20n1. It includes meetings, worker-related issues, presentations, and training. The days would, of course, still contain the usual, ongoing activities as well.

| Date | Activity |
| --- | --- |
| Sept. 4 | Reviewed holiday and summer coverage with assistant director and supervisor |
| | Reviewed anticipated November–December–January holiday schedule and coverage |
| Sept. 6 | Regular QI meeting; presented results of study documentation of pediatric in-patient admission having infection present at admission |
| | Fire drill (unplanned) |
| Sept. 7 | Assessed remote storage—legacy files; made recommendations to compliance officer, research coordinator, medical staff's clinical documentation committee |
| | Gave presentation to Women's Auxiliary regarding personal health records |
| Sept. 13 | Briefed assistant director and supervisors about educational opportunities and coached them regarding briefing their unit employees |
| | Discussed with HR department worker's request to "cash out" unused vacation days |
| | Briefed assistant director and supervisors regarding being away from Sept. 17 through 20 at training conference |
| Sept. 14 | Briefed assistant director and supervisors regarding job analysis project |
| Sept. 15 | Annual Main Street Run fund raiser—attended with department volunteer relay team |
| Sept. 17–20 | Out of office all week; attending Healthcare Tech conference |
| Sept. 18 | Met with panel of presenters and gave presentation on interoperability concerns |
| Sept. 14 | Implemented new Casual Friday dress code, effective Oct. 1 |
| | 35% of day shift: late (2.5 hours) due to area transit failure. |
| | CEO directive received: option to charge to personal leave, or take shortened lunch break; overtime option authorized; shuttle bus service at 3:00 P.M., 5:00 P.M., and 7:00 P.M. |
| | Regular clinical documentation committee meeting: feedback regarding new dictation-transcription and voice recognition system |

| Date | Activity |
|---|---|
| | Final budget close out—last fiscal year |
| Sept. 24 | Hurricane watch; schedule adjustments anticipated; on-call workers alerted |
| | Safety and disaster preparedness meeting: noon and 4:00 P.M. |
| Sept. 26 | Retirement lunch (on site) for senior vice-president—finance department |
| | Monthly meeting: department heads' peer group; gave presentation on STEM-H trends |
| | Follow-up meeting with assistant director and supervisors regarding November–December–January holiday coverage plans; issued memo to all department employees regarding their requests, and due date |
| | Preparation for clinical affiliation student's arrival October 1 |
| Sept. 27 | Unannounced internal audit regarding employee roster. Payroll, employee status, vacation, holiday, sick leave usage. |
| | Flooded basement: remote storage area |
| | Processed voluntary resignation form: department secretary |
| | Interviewed two prospective candidates for secretary |
| | Regular monthly meeting: safety and disaster preparedness committee; preparation for annual disaster drill on October 15 |
| Sept. 28 | Renewed contract with transcription service (1 year) |
| | Enrolled in formal course: project manager certification |

# Appendix 15-B

## Calendar for Wheel Book and Case Problems

### January

| Su | Mo | Tu | We | Th | Fr | Sa |
|----|----|----|----|----|----|----|
|    | **1** | 2 | 3 | 4 | 5 | 6 |
| 7 | 8 | 9 | 10 | 11 | 12 | 13 |
| 14 | **15** | 16 | 17 | 18 | 19 | 20 |
| 21 | 22 | 23 | 24 | 25 | 26 | 27 |
| 28 | 29 | 30 | 31 |   |   |   |

### February

| Su | Mo | Tu | We | Th | Fr | Sa |
|----|----|----|----|----|----|----|
|    |    |    |    | 1 | 2 | 3 |
| 4 | 5 | 6 | 7 | 8 | 9 | 10 |
| 11 | 12 | 13 | 14 | 15 | 16 | 17 |
| 18 | **19** | 20 | 21 | 22 | 23 | 24 |
| 25 | 26 | 27 | 28 |   |   |   |

### March

| Su | Mo | Tu | We | Th | Fr | Sa |
|----|----|----|----|----|----|----|
|    |    |    |    | 1 | 2 | 3 |
| 4 | 5 | 6 | 7 | 8 | 9 | 10 |
| 11 | 12 | 13 | 14 | 15 | 16 | 17 |
| 18 | 19 | 20 | 21 | 22 | 23 | 24 |
| 25 | 26 | 27 | 28 | 29 | 30 | 31 |

### April

| Su | Mo | Tu | We | Th | Fr | Sa |
|----|----|----|----|----|----|----|
| 1 | 2 | 3 | 4 | 5 | 6 | 7 |
| 8 | 9 | 10 | 11 | 12 | 13 | 14 |
| 15 | 16 | 17 | 18 | 19 | 20 | 21 |
| 22 | 23 | 24 | 25 | 26 | 27 | 28 |
| 29 | 30 |   |   |   |   |   |

### May

| Su | Mo | Tu | We | Th | Fr | Sa |
|----|----|----|----|----|----|----|
|    |    | 1 | 2 | 3 | 4 | 5 |
| 6 | 7 | 8 | 9 | 10 | 11 | 12 |
| 13 | 14 | 15 | 16 | 17 | 18 | 19 |
| 20 | 21 | 22 | 23 | 24 | 25 | 26 |
| 27 | **28** | 29 | 30 | 31 |   |   |

### June

| Su | Mo | Tu | We | Th | Fr | Sa |
|----|----|----|----|----|----|----|
|    |    |    |    |    | 1 | 2 |
| 3 | 4 | 5 | 6 | 7 | 8 | 9 |
| 10 | 11 | 12 | 13 | 14 | 15 | 16 |
| 17 | 18 | 19 | 20 | 21 | 22 | 23 |
| 24 | 25 | 26 | 27 | 28 | 29 | 30 |

### July

| Su | Mo | Tu | We | Th | Fr | Sa |
|----|----|----|----|----|----|----|
| 1 | 2 | 3 | **4** | 5 | 6 | 7 |
| 8 | 9 | 10 | 11 | 12 | 13 | 14 |
| 15 | 16 | 17 | 18 | 19 | 20 | 21 |
| 22 | 23 | 24 | 25 | 26 | 27 | 28 |
| 29 | 30 | 31 |   |   |   |   |

### August

| Su | Mo | Tu | We | Th | Fr | Sa |
|----|----|----|----|----|----|----|
|    |    |    | 1 | 2 | 3 | 4 |
| 5 | 6 | 7 | 8 | 9 | 10 | 11 |
| 12 | 13 | 14 | 15 | 16 | 17 | 18 |
| 19 | 20 | 21 | 22 | 23 | 24 | 25 |
| 26 | 27 | 28 | 29 | 30 | 31 |   |

### September

| Su | Mo | Tu | We | Th | Fr | Sa |
|----|----|----|----|----|----|----|
|    |    |    |    |    |    | 1 |
| 2 | **3** | 4 | 5 | 6 | 7 | 8 |
| 9 | 10 | 11 | 12 | 13 | 14 | 15 |
| 16 | 17 | 18 | 19 | 20 | 21 | 22 |
| 23 | 24 | 25 | 26 | 27 | 28 | 29 |
| 30 |   |   |   |   |   |   |

### October

| Su | Mo | Tu | We | Th | Fr | Sa |
|----|----|----|----|----|----|----|
|    | 1 | 2 | 3 | 4 | 5 | 6 |
| 7 | **8** | 9 | 10 | 11 | 12 | 13 |
| 14 | 15 | 16 | 17 | 18 | 19 | 20 |
| 21 | 22 | 23 | 24 | 25 | 26 | 27 |
| 28 | 29 | 30 | 31 |   |   |   |

### November

| Su | Mo | Tu | We | Th | Fr | Sa |
|----|----|----|----|----|----|----|
|    |    |    |    | 1 | 2 | 3 |
| 4 | 5 | 6 | 7 | 8 | 9 | 10 |
| **11** | **12** | 13 | 14 | 15 | 16 | 17 |
| 18 | 19 | 20 | 21 | **22** | 23 | 24 |
| 25 | 26 | 27 | 28 | 29 | 30 |   |

### December

| Su | Mo | Tu | We | Th | Fr | Sa |
|----|----|----|----|----|----|----|
|    |    |    |    |    |    | 1 |
| 2 | 3 | 4 | 5 | 6 | 7 | 8 |
| 9 | 10 | 11 | 12 | 13 | 14 | 15 |
| 16 | 17 | 18 | 19 | 20 | 21 | 22 |
| 23 | 24 | **25** | 26 | 27 | 28 | 29 |
| 30 | 31 |   |   |   |   |   |

## January

| Su | Mo | Tu | We | Th | Fr | Sa |
|----|----|----|----|----|----|----|
|    | **1** | 2 | 3 | 4 | 5 |  |
| 6 | 7 | 8 | 9 | 10 | 11 | 12 |
| 13 | 14 | 15 | 16 | 17 | 18 | 19 |
| 20 | **21** | 22 | 23 | 24 | 25 | 26 |
| 27 | 28 | 29 | 30 | 31 |  |  |

## February

| Su | Mo | Tu | We | Th | Fr | Sa |
|----|----|----|----|----|----|----|
|    |    |    |    |    | 1 | 2 |
| 3 | 4 | 5 | 6 | 7 | 8 | 9 |
| 10 | 11 | 12 | 13 | 14 | 15 | 16 |
| 17 | **18** | 19 | 20 | 21 | 22 | 23 |
| 24 | 25 | 26 | 27 | 28 |  |  |

## March

| Su | Mo | Tu | We | Th | Fr | Sa |
|----|----|----|----|----|----|----|
|    |    |    |    |    | 1 | 2 |
| 3 | 4 | 5 | 6 | 7 | 8 | 9 |
| 10 | 11 | 12 | 13 | 14 | 15 | 16 |
| 17 | 18 | 19 | 20 | 21 | 22 | 23 |
| 24 | 25 | 26 | 27 | 28 | 29 | 30 |
| 31 |  |  |  |  |  |  |

## April

| Su | Mo | Tu | We | Th | Fr | Sa |
|----|----|----|----|----|----|----|
|    | 1 | 2 | 3 | 4 | 5 | 6 |
| 7 | 8 | 9 | 10 | 11 | 12 | 13 |
| 14 | 15 | 16 | 17 | 18 | 19 | 20 |
| 21 | 22 | 23 | 24 | 25 | 26 | 27 |
| 28 | 29 | 30 |  |  |  |  |

## May

| Su | Mo | Tu | We | Th | Fr | Sa |
|----|----|----|----|----|----|----|
|    |    |    | 1 | 2 | 3 | 4 |
| 5 | 6 | 7 | 8 | 9 | 10 | 11 |
| 12 | 13 | 14 | 15 | 16 | 17 | 18 |
| 19 | 20 | 21 | 22 | 23 | 24 | 25 |
| 26 | **27** | 28 | 29 | 30 | 31 |  |

## June

| Su | Mo | Tu | We | Th | Fr | Sa |
|----|----|----|----|----|----|----|
|    |    |    |    |    |    | 1 |
| 2 | 3 | 4 | 5 | 6 | 7 | 8 |
| 9 | 10 | 11 | 12 | 13 | 14 | 15 |
| 16 | 17 | 18 | 19 | 20 | 21 | 22 |
| 23 | 24 | 25 | 26 | 27 | 28 | 29 |
| 30 |  |  |  |  |  |  |

# Index

## A

Accountable care organizations (ACO), 12
Accounts, system of, 174
Accrediting standards, 6–7
Adaptation
    employee, to organizational life, 217–218
    organizational, 55–56
Affiliation, clinical, program and contract, 208–209
After-action report, 165, 291
Age Discrimination in Employment Act, 92
Agreement, collective bargaining, 238
    sample, 240–247
American Health Information Management Association (AHIMA), 24–26, 47, 96, 292
American Hospital Association, 5
Americans with Disabilities Act (ADA), 92, 314
Annual congressional budget allocations, 12–13
Annual report, 270, 281–282
    executive summary of, 270–271, 283
Appeal, disciplinary action, 237
Appraisal, performance
    See Performance appraisal
Appreciative inquiry, 222–223
    motivational aspects of, 222–223
    process of, 222
Assets and information, organizational, use of, 197
Audit findings and corrective actions, 188
Audit, general, 188
Audit committee, 188
Authority
    charismatic, 73
    consent theory of, 72–73
    cultural expectations of, 74
    by default, 75
    of facts, 74, 75
    formal, organizational, 73–74
    functional, 74
    holders, characteristics of, 75
    importance of, 71–72
    and law of the situation, 74–75
    manager's use of sources of, 75
    rational-legal, 73
    restrictions on use of, 75–76
    splintered, in split-reporting, 119–120
    traditional, 73
Autocratic leadership, 81

## B

Barnard, Chester, 72–73, 92
Barriers to communication, 253, 264–265
Barth, Carl G. L., 3
Benchmarking, 296–297
    sample studies, 297–299
    sources of measures for, 297
Benefits administration, 307
Boutique care, 2
Boyd cycle
    See OODA loop
Budget(ing)
    approaches to, 175–176
    capital, 178, 180
    context of, 169
    cutting, 186
    and general audit, 188
    implementation of, 178, 179
    issues, 189–191
    justification of, 185–186
    maintenance, 181–182
    milestone, 173
    periodic moving, 173
    periods, 172–173
    personnel, 183–185
    process, 176–177
    requisites of, 172
    review and approval of, 177–178
    sample, 188–192
    staff development, 182–183
    supplies, 180–182
    types of, 173–174
    uses of, 172
    variances, 186–188
Bureaucracy, 43–44
Bureaucratic imperialism, 52–54
Bureaucratic leadership, 81
Business plan(ning)
    content of, 274
    independent practice for, 272–274

## C

Calendar for wheel book and case problems, 340–341
Capital budget, 178, 180
Care
    levels of, 5–6
    patterns of, 4, 292
Career development, 26–27
    healthcare professional and, 333–337
Caregiver, family as, 3
Cause-effect chart, 301
Centers for Disease Control and Prevention, 24
Centers for Medicare and Medicaid Services (CMS), 7
Chairperson, committee, 156–158
    chairing meetings, 156–157
    duties of, 156
    follow-up by, 157–158
    selection of, 156
Change
    addressing directly, 29
    constancy versus, 27
    control of responses to, 29–30
    effective management of, 31
    manager, as agent of, 19
    the manager and, 69–70
    organizational, as cause for resistance, 28
    and resistance to, 27–31, 329–331
    successful, illustrations of, 19–27
Change agent, the manager as, 19
Checks-and-balances system, 151
Civil Rights Act of 1964, 92, 314, 316
Civil Rights Act of 1991, 314
Classification of organizations, 41
    authority structure, 41
    genotype, 41–42
    prime beneficiary, 41
Clientele network, the, 44–45
    for physical therapy unit, 51–52
Clients, 2–3, 45–46
Clinical affiliation, program and contract, 208–209
Co-optation, organizational survival and, 54–55
Co-opted groups, 54–55
Coalitions, health care and community, 50–51

Collaborative partnerships, 4, 5
Collective bargaining agreement, sample, 240–247
Commitment, top management, 289–290
Committee(s)
 ad hoc, 149
 audit, 188
 chairperson, 156–158
 effectiveness of, enhancing the, 153–156
 limitations of, 152–153
 meeting, minutes for, 158–161
 member orientation, 158
 nature of, 149–150
 paralysis, 163
 permanent, 149
 as plural executive, 149–150
 purposes and uses of, 147–152
 review of, periodic, 155–156
 scope, function, and authority, 154
 size and composition of, 154–155
 as task force, 150
 and teams, 167
Communication
 addressing groups, 253–254
 barriers to, 253, 264–265
 components of, 252
 defined, 250
 e-mail and, 251–252
 face-to-face, 250–251
 the manager and, 250–252
 methods of improving, 252–253
 non-verbal, 252
 organizational, 262–266
 the telephone and, 251
 tools for, 263–264
 verbal (oral), 252
 voice mail and, 251
 written, 251, 255–262
Compensation
 *See* Wage and salary administration
Comprehensive entries, 338–339
Concierge care, 2
Conduct and behavior, standards of, 196–198
Confidentiality, patient, 198
Conflict
 arena for, 231
 basic, 227–228
 hidden agenda and, 228
 of interest, 196–197
 model with example, 227
 organizational, 227–232
 participants in, 230
 sources of, 228–230
 strategies for addressing, 231–232
 study of, 227
 to whistleblower action, 232
Constraints on planning, 91–92
Consultant, practitioner as a, 139
Consultative leadership, 82

Continuous quality improvement (CQI), 287, 291
Contract, health information consultant, 140–145
Contract management, 122–123
Contract services, 128–129
Contractor, independent, 139
Contracts, reports and guidelines for, 139–140
Controlling
 basic process of, 294
 benchmarking in, 296–299
 characteristics of, 292–293
 defined, 292
 introduced, 15–16
 strategies for, 295–296
 tools of, 297–301
Controls, characteristics of adequate, 294–295
Conventional organizational chart, 131
Corporate culture, 57–58
 committees and teams, 147
 concept of, 57
 fiscal management, 169
 and planning, 92
Cost center, 174–175
Cost comparison, 186
Critical cycle, the, 301–302
Cross-training, 29
Cultural expectations of work, 220
Customer, department division by, 124

**D**

Data mining, 9
Data warehousing, 9
Day-to-day actions, 319
Decision(s)
 alternatives, evaluating, 112, 113
 continuing assessment of, 113–114
 importance of, evaluating, 111–112
 reversibility of, 111
 satisficing and maximizing, 112–113
 tree, 115–116
Decision making, 16, 111–116
 decision tree, 115–116
 devil's advocate in, 114
 factor analysis matrix for, 114–115
 impact and probability, 111
 root and branch, 112
 tools and techniques of, 114–116
Delegation
 guidelines for, 76–78
 importance of, 76
 pitfalls of, 77
Department of Health and Human Services (DHHS), 7, 24
Departmental philosophy, 96
Departmentation, 123–125
 temporary, 126–127
Development, employee, 193

Direct expenses, 185, 186
Directing, 16
Directives, orders and, 266
Discharge, 234–237
 form for, 236
Disciplinary action, appeal of, 237
Discipline, 232–237
 defined, 232
 documentation of, 311–312
 human resources involvement in, 310–311
 manager's role in, 232–233
 progressive, 233–237
Display charts, TQM, 301
Dissatisfiers, motivational effects of, 221
Distinctive leadership actions, 87
Diversity, 206, 207
Documentation, disciplinary, 311–312
Due diligence review, 274–275

**E**

E-mail, 255–256
 guidelines for, 255–256
 policy, 199
 use of, 198–200
Elder care, 278
Electromation decision, 162–163
Electronic health record (EHR), 24–26, 80
Emergency preparedness, 291
Emergency service, 2
Employee
 development, 193
 health, 307
 orientation, 194–200
 political activity, 198
 relations, 307
 relationships, 197
 satisfaction, 292
 selection, 218
 strategies for motivating, 220–222
Employer-employee relationship, 128
Employment, 307
Employment laws, 305
Employment office, 304
Equal Employment Opportunity Commission (EEOC), 314
Equal Pay Act, 313
Evaluation, employee
 *See* Performance appraisal
Excellence, 287, 288

**F**

Factor analysis matrix, 114–115
Fair Labor Standards Act (FLSA), 137, 313
Family and Medical Leave Act (FMLA), 314

Fayol, Henri, 37
Feedback, 39, 40
Fixed budget, 173
Flattening, organizational, 304, 305
Flextime, 129
Flowchart
    symbols for, 300, 301
    types of, 299–300
    uses of, 300
Follet, Mary Parker, 74
Formal co-optation, 54
Fraud and abuse, prevention of, 21
Full-time equivalent(s) (FTE), 183, 184
    calculation of, 184
Function, departmental division by, 124
Functional authority, 122
Functional objectives, 98–99

**G**

Gantt, Henry L., 36, 298
Gantt chart, 298, 299
    examples of, 299, 300
Gatekeeper, primary care physician as, 11
Gilbreth, Frank and Lillian, 36
Goals, organizational, 97
Goal succession, multiplication and
    expansion, 56
Grievance procedure, excerpts, 231
Group deliberations
    advantage of, 150–151
    guidelines for, 165–167
Guidelines for contracts and reports,
    139–140

**H**

Hawthorne effect, 36
Health information exchange, 9
Health Information Technology for
    Economic and Clinical Health
    Act, the, (HITECH), 290
Health Insurance Portability and
    Accountability Act of 1996
    (HIPAA), 11
    the department manager and, 23–24
    as extensive change, 21
    future of, 23–24
    organizational effects of, 22–23
    and physical layout, 23
    privacy official for, 23
    Privacy Rule of, 22–23
    Title II of, 21–22
Health insurance proposals, 33
    template for assessing, 33
Health maintenance organization
    (HMO), 11
Health Maintenance Organization Act of
    1973, 11

Healthcare
    Affordable Care Act and, 13
    network designation, 13
    organization, dual pyramid
        form in, 123
    organizations, classification of, 42–43
    regional pricing for, 13
    reimbursement, 10
    technology, impact of, 8–10
    unions, 238–239
Healthcare professional as manager,
    333–337
    balancing management with
        profession, 324
    employee problems and, 331
    methods improvement and, 331
Healthcare programs, 97
Heritage statement, 95
Hibernation, organizational, 55–56
High-skill professional, the, 326–327
Histogram, 301
History of management, 36
Hospice care, 6
Hostile work environment, 316–317
Human resources
    for assistance with, 308
    department of, 303–304
    directions in, 305–306
    discipline, role in, 310–311
    and documentation, 311–312
    employment law and, 312–316
    functions of, 307
    job descriptions and, 309
    learning about, 306–308
    and legalistic environment, 316–318
    manager's input to, 311
    nature of function, 306
    and performance appraisal, 310
    as personnel department, 303
    reporting relationship of, 306–307
    securing help from, 308–309
    as staff function, 304
    and training, 311
    and workplace violence, 315–316

**I**

Identify theft, medical, 291–292
Improvement
    failure of, 293–294
    quality, 287
In-service training, 182–183
Incremental budgeting, 175
Independent contractor, 139
Indirect expenses, 185, 186
Influence, concept of, 71
Informal co-optation, 54
Informatics standards, 9–10
Initiatives, performance improvement,
    289

Integration into organization, techniques
    for fostering, 218–219
Interest, conflict of, 196–197
Internal Revenue Service (IRS), 128
Internet
    policy, 199
    use of, 198–200
Interpersonal relationships, 85

**J**

Job description, 133–138
    content and format, 134–136
    in employee development and
        retention, 138
    in employee selection, 137–138
    example, 135
    job analysis and, 133–134
    job rating and classification in,
        136–137
    recruiting and the, 137
    updating, 309
    uses of, 138
Job rotation, 204
Joint Commission, The (TJC), 5
Joint venture, 4, 5

**K**

Know your organization, 67

**L**

Labor-Management Relations Act
    (Taft-Hartley), 92
Labor relations, 307, 313
Labor union trends, 238
Laissez-faire leadership, 82
Language, specialized professional,
    331–332
Laws
    employment, 305
    health care, 6–7
    wage and hour, 313
Leader(s)
    plan of action of, 80–81
    sources of, 78
Leadership, 69–87
    autocratic, 81
    bureaucratic, 81
    communicating style, 83–84
    consultative, 82
    continuum of styles, 82–83
    data-driven approach, 86–87
    defined, 78
    distinctive actions, 87
    factors influencing style, 83
    formal and informal, 78

functions of, 80
and the healthcare professional, 328–329
laissez-faire, 82
opportunities for growth, 86–87
participative, 81–82
paternalistic, 82
personal, 85–86
qualities of, 79–80
roles, 88
seeking positions of, 78–79
situational, 84–85
styles of, 81–82
values, 86
wheel book relation, 87–88
Letters, memos and, 258–262
Levels of care, 5–6
Life cycle, organizational, 58–63
Life cycle model, 63–65
Lindblom, Charles, 112
Line and staff, 121–123
    authority in, 122
    interaction of, 122

# M

Managed care, 11–12
Management
    as art and science, 16–17
    changes, as cause of resistance, 28–29
    contract, 122–123
    effectiveness, ego barrier to, 324–325
    functions of, 15–16
    generalist, 321–324
    history of, 36
    human relations approach to, 36–37
    inventory of personnel, 138–139
    operations research approach to, 37
    scientific, 36
    as second career, 321
    span of, 120–121
    style, 329
    systems approach to, 37–40
Management by objectives (MBO), 94
Management engineering, 289
Management Reference portfolio, 65–67
    concept and use, 65–69
    content, 320
    examples
        budget, 176
        teams and committees, 167
Manager
    and change, 69–70
    as change agent, 19
    and communication, 250–252, 264
    effective, characteristics of, 16–17
    healthcare practitioner as, 15, 16
    and human resources help, 308–309
    leadership accomplishment, 87
    the professional as a, 321–324

project, 104
    supporting skills for the, 336–337
    wheel book, 17–18, 87–88
Master budget, 174
Matrix organization, 126
Mayo, Elton, 36
Medicaid, 10, 13
Medical cost-sharing model, 12
Medicare, 10
Meeting
    general guidelines for, 254–255
    staff, 254
Meeting minutes, committee, 158–159
    contents of, 159–161
    preparation of, 159
Memos, letters and, 258–262
Mentoring, 207–208
Merger(s), 4–5
    defined, 4
Methods, 103
Middle managers, 257
Milestone budgeting, 173
Mission, organizational, 94–97
Motivation
    appreciative inquiry and, 222–223
    in critical incidents, 221–222
    and downsizing, 223–226
    employee, strategies for, 220–222
    general, 217–219
    theories of, 219–220
Motivational strategies, 221
Motivators, true, 220–221
Moving budget, periodic, 173

# N

National Labor Relations Act (NLRA), 162, 313
    1975 amendments to, 238
National Labor Relations Board (NLRB), 162
Non-verbal communication, 252
Number, departmental division by, 124

# O

Objectives
    functional, 98–99
    organizational, 97–98
Occupational and Safety Health Act, 92
OODA loop, 113
Oral warning, 233–234
    form for, 234
Orders
    and directives, 266
    verbal versus written, 266
Organization(s)(al)
    adaptation, 55–56
    adversaries to, 49–50

advisers to, 48–49
associates of, 47–48
by authority structure, 41
classification of, 41–42
conflict, 227–232
contract services, 128–129
controllers of, 49
dual pyramid form of, 123
employee identification with, 219
flattening, 304, 305
flexible options for worker
    scheduling, 129
flextime, 129
form, consequences of, 44
formal versus informal, 40
by genotypic characteristics, 41–42
health care, 42–43
hibernation, 55–56
life, adaptation to, 217–218
life cycle, 58–63
matrix, 126
objectives, 97–98
outsourcing, 127–128
prime beneficiary, 41
restructuring, 4, 26
structure, flexibility in, 126
suppliers to, 46–47
supporters of, 48
telecommuting, 129–130
temporary agency services, 127
temporary departmentation, 126–127
as total system, 35–36
values, 94–97
Organizational chart, 130–133
    arrangements of, 131–132
    examples of, 132
    limitations of, 131
    preparation of, 132–133
    types of, 131
    uses of, 130–131
Organizational communication, 262–266
    barriers to, 264–265
    formal, 262
    informal, 263
    tools for improving, 263–264
Organizing, 15, 16
    concepts and principles of, 118–120
    defined, 117
    the process of, 117–118
Orientation, employee, 194–200
    departmental, contents and checklist
        general, contents and checklist, 195
Orphan activities, 124–125
Outsourcing, 127–128

# P

Pareto, Vilfredo, 113
Pareto chart, 301

Pareto principle, 113
Participative leadership, 81–82, 290
Partnerships, collaborative, 4, 5
Paternalistic leadership, 82
Patient
    confidentiality, 198
    privacy, 291–292
    safety, 291
    satisfaction, 292
Patient Protection and Affordable Care
        Act of 2010, 31–32
Patient Safety and Quality Improvement
        Act of 2005, 290
Patient Self-Determination Act of 1990,
        20–21
Patterns of care, 292
Payroll, 307
Performance appraisal, 310
Performance improvement
    focus of studies of, 290–292
    initiatives, 289
Personal health record (PHR), 8–9
Personnel budget, 183–185
Personnel department
    See Human resources
Philosophy
    departmental, 96
    proceduralized, 288–289
Physical therapy unit, clientele network
        for, 51–52
Plan(s)
    in anticipation of unknown, 94
    business, content of, 274
    business, independent practice,
        272–274
    changes and updates to, 93–94
    characteristics of effective, 92–93
    long-range, excerpt, 202
    strategic, 268–270
    types of, 94
Plan of correction (POC), 275–277
    characteristics of, 89–90
    constraints on, 91–92
    defined, 89
Planning
    examples of variables in client
        characteristics, 93-95
        correctional facilities, 93
        homeless shelters, 93
        industrial clinics, 93
        truck stop dispensaries, 93
    importance of fact finding, 93
    limiting factors on, 92
    participants in, 90, 294
    the process of, 90–91, 110
    project, 104
Plural executive, committee as, 149–150
Policies
    changes in, as cause of resistance, 29
    e-mail and Internet, 199
    examples of, 100–101

sources of, 99–100
    wording of, 100–101
Political activity, employee, 198
Position description
    See Job description
Power, concept of, 70–71
PPBS approach, 175
Privacy, patient, 291–292
Privacy Rule, HIPAA, 22–23
Problem-solving, team-oriented, 289
Procedure(s), 101–103
    development of manual, 103
    example, 103
    grievance, excerpts, 231
    manual format, 101–103
Process, departmental division by, 124
Product, departmental division by, 124
Professional, health care
    career development for, 334–335
    and change, 329–331
    credibility of superior of, 327–328
    dedication and, 335–336
    as a functional specialist, 322
    and goal alignment, 336
    high-skill, problems with, 326–327
    language of, 331–332
    leadership and the, 328–329
    management style and the, 329
    as manager, 330–331
    as scarce resource, 325–326
Professional temps, 127
Progressive discipline
    counseling in, 233
    discharge in, 234–237
    infractions in, guidelines for, 237
    oral warning in, 233–234
    suspension in, 234–237
    written warning in, 234, 235
Project
    major elements and examples, 104–110
    manager, 104
Project planning, 104
Project proposal, major, 270–272
    background for, 271
    content of, 271–272, 284–286
    development officer, role of, 271

**Q**

Quality
    assurance, 289
    control, 289
    improvement, 289, 290

**R**

Range of service, 5–6
Recruiting, 307, 309

Recruitment process, 137
Reduction-in-force (RIF), 223
Referral practices, 197–198
Regional Health Information Exchanges
        (RHIE), 25
Regulations, healthcare, 6–7
Reimbursement, healthcare, 10
Reimbursement systems
    fraud and abuse in, 14
    weaknesses of, 14
Resistance to change
    addressing with employees, 30
    causes of, 27–29
    the professional and, 329–331
Responsibility center, 175
Restructuring, organizational, 4, 26
Retainer-fee care, 2
Revenue cycle, the, 170–171, 291
    and cash, 171
    revenue sources, 171
Review, due diligence, 274–275
Robotic technology, 8
Roethlisberger, F. J., 36
Rules, 103–104
    work, 218
Run chart, 301

**S**

Safety, patient, 291
SBAR method, 265
Scattergram, 301
Scheduling, specific, 125–126
Scientific management, 36
Self-directed work teams, 289
Service, range of, 5–6
Sexual harassment, 210–212, 314–315
Simon, Herbert, 72
Situational leadership, 84–85
Six Sigma, 295
Social and ethical factors, 14
Social media policies and practices,
        256–258
Social networking, 199–200
Software licensure, 182
Sound fiscal management, 169–170
Span of management, 120–121
    determinants of, 120–121
Speaking to groups, 253–254
Split-reporting relationship, 119–120
Staff meeting, 254
Staffing, 16
Staffing flexibility, 127
Standards
    accreditation, 6–7
    of conduct and behavior, 196–198
    control, types of, 295
    informatics, 9–10
Step budget, 173–174

Strategic plan(ning)
  content of, 268
  process of, 269–270
Strategies, motivational, 221
Structuralism, 37
Style, leadership, 82–84
Succession plans, 93
Suppliers, 46–48
Support services, management, 3–4
Supportive work environment, 317–318
Surveyor report, 276
Survival strategies, organizational, 52
Suspension, 234–237
  form for, 235
SWOT analysis, 264, 269
Systems approach to management, 37–40

## T

Taft-Hartley Act, 92, 313
Task force, 150
Taylor, Frederick, 36
Team(s)
  as compared with committee, 161–162
  Electromation decision and, 162–163
  legal issues with, 162
  precautions for using, 15
  proper focus of, 164–165
  shortcomings of, 163–164
  work, self-directed, 289
Team-oriented problem solving, 289
Technology, impact of, 8–10
Telecommuting, 129–130
Telephone, communication via, 251
Temporary agency services, 127
Territory, departmental division by, 124
Theories of motivation, 219–220
Thriving organization, 287–288
Throughputs, 39
Time, departmental division by, 124
Title VII
  See Civil Rights Act of 1964

Tools of control, 297–301
Top-level management, 170
Total quality management (TQM), 161, 288, 292, 295
Training, 200–207
  and diversity, 206, 207
  evaluating outcomes of, 205
  implementation of program, 205
  job rotation as, 206
  justification of budget for, example, 206
  methods and techniques, 204
  module content, 203–204
  needs, identifying, 200–203
  resources for, 205–206
Trends, health care, 3–4

## U

Unions, health care, 238–239
Utilization review, 14

## V

Values
  leadership, 86
  organizational, 94–97
Variable budget, 173
Variances, budget, 186–188
  analysis of, 187–188
Verbal (oral) communication, 252
Violence, workplace, 315–316
Virtual health, 10
Vision, organizational, 94–97
Voice mail, 251

## W

Wage and hour laws, 313
Wage and salary administration, 307
Wagner Act

See National Labor Relations Act (NLRA)
Warning, oral, 233–234
Warning, written, 234, 235
Weber, Max, 37, 43, 73
Wheel book, 338–339
  concept and definition, 17
  format, 17
  manager, 17–18, 87–88
  uses of, 17
Whistleblower actions, 232
Work
  cultural expectations of, 220
  habits, 85–86
  rules, 218
Work teams, self-directed, 289
Worker scheduling, flexible options for, 129
Workplace violence, 315–316
Written communication
  audience for, 258–259
  basic, 251
  e-mail and, 255–256
  editing of, 260
  formal, 262
  functions of, 258
  habits affecting, 260–261
  importance of, 255
  memos and letters and, 258–262
  samples, right and wrong, 261–262
  simple words in, 259
  unneeded words in, 259
Written report, 140

## Z

Zero-based budgeting, 175–176
*Zone of acceptance,* 72, 75, 76
*Zone of indifference,* 72